Anatomy in
Diagnostic Imaging

Dedicated to our inquiring students

Anatomy in Diagnostic Imaging

Peter Fleckenstein

Emeritus Chief Radiologist
and Lecturer of Radiological Anatomy
University of Copenhagen
Denmark

Jørgen Tranum-Jensen MD

Professor of Anatomy
Panuminstituttet
University of Copenhagen
Denmark

Co-author:

Peter Sand Myschetzky MD

Chief Radiologist
Department of Radiology
Gentofte Hospital
University of Copenhagen
Denmark

THIRD EDITION

WILEY Blackwell

Registered office: John Wiley & Sons, Ltd, The Atrium, Southern Gate, Chichester, West Sussex, PO19 8SQ, UK

Editorial offices: 9600 Garsington Road, Oxford, OX4 2DQ, UK
      The Atrium, Southern Gate, Chichester, West Sussex, PO19 8SQ, UK
      111 River Street, Hoboken, NJ 07030-5774, USA

For details of our global editorial offices, for customer services and for information about how to apply for permission to reuse the copyright material in this book please see our website at www.wiley.com/wiley-blackwell

Library of Congress Cataloging-in-Publication Data

Fleckenstein, Peter, author.
  Anatomy in diagnostic imaging / Peter Fleckenstein, Jørgen Tranum-Jensen; co-author,
Peter Sand Myschetzky. – Third edition.
      p. ; cm.
  Includes index.
  ISBN 978-1-4051-3991-5 (pbk.)
  I. Tranum-Jensen, Jørgen, author. II. Myschetzky, Peter Sand, author. III. Title.
  [DNLM: 1. Anatomy–Atlases. 2. Diagnostic Imaging–Atlases. QS 17]
  RC78.7.D53
  616.07'54022–dc23
                                   2013049538

A catalogue record for this book is available from the British Library.

Cover image: courtesy of Peter Fleckenstein and Jørgen Tranum-Jensen
Cover design by Sarah Dickinson

Set in 10/13.5 pt Meridien by Toppan Best-set Premedia Limited
Printed and bound in Singapore by Markono Print Media Pte Ltd

1 2014

Preface to the third edition

Almost 20 years have passed since the first edition of *Anatomy in Diagnostic Imaging* was published, and encouraged by the receipt of the second edition we felt it was time to prepare this third edition, maintaining the scope of the previous editions, as an all-round reference collection of fully interpreted normal images, addressing students as well as professional medical personnel working with diagnostic imaging.

We have made a special effort to elaborate on MR imaging of the major joints, shoulder, elbow, hip, knee and ankle imaged in two or three planes. A CT series of the skull has been added and the CT series of the brain has been replaced by a new series. The section on obstetric ultrasonography has been considerably expanded to cover all standard examinations performed during a normal pregnancy. Further, we have added an MR series of the orbit and a new series of the lumbar spine, and other images have been supplemented or replaced.

The introductory chapter has been revised and updated, still with the scope that it should be nothing more than an understandable introduction to the imaging techniques and principles presented in the book.

Acknowledgements

During the preparation of the third edition we have again profited from the generous help of many colleagues: Connie Jørgensen, Rigshospitalet, Copenhagen; Anne-Mette Leffers, Hamlet Private Hospital, Copenhagen; Peter Oturai, Rigshospitalet, Copenhagen; Henrik Lundell, Hvidovre Hospital, Copenhagen and Martin Vinten, Glostrup Hospital, Copenhagen, together with colleagues and staff at the X-ray Department of Gentofte Hospital, and our thanks also go to photographer Keld Ottosen, Department of Cellular and Molecular Medicine, University of Copenhagen for skillful help with the photographic plates.

We also wish to thank Wiley Blackwell for their excellent collaboration and patience during the preparation of this third edition.

Finally, we cannot sink deeper into the bottomless debt of gratitude to our families for allowing us again to spend countless, but exciting hours preparing this third edition.

Peter Fleckenstein
Jørgen Tranum-Jensen
Peter Sand Myschetzky

Contents

Principles and Techniques in Diagnostic Imaging

Several physical principles are utilized in diagnostic imaging to visualize the structure, composition and functions of the living body. An elementary understanding of the imaging techniques and the basic physical principles is a prerequisite for full recognition of the diagnostic possibilities and for thorough and critical image interpretation.

This chapter is an introduction to the basic physical principles, the techniques and the concepts used in diagnostic imaging, avoiding undue technical details and strenuous mathematical formalisms.

Techniques

X-ray
CT
MR
Ultrasound
Scintigraphy

Techniques based on X-rays

The generation and nature of X-rays

X-rays occupy a range within the electromagnetic wave spectrum. For purposes of diagnostic imaging, useful wavelengths are between 0.06 and 0.006 nm. Unlike visible light, X-rays cannot be deflected by lenses or analogous devices. Diffraction and wave optics can therefore largely be ignored in diagnostic imaging with X-rays. It is useful to picture X-rays as linearly propagating streams of indivisible quanta of energy, *photons*. Accordingly, X-rays are commonly characterized by their photon energies rather than by their wavelengths or their wave frequency. Because X-rays are generated by conversion of the energy acquired by electrons accelerated through an electric field in the kilo-volt (kV) range, the convenient unit for X-ray photon energies is the kilo-electron-volt (keV); the diagnostic relevant range being 20–200 keV (Figure 1).

The propagation velocity (c) of electromagnetic waves is constant (*in vacuo*): 3×10^{17} nm × sec^{-1}, and relates to wavelength (λ) and frequency (v) by: $c = \lambda \times v$.

Electromagnetic waves are emitted as discrete quanta of energy (photons). The energy (E) of a photon relates to its frequency (v) by: $E = h \times v = \dfrac{h \times c}{\lambda}$, where h is Planck's constant. If energy is expressed in keV and wavelength (λ) in nanometers, the relation becomes: $E = \dfrac{1.24}{\lambda}$.

One electron volt (eV) is the energy acquired by an electron accelerated through a gradient of one volt. 1000 eV = 1 keV.

The X-ray tube

The source of X-rays for diagnostic imaging is *the X-ray tube* (Figure 2) in which a narrow beam of electrons, emitted from an electrically heated tungsten filament (the cathode), is accelerated *in vacuo* and focused electrostatically to impinge the target anode that emits a small fraction (0.2–2%) of the incident electron energy as X-rays. The rest of the energy dissipates as heat in the anode, which usually is made from a tungsten alloy with high thermal stability, shaped as a disc and rotating at high speed to spread the thermal load evenly over a large area.

The energy (wavelength) of the X-rays generated by the tube is primarily controlled by adjustment of the electrical potential difference between the cathode and the anode, *the accelerating voltage*. The high voltage is generated by rectification and high voltage transformation of common 50–60 Hz alternating current (AC) which has been converted up to some 50,000 Hz AC. Evening-out is incomplete and the high voltage is rippled. The ripple is expressed as the difference between the peak and the minimum voltage in per cent of the peak voltage and mounts to 5–10% in most high voltage generators. The high voltage setting of an X-ray unit usually refers to the peak voltage and is denoted *kVp* to indicate this fact.

The intensity of X-rays produced by the tube at a given voltage setting is determined by the number of electrons hitting the anode, that is, the current carried by the electrons through the vacuum from the cathode to the anode, termed *the beam (or tube) current* and expressed in milliamperes (mA). For accelerating voltages above some 40 kV (the saturation voltage), the beam current is largely determined by the cathode filament temperature only and can be regulated by the filament heating current supply.

The quantity (dose) of X-rays delivered by the tube is proportional to the time the beam current flows and is conveniently expressed as milliampere seconds (*mAs*).

The X-ray photons emitted by the anode distribute with varying intensity over a spectrum with a maximum set by the peak accelerating voltage of the tube. Thus, the X-ray beam is polychromatic. Even if the accelerating voltage is constant (not rippled) the beam is still highly polychromatic due to the nature of the process by which X-rays are generated at the anode ("*bremsstrahlung*"), not to be elaborated here.

Photons with energies below some 20 keV are useless for most radiography purposes because they cannot penetrate the body parts examined. Still they are harmful because their energy is absorbed superficially in the irradiated tissue, especially the skin. Insertion of thin aluminum or copper plates, *filters*, in the path of the X-ray beam removes these unwanted low energy photons (Figure 3). The mean photon energy thereby increases; the beam is said to be *hardened*. Mammography employs the lowest photon energies in diagnostic X-ray imaging, around 25–30 keV, in order to optimize detection of the very small differences in X-ray absorption between normal and cancerous tissue.

The X-ray tube is surrounded by a lead shield with a window that permits passage of the X-rays. The size and shape of the window, *the aperture*, can be varied by means of adjustable *diaphragms* (Figure 2). The X-rays radiate from the tube as a diverging bundle originating from the area on the anode hit by the electron beam, *the "focus"*, and limited by

Anatomy in Diagnostic Imaging, Third Edition. Peter Fleckenstein and Jørgen Tranum-Jensen.
© 2014 Peter Fleckenstein, Jørgen Tranum-Jensen and Peter Sand Myschetzky. Published 2104 by John Wiley & Sons, Ltd.

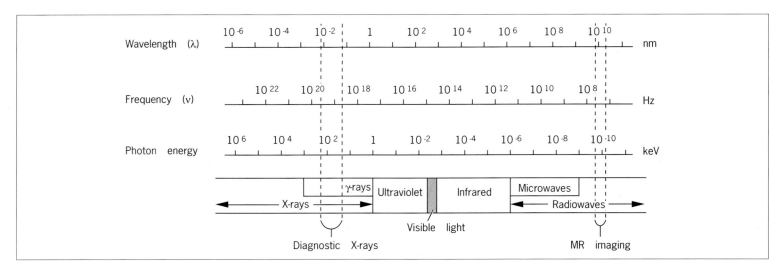

Figure 1 The electromagnetic wave spectrum, given by wavelength, frequency and photon energy.

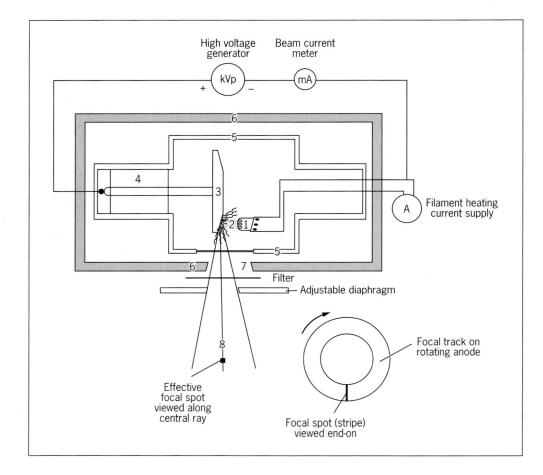

Figure 2 Diagrammatic presentation of the basic elements of a diagnostic X-ray tube. Details of circuitry are not given.
1: Cathode filament
2: Electron beam
3: Rotating anode
4: Anode motor drive
5: Vacuum tube
6: Lead shield
7: Window
8: Central ray

the tube exit aperture. The axis of the bundle is called *the central ray*, and the focus viewed along this axis is called *the effective focal spot*. The smaller this spot, the better the resolution in the radiograph. They are mostly in the order of 1 mm² or less; in mammography down to 0.1 mm² which allows detection of the tiny calcium deposits often found in malignant mammary tumors.

The X-ray beam should always be restricted by the diaphragms to illuminate the minimally required area of the body to minimize radiation exposure. This adjustment is called *collimation*.

Interactions of X-rays with matter

At the X-ray energies applied in diagnostic imaging, three types of interaction are to be considered: elastic scatter, the photoelectric effect, and inelastic (Compton) scatter.

Elastic scatter is an interaction whereby photons undergo a change of direction without loss of energy. This type of scatter takes place at all diagnostically relevant photon energies, but accounts for only a few per cent of the total scatter.

The photoelectric effect (Figure 4) is an interaction in which the incident X-ray photon delivers all of its energy to an

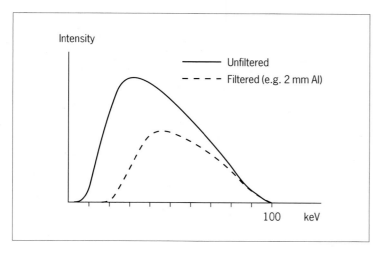

Figure 3 The effect of filtering on the distribution of photon energies in the X-ray beam from a 100 kVp tube.
Even the unfiltered beam has been "filtered" by passage through the wall of the X-ray tube whereby the lowest energies have been rejected. Additional filtering lowers the overall intensity, but increases the mean photon energy.

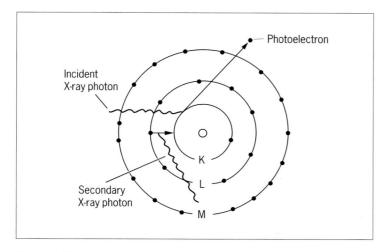

Figure 4 The photoelectric interaction.

atom which in turn releases this energy in the form of an electron, a *photoelectron*, which is ejected from one of the inner electron shells of the atom at high speed. An electron from one of the outer shells soon "falls in" to fill the vacancy, and energy is concomitantly released in the form of a new X-ray photon, emitted in a random direction and with an energy that is characteristic for the particular element. This secondary photon is of lower energy than the exiting photon. It may emerge as secondary radiation from the object, but is mostly absorbed by new interactions. The atom is left ionized, and the released electron collides with other atoms and causes a large number of secondary ionizations. The photoelectric effect is strong when the incident photon energy is just moderately higher than the binding energy of an inner shell electron. Only the two electrons in the innermost shell, the K-shell, have binding energies sufficiently high to engage in photoelectric interactions within

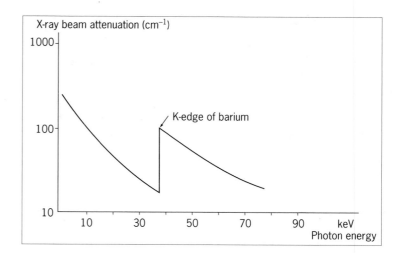

Figure 5 The K-edge effect.
X-ray absorption increases steeply at photon energies equal to the binding energy of the K-shell electrons of an element, a so-called K-edge.

Table 1

Element	K-edge (keV)
Carbon	0.3
Nitrogen	0.4
Oxygen	0.5
Phosphorus	2.1
Calcium	4.0
Iodine	33.2
Barium	37.4
Lead	88.1
Iron	7.1

the diagnostically relevant X-ray energy range. The photon energy, just sufficient to release a photoelectron from the K-shell, is denoted a *K-edge*, because the X-ray attenuation increases steeply as a threshold phenomenon at this energy level (Figure 5). The K-edges have characteristic values for different elements (Table 1). In soft tissues composed of lighter elements (C, N, O), photoelectric attenuation becomes quantitatively unimportant at photon energies above some 35 keV. Because the binding energy of K-shell electrons is higher for higher elements (such as calcium), the photoelectric effect remains quantitatively important for bone imaging up to some 50 keV. Barium and iodine have their K-edges at 37 keV and 33 keV, respectively. It is these high K-edges that are utilized when barium and iodine are used in contrast media.

The inelastic (Compton) scatter (Figure 6) results from interaction of X-ray photons with outer shell electrons which are ejected (recoil electrons) to leave the atom ionized, while the incident photon proceeds with reduced energy and a change of direction. An X-ray photon may engage in several such events of inelastic scatter on its path through an object,

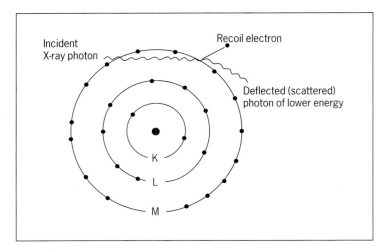

Figure 6 Inelastic (Compton) scatter.

eventually giving up all of its energy, that is, it becomes absorbed in the tissue. Compton scatter accounts for most of the scatter in diagnostic radiology. It depends primarily on the number of electrons per unit volume of tissue, and this in turn correlates almost linearly with the mass density of the tissues. It is independent of atomic number, and this is why the contrast of bone relative to soft tissues decreases at higher X-ray energies, where the photoelectric effect disappears.

Both the photoelectric effect and inelastic scatter result in a loss of electrons from atoms. This may cause the breakage of chemical bonds, and because the ionized atoms (notably those of C, N and O) are chemically highly reactive, new chemical bonds are established that are alien to the tissue. It is the X-rays' ability to cause ionizations that includes them in the family of *ionizing radiation*, and it is these ionizations and their derived chemical reactions that cause the biological damage of such radiation.

Units of absorbed dose and biological effect of ionizing radiation

The quantity of energy absorbed by a tissue is expressed in unit *gray* (Gy), one gray being equal to absorption of 1 joule kg^{-1}. The former unit of absorbed dose, *rad*, relates to gray by 1 Gy = 100 rad.

A practical measure of the biological effects (damage) of ionizing radiation (the *equivalent dose*) is given in unit *sievert* (Sv) which is the absorbed dose in gray multiplied by a "quality (weighting) factor" for the specific type of radiation in question. The quality factor for diagnostic X-rays and γ-emitting isotopes is around 1, while it is 10–20 for α-radiation and 1–2 for β-radiation, dependent on its energy. Though α- and β-radiation penetrate tissues poorly they can inflict serious damage if delivered by isotopes present within the body and perhaps even concentrated in particular tissues, for example in bone marrow. The former unit for equivalent dose, *rem*, relates to sievert by 1 Sv = 100 rem.

The differential ability of various tissues to scatter and absorb X-ray photons, no matter by which mechanisms, is given by their *linear attenuation coefficient* (cm^{-1}) which expresses the fractional reduction in beam intensity along a linear beam path after passage through one centimeter of the tissue. The linear attenuation coefficient of a given tissue varies with the X-ray photon energy, being high for lower energies where the photoelectric effect prevails and leveling off for higher energies where Compton scatter dominates, and hence the mass density rather than the atomic composition of the tissue becomes the prime determinant of attenuation (Figures 7 and 8).

Conventional imaging with X-rays

The basic set-up for conventional imaging with X-rays is very simple (Figure 9). The X-ray tube focal spot acts as a point source. The body part examined is composed of structural elements with different transparencies (attenuation coefficients) for X-rays, and the image appears as a 2D projection of the 3D object, much like a shadow figure, following the simple geometric rule of central projection. Thus, X-ray imaging is very different from optical imaging which implies a distinct focal plane in the object and a distinct image plane.

The bundle of collimated and filtered X-rays leaving a correctly adjusted tube has approximately the same intensity throughout a cross-section of the bundle. Accordingly, the intensity decreases proportionately as the square of the distance from the focal spot. The streams of linearly propagating X-ray photons ("rays") are variously attenuated by scatter and absorption along different linear paths through the object, depending on the thickness, the density and the elemental composition of the structural details passed. The emerging bundle of X-rays, modulated during passage through the object, conveys information in the form of variations in beam intensity within a cross-section of the bundle. This modulated bundle of X-rays is sometimes referred to as *the aerial image*, which may be recorded on a photographic film, a fluorescent screen or a digital image recorder inserted anywhere across the bundle.

Imaging geometry

It follows from the principle of central projection that *the image is always magnified*. The magnification increases when the object-to-film distance (OFD) is increased, and the magnification decreases when the focus-to-object distance (FOD) is increased (Figure 9). This implies that relative dimensional distortions are inherent in the image because structural details located closer to the focus are magnified more than details from a more remote location within the object (Figure 9B). This effect becomes more pronounced the thicker the object is relative to the focus-to-film distance. Inherent in the imaging principle is also that structural elements along the same linear

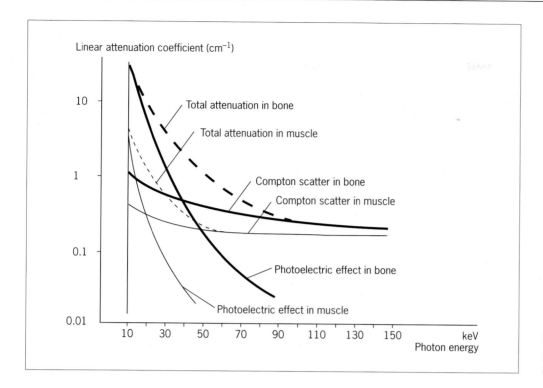

Figure 7 The relative contribution of the photoelectric effect and of Compton scatter to attenuation of X-rays in bone and muscle.

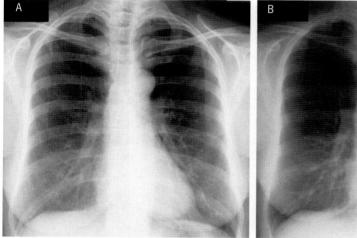

Figure 8 The effect of X-ray energy on image contrast between bone and soft tissues. Image (A) is recorded with a voltage setting at 50 kVp, (B) at 150 kVp. The lower beam energy in (A) yields higher contrast between bone and soft tissues, because of the contribution of photoelectric interactions in bone imaging at low kVp.

path are all superimposed, and information on their relative depth in the object is not contained in the image.

The contour sharpness of an imaged object (e.g. a trabecula of bone) is highly dependent on the size of the focal spot as well as the OFD relative to the FOD; the shorter the OFD and the longer the FOD, the sharper the contour. The width of the contour blurring, *the penumbra*, is equal to the projected image of the focal spot through a tiny pinhole at the position of the object (Figure 10). The shorter the FOD and the longer the OFD, the wider the penumbra becomes.

Scattered radiation

The interaction of the incident X-rays with the object causes random scatter of X-ray photons. This scatter is, on the one hand, a major contributor to the linear ray attenuation on which X-ray imaging is based, but is on the other hand a nuisance if the scattered photons reach the image recorder (film) because they spread randomly as noise over the field and impair image contrast and resolution. Thus, preventing scattered X-rays from reaching the film is a major concern in radiology. One or more of the following measures are employed to this end:

1 Collimation of the beam to that minimally necessary for imaging the object in question, thereby eliminating scattered radiation from irrelevant structures. This is an important measure also from a radiation hygienic point of view.

2 The length of the beam path through the body part examined may be reduced by appropriate positioning,

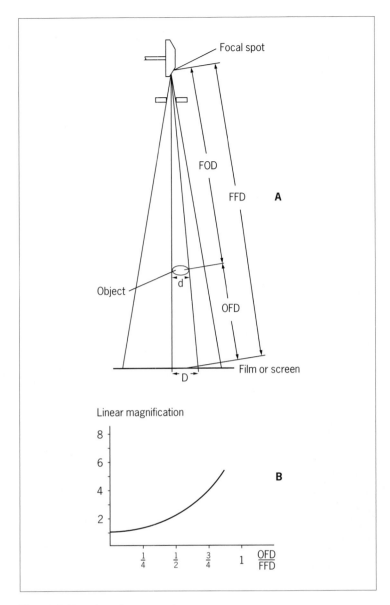

Figure 9 X-ray imaging geometry.

(A) Linear magnification $M = \dfrac{D}{d} = \dfrac{FFD}{FOD} = \dfrac{FFD}{FFD - OFD}$

(B) Magnification as a function of the object-to-film distance (OFD) relative to the focus-to-film distance (FFD).

sometimes supplemented with compression as used in mammography.

3 Increasing the air gap between the object and the film causes more of the scattered photons to miss the film. Magnification is thereby increased, but this may be compensated by an increase of the focus-to-object distance.

4 Choosing an appropriate kVp setting relative to the elemental composition of the object in order to maximize photoelectric interactions (in, for example, bone and contrast media) greatly improves contrast.

5 An effective and commonly applied measure to exclude scattered photons is the use of *grids* inserted in the beam path in front of the film. Grids are built from closely spaced

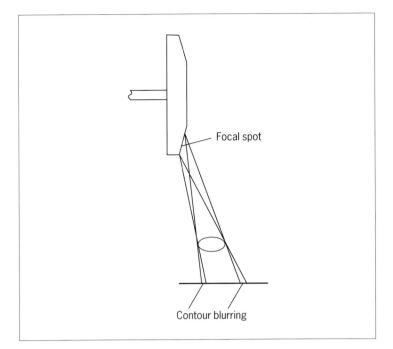

Figure 10 The influence of focal spot size on image sharpness.

thin lead strips interspersed by a material that is freely permeable to X-rays. The lead strips will absorb X-rays which are not arriving parallel or nearly parallel to the strips. The strips may be arranged at angles to match the direction of the unscattered X-rays throughout the image plane (Figure 11). The grid superimposes fine parallel lines on the image. For some applications this is tolerable, for others it is not, and the lines are then eliminated by transversal motion of the grid during exposure of the film. The mechanical device used to guide this motion is designated a *Bucky grid*.

Conventional X-ray tomography

Tomography means "drawing of a section" and denotes a special X-ray technique to image only structures contained in a predetermined plane of interest within the body part examined, while structures above and below this plane are blurred out. The basic principle of conventional tomography is, during the exposure, to move the X-ray tube and the film cassette synchronously but in opposite directions relative to a stationary axis which determines the tomographic plane (Figure 12). The movements may be just straight line translational or may follow more complicated paths. The angular movement relative to the axis, *the tomographic angle*, determines the thickness of the tissue "slice" to be imaged sharply. The larger the angle, the thinner the slice.

Conventional tomography is now replaced by computed tomography (CT, see below) for most purposes, but special machines that produce a panoramic image of a curved plane have been constructed for special purposes, best known from *orthopantomograms* of the dental arches.

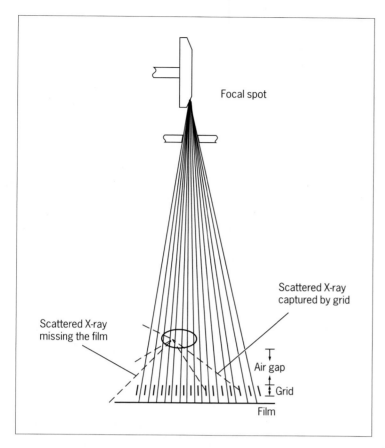

Figure 11 Exclusion of scattered radiation by air-gap and grid. The depicted grid is of the "focussed" type with angled lamellae, designed to a certain film-to-focus distance.

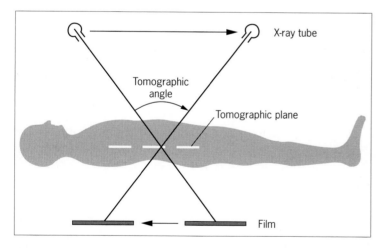

Figure 12 Principle of conventional X-ray tomography.

X-ray films

Films for X-ray imaging are manufactured to optimize their efficiency as detectors of X-ray photons. This is achieved with special photographic emulsions layered on both sides of the film base. This double coating slightly reduces the resolution of the film and for special purposes where high resolution is essential (e.g. in mammography), single coated films are used. The efficiency of X-ray photons to expose the photographic emulsion is only moderate, but is increased up to a factor of 100 by sandwiching the film between two layers of *intensifying screens* within the film *cassette*, which is a light-proof, but X-ray-transparent box containing the film. The intensifying screens are thin foils that are freely permeable for the X-rays and contain a substance that emits multiple lower energy photons (within the visible light spectrum) when hit by a single high-energy X-ray photon.

The performance of an X-ray film (with associated intensifying screens) as a recorder of the X-ray image is expressed in the *characteristic curve* for the film (Figure 13). The characteristic curve varies with the kVp setting and the development conditions applied. The two key parameters of the film are the *speed* and the *contrast*. The speed denotes the exposure needed to reach a specific optical density (O.D.), usually 1. The contrast is given by the slope of the linear part of the characteristic curve, denoted *gamma* (γ), and it expresses the exposure range which will be displayed on the gray-tone scale between white and black. The lower the gamma, the larger the exposure range to be covered, but the smaller will be the difference on the gray-tone scale between closely spaced doses of exposure, that is, less image contrast between two structures that transmit the X-rays with only a small difference in attenuation.

The classical X-ray film is now rapidly being replaced by various image recording systems that provide the images in digital format, so-called digital radiography (see below).

Fluorescent screens and image-intensifying tubes

The image conveyed by the X-ray bundle emerging from the patient may be viewed directly on a screen coated with a substance, a *"phosphor"*, which emits visible light (fluoresces) when hit by X-rays. Observation of the X-ray image on such a screen is called *fluoroscopy*. The advantage of fluoroscopy is that motion may be observed directly, for example the act of swallowing contrast media through the pharynx and down the esophagus. The light yield of such screens is rather low, and quite high patient doses of X-rays are needed to obtain an image of sufficient brightness to be viewed directly with the naked eye. Formerly, radiologists spend long hours in dim light viewing such screens. Fluoroscopy was greatly improved by the advent of *the image intensifying tube* (Figure 14). The input screen of this tube receives the X-rays from the patient and emits multiple lower energy photons from a phosphor. These photons in turn elicit release of electrons from an adjacent photocathode layer. These electrons are accelerated through a high voltage gradient along the tube and are at the same time focused by an electrostatic lens arrangement to hit a smaller screen at the other end of the tube. This screen is coated with a phosphor that emits visible (yellow-green) light with high efficiency when hit by electrons. The gain in screen brightness, the intensification, from the input to the output screen is in the order of several thousand-fold. The image on the output screen is usually viewed with a video camera and displayed on a TV monitor.

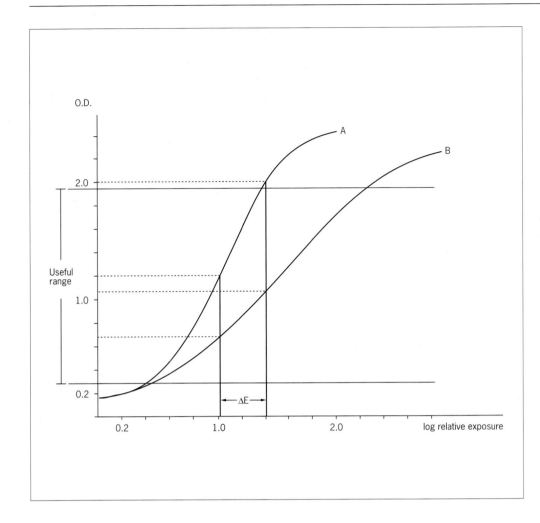

Figure 13 Characteristic curve of two different films.
Film A has a higher speed (is more sensitive) than film B. Film A also gives more contrast than B because a given narrow exposure range (ΔE) is differentiated over more gray tones by film A. Film B, on the other hand, will display a broader exposure range within the useful range of film densities (O.D. ~ 0.25–2.0).
The optical density (O.D.) of a transparent object, e.g. an X-ray film viewed on a light box, is defined by

$$O.D. = \log\frac{I_e}{I_i}$$

where I_i and I_e denote the intensity of incident and transmitted light, respectively. Thus, an O.D. of 2 means that only 1/100 of the incident light from the box is transmitted, which means nearly black.

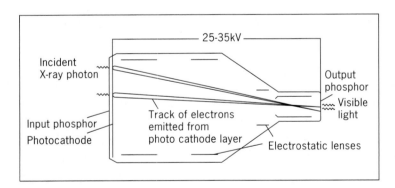

Figure 14 The basic design of an image intensifier tube. For explanation, see text.

Digital radiography

Instead of using a photographic emulsion the image may be recorded on plates, *imaging plates*, coated with a material, a *storage phosphor* (barium fluorohalides), which retains some of the incident X-ray energy as a latent image, analogous to the latent image of a classical photographic emulsion before development. When exposed to light of long wavelength (e.g. red laser light) the energy stored in the phosphor is released as light of short wavelength, a phenomenon known as *photostimulated luminescense*. When such an imaging plate

is scanned with a sharply focused red laser beam and the luminescence picked up in a photomultiplier, a digitalized image may be constructed point by point from the photomultiplier output signal (Figure 15). In the resultant image, each image point (pixel) corresponds approximately to an area the size of the focused laser beam.

A digitized image may also be recorded directly on a *direct flat panel detector* (Figure 16) made up from a layer of amorphous selenium that produces charge pairs (+/−, where the minus sign equals free electrons) when hit by X-ray photons. An electrical field laid across the selenium layer drags the electrons in linear paths onto a thin film of discrete detectors deposited in a 2D array on a glass substrate. Each detector corresponds to a pixel in the final image. The detectors store charge proportionate to the number of electrons received which again is proportionate to the number of X-ray photons received by the overlying selenium layer. The size of each detector is in the order of $100 \times 100\,\mu m$ and contains a capacitor for storage of charge and a thin film transistor (TFT) switch for read-out of the charge captured by each pixel. Other flat panel detectors are based in indirect release of electrons where the incident X-rays first hit a phosphor which releases visible light photons, which in turn release electrons from a photocathode layer, analogous to the process in the input screen of an image intensifier tube.

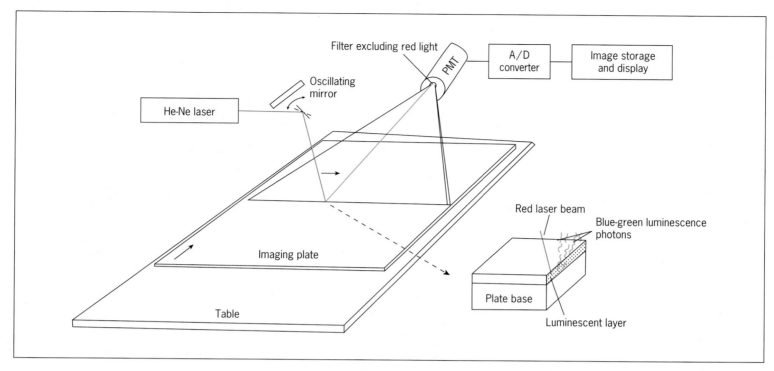

Figure 15 An imaging plate based on photo-stimulated luminescence.
The latent X-ray image is stored in the luminescent layer of the plate. The plate is advanced on a table and scanned by a narrowly focused red laser beam which elicits release of blue-green light from the plate, proportionate to its X-ray exposure at each point along the scanned lines. The emitted (blue-green) light is picked up by a planar fiber-optic conductor and fed into a photomultiplier tube (PMT). A filter prevents red laser light from reaching the PMT. After reading of the plate the latent image is erased by exposure to strong bright light, and the plate can then be reused.

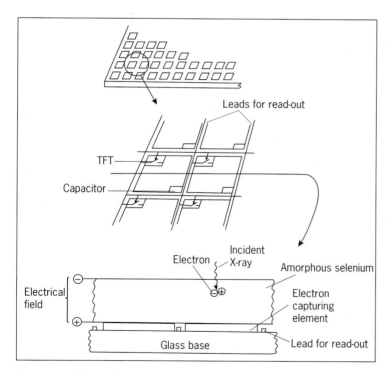

Figure 16 A direct flat panel detector.
Each detector element consists of an electron capture area, a capacitor and a thin film transistor (TFT) switch. The aerial image hits a layer of amorphous selenium which releases free electrons when hit by X-ray photons. The free electrons are drawn in straight paths onto the detector elements by an electrical field. The accumulated electrical charge is stored in the capacitor. A net of leads operates the TFT switches during read-out of the charge stored by each element.

A major advantage of the detector systems used for digital radiography is that their characteristic curve is linear and has a greater dynamic range, that is, extends over a much broader range of exposures (Figure 17). Further, the image data may be manipulated, for example to enhance the contrast at edges and to subtract background.

Digital subtraction X-ray imaging

The principle of image subtraction is especially applied in angiography. It involves the recording of one plain image before and followed by a sequence of images during and after intravascular injection of a contrast medium. The first image is used as a "mask" with reversed contrast. When this mask is superimposed on one of the following images all the image details that were stationary between the exposures cancel out leaving only those structures (e.g. arteries) that were delineated by the contrast medium in the second image. The contrast of the resultant subtracted image may be increased to display the vascular ramifications with great clarity.

The success of image subtraction is heavily dependent on effective immobilization of the body part examined so that the two images are truly identical except for the injected contrast. This condition implies that the heart can only be imaged by digital subtraction if the exposures are triggered on exactly the same point in the ECG. For imaging of gastrointestinal vessels the peristalsis is temporarily arrested by pharmacological means.

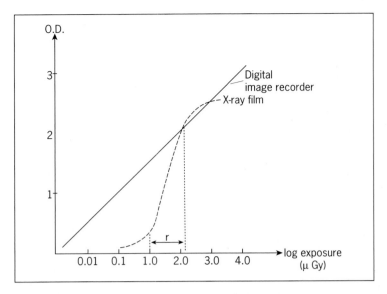

Figure 17 The characteristic curve of a digital imaging plate or a flat panel detector compared to a classical X-ray film.
The sensitivity is strictly linear and covers a range 3–4 decades broader than classical X-ray films.
r: useful exposure range of an X-ray film.

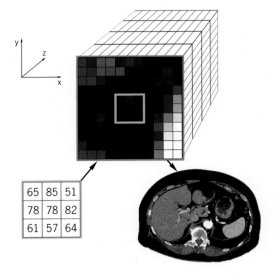

Figure 18 An image composed of pixels, each representing a volume element, a voxel.
The yellow frame (lower left) contains 9 pixels, each representing a volume of tissue (a voxel) with a calculated CT number. According to these numbers, each pixel has been assigned a gray-tone. Together the collection of all the pixels make up the image (lower right). The depth (z) of the voxel equals the section thickness. For computation of images maintaining the same resolution at any angle through a stack of images, voxels must be cubic (x = y = z).

The principle of image subtraction may also be applied to two images recorded in rapid succession, but at different kVp settings (e.g. at 50 and 150 kVp) in order to enhance or reduce the contrast of structures whose attenuation coefficients change significantly between the two kV settings, for example of bones or contrast media. This procedure is called *dual energy subtraction*. The same principle is utilized in *DXA (DEXA) scanning* (dual energy X-ray absorptiometry) where the patient is scanned linearly with a thin fan of X-rays alternating between the two different photon energies. An X-ray detector measures the transmission of each of these energies. A computer calculates the mineralization of the bones and constructs an image. The mineralization can be expressed as *bone mineral content* (BMC), in $g\,cm^{-1}$, that is, the total mineral content in a 1-cm-thick slice of the bone, or as the average *bone mineral density* (BMD), in $g\,cm^{-2}$, that is, BMC divided by the width of the slice in centimeters.

Computed X-ray tomography

A computed X-ray tomogram, a *CT image*, is a squared matrix of picture elements, *pixels*, each representing a small volume element, a *voxel*, within an imaginary "section" or "slice" of the body part examined (Figure 18). The average linear attenuation coefficient of each voxel has been derived by computation from a series of measurements collected by the CT scanner, and has been assigned a gray-tone value linearly related to its magnitude. Highly attenuating structures like compact bone, are shown in white and slightly attenuating structures like air, are shown in black, that is, as they would appear in conventional X-ray imaging. Thus the CT image is

a map of the spatial distribution of calculated X-ray attenuation coefficients.

The resolution of a CT image is in principle determined by the size of the image matrix, relative to the imaged area, the *field of view* (FOV). Matrices used for diagnostic imaging usually range from 128×128 to 1024×1024 with 512×512 (i.e. 262144 pixels) being a commonly used matrix. Applied to a $40 \times 40\,cm$ FOV, the pixel size becomes $0.8 \times 0.8\,mm$. Had this matrix been applied to a $20 \times 20\,cm$ FOV, the pixel size would become $0.4 \times 0.4\,mm$. In practice, the true resolution is less.

When the pixel size is decreased, the signal from each voxel (pixel) as well as the signal-to-noise ratio also decrease. The signal-to-noise ratio of a photon signal is $N/N^{1/2}$, where N is the number of photons counted (Poisson statistics). This means that if the pixel size is decreased, the sampling time or the dose rate must be increased to obtain a true improvement of resolution.

The CT scanner

The basic design of a commonly used CT scanner is shown in Figure 19. The X-ray tube is set in motion on a circular rail, *the gantry*, surrounding the patient who is positioned on a couch centrally in the gantry. The X-ray beam is collimated to a fan that intersects the patient. The angular width of the fan determines the field to be imaged and is commonly about 60° to cover the full cross-section of the patient's torso. The intensity of the X-rays after passage of the patient is recorded by a closely spaced array of detectors mounted on the same frame as the X-ray tube to ensure that it rotates in exact

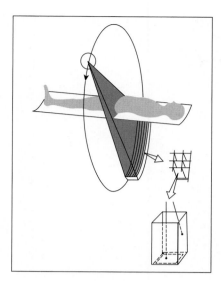

Figure 19 The basic design of a multislice CT scanner. The X-ray tube rotates in synchrony with the detector array which is composed of a large number of parallel rows of detectors recording the intensity of X-rays having passed through the patient in multiple directions during a turn of the tube and detector assembly. Each of the X-ray capturing detectors are shielded by a collimator that permits only X-rays coming in a straight line from the focal spot of the X-ray tube to reach the detector.

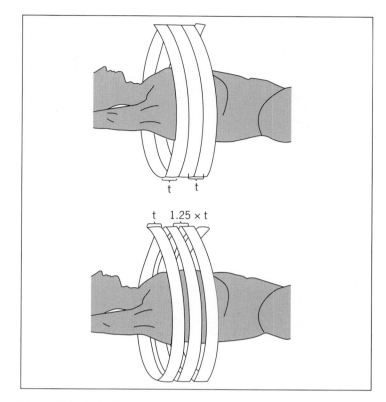

Figure 20 Helical CT scanning. The patient is lying on the couch which moves at constant speed through a multislice scanner. If the couch during one 360° revolution of the X-ray tube moves the same distance as the width of the detector array (t), the pitch equals t; the pitch factor is one (upper figure). If the couch moves 25% faster, the pitch factor becomes 1.25, that is, the sections are spaced by a slice of tissue, one fourth of the section thickness, not being imaged (lower figure). A pitch factor of less than one means that the sections overlap.

synchrony with the tube. During one revolution of the X-ray tube the detectors record the intensity of transmitted X-rays along a very large number of linear paths, in the order of one million or more measurements. In the latest generation of scanners several rows of detectors are mounted parallel to each other, allowing simultaneous acquisition of data from several adjacent slices during one revolution of the X-ray tube, the so-called *multislice technique*. The number of simultaneously recorded slices may be over a hundred, in some scanners even 320, all recorded during one revolution in less than a second. For a detector width of 0.5 cm, a 320-slice helical scanner will cover a 16-cm-thick "slice" of the patient. The detectors are shielded by narrow collimators that only allow X-rays coming in straight line from the X-ray tube to reach the detector.

The kVp of the X-ray tube is set so high (120–140 kV) that inelastic (Compton) scatter is the only quantitatively important process that attenuates the beam. This implies that the CT image can, with good approximation, be read as a map of tissue mass densities.

In earlier ("third generation") designs the detectors were mounted on the gantry opposite the X-ray tube and set to follow in synchrony the circular motion of the tube. The couch was moved in steps between each collection of a 360° series of measurements, that is, the measurements were sampled from planar slices. Today, the couch is set to move continuously at constant speed. Data are thereby collected from a helical "slice" of the patient, so-called *helical ("spiral") scanning*, which has reduced the time for an examination considerably. Data for construction of a planar image from

helical sampling are obtained by interpolation between adjacent spiral sections. The *pitch* denotes the distance travelled by the couch relative to the section thickness during one revolution of the tube. Thus, a pitch of one means that for collection of data for a 5 mm slice the couch has moved 5 mm; had it moved 10 mm the pitch would be two (Figure 20). At pitch values above one the topographical definition of the imaged structures becomes increasingly imprecise and small structural details may be overlooked if located in the tissue separating the helical slices, just as with planar sampling. Pitch values below one means that the slices overlap, that is, over-sampling which improves resolution.

The CT scanner may also be used to collect an image similar to a conventional X-ray image if the X-ray tube and the detector array are kept stationary while the patient, lying on the couch, is moved longitudinally through the gantry. Such a *"scout view"* (*scanogram*) is usually taken at the beginning of an examination and used for planning of the following tomographic sequence and as a reference on which the positions of the tomograms are indicated.

To overcome *movement artifacts* in cardiac CT imaging, the data sampling may be gated on the ECG to within a particular phase of the cardiac cycle. Respiratory movement artifacts

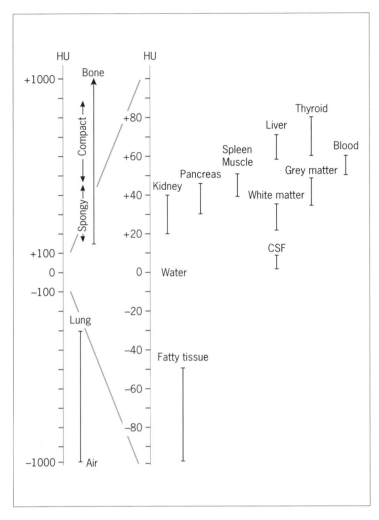

Figure 21 The Hounsfield scale.
Approximate CT numbers of some tissues and organs are indicated.

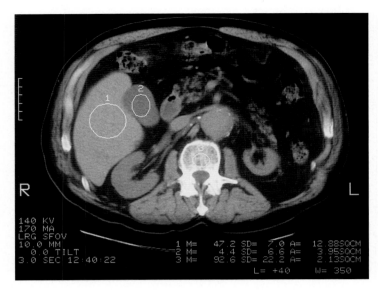

Figure 22 CT image of abdomen.
R and L denote patient's right and left. A centimeter scale to the left in the image gives the linear calibration. The image is displayed with settings of level and window of 40 and 350, respectively. The X-ray tube has been operated at 140 kVp with a tube current of 170 mA. The tomographic slice thickness is 10 mm, and the data to construct the image have been collected over a period of 3 seconds. Three locations have been selected for display of numerical figures of X-ray attenuation. Location I is in the liver and has an area of 12.88 square centimeter, and an average CT number of 47.2 with a standard deviation (SD) of 7.0. Location 2 is in the gall bladder, location 3 is in the cancellous bone of a vertebral body. Note the high SD of the latter. Atherosclerotic calcifications are present in the aorta and right renal artery.

are overcome by asking the patient to suspend breathing during the short period of data acquisition.

Image construction

The attenuation of X-rays recorded along one of the numerous paths through each section is the sum of contributions from all the voxels passed, and all the voxels in the section have been intersected by a multitude of beam paths. By a computational procedure known as *filtered back projection*, the average linear attenuation coefficient of each voxel can now be calculated. The attenuation coefficients are calculated relative to that of water and for convenience multiplied by a constant to make them large whole numbers. The coefficient for water is by definition zero, and the constant is chosen so that the coefficient for air becomes −1024 (2^{10}). (Formerly the coefficient for air was set to be −1000, the difference having little practical importance.) This brings bone to values of up to around +2000 for the most compact types of bone. The scale of attenuation coefficients spanning 4024 units (−1024 to +3000) is the *Hounsfield scale,* and one unit is called a *CT number* or a *Hounsfield unit* (HU). The scale is shown in Figure 21, where the values of some tissues are given. The

scale is to some extent instrument specific depending on, among others, the accelerating voltage and the beam filtering applied. An area of a particular tissue may be selected on the CT image with a cursor to determine its average CT number and its standard deviation (Figure 22). In clinical practice a structure/tissue that is imaged with low opacity is called *hypodense*, that is, it attenuates the X-rays less than the surrounding structures/tissues. The opposite is *hyperdense*.

The human eye cannot discriminate more than about 20 steps on a gray-tone scale from black to white. Because many tissues differ by only a few Hounsfield units they will only be differentiated in the image if a small range of the Hounsfield scale is displayed on the gray-tone scale. The number of Hounsfield units displayed is denoted *the window width* (W) and the midpoint value of the window is denoted *the window level* (L). If the window is chosen to cover, for example, 100 units to be discriminated on a 20-step gray-tone scale each step will cover 5 units. All voxels with a CT number higher than the upper limit of the window will be displayed in white, and all below will be in black. The effect of varying the window width around a fixed level, and of varying the level with a fixed window is shown in Figure 23. It is obvious that the window and level must be chosen appropriately for discrimination of different tissues of interest. Certain combi-

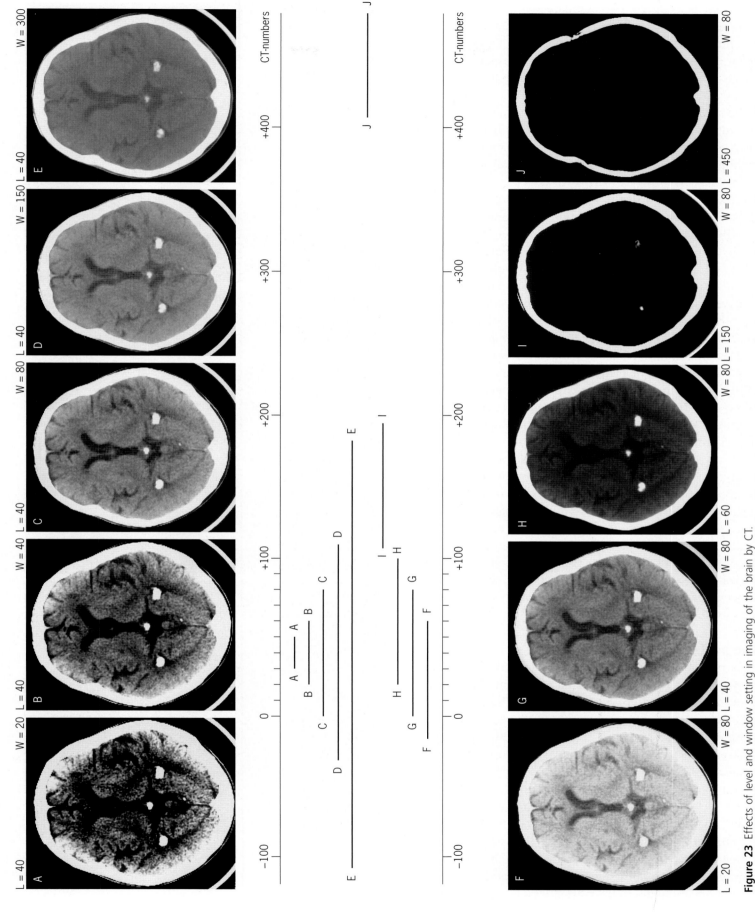

Figure 23 Effects of level and window setting in imaging of the brain by CT. The upper panel shows the tomogram displayed with a constant level (40) and increasing window from left to right. The lower panel shows the tomogram displayed with a constant window (80) and increasing level from left to right. Note calcifications in pineal body and choroid plexus.

nations may be referred to as standard *bone settings*, *soft tissue settings*, and *lung settings*, etc. (Figure 24).

It is important to bear in mind that the CT number of a voxel and the derived gray-tone of the corresponding pixel is set by the average attenuation within that voxel. This imaging principle implies that the dimensions of a structure may be appreciably distorted, especially where tissues of widely differing CT numbers meet, for example bone and brain. If a voxel contains say 10% dense bone and 90% brain by volume, the average CT number may be around 120. If now the image is displayed with a window of 100 and a level of 40, the upper limit of the window will be at 90, and the pixel is consequently shown in white which means that the bone will appear thicker than it is. If the level was raised to 150, the CT numbers differentiated on the 20-step gray-tone scale would span from 100–200, that is, it would include the voxel of 120 which would be displayed as a dark gray pixel as if it were all brain. Such dimensional distortions in CT images are referred to as *the partial volume effect*, which become more disturbing the thicker the sections are because more different tissues may become included in the voxel. The effect is very pronounced also at the borders between airways and air. Thus the diameter of a bronchus will appear too small with a setting that resolves the smaller lung vessels. Note also on Figure 23F–J how the apparent thickness of the skull decreases from left to right.

As X-rays penetrate tissues they become increasingly "hardened", because the lower energy photons are preferentially absorbed and scattered. The linear attenuation coefficient therefore decreases. The computing program of the CT scanner takes this effect into account, albeit on the basis of expected averages. If a piece of metal, for example a dental filling, is included in the section, gross artifacts arise, so-called *beam-hardening artifacts*. Such artifacts may be seen also in soft tissues encased in thick bone, for example in the posterior cranial fossa.

Image post-processing

A stack of consecutive 2D images of axial sections contains information of the HU value of all voxels in the scanned volume. Provided the voxels are isotropic, that is, are tiny cubes, arbitrarily chosen planar or curved sections through the volume can be calculated to the same resolution as the original axial sections. This procedure is known as *multiplanar reformation* (*MPR*).

If an image is constructed by summation of all the attenuation coefficients of all the voxels encountered by imaginary parallel "rays" traversing the whole stack, the result is a 2D image analogous to a conventional X-ray. If instead the image is composed only from the voxels with the highest HU value encountered by each of the imaginary beams, the result is an image enhancing high-contrast structures, for example calcifications and contrast-filled vessels. The procedure is known as *maximum intensity projection* (*MIP*). When applied not to the whole stack, but to a selected number of consecutive images,

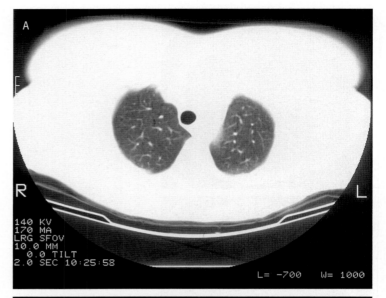

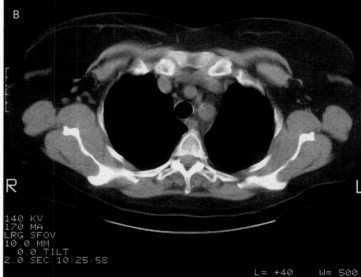

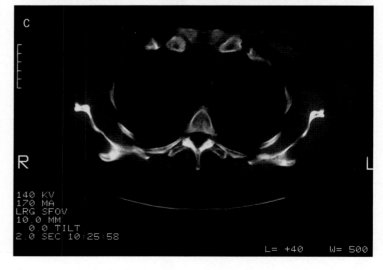

Figure 24 Standard "tissue settings" in a CT slice of the thorax. Upper frame (A): "Lung settings" (L = −700/W = 1000). Middle frame (B): "Soft tissue settings" (L = 40/W = 500). Lower frame (C): "Bone settings" (L = 250/W = 500).

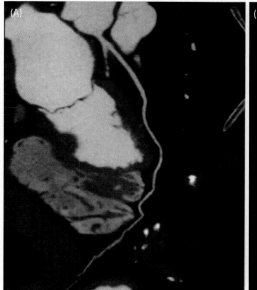

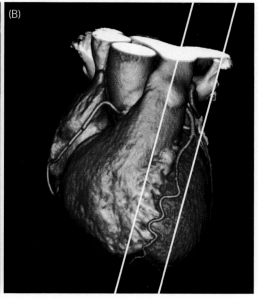

Figure 25 Example of maximum intensity projection, MIP (A) and volume rendering (B) of the heart.
(A) is a MIP of an oblique slice of the heart imaged in (B), where the approximate slice location and thickness is indicated. (B) is a volume-rendered image, permitting only voxels with CT numbers characteristic of heart muscle and of contrast medium to contribute to the image.

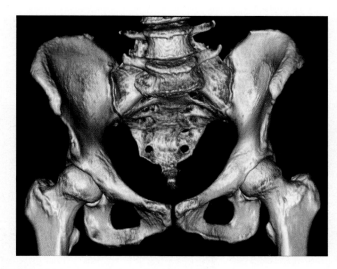

Figure 26 Volume rendering of pelvis and hips.
The image is computed only from voxels having CT numbers characteristic of bone.

representing a slab of the total volume and containing a structure of interest, improved visualization of details is obtained (Figure 25).

If the whole set of HU values for all the voxels in a volume is displayed in a histogram certain values may be excluded from the image, for example all voxels below −100 HU, which means that fat and air-filled lung tissue will not be visualized. Similarly, dense bone may be excluded from contribution to the image. The range of HU values selected to contribute to the image may be assigned different colors and opacities, thereby improving the visualization of, for example, contrast-filled vessels.

The exclusion threshold may also be set so high that only bone is imaged (Figure 26). These techniques which are based on selective inclusion together with color and opacity coding from the whole set of voxels are denoted *volume-rendering* techniques (Figure 27).

It is possible also to construct *surface-rendered* images which include only voxels located where steep gradients in the HU values of nearby voxels occur, for example from tissue to air as in virtual colonoscopy (Figure 28).

Volume-rendered images can be constructed corresponding to any angle of view of the data set, and provided there is sufficient computer power, the structure may be set to rotate slowly on the screen. Addition of a virtual light source adding shades to the object improves the 3D presentation.

X-ray contrast enhancing media

Contrast media are used to either increase or to decrease the X-ray attenuation coefficient of a tissue or an organ in order to make it stand out in positive or negative contrast relative to its surroundings.

All positive contrast media now in use contain iodine or barium. These elements have K-absorption edges at 33 and 37 keV, respectively (Figure 5 and Table 1). This means that they effectively absorb X-ray photons by photoelectric interaction in the 33 (37) to about 55 keV range, which is well represented in the beam from an X-ray tube operated at 80–100 kVp. At high kVp settings, for example 150 kV, the positive contrast effect of these elements is considerably lowered because Compton scatter then dominates. So, when the concentration of contrast medium is low, lower voltage settings are generally used in conventional X-ray imaging.

Barium
Barium is used as suspensions of fine particles of barium sulfate for imaging of the alimentary tract. Formulations differ with respect to barium content, viscosity, and "stickiness", according to purpose.

The pharynx and esophagus may be examined by fluoroscopy during the act of swallowing a gulp of barium suspension.

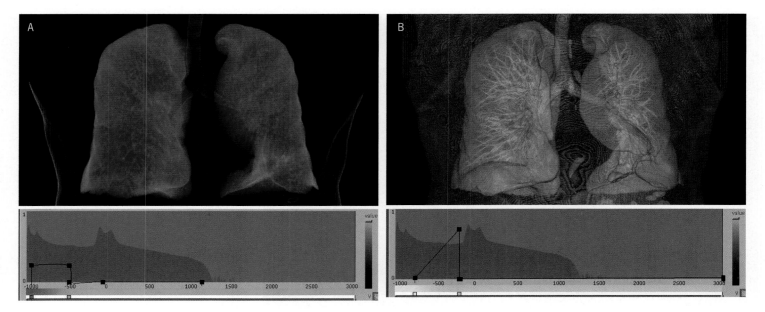

Figure 27 Volume rendering of the lungs.
(A) The lower panel shows a histogram of the CT numbers of all the voxels in the scanned body part, extending from −1000 (air) to dense bone (+1300). Only the voxels indicated by the rectangle to the left have been permitted to contribute to the image and are color coded as indicated on the color scale under the histogram. (B) The triangle to the left indicates the range of CT numbers (−800 to −225) selected to contribute to the image, however of increasing transparency towards the lower values as seen on the color scale below. The result is that the lung tissue appears transparent permitting imaging of the embedded bronchial tree.

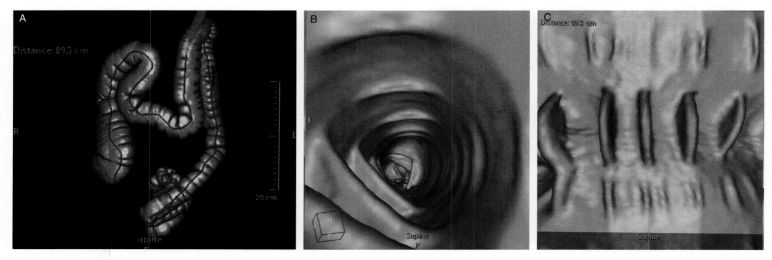

Figure 28 Virtual colonoscopy.
Frame (A) shows a surface-rendered image of an air inflated colon. The path of the virtual colonoscopy is indicated by the red line. The blue arrow indicates the direction of view into the stretch of transverse
colon indicated by yellow and imaged in (B). The distance from anus is shown to the left. The image (C) is a so-called filet view of (B) where the colon has been cut open to allow "face-on" inspection of the mucosal surface.

The stomach, duodenum and small intestine may similarly be examined after ingestion of a barium meal. For examination of the stomach, sodium bicarbonate is often added to the suspension in order to produce an image where the sticky suspension lines the wall of the stomach which has been distended by carbon dioxide gas liberated from the bicarbonate. This is a so-called *double contrast examination*, where gas serves as the negative double contrast agent. This examination may yield fine resolution of details in the gastric mucosal surface. Barium suspensions given as *enemas* are used for examination of the rectum, the colon and the terminal ileum, often combined with insufflation of air to produce a double-contrast image for improved visualization of mucosal details.

Iodine

Iodine is used in stable covalent binding to various organic molecules. The development of atoxic and *water soluble, iodinated contrast media* that are tolerated by intravascular and subarachnoid injection, and which are rapidly cleared by renal excretion, was a major breakthrough in radiology.

From a practical point of view, and disregarding details of their chemistry, the water-soluble contrast media are commonly grouped into *ionic* versus *non-ionic* and *high-osmolality* versus *low-osmolality* media.

The contrast enhancement produced by any of the media is determined by the number of iodine atoms encountered by an X-ray photon along a linear path through the object. If the path is short, for example across a small vessel or duct, the concentration of the medium must be correspondingly high. This may often be achieved only at concentrations of the medium well above normal plasma osmolality ($300\,\text{mOsm}\,\text{kg}^{-1}$), for some applications going as high as $1500\,\text{mOsm}\,\text{kg}^{-1}$, which frequently causes adverse reactions. This problem is especially pronounced with ionic media because they dissociate to produce two or more osmotic effectors in solution. By various non-ionic substitutions and by increasing the number of iodine atoms per molecule it has become possible to develop *non-ionic, low-osmolality contrast media* which have become especially useful for angiography. It is possible using these media to keep the intravascular osmolality below some $500\,\text{mOsm}\,\text{kg}^{-1}$ or less in high-resolution angiography.

A major concern in *urography* is that the contrast medium should have a high renal clearance rate, resulting in a high urinary concentration. The media may be given by slow intravenous injection and in lower concentrations. The intravascular osmolality may therefore be kept low even with ionic media.

Water-soluble, iodinated contrast media can be used for a variety of other purposes, for example sialography, dacryocystography, direct pyelography and cystography, hysterosalpingography, cholangiography, arthrography, and bronchography. They are used also to visualize the gastrointestinal canal, especially in CT imaging.

Gas

Air or carbon dioxide are used as *negative contrast media*. Their use in combination with barium for gastrointestinal double-contrast examinations has already been mentioned.

Techniques based on nuclear magnetic resonance

Principles of MR scanning

The nuclear magnetic dipole moment

An electrical charge which has an angular momentum, a *spin*, creates a *magnetic dipole moment* aligned with the axis of spin. This applies to electrons and protons which both have a spin and a charge, but also to neutrons because the component electrical charges of this particle are non-uniformly distributed within its volume. Two identical and closely packed particles, for example two protons or two neutrons within an atomic nucleus, will align their spins so as to cancel out their magnetic dipole moments. Therefore, only nuclei with an odd number of protons and/or neutrons possess a magnetic dipole moment for the nucleus as a whole. Among the biological relevant atomic nuclei with magnetic dipole moments, that of hydrogen, ^{1}H, the single proton, is by far the quantitatively dominating species, and it is also ubiquitously present in living matter. Some isotopes of other biologically relevant elements, for example ^{13}C, ^{23}Na and ^{31}P, also have magnetic dipole moments and are utilized experimentally. ^{19}F may be used as a molecular label, for example on drugs and metabolites.

Nuclear magnetic resonance imaging (MRI or just "MR") is based on manipulation of nuclear magnetic dipole moments by means of externally applied magnetic fields and subsequent recording and analysis of the radio signals emitted from the nuclei in response to these manipulations. The phenomenon of nuclear magnetic resonance (NMR) has long been exploited as a fruitful analytical tool in chemistry. The development of diagnostic imaging techniques based on NMR required the construction of apparatuses for generation of strong and uniform magnetic fields, large enough to accommodate a whole person, and development of methods to resolve the topological origin of complex radio signals emitted from within the body.

Because virtually all diagnostic MR imaging thus far has been concerned with NMR of protons (hydrogen), the following account will refer to the proton, but the principles and concepts apply to any nucleus with a magnetic dipole moment.

The MR scanner

The basic components of an MR scanner are shown in simplified form in Figure 29. The *main magnet* produces a very strong and homogenous field of 0.1–3 T (7 T in some special scanners) inside the bore of the magnet. This field must be extremely stable in time and is commonly produced with superconducting coils cooled with liquid helium. Some

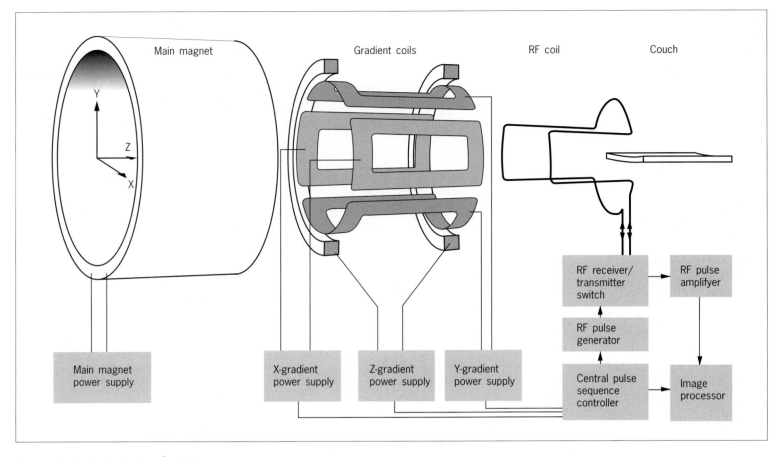

Figure 29 The basic design of a MR scanner.

Tesla

Magnetic field strength is measured in unit *Tesla* (T). One Tesla is defined as the field which exerts a force of 1 Newton (N) on a one metre length of conductor carrying one ampere (A) of current perpendicular to the magnetic field. Tesla relates to unit *gauss* by 1 T = 10,000 gauss. For comparison, the magnetic field strength at the Earth's surface is $30 - 70 \times 10^{-6}$ T (0.3–0.7 gauss), highest at the poles.

---

smaller MR scanners employ resistive coils, others are constructed over permanent, ferromagnetic magnets, but none of these can produce fields as strong and stable as those based on superconducting coils. A main reason to apply strong fields is that the signal-to-noise ratio in the radio signals used to construct the MR image thereby improves.

A whole body MR scanner is voluminous and expensive and not needed for many purposes. Smaller scanners just big enough to accommodate an arm, a leg, or a head have therefore also been developed.

Inside the bore of the magnet are installed three sets of coils used for production of *magnetic field gradients*, one in the direction of the main field (the Z-axis) and two perpendicular to this (the X- and Y-axis). The gradient field strengths over the entire patient are less than 1% of the main field strength and can be rapidly varied in time. Inside the gradient coil assembly is mounted a *radiofrequency* (RF) *transmitter/receiver coil*. For some applications, a small, separate receiver coil, molded to the surface contour of the body part examined, denoted a *surface coil*, is placed directly on the surface of the body. This improves the signal-to-noise ratio and the resolution in the final image, but limits the volume that can be examined.

The patient is finally installed on a couch centrally in the bore. A *pulse sequence controller* operates the gradient coil power supplies and the transmitter-receiver switch of the RF coil through the complex sequences used for the various MR imaging modes. The received RF signals are analyzed by Fourier transformation and spatially decoded in the image processor to be displayed as an image, which is a map of the amplitude of RF signals emitted from small volume elements, *voxels*, in an imaginary slice of the patient.

Proton magnetization

When a proton is exposed to a steady external magnetic field, a force will act on its magnetic dipole moment so as to orient it parallel with the external field, but, due to the spin, it does not swing in as a compass needle would do. Instead it performs a maintained circular movement, called *precession*, in which its own axis of spin rotates at an angle around another axis that is parallel with the external field, much like a toy spinning top in the gravitational field (Figure 30). The magnetic dipole moment of the precessing proton has a magnitude and a direction and may therefore conveniently be expressed by a vector. This vector may be resolved in one component aligned with the axis of precession, "the longitudinal component", and a second component, oriented perpendicular to the external field and rotating with the frequency of precession, the "transverse component" (Figure 30).

The frequency of precession, the *Larmor frequency*, is linearly related to the strength of the external field as expressed by the Larmor equation. The precessional frequency of protons is $42.58 \, \text{MHz T}^{-1}$, a constant denoted the *gyromagnetic ratio* (γ) of the proton (hydrogen). The Larmor frequency is actually not exactly the same for all protons, but differs by a few ppm depending on the chemical bonds they have established. Thus, the Larmor frequency of protons in water and in aliphatic fatty acid chains differs by about $3 \, \text{ppm}$ ($\sim 130 \, \text{Hz}$) in a $1 \, \text{T}$ field. Such differences are designated *chemical shifts*. The chemical shifts may cause positional shifts of fat relative to water along the direction of the frequency encoding gradient in some imaging sequences.

The Larmor equation

The Larmor frequency $\omega = \upsilon_L \times 2\pi = \gamma \times T$, where ω is the angular velocity, υ_L is the frequency of precession, γ is the gyromagnetic ratio and T is the field strength in Tesla.

Some gyromagnetic ratios in MHz T^{-1}:

^{1}H: 42.58 ^{13}C: 10.71 ^{23}Na: 11.27 ^{31}P: 17.25

Exposed to the external field, the spin of the proton may be at one of two discrete energy levels, according to principles of quantum mechanics, not to be elaborated here. At the low spin-energy level the longitudinal component of the magnetic vector points in the same direction as the external field, at the high energy level it points in the opposite direction (Figure 31). The fractional distribution of protons between these two states depends on the temperature and the strength of the external field. Even at the high field strengths applied in diagnostic imaging (0.1–2 T), the net magnetization of protons at 37° C is weak with only a small surplus of protons (a few ppm in a 1 T field) being at the low spin-energy level. The net magnetization may, just as the magnetic dipole moment of the individual protons,

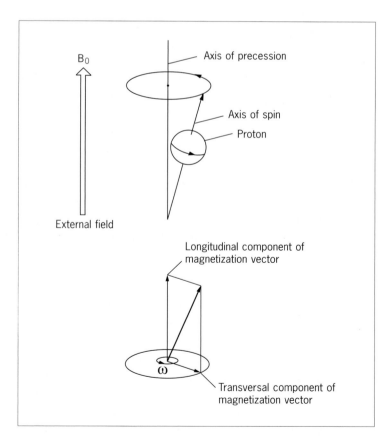

Figure 30 Proton spin and precession.

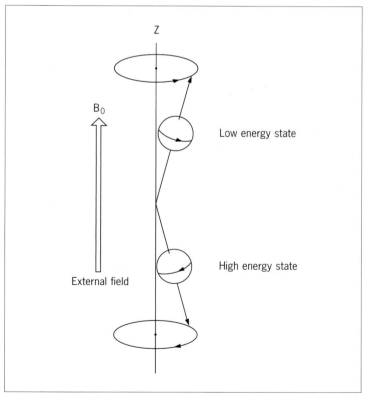

Figure 31 Illustration of proton spin levels.

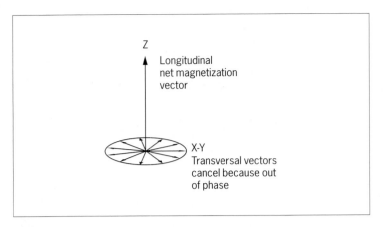

Figure 32 Pictorial representation of the net magnetization vector.

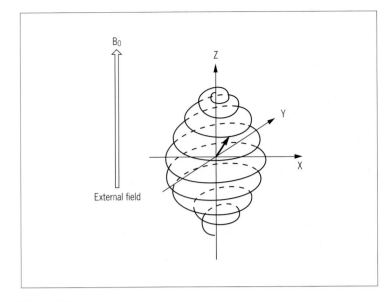

Figure 33

Diagrammatic illustration of the gradual change of the net magnetization vector under the influence of an increasing input of energy, delivered by RF-waves at the Larmor frequency.

conveniently be described by a vector (Figure 32). It is important to note that this *net magnetization vector* represents the statistical equilibrium of a huge population of protons which are constantly influenced by thermal (Brownian) motion, and shifting between the two spin-energy levels. This equilibrium net magnetization vector is aligned parallel (longitudinal) to the external field. The transversal, rotating vectors of the individual protons cancel out because they are out of phase in the equilibrium state.

Resonance

When a body part/tissue has been installed in the strong, steady and uniform field of the MR scanner, the equilibrium state, represented by the net magnetization vector becomes established within seconds. This equilibrium may be disturbed and shifted by a pulse of electromagnetic waves (photons) at the Larmor frequency of the protons (42.58 MHz in a 1 T field) entering perpendicular to the main field. This frequency is within the radiofrequency (RF) region of the electromagnetic wave spectrum (Figure 1). Only RF waves of exactly this frequency will transfer energy by *resonance* to the precessing protons. In principle, a bar magnet oriented perpendicular to the main field and rotating at 42.58×10^6 revolutions per second would do the same job. This transfer of energy by resonance has *two* effects on the precessing protons.

Firstly, protons at the low spin-energy level, having absorbed the energy of a RF photon, shift to the high energy state accompanied by a shift in the direction of their magnetic dipole moments. Accordingly, the magnitude of the *longitudinal net magnetization vector* decreases as more and more protons shift to the high energy state. At a certain RF energy input the longitudinal vector disappears. By further input of RF energy a surplus of protons is lifted to the high spin-energy state whereby the longitudinal vector reappears, but now in the opposite direction.

The second effect of the RF pulse is to force the protons into coherent ("in phase" or "synchronous") precession. This

is manifested by the appearance of a *transverse net magnetization vector* that rotates with the Larmor frequency.

The net magnetization vector is at any given time the resultant of the longitudinal and transverse magnetization vectors. Thus, with an increasing RF energy input, the longitudinal vector decreases and the transverse vector grows. The net magnetization vector is therefore tilted more and more towards the transverse orientation while rotating at the Larmor frequency (Figure 33). The angle between the direction of the main field and the net magnetization vector is denoted *the flip angle*. An RF pulse delivering just enough energy to tilt ('flip') the net magnetization vector into the transverse orientation is called a *90° pulse*. An RF pulse twice this magnitude will cause the reappearance of the longitudinal vector, but in the opposite direction, relative to the main field. Such a pulse is called a *180° pulse* and the protons are said to be *saturated*. RF energy inputs between a 90° and a 180° pulse are said to produce *partial saturation*. The duration of the excitatory RF pulses used in MR imaging is in the order of a few milliseconds, to give an idea of the timescale.

Relaxation

When the RF pulse is turned off, the excited protons return over a period of time to the initial equilibrium state. This process is called *relaxation*. Now, importantly, the recovery of longitudinal magnetization and the decay of transversal magnetization follow different and independent time courses, both according to simple exponential functions, but with different time constants, denoted *T1* for the recovery of longitudinal magnetization, and *T2* for the decay of transversal magnetization. T1 is the time at which the longitudinal magnetization has recovered 63% of its equilibrium magnitude.

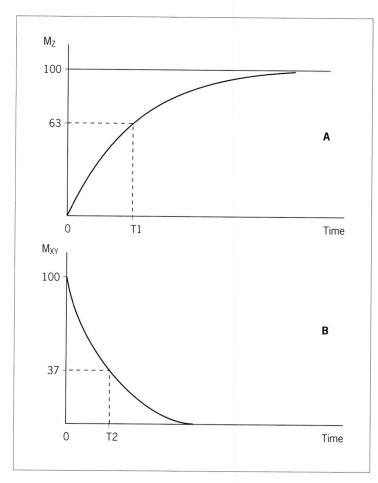

Figure 34

(A) The exponential recovery of the longitudinal net magnetization vector (MZ) after termination of a 90° RF pulse at time 0.

The magnitude of $MZ = M_0(1 - e^{-t/T1})$,

where M_0 is the magnitude of the net magnetization vector at equilibrium. T1 is the time constant of the recovery process.

At t = T1; $MZ = M_0 \times \left(1 - \dfrac{1}{e}\right) = M_0 \times 0.63$

(B) The exponential decay of the transversal, rotating net magnetization vector (M_{XY}) after termination of a 90° RF pulse at time 0.
The magnitude of M_{XY} as a function of time (t) is given by:

$M_{XY} = M_0 e^{-t/T2}$,

where T2 is the time constant of the decay process.

At t = T2; $M_{XY} = M_0 \times \dfrac{1}{e} = M_0 \times 0.37$

T2 is the time taken for the induced transversal magnetization to decay by 63% (to 37%) of its maximum strength (Figure 34). The two relaxation processes reflect two types of interactions between the precessing protons and their surroundings.

Recovery of longitudinal magnetization implies loss of energy whereby those protons that were lifted to the high spin-energy state by the RF pulse give up this energy and fall back. This loss of energy is largely of thermal nature with a molecular basis in random collisions with surrounding molecules, collectively called "the lattice". The longitudinal relaxation process is therefore, according to its nature referred to as the "*thermal relaxation time*" or the "*spin-lattice relaxation time*".

Decay of transverse magnetization implies loss of phase coherence among the precessing protons. This process has its origin in mutual magnetic interactions between the protons, and between the protons and local field inhomogeneities, for example due to the presence of other atoms with magnetic dipole moments and protons precessing at other frequencies due to chemical shifts or due to inhomogeneities/instabilities in the external field. Because interaction between nuclei with different spins is a major contributor to the transversal relaxation process, this is often referred to as the "*spin–spin relaxation time*". In pure liquids, characterized by mobile molecules, intrinsic and local field variations are rapidly fluctuating and tend to average out. In solids, molecules are more fixed and local intrinsic field inhomogeneities therefore more permanent, causing protons to systematically dephase. Therefore T2 tends to be short (milliseconds) in solids and long (seconds) in liquids.

T1 will always be longer than T2, but, especially in liquids, they may approach the same value. Tissues may, simplified, be regarded as complex mixtures of solids, solutes in solvent (water) and lipids which at body temperature are somewhere in between solid and liquid. Water and the fatty acid chains of lipids are by far the dominating contributors to the proton MR signals utilized in diagnostic imaging. The other elements may be regarded as elements in a complex "lattice" which shapes the thermal relaxation, expressed by T1, and which creates the local (intrinsic) field inhomogeneities which shape the spin–spin relaxation, expressed by T2. T1 and T2 of a given tissue therefore become sort of averages. Increasing the field strength always increases T1 while T2, in some tissues is largely unaffected, and in others increasing. Actual figures for T1 in a 1 T field varies between different soft tissues from about 200 msec in fatty tissue to about 800 msec in gray matter of the brain. For comparison T1 of pure water is about 2500 msec and about 2000 msec in cerebrospinal fluid (CSF). T2 similarly varies from about 40 msec in liver and muscle to about 90 msec in pure fat and white matter of the brain and about 300 msec in CSF. The chemical shift (~3 ppm) between protons of water and protons of fatty acids causes especially rapid decay of transverse magnetization in tissues where fat and "watery" tissue is intimately mixed, for example in bone marrow. Dense bone contains too few mobile protons to yield detectable MR signals in diagnostic imaging.

The concentration of protons, detectable by MR imaging in a tissue is denoted the *proton spin density* or just "*proton density*" the latter term ignoring that some protons contribute little or nothing to the signal. MR imaging is directed at detection and visualization of differences in spin density and parameters such as T1 and T2 between different tissues and

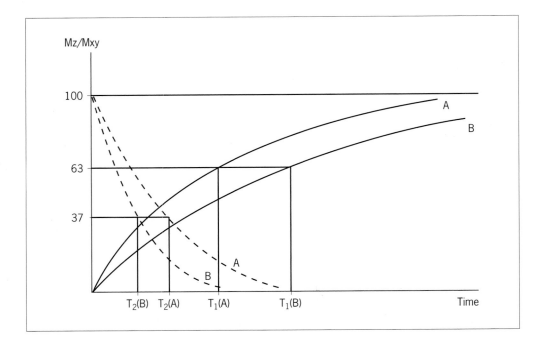

Figure 35 Recovery of longitudinal magnetization (M_Z, full lines) and decay of transversal magnetization (M_{XY}, broken lines) in two tissues, A and B. Tissue A has the shortest T1 and the longest T2.

fluids within the body (Figure 35), denoted *proton spin density, T1-,* and *T2 weighted imaging*.

During the period of relaxation of the magnetized tissue an electromotive force can be induced in an appropriately situated receiver coil as an RF signal in synchrony with the precessing protons. This RF signal is analyzed and decoded to be displayed as an image. Importantly, only protons that precess in phase give rise to detectable radio signals. This means that the induced radio emission from a volume element (voxel) ceases when the transversal component of the net magnetization vector in that volume has decayed, even though the longitudinal component has not yet recovered. Thus to detect differences between tissues in T1, and also to fully exploit differences in T2, complex excitatory pulse sequences are applied, to be detailed in due course. Importantly, fully saturated protons, that is, the longitudinal magnetization vector has been fully reversed by an 180° RF pulse, do not emit a radio signal.

The spin-echo phenomenon

Loss of phase coherence, "dephasing", means loss of RF signal. Part of this loss is due to the spin–spin relaxation expressed by T2, which is an inherent property of the material/tissue. The observed rate of decay of phase coherence, denoted T2*, is always faster because of inhomogeneities in the magnetic field. The latter is an "external" disturbance of the measurement, the effect of which can be cancelled by the spin-echo maneuver, explained in Figure 36, where the magnetization vectors for convenience are depicted in a coordinate system that rotates at the Larmor frequency to allow visualization of small differences in precessional frequency among the protons. Imagine that we ourselves sit in the rotating coordinate system and therefore see the X-,

Y- and Z-axis stationary. The spin-echo maneuver effectively cancels out that part of the dephasing which is due to field inhomogeneities, provided they are stable over the time taken to produce the echo (*TE*).

If two echoes are produced by two 180° pulses spaced in time after the first excitatory 90° pulse and the first echo is sampled shortly after the excitation (short TE) before differences in T2 relaxation time weaken the signal this echo will produce an image of proton densities in the tissues. A second echo sampled with a long TE will produce an image showing differences in T2 between tissues. The time between two excitatory 90° pulses, the repetition time, is denoted *TR*. Nearly all contemporary imaging sequences are based on sampling of echo signals.

Gradient echoes

An alternative method used to produce refocusing of dephasing protons (i.e. echoes) utilizes the effect of reversal of the longitudinal magnetic gradient, so-called *gradient echoes*. This maneuver is applied in fast imaging sequences using small flip angles (e.g. 30°) thereby shortening TE and shortening the period needed for recovery of the longitudinal magnetization (T1). Because the flip angle is small RF pulses can be applied at much shorter intervals compared to spin-echo sequences (shorter TR), and it is not necessary to await full recovery of longitudinal magnetization because several excitatory RF pulses can be applied before the protons saturate. The combination of small flip angles and gradient echoes are commonly termed *FLASH* (*fast low angle shot*) sequences. They have the virtue of speed, many times faster than spin-echo sequences, but at the price of reduced resolution, because the gradient echo maneuvers do not restore the distortions caused by field inhomogeneities and the

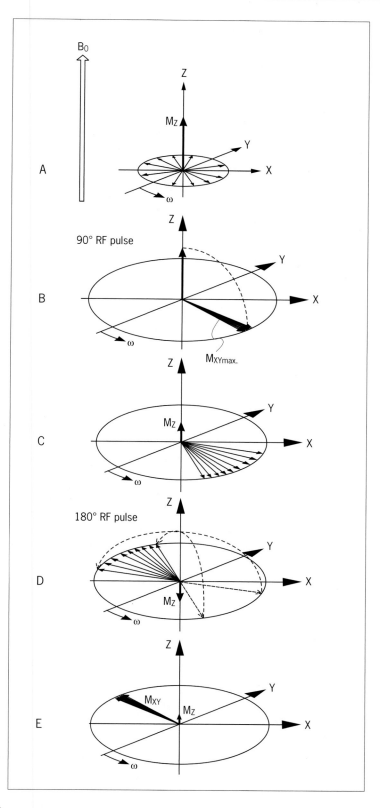

Figure 36 The spin-echo phenomenon

(A) In the equilibrium state all the transverse (M_{XY}) components of the proton magnetization vectors are out of phase. The sum of the longitudinal components (M_Z) is aligned with the main field (B_O). Omega (ω) marks the angular velocity of precession.

(B) A 90° RF pulse aligned with the X- or Y-axis flips the longitudinal vector into the transverse plane and forces the transverse components of the proton magnetization vectors to precess in phase. The single resultant M_{XY} vector is large and emits a strong radiosignal at the Larmor frequency.

(C) After termination of the 90° pulse the transverse component begins to fan out due to small differences in precessional frequency of the individual protons, i.e. T2* relaxation. At the same time the longitudinal vector begins to grow up due to T1 relaxation.

(C) A 180° RF pulse applied at time TE/2 reverses the longitudinal vector and the direction of precession so that the faster precessing protons begin to catch up with the slower, i.e. the fan of vectors closes again.

(E) At time TE (time of echo = 2 × TE/2) the transverse components of the proton magnetization vectors have regathered ('refocussed') and emit again a strong radiosignal, however reduced by the T1 relaxation which has taken place over the TE period.

signal-to-noise ratio is smaller because the emitted RF signals are weaker due to the small flip angle which produces less transverse magnetization. The FLASH sequences are because of their speed particularly useful for imaging of moving objects like the heart and gut with peristalsis. By these fast sequences it has become possible to collect data for one slice in one second or less, opening up for real time (live) MRI.

MR contrast agents

The relaxation times (T1 and T2) of a tissue will be shortened if a paramagnetic substance is targeted to the tissue. The paramagnetic substance acts as a disturbing admixture of strong magnetic dipoles due to unpaired electrons in their atoms. This effect is utilized in MR imaging using the rare earth element *gadolinium* (Gd), which shortens T1 strongly and therefore provides improved contrast in T1 weighted imaging. Gadolinium is highly toxic in free form, but can be firmly trapped by various chelators long enough to be nearly quantitatively excreted in urine, provided renal function is normal or near normal. Several such chelators are presently on the market. The Gd contrast media are particularly useful in the CNS because they will not pass the normal blood–brain barrier and can therefore be used to detect lesions of this barrier, for example caused by tumors. They are also used for angiography, for mapping blood perfusion in organs and for urological examinations analogous to the use of contrast media in conventional X-ray and CT imaging.

Negative contrast media produce signal voids. Iron oxide particles effectively produce local field inhomogeneities and belong to this category. It has limited use in gastrointestinal MR imaging. Air gives no MR signal and may be used for examination of rectum and colon.

Obtaining spatial (topographic) resolution of MR signals

The final MR image is, as the CT image, a squared matrix of *pixels*, each representing a small volume element, a *voxel*, within an imaginary "slice" of the patient. Each pixel has been assigned a gray-tone value proportional to the amplitude of the radio signal emitted from the corresponding voxel in a defined period of time following a sequence of RF excitations, chosen to maximize differences between tissues with respect to a particular parameter, for example T1 or T2.

To obtain the required spatial resolution, three coordinates need to be known for each voxel. To select the position of the tomographic section (the first coordinate, Z), a magnetic field gradient is established along the patient (Figure 37A). In consequence of this gradient, a given radiofrequency will elicit resonance only in protons located within a narrow cross-section of the gradient/patient. Changing the frequency of the excitatory RF pulse will move the cross-section to another position along the gradient where it matches the Larmor frequency of the protons. The steeper the gradient

and the narrower the frequency bandwidth of the RF pulse, the thinner the slice to be excited by resonance at the Larmor frequency. Usually the gradient and the bandwidth is adjusted to excite a slice 0.5–5 mm thick, depending on the purpose. This *slice selecting gradient* is present during the period of the exciting RF pulses and defines the position of the tomographic section.

The two additional coordinates (X and Y), needed to define the voxel, are obtained by applying two additional weak gradients, the phase encoding gradient and the frequency encoding gradient.

The phase encoding gradient is applied perpendicular to the slice selecting gradient, and is switched on for only a very short period of time (3–5 msec) after the excitatory RF pulse has been switched off. It has the effect of producing a continuous change in precessional phase across the slice, so that a particular phase corresponds to a particular row of voxels (vertical row in Figure 37B).

The frequency encoding gradient is applied at right angles to both the slice selecting gradient and the phase encoding gradient. It is switched on after the phase encoding gradient has been switched off, and is maintained during the period where the RF signals are sampled, and is therefore also denoted the *"read out gradient"*. This gradient will have the effect of establishing a continuous increase in precessional (Larmor) frequencies from one edge of the section to the other, so that a particular frequency derives from a particular row of voxels across the slice (horizontal row in Figure 37B).

Commonly used image matrices are 256×256 and 512×512 pixels. To achieve the same resolution in the X- and Y directions, the image must accordingly be constructed from 256 or 512 data samples, recorded with 256 respectively 512 different settings of the phase encoding gradient. This is the main reason for the long data acquisition time in MR- compared to CT imaging.

The very principle of obtaining spatial resolution by the use of three magnetic field gradients has the inherent problem that they all produce phase changes, the two of them counteracting the unambiguity of the intended phase change produced by the phase encoding gradient. Also the field inhomogeneity caused by the gradients increases the rate of dephasing, that is, shortens T2. These effects are compensated for by applying an appropriately timed gradient in the reverse direction in order to counterbalance the precessional changes produced by the other. The slice selecting gradient is balanced by a reversed gradient of the same magnitude and a duration corresponding to the duration of the RF pulse. The signal sampling takes place in the middle of the period the frequency encoding gradient is switched on, and the balancing gradient of opposite direction is applied prior to the signal sampling and is of half the duration in order to hit the point of balance at the time of signal sampling. The timing of the sequence of RF pulses, gradient activation and signal sampling is pictured in Figure 38, showing a spin-echo imaging sequence.

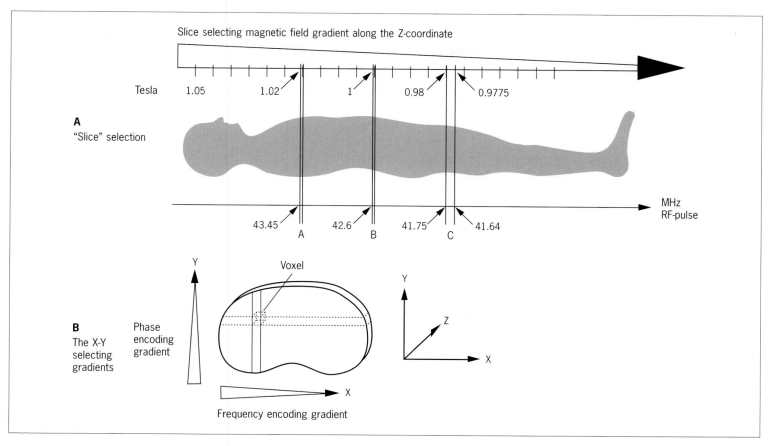

Figure 37 Principle of spatial resolution.
A thin slice (A) will be excited by an RF-pulse of e.g. 43.45 MHz. Changing the RF-pulse to 42.6 MHz moves the excited section to position B. If the RF-pulse has a bandwidth from 41.64 to 41.75 MHz, a thicker slice at position C becomes excited.

Now, the complex radio signals emitted by the excited cross-section of the patient is picked up by the receiver coil and subjected to a Fourier analysis which means resolution into a number of component elementary sine waves. The frequency and phase of each of these elementary waves define together the coordinates of the voxel from which the waves originated. The amplitude of the elementary wave can now be assigned a gray tone proportional to its magnitude and is displayed as the corresponding pixel in the image. By convention, high signal amplitudes are displayed towards white and low amplitudes towards black on the gray-tone scale. As in CT imaging, the scale has about 20 steps, and the "window width" and the "window level" can be varied. In clinical practice, a tissue with low signal intensity (dark) relative to its surroundings is called *hypointense*, opposite to *hyperintense*. Sometimes additional color encoding is used.

The three gradients used to obtain spatial resolution of the MR signals can be interchanged so that axial, sagittal and coronal sections may freely be produced without moving the patient. Also, as with CT, any oblique section may be calculated from the data set, provided the series of sections are not spaced. It is also possible to excite and sample radio signals from several appropriately spaced sections to speed up the collection of a long series of sections, known as *multislice imaging*, which may shorten the total examination time by a factor 10. Nevertheless, the collection of data for a conventional MR examination takes several minutes.

The many repetitions of the imaging sequence, each time with a new setting of the phase encoding gradient, greatly prolongs the sampling of the data needed to compute the image. To reduce the sampling time, imaging sequences have been developed where a train of echoes, each with a different setting of the phase encoding gradient, is produced by a series of 180° pulses following the initial 90° pulse of a spin-echo sequence. These sequences, known as *fast* or *turbo spin-echo sequences*, considerably shorten the data acquisition time, but imply an averaging of signals over the course of the T1 recovery curve. This affects the interpretation of image contrast relative to classical spin-echo imaging. Analogous techniques employing gradient echoes with reduced flip angle also greatly speed up the data acquisition time.

Flow effects and movement artifacts in MR imaging

Flow in blood vessels and CSF may influence MR imaging in very complex ways. Depending on the RF pulse sequence applied, the presence of flow may give rise to weaker or stronger signals than expected. Without going into detail it appears clear that fast flow perpendicular to the section may have the effect of carrying away those protons that should have given a signal during the RF signal sampling period. The

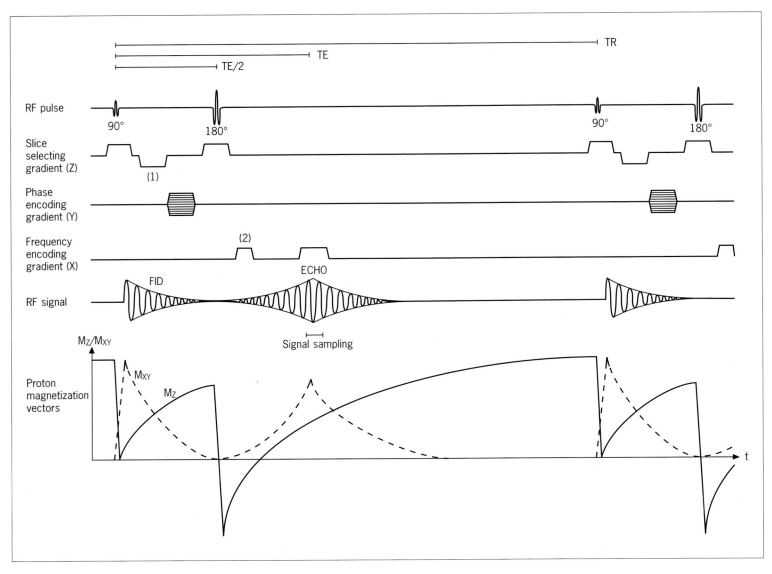

Figure 38 The standard spin-echo pulse sequence.
This sequence begins with a 90° RF pulse, applied when the slice selecting (Z-) gradient has been switched on. The following period of Z-gradient reversal (1) compensates for the dephasing caused by the slice selecting gradient during the RF pulse period. The 90° pulse elicits a RF signal, produced by the M_{XY} magnetization vector depicted in the lower panel (and in Fig. 36B). This signal decays exponentially, the so-called *free induction decay* (FID). At time TE/2 the slice selecting gradient is again switched on and a 180° RF pulse is sent in (conf. also Fig. 36D). This has the effect of refocussing the dephasing M_{XY} vectors to produce an echo signal at time TE, rising and falling exponentially. The echo signal is normally sampled around its midpoint. This RF signal has been encoded along the X- and Y-axis by two additional gradients. The X-gradient (the 'read out gradient'), which is active during signal sampling, has been preactivated (2) to compensate for the dephasing it produces. The preactivation is in this sequence positive because the phases have been reversed by the 180° pulse, otherwise it should have been negative. The multiple horizontal bars in the symbol for the phase encoding (Y-) gradient indicate that this gradient is given a new strength, each time the sequence is repeated at TR (time of repetition) until enough sequences have been run to compute the image, usually 256 times. The intentional phase changes produced by the Y-gradient are of course not compensated for by gradient reversal.

vessel therefore becomes signal void and its lumen is displayed black in the image.

In other situations, pre-excited protons may be carried into the section by flow. This may be the case in a series of images/slices taken in rapid succession where blood with already excited protons flows into the next slice and becomes further excited and so on until they become fully saturated and therefore become signal void. Blood flowing in the opposite direction does not become saturated because it flows into slices that have not been excited before. This explains why

arteries and veins where blood flows in opposite directions often become imaged with opposite contrast. If the slices on both sides of the slice to be imaged have been pre-excited with a 90° RF pulse, then the blood of arteries and veins flowing into the imaging slice will all become fully saturated by the imaging 90° excitation pulse and will accordingly become signal void.

Flow in the plane of the section may disturb the spatial X-Y encoding/decoding and give rise to artifacts. Wherever flowing blood is imaged one must anticipate that the signal intensity from the blood may be spurious and that peculiar positional artifacts may be present. These are often seen as blurred streaks through the vessel, extending across the image in the direction of the phase encoding gradient.

Movement artifacts are much more of a problem than in CT, because MR data acquisition times are in general considerably longer. For proper cardiac imaging, the data collection has to be gated on the ECG. Also gating on the respiratory cycle may be necessary. Finally, and regrettably, intestinal peristalsis often degrades the resolution in abdominal MR imaging.

MR Angiography (MRA)

Various techniques have been developed to selectively detect flowing protons for the production of angiograms without the use of contrast media.

There are two methods in current use:

The *time-of-flight* (TOF) method is based on suppression of signals from stationary tissue by presaturation of protons with a $180°$ RF pulse. Protons carried by new blood flowing into the presaturated tissue are then exposed to an RF pulse producing a less than $90°$ flip angle (e.g. $45°$) and the RF signals are picked up by a fast, repeated series of gradient echoes, followed by a new $45°$ pulse and so on (short TR) until a series of images has been collected. The $45°$ pulses will maintain saturation of the stationary protons. However, blood flowing in the plane of the imaged slab becomes gradually saturated by the repeated $45°$ RF pulses, posing a limit to the thickness of the slabs that can be imaged. There are methods to extend this limit of TOF-MRA, not to be elaborated here.

The *phase-contrast (PC)* method employs phase encoding in three directions (X, Y and Z). A proton that has moved between the time of encoding and signal sampling can then be identified by having a phase encoding different from its static surroundings. By adjustment of the gradient strengths it is possible to distinguish between fast and slow flow and thereby produce separate arteriograms and venograms. The phase contrast method (PC-MRA) allows detection of flow in all directions, but the data acquisition time is long.

All non-contrast MRA techniques have limitations, therefore, in clinical practice, MR contrast media are widely used.

MR imaging modes and pulse sequences

There are three basic MR imaging modes used in diagnostic practice:

1 *Proton spin-density weighted imaging* is directed at visualizing differences between tissues in their density of protons, irrespective of their differences in chemical bonds and differences in T1 and T2. However, some protons do not contribute to the image because their mobility is restricted, for example in bones and tendons. Therefore in clinical imaging the term *proton spin-density* should be preferred over "proton density" to indicate that the signal does not reflect the true proton density of a tissue. The contrast between pixels can then be translated into differences in proton spin-density between voxels.

2 *T1 weighted imaging* is directed at visualizing differences between tissues in the recovery time of the longitudinal equilibrium magnetization after it has been disturbed by an RF pulse. The difference between voxels in T1 is displayed in the image as differences between pixels. T1 weighted images generally give the best all-round anatomical resolution.

3 *T2 weighted imaging* is directed at visualizing differences between tissues in the decay time of transverse magnetization after it has been induced by an RF pulse. Thus, differences in T2 between voxels are displayed in the image as contrast between pixels. T2 weighted images are particularly useful for distinction of fluids, like CSF. Pathological changes are often accompanied by fluid accumulation (intra and/or extracellular edema) in the tissue, and therefore show up clearly in T2 weighted images.

Besides the above three basic imaging modes there are many others, less often used in clinical practice. Only two will be mentioned here:

MR spectroscopy

The small changes in precessional frequency of protons depending on the chemical bonds they are engaged in, the so-called *chemical shifts*, which characterize the molecule, allow the concentration of a particular molecule to be determined relative to the concentration in the surroundings by MR techniques, not to be detailed here. In principle it is possible to determine the relative concentration in each single voxel, but normally a collection of, say 64 voxels are sampled. The relative concentrations of, for example, lactate may then be color coded and superimposed on the MR image of a slice of the organ. Apart from experimental studies it is mostly used for diagnosis in the CNS, where, for example, lactate accumulation indicates hypoxic regions. Other molecules accumulate in certain tumors, and others are characteristic for necrotic tissue.

Diffusion weighted imaging

This imaging mode visualizes the diffusional mobility of protons in the tissue, water being the dominant carrier of diffusible protons. Diffusional mobility is a parameter basically different from T1, T2 and proton spin-density weighted imaging. Diffusion is the result of random thermal movements of molecules. If not restricted by barriers a cluster of molecules would spread spherically from an origin. However, the cell membranes in a tissue act as barriers, restricting the mobility of both intra- and extracellular molecules. In a tissue suffering intracellular edema, as seen in the early phases of anoxia, the extracellular space becomes narrowed, whereby the mobility of extracellular molecules becomes restricted. The diffusional mobility of molecules in a tissue is expressed as the net displacement of molecules per second across an area of $1\,mm^2$, termed the *apparent diffusion coefficient (ADC)*. Due to the presence of barriers the ADC will differ in different directions, notably in tissues having a predominant directionality of barriers as is the case in bundles of nerve fibers, especially marked if the fibers are myelinated, that is, are wrapped in several layers of cell membrane.

The ADC is determined by a method basically similar to MR phase contrast angiography (PC-MR), mentioned earlier, but at a micro scale, by using thin sections and fast imaging sequences for determination of proton spins that have moved small distances into surroundings which have a different phase encoding. This way differences in directional mobility can be determined relative to the X, Y and Z axes. After color coding relative to these axes a *diffusion tensor image* can be constructed and displayed as a map of differences in directional mobility within a section. The technique has proved particularly useful for imaging the directionality of nerve fibers in white matter of the CNS (Figure 39). The mapping may be extended in three dimensions by selecting a small volume of tissue, in for example the cerebral cortex, and tracking the neighboring voxel having the same tensor directionality and so on through the whole stack of sections, thereby mapping conduction tracts through all the levels in the CNS (Figure 40).

Basic MR pulse sequences

This section summarizes the main points of importance to MR imaging and exemplifies their use in some pulse sequences. A wealth of pulse sequences, some of which are quite complicated, have been developed over the years. It is beyond the scope of this text to deal with more than a few of the simpler examples.

In the equilibrium state no radio signals are emitted from the tissues that have been magnetized by the main field. This is because the longitudinal magnetization vector is aligned with the main field, and because the rotating transversal vectors of the individual protons are completely out of phase and therefore cancel each other. Radio signals are emitted only when the net magnetization vector has a rotating transversal component, that is, a sufficient number of protons must precess in phase to produce a detectable radio signal.

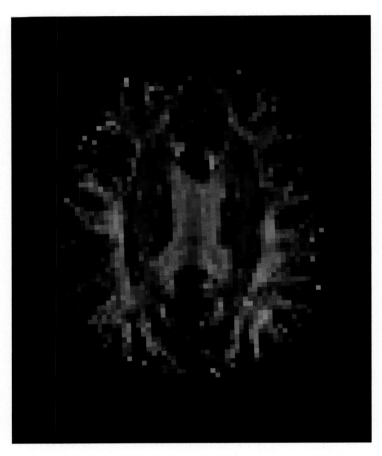

Figure 39 Diffusion weighted MR image of a transverse section of the brain.
The tensors indicating the direction of spatially restricted diffusion are color coded so that voxels with free diffusional mobility in transverse direction are red, those with cranio-caudal mobility are blue, and those with dorso-ventral mobility are green. The collection of red voxels in the middle of the image represents the corpus callosum. Lateral to this is the corona radiate in blue, and lateral to this are bundles of association fibers in green.

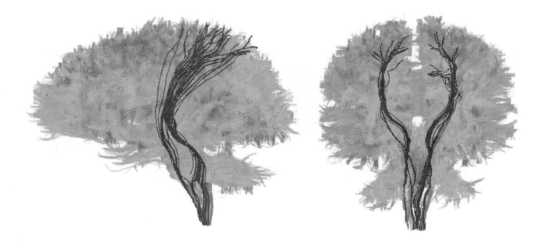

Figure 40 Mapping of conduction tracts between cerebral cortex and spinal cord. For explanation see text.

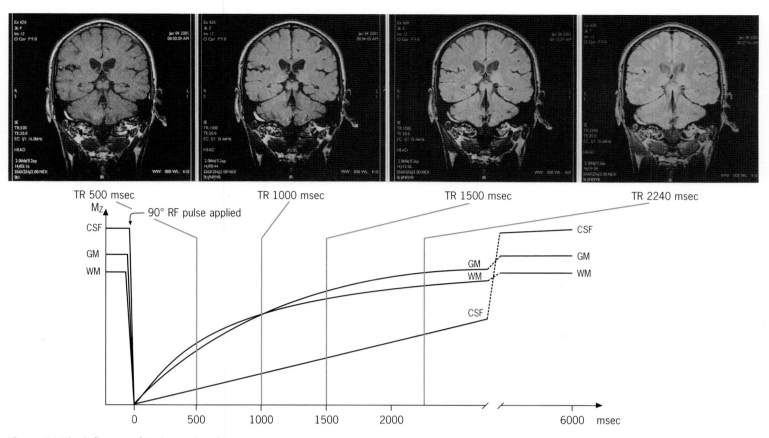

Figure 41 The influence of T1 in a spin-echo sequence.

The graph shows the approximate time course of recovery of longitudinal magnetization (M_Z) in cerebrospinal fluid (CSF), grey matter (GM) and white matter (WM) following a 90° RF pulse at time 0. The approximate relative proton density of these materials is indicated on the M_Z-axis. A spin-echo with a short TE (20 msec) has been produced at 500, 1000, 1500 and 2240 msec after the 90° pulse. The short TE has the effect that T_2 relaxation does not significantly influence the signal strength which accordingly reflects the level of recovery of longitudinal magnetization, ruled by T1 of the materials. The resulting images are shown in the upper panel, all displayed with the same setting of imaging window and level, allowing assessment of relative signal strength between images.

At 500 msec the overall signal strength is low, the signal from WM being a little higher than that from GM, while the signal from CSF in the ventricles is very low. This image reflects most clearly the differences in T1 and is accordingly a *T1 weighted image*. At 1000 msec the signal from WM and GM equals. At 1500 msec the signal from GM has risen above WM, and even more so at 2240 msec. At this time GM and WM are both approaching equilibrium, and the signal strengths reflect the proton spin density of WM relative to GM, but not to CSF which is still far from equilibrium and produce a relatively low signal due to its very long T1.

At about 5000 msec the CSF would similarly have approached equilibrium. A spin-echo pulse sequence with a TR of 5000 msec and a TE of 20 msec, a so-called *saturation recovery pulse sequence* would therefore reflect the relative proton spin density of all the tissues/fluids. However, such long values of TR are not used in practice because the long data acquisition time required becomes impractical. The sequences with shorter TR used for the images in the upper panel are all *partial saturation recovery sequences*.

To obtain radio signals specifically related to the proton spin density, the T1 or the T2 parameters of the tissues, it is necessary to employ variously timed excitatory RF pulse sequences. These pulse sequences are repeated until enough signals are collected to compute the image. Usually, 2 to 4 independently sampled sets are averaged to produce high-quality images.

Figures 41 and 42 explain how the timing of TR and TE in a spin-echo sequence influences the relative signal strength from different tissues, exemplified by brain imaging, and how T1, T2 and proton density weighted images can be produced by proper choice of timing. Figures 36 and 38 may be consulted for more details on the principle of the spin-echo sequence. Instead of using 90° RF pulses to elicit the echoes, gradient reversals may be used to elicit gradient echoes (see p. 24).

Recordings of T1 weighted images employ a short TR (time of repetition) of 200–700 msec, and a short TE (time to echo) of 15–30 msec. Opposite T2 weighted recordings employ a long TR, 2000–3000 msec, and a long TE, 80–200 msec. An image recorded with a long TR and a short TE is called a *proton spin-density weighted* (or sometimes an *intermediately weighted image*), because the signal reflects the relative proton spin-density of most tissues, though not of CSF because of its very long T1.

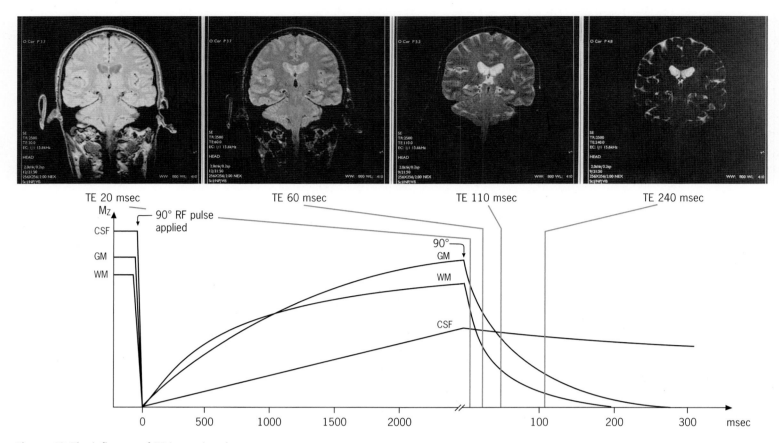

Figure 42 The influence of T2 in a spin-echo sequence.

The graph shows (analogous to Fig. 41) the recovery of longitudinal magnetization in WM, GM and CSF up to 2500 msec following an initial 90° RF pulse. At 2500 msec (TR) another 90° pulse is applied. The curves to the right of this point in time show (on an extended time scale) the approximate time course of decay of the transverse magnetization vectors, ruled by the T2 of the tissues/CSF. At 10, 30, 55 or 120 msec (TE/2) after the 90° pulse, a 180° RF pulse is applied and the resulting echos (conf. Fig. 36) are sampled at 20, 60, 110 and 240 msec (TE). The 90° pulses are repeated every 2500 msec (TR) until sufficient data are collected to compute an image. The resulting images are shown in the upper panel.

At a TE of 20 msec the signals from GM and WM are high, because the T2 relaxation is still only moderate. The signal from CSF is lower because the TR is short relative to the T1 of CSF.

At a TE of 60 msec the fast T2 relaxation in WM and GM has markedly lowered the signal strength from these tissues, the WM signal has already fallen below that of CSF.

At a TE of 110 msec the WM and GM signals have fallen well below CSF. This image which clearly display the differences in T2 between the tissues/CSF is a *T2 weighted image*.

At TE of 240 msec signal remain only in CSF due to its long T2.

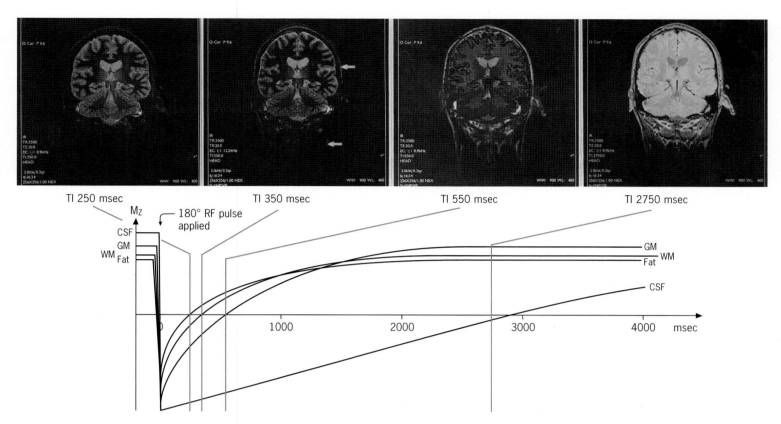

Figure 43 The inversion recovery pulse sequence.

The graph shows the the approximate time course of recovery of longitudinal magnetization following a 180° RF pulse which has inverted the longitudinal net magnetization vector of the different tissues relative to the main field. During recovery of the inverted net longitudinal magnetization it becomes zero at one point in time. Because the rate of recovery is different: fat faster than WM – faster than GM – faster than CSF, the time at which the net longitudinal magnetization turns zero is different for the different tissues. This "null time" is for each tissue identified as the point where its graph of recovery crosses the abscissa. When a 90° pulse is applied at this time (the 'inversion time,' TI), and an echo signal is produced by a 180° pulse in rapid succession, the "nulled" tissue will produce no signal. The upper panel displays the images produced with inversion times (TI) of 250, 350, 550 and 2750 msec, and the same short TE of 20 msec. TR is chosen long, 3500 msec, to allow full recovery of the tissues between the inverting pulses (except for CSF). Note that the signals from the different tissues depend on the numerical value of the vectors, not their direction.

At TI 250 msec the signal from subcutaneous fat is virtually zero, and the signal from WM is weak, while GM and CSF produce clear signals.

At TI 350 msec WM is signal void while a weak signal has appeared in the subcutaneous fat and in fat between neck muscles (arrows). At the same time the GM signal has weakened while the CSF signal stay nearly constant.

At TI 550 msec GM has become signal void while the signal from WM has reappeared and the signal from fat has grown stronger.

At TI 2750 msec all the tissue signals have reached their maximum while the CSF signal is now around its point of "nulling".

The inversion recovery pulse sequence

This pulse sequence extends the period of T1 recovery and may be used for production of strongly T1 weighted images, but is especially used to selectively suppress the signal from particular types of tissue, for example fat, which may hide the signals from small embedded structures like nerves that differ only little in the value of T1, but may be differentiated in this sequence because the period for T½ (τ) recovery is extended. Used this way the sequence is denoted a *fat suppression sequence*, also known as *STIR* (short tau inversion recovery). The inversion recovery sequence is explained and exemplified by brain imaging in Figure 43.

Techniques based on ultrasound reflection

Clinical imaging with ultrasound, *ultrasonography* (sonography/diagnostic ultrasound), is based on emission of high frequency sound waves and recording of echoes produced by reflection as the sound waves travel through the tissues and organs examined. The basic elements of an ultrasonography unit is a *transducer* which functions both as transmitter and receiver of ultrasound waves, an *ultrasound pulse generator*, an ultrasound *beam former*, a transmit/receive switch, a processor of received signals, and an image display unit.

The generation and nature of ultrasound

Ultrasound waves are *mechanical* waves, bound to propagate in matter. Their propagation through a material has its basis in coherent oscillatory movements of the constituent molecules, considered as particles, *longitudinal* to the direction of propagation of the sound wave front. The material is conveniently viewed as being composed of small units of mass, "*sound particles*", that need not have a uniform molecular composition, which they seldom do have. The individual particles oscillate about an equilibrium position fixed in space, like balls elastically suspended between two springs. The number of oscillations undergone by the particles in one second is the frequency of the sound in unit *Hertz* (Hz). The coherent particle oscillations spread through the material by mechanical transfer of kinetic energy from one particle to the next giving rise to alternating bands of compressions and rarefactions that propagate through the material with a *propagation velocity* which is constant and specific for the material. The distance between successive compressions (or rarefactions) is denoted the *wavelength* of the sound. Thus, the propagating sound waves are characterized by their frequency (v), wavelength (λ) and propagation velocity (c) through the relation $c = v \times \lambda$, as are other types of waves.

The frequencies utilized in ultrasonography are in the 2–18 MHz range (1 MHz = 10^6 Hz), for special purposes, for example in ophthalmology and dermatology up to 40 MHz. The propagation velocity (the speed of sound) in soft tissues, blood and water varies by only a few per cent around an average value of 1540 m × sec^{-1}, with corresponding wavelengths of about 0.75 mm at 2 MHz, decreasing to about 0.1 mm at 16 MHz. The propagation velocity is much higher in dense bone (about 3500 m × sec^{-1}) and much lower in air (300 m × sec^{-1}).

The property of a material that determines the velocity (c) is the *acoustic impedance* (Z) which relates to the mass density (ρ) and the modulus of elasticity/stiffness (E) through the relation:

$$Z = \sqrt{\rho \times E} = \rho \times c$$

It is the small differences in Z between different soft tissues which are utilized in ultrasonography.

It is important to distinguish the propagating acoustic wave phenomenon from the coherent oscillatory motions of the individual particles in the material. The maximum velocity of the particles, as they pass their equilibrium positions, relates to the energy transported by the acoustic wave through the material. At the energy inputs applied in ultrasonography, the maximum particle velocities in soft tissues are only 3–4 cm × sec^{-1} or less, and the excursion to either side of their equilibrium positions, denoted the *elongation*, is in the order of 2 nm (nanometer) or less, not to be confused with the wavelength (λ) of the sound.

The ultrasound transducer

The source of ultrasound for diagnostic imaging is the piezoelectric ultrasound transducer (Figure 44). The key component of this assembly is a disc of a special ceramic material made up of orderly aligned molecules that have the property of being electrical dipoles. A thin layer of electrically conducting metal has been plated onto both sides of the disc, so that an electrical field (in the order of 150 volts) can be set up across the disc, which is often termed the "*crystal*". In response to an electrical field the molecular dipoles realign, and the disc consequently changes its thickness. When a high-frequency alternating voltage is applied, the disc oscillates and these oscillations become particularly forceful and uniform at a particular frequency, *the resonance frequency*. When the voltage is turned off, the crystal continues to oscillate at its resonance frequency, which is determined by the thickness of the disc. The "backing material" in the transducer assembly quickly damps this "after ringing". It is

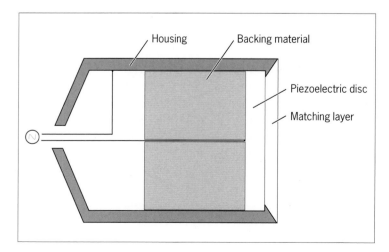

Figure 44 The basic design of an ultrasound transducer.

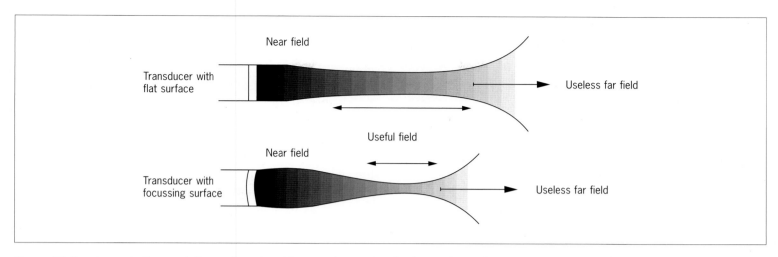

Figure 45 The shape of ultrasound "beams" produced by an unfocussed and a focussed transducer.

essential that the ultrasound impulse lengths are extremely short (in the order of 1 μsec), because the axial ("depth") resolution decreases for increasing spatial pulse length. Reduction of the wave length (i.e. increased frequency) also reduces the spatial pulse length and improves resolution.

The transducer is covered by a thin "matching layer" of a material with an acoustic impedance in between that of the ceramic disc and that of the skin. When the transducer is held against the skin the acoustic impedance is further improved by a watery gel spread in advance over the skin.

The piezoelectric transducer functions also in the reverse direction as receiver of ultrasound echoes. The receiving period is much longer (some hundred μsec) than the transmission period to give time for capture of echoes stemming from deeply located structures. When the receiving ("listening") transducer is hit by incoming ultrasound waves the disc becomes slightly deformed and electrical potentials in the order of 2 μvolts are set up across the disc. These electrical signals are the ones used to construct the image.

For simplicity a scanner with only one transducer element is considered first. The ceramic disc of the transducer acts as a vibrating piston producing a "beam" of ultrasound waves (Figure 45). If the disc is circular and plane the beam becomes almost rod-shaped out to a certain distance from the disc, the "near field" or Fresnel zone, and the beam intensity falls off steeply along the edge of the beam. This is the useful part of the beam. At a certain distance from the crystal the beam spreads out in a cone, the "far field" or Fraunhofer zone, which is not useful for imaging. The physics governing the shape of the beam is rather complex, but depends primarily on the diameter of the crystal and the sound frequency. The disc may be concave shaped or an acoustic lens may be inserted to make the beam converge towards a focus, but this reduces the length of the useful field (Figure 45). The lateral resolution depends on the width of the beam. Focusing improves resolution, but reduces the thickness of tissue imaged.

It should be noted that when the transducer is used for imaging, the waves are sent off in very short "trains" followed by a pause where the transducer "listens" to echoes. The spatial length of a train is 2 mm or less, but follows the path of the continuous beam as a propagating cross-section of it.

Interactions of ultrasound with matter

At all ultrasound frequencies and intensities applied in diagnostic imaging, three types of interactions are relevant: *absorption*, *reflection*, and *diffuse scatter*, all contributing to *attenuation* of the ultrasound beam intensity. Additionally, refraction and diffraction phenomena take place, but they are of minor practical significance. At beam intensities much higher and of longer duration than those used for imaging, various destructive effects take place in the tissue, not to be elaborated on here.

Absorption

Absorption of ultrasound in tissues means transfer of kinetic energy from the coherent particle oscillations into disordered particle motions, that is, *heat*, caused by internal friction between the constituent molecules of the tissue. Absorption is the dominant contributor to ultrasound beam attenuation. The intensity of the beam decays exponentially with distance and is therefore conveniently expressed in *decibels* (dB). Additionally, absorption increases linearly with the frequency in soft tissues. On average the absorption mounts to 1 db cm^{-1} MHz^{-1}. Thus, at a depth of 10 cm the intensity of a 5 MHz beam has been reduced by 50 dB, that is, a 100 000-fold reduction.

Decibel (dB) is a measure of relative intensities of sound defined as: $dB = 10 \times \log\frac{I_2}{I_1}$, where I_1 is the intensity of the beam as it leaves the transducer and I_2 is the intensity of the beam after travelling to a given depth, or of echoes reaching the listening transducer.

The intensity of a sound beam is the energy flux per unit area perpendicular to the beam; commonly expressed as watt (W) cm^{-2}. 1 W equals 1 joule per second.

Considering that an echo from this depth will have to travel another 10 cm back to the transducer, the signal will have decayed by about 100 dB relative to an echo received from a structure superficially in the skin. A signal reduced this much is virtually useless. Therefore for imaging of deep structures, for example in the abdomen, lower frequencies are used, but this is at the expense of resolution. Absorption in urine is significantly lower than in soft tissues. A filled bladder may therefore be utilized as an *"acoustic window"* to pelvic viscera.

Reflection

When the propagating ultrasound wave front encounters an interface between two tissues of different acoustic impedance, part of the energy is reflected as an echo. If the acoustic impedances of the two tissues are identical, no echo is produced. If the difference is very large, as between soft tissue and bone or air, virtually all the wave energy is reflected, producing a strong echo and an *"acoustic shadow"* behind the bone or an air-filled organ. This effect makes it impossible to image the adult brain through the skull, while a neonatal brain may be imaged excellently through the fontanelles. It also makes it impossible to image lungs and air-filled intestines.

It is primarily the reflections – echoes – from interfaces between tissues of small or moderate differences in acoustic impedance that are utilized in ultrasonography. If the interface is perfectly smooth and of sufficient size, the wave is reflected as by a mirror, denoted *specular reflection* (Figure 46A). This implies that if the interface is at an angle to the beam, the echo may miss the transducer. Thus, very smooth surfaces, for example an umbilical cord, will be imaged only where parts of its surface are perpendicular to the beam. If, however, the surface is ruffled, the reflected wave takes different directions, and part of it may reach the receiving transducer (Figure 46B). This is why curved organ surfaces are usually imaged, albeit with decreasing contrast the more steeply the surface is angled relative to the beam.

Structures producing echoes are bright looking and said to be *echogenic* and differences in *echogenicity* of tissues producing more echoes relative to the surroundings are said to be *hyperechoic* or *hyperdense*, the opposite being *hypoechoic/hypodense*.

Diffuse scatter

When the ultrasound wave encounters a finely rippled surface or corpuscles which are small relative to the

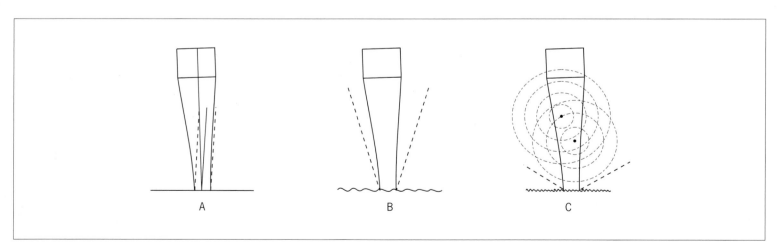

Figure 46

(A) Specular reflection.
  The angle of incidence equals the angle of reflection. If the angle deviates more than little from perpendicular, the reflected sound waves will miss the transducer.

(B) Reflection from a ruffled surface.
  The reflected waves spread over an angle so that only a smaller fraction reaches the transducer.

(C) Diffuse scatter.
  Small corpuscles or a finely rippled surface will spread the sound waves in all directions so that only a very small fraction returns to the transducer.

wavelength, for example small blood vessels, and the acoustic impedance differs from the surroundings, the corpuscles give rise to diffuse scatter in the form of spherical waves originating from the corpuscles (Figure 46C). Only a very small fraction of these waves reaches the transducer, but they contribute to the finely speckled appearance of parenchymatous organs like the liver, spleen, kidney, and uterus, as well as skeletal muscles.

Small air bubbles are effective producers of diffuse scatter. Following compression by the incoming sound wave they vibrate and give rise to circular sound waves whose frequencies are integers of the frequency transmitted by the transducer, so-called *harmonic frequencies* or *harmonics*.

Ultrasound imaging modes

Assuming a constant velocity of sound ($1540\,\mathrm{m} \times \sec^{-1}$) in soft tissues – and this is almost true – the time taken from a $1\,\mu\sec$ pulse until receipt of an echo can be directly translated into twice the distance to (and from) the reflecting surface. This is precisely analogous to what a fisherman does when he estimates the depth of a shoal of herring with his sonar. Time to receipt of echo from 10 cm depth will be some $130\,\mu\sec$, so the time resolution needs to be accurate.

The echoes received from a stationary transducer may be displayed on an oscilloscope trace as deflections proportional to the magnitude of the echoes. This is denoted amplitude mode, or *A-mode imaging* (Figure 47A). Instead of deflections, the intensity of the oscilloscope beam may be modulated along the trace to produce dots of different brightness. This is denoted brightness mode, or *B-mode imaging* (Figure 47B). If the distance to the reflecting objects changes over time, then the dots will move back or forth along the oscilloscope trace. So, if the trace is recorded on a strip chart recorder, curves will be drawn that show the motion of the reflectors as a function of time. This is denoted motion mode, or *M-mode* imaging, which is used especially in cardiology for the study of, for example, valve motions (Figure 47M).

None of the above modes produce real images. If, however, the transducer beam is set to scan back and forth at a constant angular speed around 20 times per second, and if the echoes are displayed in B-mode along a line that sweeps over the video screen synchronously with the transducer, then a real time tomographic image, a *2D B-mode image*, is produced from the ultrasound echoes (Figure 47 Sector).

Transducer designs

The angular sector scanning mode may be produced with a mechanical construct that involves moving parts (Figure 48A), but is now almost universally replaced by solid state assemblies of multiple transducers, so-called *linear (or curvilinear) array transducers*. Each transducer element is rectangular and very thin (typically less than half the wavelength of

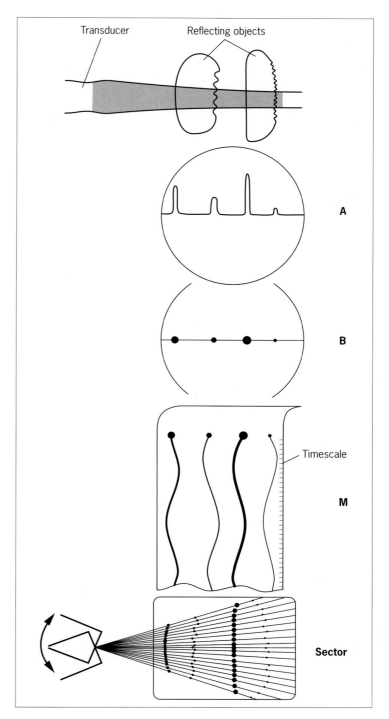

Figure 47 Ultrasound imaging modes.
Ultrasound beam passing various reflecting surfaces.
A-mode display, "amplitude mode".
The echoes are displayed on an oscilloscope screen as deflections with amplitudes and positions corresponding to the reflecting surfaces.
B-mode display, "brightness mode".
The echoes are displayed as dots with brightness and positions corresponding to the reflecting surfaces.
M-mode display, "motion mode".
The echoes are recorded in the B-mode on a strip chart. If the reflecting surfaces move, their movements are recorded as waving curves. Periodicity and amplitude of movements are clearly visualized.
Sector scanning, real-time tomographic mode.
The echoes are displayed in the B-mode on a videoscreen as the transducer scans back and forth through an angle (a "sector").

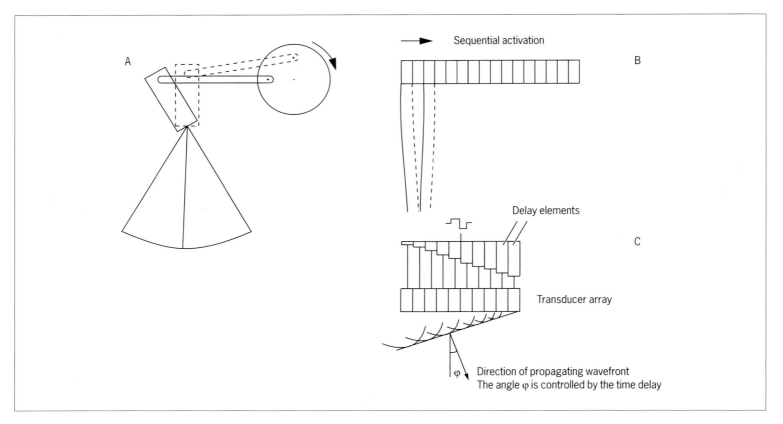

Figure 48 Ultrasound scanning principles.
(A) Simple mechanical device to produce sector scanning.
(B) Linear transducer array.
(C) Phased array transducer.

the sound produced) so that a large number (e.g. 25 per cm) of closely spaced elements can be accommodated in the array.

A linear array may be operated following two different principles:

A group of, for example, 20 elements are activated simultaneously and produce a short wave train which is shaped as if it originated from a single transducer. While the train travels into the tissues, a larger number of elements listen for echoes. The next group of 20 transducer elements to be fired overlap the first group with, for example, 4 elements, and so on along the full length of the array, the resulting image being rectangular (Figure 48B).

Another way of operating a linear array is as a *phased array* where the elements of the array are activated with a tiny delay between neighboring elements. The wave fronts emitted from the elements are therefore out of phase and will mutually interfere to produce a plane wave front propagating at an angle (φ) to the transducer (Figure 48C). In the subsequent receive period all elements contribute. In the next activation the delay between activation of neighboring elements is slightly changed. If decreased the angle φ will be smaller. This way the transducer assembly can be set to scan (sweep) and image a trapezoidal sector, the scanner front being the short side of the rectangle. The timing is further refined to produce wave fronts that are distally

concave, so that the beam is focused at selected depths, where the resolution will be at its maximum. Two or more maxima may be selected at various depths, by shifting the focus between each sweep and superimposing the images of two or more sweeps. This, however, is at the cost of frame speed. The electronic circuits steering the delays and the shift between transmit and receive periods is known as the *beam former*.

To compensate for the exponential loss of energy in the transmitted wave front and in the reflected echoes all ultrasound scanners are equipped with a facility termed the *time-gain-control* (TGC), which is an amplifier that amplifies the signals relative to their timing and inverse to the exponential decay due to absorption. This compensation is based on average decays, and most scanners have controls to enhance or reduce the amplification of signals at certain depths, selected by the operator. Also, electronic *edge enhancement* can aid the visualization of some structures.

A variety of transducer constructs have been developed for special purposes, for example for transvaginal scanning of the uterus, transrectal scanning of the prostate, transesophageal scanning of the heart and for endovascular scanning during insertion of stents.

Transducers for rapid sampling of a series of images without moving the transducer are used for 3D reconstructions (3D stationary images) using similar computational procedures as used in CT scanning. Such reconstructions have become widely used in obstetrics, because the interface between the amniotic fluid and the fetal skin is sharp and ideal for surface rendering. Special fast phased array scanners with thousands of transducer elements can produce live 3D images, called 4D scanning.

Transducers which amplify echoes with higher order *harmonics* (i.e. waves with frequencies that are whole integers of the transmission frequency of the transducer) are especially used for examinations with microbubble contrast agents, due to their high emission of harmonics. These transducers may also improve "ordinary" ultrasonographic imaging by reduction of some artifacts arising close to the transducer by mechanisms not to be elaborated on here.

The Doppler shift and Doppler imaging

Sound reflected from an object moving away from the transducer will return to the transducer with increased wavelength (decreased frequency), and conversely with an increased frequency if the object is moving towards the transducer. Such shifts in frequency are called *Doppler shifts*, the magnitudes of which are ruled by the equation:

$$\Delta f = f_i - f_r = \frac{v}{v + c} \times 2 \times f_i$$

Where Δf is the Doppler shift, f_i is the frequency of the transducer, f_r is the frequency of the reflected sound, v is the velocity of the reflector, and c is the velocity of sound in soft tissues (1540 m sec^{-1}). With a 5 MHz transducer and blood flowing towards the transducer at a speed of 30 cm sec^{-1}, the Doppler shift mounts to 1.95 kHz to give an idea of the magnitude of such shifts. If the flow is at an angle (φ) to the ultrasound beam, the measurement has to be corrected by the cosine of φ. Because the measured blood flow velocities are small compared to the velocity of the sound waves, v can be ignored in the denominator.

Rearranged, simplified and corrected for φ the formula becomes:

$$v = \frac{\Delta f \times c}{2 f_i \times \cos \varphi}$$

The smaller the angle φ, the more accurate the flow measurement will be.

Blood flow velocities are generally measured with a *duplex scanner* where one of the channels (transducer elements) is chosen to measure the Doppler shift in A-mode while the other channels record a usual 2D B-mode image. The direction of the A-mode channel is indicated by a line on the image, and the measuring depth along this streak is selected with a cursor, so that only Doppler shifted reflections coming in with a time delay corresponding to this depth along the line will be analyzed. This measuring site can be positioned with high precision, and the spectrum of Doppler shift frequencies as a function of time is displayed together with the 2D B-mode image (Figure 49).

Color flow imaging

The Doppler shift may be utilized to produce images where blood vessels in general are imaged with a color coding in a selected smaller area of an M-mode image (Figure 50). The principle of the method is that consecutive trains of echoes coming in along the scan lines passing through the selected area are compared and analyzed for small differences in the frequency (or the position) of echoes indicating that the echoes stem from moving objects. Movements away from or towards the transducer are distinguished and color coded accordingly, for example so that objects (blood) flowing towards the transducer are coded in red and in blue for movement away from the transducer.

Ultrasonographic contrast media

Bubbles tiny enough to pass blood capillaries, that is, <8 μm, are used to enhance the echogenicity of the circulating blood. Simple air bubbles, small enough for the purpose, may be produced by forcefully passing physiologic saline back and forth between two syringes shortly before being given as an intravenous injection. However, simple air bubbles are not stable and disappear rapidly in the circulation. A number of stabilized bubble formulations have been developed, based on shielding of the bubbles with a coat of a biodegradable material, for example denatured albumin or various lipids. The stability and echogenicity of the bubbles has been further improved by the use of other gasses than air, for example octafluoropropane.

These contrast media strongly enhance the echogenicity of blood and make highly vascularized tissues stand out relative to less vascularized tissues, which may aid in the identification of cancer tissue which is often more vascularized than the normal tissue it is derived from. In cardiac imaging these contrast media may increase the echogenicity of left ventricular blood and aid in the detection of septal defects, and they are valuable for the detection of mural thrombi by enhancing the difference in echogenicity of liquid and clotted blood which do not take up the bubbles.

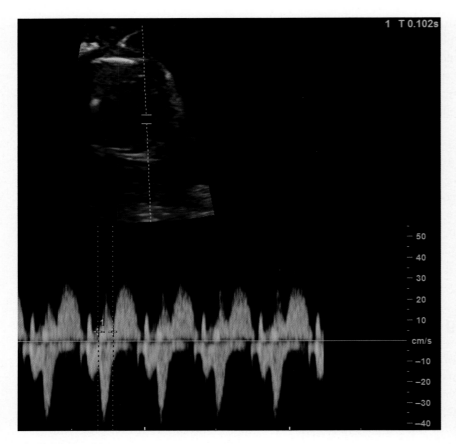

Figure 49 Duplex scanning of fetal heart.
The site for measurement of blood flow is selected on the ultrasonogram and indicated by two parallel lines on the track from the transducer element selected for the Doppler measurement. The lower panel displays the spectrum of Doppler shifts as a function of time (in cm/s) recorded from which the magnitude and direction of blood flow recorded over five cardiac cycles can be read. The downward-directed flow stems from the inflow of blood from the atrium, initially passive, then forced by atrial contraction (sharp downward peak). The broad upward peak represents aortic outflow. The distance marked "1" represents the atrio-ventricular conduction time.

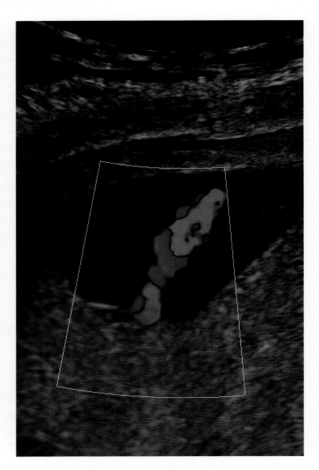

Figure 50 Color flow Doppler imaging of the umbilical cord.
The direction of blood flow in the umbilical vein and the arteries is opposite and has accordingly been color coded opposite in blue and red.

Techniques based on radioisotope emissions

Scintigraphy

Diagnostic scintigraphic imaging involves the following basic elements: a suitable *radioisotope* given in an appropriate *chemical and pharmaceutical formulation* that assigns it a specific target within the body, and a *recording system*, which can map the distribution of the radioisotope, for most purposes being *the gamma camera*.

Suitable radioisotopes

Radioisotopes used for most routine diagnostic imaging are emitters of γ-photons with energies in the 80–200 keV range, that is, equivalent to usual diagnostic X-ray photon energies (Figure 1). The designations γ-rays and X-rays refer to the origin of the photons: X-rays derive from processes confined to the electron shells of atoms, while γ-rays arise from processes in the nuclei of certain unstable isotopes.

The photons of γ-radiation have discrete energies specific to the nuclear reaction they derive from, that is, the radiation is monochromatic, while photons from an X-ray tube are polychromatic in a continuous spectrum. The monochromaticity of γ-emissions is important because it can be utilized to distinguish the origin of γ-photons by analysis of their energies.

Photons with energies in the range mentioned earlier penetrate tissues very well and therefore easily escape the body to be recorded by an external detector.

Radioisotopes that emit β^-- and α-radiation are generally useless for diagnostic imaging because these types of radiation are effectively absorbed in the tissues, and also because their radiations elicit much secondary ionization, that is, cause biological damage. Some radioisotopes which emit favorable γ-radiation must be rejected because their decay products are harmful β^--emitters. Positron (β^+)-emitters have special applications (PET) to be briefly touched upon at the end of this chapter.

Clearly, the radiation dose received by the patient must be kept to a minimum. For this reason the *half-life* (T½) of the radioisotope should be so short that the needless radiation received after the examination soon levels off. A T½ of half to twice the time needed for performing the clinical examination may be considered appropriate. In some applications the elimination becomes further accelerated by renal excretion or respiration. In general, the radiation received by the patient during scintigraphic examinations is about equal to that of X-ray examinations.

Further requirements of an ideal radioisotope are that it should be atoxic in the doses required, and that it should have chemistry favorable for binding to pharmaceuticals, allowing its targeting to specific tissues and organs in the body. Finally, it should be readily available at a reasonable cost. Radioisotopes that meet these demands and which accordingly are used in diagnostic practice include ^{67}Ga (T½ ~ 78 hours), ^{81m}Kr (T½ ~ 13 sec), ^{99m}Tc (T½ ~ 6 hours), ^{123}I (T½ ~ 13 hours), and ^{133}Xe (T½ ~ 5 days). Several others are available and are used alternatively or for special purposes.

Pharmaceutical formulations

For most purposes, radioisotopes are used in specific chemical formulations or attached as a label to a pharmaceutical in order to target the isotope to a special tissue, a metabolic pathway or a physiologic/pathophysiologic phenomenon.

^{123}I is used for thyroid scintigraphy given as iodide. ^{81m}Kr and ^{133}Xe is inhaled as a gas for examination of lung ventilation. ^{99m}Tc takes up a dominant position in diagnostic imaging because its half-life is ideal, and the emitted γ-photon has an energy (140 keV) that penetrates tissues very well and is favorable for detection with a gamma camera. The decay product ^{99}Tc decays further with β^--emission to a stable ruthenium isotope, but the half-life of this transition is so long (2×10^5 years) that it is biologically unimportant. ^{99m}Tc is readily available from a generator (a $^{99}_{42}$Mo -"cow", which can be milked every day) in the form of pertechnetate (TcO4$^-$) which has a chemistry that is favorable for a number of coupling reactions. Thus ^{99m}Tc may be used coupled to phosphonate compounds for bone scintigraphy (Figure 51), to HIDA for biliary scintigraphy, to mercaptoacetyl-triglycin (MAG3) for renography, to albumin-aggregates for perfusion studies, for example lung perfusion; coupled to colloids for labeling of macrophages in liver, spleen, and bone marrow, and coupled to glucoheptonate or hexametazime for brain scintigraphy, to mention a few applications.

The gamma camera

The basic design of a gamma camera, as used for diagnostic scintigraphic imaging, is shown in Figure 52. The γ-photon detector is a large single crystal of sodium iodide, doped with thallium. A collimator consisting of a lead plate with numerous closely spaced holes is mounted in front of the crystal. The holes may be parallel or they may be diverging towards the patient in order to obtain a larger field of view or converging to produce an enlarged image with more details. The collimator absorbs γ-photons which do not travel parallel or nearly parallel with the axis of the holes. Thus, the collimator defines, for each point in the crystal, the direction of incident γ-photons.

When hit by γ-photons, the crystal emits (scintillates) quanta of blue light proportional to the energy of the incident γ-photon. The evoked light emission is picked up by a hexagonal array of up to about a hundred photomultipliers mounted in tight optical contact with the back of the crystal. The photomultiplier signals are fed into a computer which

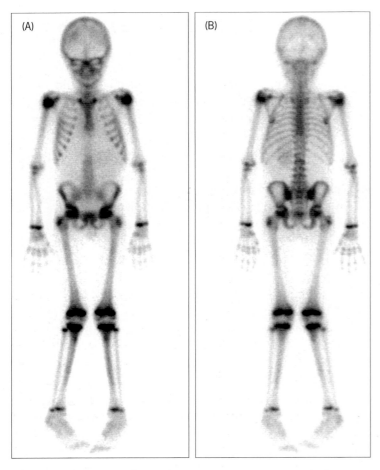

Figure 51 Whole body ^{99m}Tc-diphosphonate bone scintigrams of a six year old boy.
(A) is recorded with the boy's front in contact with the gamma camera; (B) with the back and buttock in contact. Note the high signal intensity from growth plates and other sites of growth. By comparing the two images it is clearly seen that the recorded signal intensity is dependent on the distance from the camera.

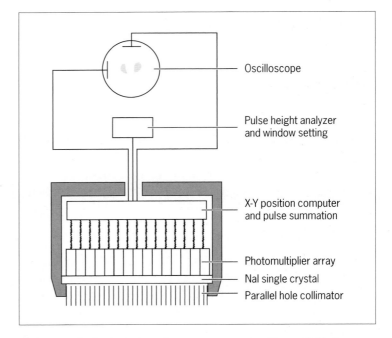

Figure 52 The basic design of a gamma camera with parallel hole collimator.

performs two basic calculations. Firstly, the position (X-Y coordinates) of the scintillation event is calculated by comparing the signal intensities from the photomultipliers to locate the source. Secondly, the "pulse height" is calculated as the sum of all the signals belonging to a single scintillation event. The sum is proportional to the energy of the incident γ-photon, which in turn is specific to the isotope. If the pulse height is lower than "expected" it is likely to derive from a γ-photon that was scattered, losing energy *en route* to the camera. An adjustable "window" is set to reject scintillations with less than, say 90% of the expected maximum pulse height. The accepted scintillations are stored and displayed on a screen where the image gradually builds up. A typical gamma camera has the capacity to process some 50,000 scintillations per second, and reasonable image quality requires some 10^6 scintillations.

The resulting scintigram is a 2D projection of the spatial distribution of the isotope within the body. Firstly, the spatial resolution falls rapidly off with distance to the camera,

because the camera discriminates only the angle of incoming photons. The resolution of a good gamma camera is only some 1.5–2 cm for an object located 5 cm from the front of the collimator. Secondly, because the intensity of γ-radiation from a given direction decreases with the square of the distance from the source, the number of photons reaching the detector from a deeply located source will be smaller than if the source was more superficially located. This difference is further augmented by the fact that a γ-photon from a deep source is more likely to be absorbed on its way, or to be scattered and lose direction and energy enough to be rejected by the collimator or the pulse height analyzer. Therefore, a scintigram will image structures close to the body surface and close to the detector with markedly better contrast and resolution than deep and remote structures (Figure 51). Therefore, in most examinations two or more scintigrams are recorded from various directions.

Single photon emission computed tomography (SPECT) and positron emission tomography (PET)

SPECT

A series of tomographic images may be obtained with γ-emitting isotopes if a gamma camera is rotated around the patient through 180° or 360° in steps of a few degrees, and data are collected at each position. By computational procedures analogous to CT imaging, 2D tomographic images and 3D reconstructions of the spatial distribution of the isotope may be produced. The data acquisition time is quite long, and the spatial resolution is in the order of one centimeter.

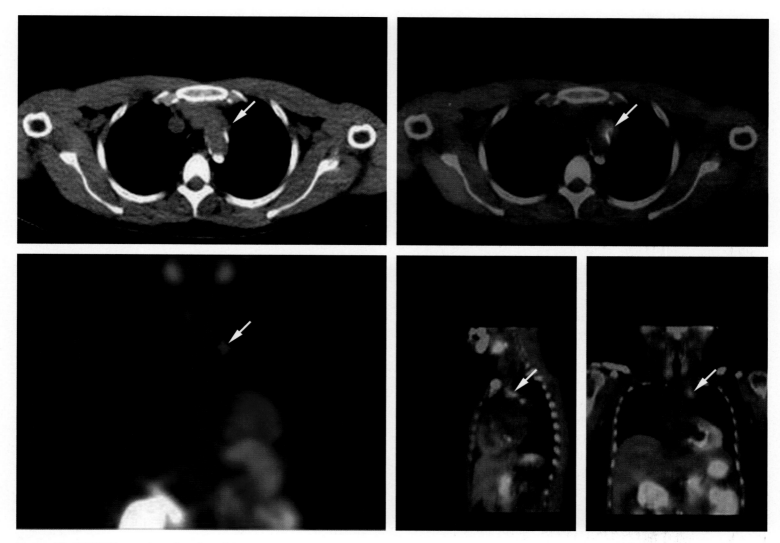

Figure 53 CT-SPECT scanning of neck and thorax.
The patient has received a dose of ^{99m}Tc-sestamibi which (among others) is taken up by the parathyroid glands. The upper left image is one image in the series of axial CT images. The lower left image is a coronal section reconstructed from the series of axial SPECT images recording the distribution of the isotope. The image at upper right is the SPECT image superimposed on the corresponding CT image and the two images at lower right are similarly superimposed sagittal and coronal images. The examination has revealed a parathyroid gland (arrows) with an aberrant location in the superior mediastinum.

PET

The radiation produced by *positron (β⁻)-emitting isotopes* is remarkable. A positron emitted from the nucleus will, after travelling a very short path (1–2 mm), be annihilated by fusion with an electron and the joint mass of the positron and the electron will thereby be converted into energy in the form of two photons, each of very high energy (511 keV) that leave the site of annihilation in exactly opposite (180°) directions.

This phenomenon is utilized for tomographic imaging (PET). The PET scanner consists of a ring of detectors, the plane of the ring defining the tomographic section. The signals received by the detectors are analyzed for coincidence, because coincidence derives from the capture of both of the 511 keV photons resulting from an annihilation event which has taken place along a straight line joining the two detectors. The signals are further analyzed for signal height and are rejected if falling below a certain set limit as with ordinary gamma cameras, and the attenuation of high-energy γ-radiation has prior to the examination been mapped in all directions through the actual patient in order to sharpen the precision in acceptance/rejection of signals. When a sufficient number of annihilation events have been recorded, it is a relatively simple computational procedure to derive a tomographic image of the isotope distribution. The spatial resolution is down to about 5 mm.

The most generally used isotope for PET scanning is ^{18}F which has a T½ of 109 minutes. It has become widely used as ^{18}F-deoxyglucose (FDG), which is taken up, but not metabolized as glucose and therefore accumulates in cells, the more glycolytically active they are. The glycolysis of malignant tumors is often highly active.

Combination of CT with SPECT or PET

In order to achieve more precise anatomical definition of the location of the isotopes imaged by SPECT or PET, the latter may be combined with CT. To ensure that the positioning of the patient is the same in the two imaging modes, the patient, lying still and quietly breathing on a couch, is passed sequentially through a CT scanner and a SPECT/PET scanner assembled into one unit sharing the same rail for the couch. After imaging in the two modes, the images can be superimposed (Figure 53).

Principles of nomenclature and positioning

The vocabulary used in diagnostic imaging to indicate planes, directions, and locations is largely identical to the established anatomical nomenclature which refers to the "anatomical standard position", that is, standing erect, arms by the sides and palms facing forwards. By tradition, in diagnostic imaging, some anatomical terms are replaced by synonymous "radiology terms", and the anatomical vocabulary has been supplemented.

Anatomical *planes* are commonly designated *sections*, with reference to tomographic imaging.

The *median section* (Figure 54A) divides the body into two halves which are symmetric on the body surface.

A *sagittal section* denotes any section parallel to the median section. The median section is sometimes denoted the mid-sagittal section.

A *paramedian section* is a sagittal section close to the median section.

A *frontal section* (Figure 54B) denotes any vertical section perpendicular to the median section. In diagnostic imaging, frontal sections are commonly denoted *coronal sections*, because they are about parallel to the plane of the coronal suture.

A *transversal section* (Figure 54C) is perpendicular to both the coronal and the sagittal sections. It is sometimes denoted a *horizontal section*, but the established term in radiology is an *axial section*, so denoted because it is the image that would be produced if a transversal slice of the body was conventionally imaged by an X-ray beam oriented along the axis of the body.

In axial MR scanning of the head, the standard tomographic planes are parallel to the *orbitomeatal plane*, which is defined by the lateral canthus of the eye and the centre of the external auditory meatus; both easy to identify. This plane is virtually identical to the anatomical *Frankfurter plane* ("German horizontal"), defined by the lower margin of the orbit and the upper edge of the external auditory meatus. In axial CT scanning of the brain it is common practice to tilt the plane so that the tomographic series start above the eyeball in order to avoid unnecessary irradiation of the lens.

In conventional X-ray imaging, the inherent magnification on an object depends on its location in the beam path between the X-ray tube focal spot and the film. Thus, on X-ray of the cranium taken with the beam entering the stern to expose a film placed behind the occiput will show the frontal sinuses at higher magnification than with the reverse beam direction. It is therefore common practice to indicate the direction of the beam path using the following terms (see Figure 55):

An *antero-posterior (a-p)* X-ray is taken with a beam entering the anterior (ventral) side of the body to expose a film/recorder placed on the posterior (dorsal) side. A *postero-anterior (p-a)* X-ray is the opposite of an a-p X-ray.

A *left lateral* X-ray is taken with a beam entering the right lateral side to expose a film placed to the left of the body. A *right lateral* X-ray is the opposite.

An *axial* X-ray is taken with a beam passing along the axis of the body (cranially or caudally) to expose a film located in a transversal plane.

A *tilted* X-ray is taken with a beam which is angled relative to a transversal plane.

An *oblique* X-ray is taken with a beam which is angled relative to a sagittal plane.

A *right anterior oblique (RAO)* X-ray is taken with the film placed on the right anterior side of the body, to be exposed by a beam entering the left dorsal side of the body.

A *left anterior oblique (LAO)* is analogous to the above with left and right interchanged.

An X-ray of the hand, wrist and lower arm is often taken with a beam entering the dorsum of the hand to expose a film below the volar face of the hand, and is denoted a *dorso-volar* X-ray. An analogous X-ray of the foot is denoted a *dorso-plantar* X-ray.

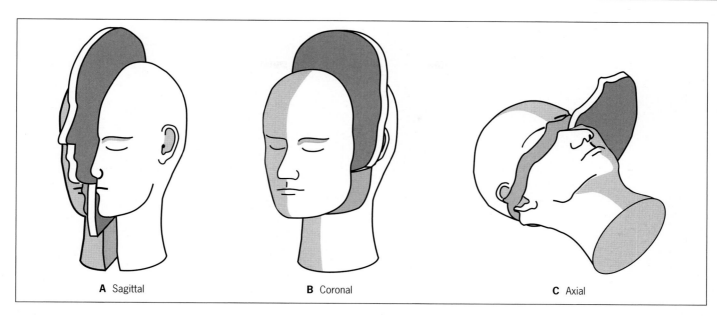

A Sagittal   **B** Coronal   **C** Axial

Figure 54 Tomographic planes.

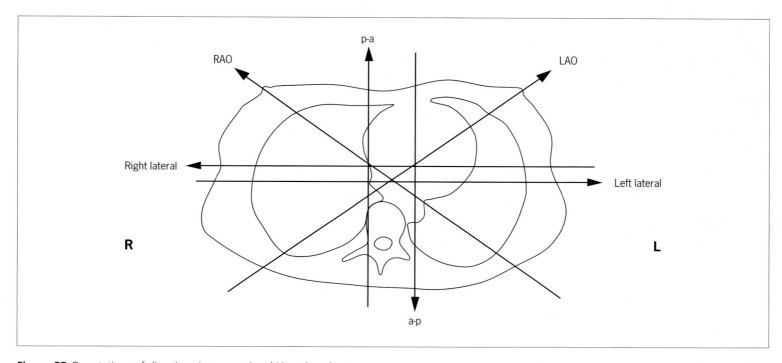

Figure 55 Denotations of directions in conventional X-ray imaging.
Arrows mark the beam direction.

Conventions of image presentation used in the atlas part of this book:

Conventional X-rays

A-p and p-a X-rays are shown as if the patient was facing the observer.

Lateral X-rays are shown with the patient's left towards the observer.

Supine and prone X-rays are shown with the patient's head towards the left or upwards.

Tomographic sections

Axial sections are seen from below. This is international convention.

Coronal sections are seen from the patient's front.

Sagittal sections are seen from the patient's left.

Nomenclature according to

Terminologia Anatomica: International Anatomical Terminology

by the Federative Committee on Anatomical Terminology (FCAT)

Thieme, Stuttgart-New York, 1998

Upper Limb

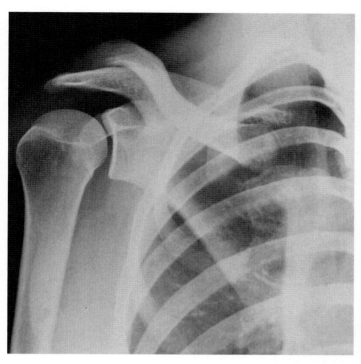
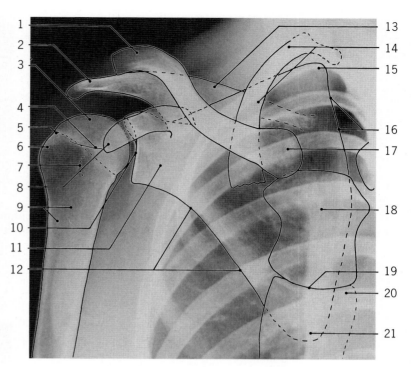

Shoulder, a-p X-ray

1: Acromial end of clavicle
2: Acromion
3: Humeral head
4: Epiphyseal scar
5: Anatomical neck
6: Greater tubercle
7: Lesser tubercle

8: Coracoid process
9: Surgical neck
10: Glenoid cavity
11: Neck of scapula
12: Lateral border of scapula
13: Spine of scapula
14: First rib

15: Superior angle of scapula
16: Medial border of scapula
17: Sternal end of clavicle
18: Manubrium of sternum
19: Sternal angle
20: Body of sternum
21: Inferior angle of scapula

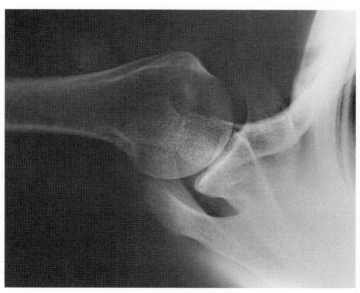
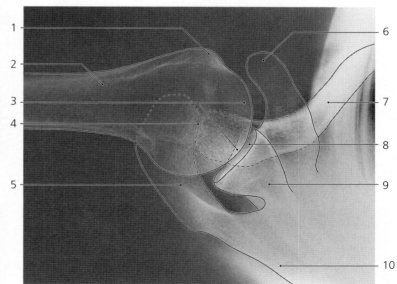

Shoulder, axial X-ray

1: Greater tubercle
2: Surgical neck of humerus
3: Humeral head
4: Acromioclavicular joint

5: Acromion
6: Coracoid process
7: Clavicle
8: Glenoid cavity

9: Neck of scapula
10: Spine of scapula

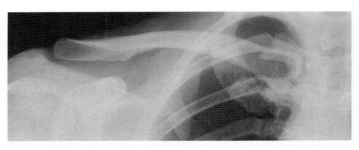
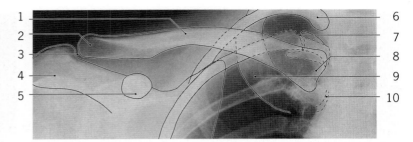

Clavicle, a-p X-ray

1: Shaft of clavicle
2: Acromial end of clavicle
3: Acromioclavicular joint
4: Acromion

5: Coracoid process
6: Second rib
7: Costotransverse joint
8: Sternal end of clavicle

9: First rib
10: Costovertebral joint

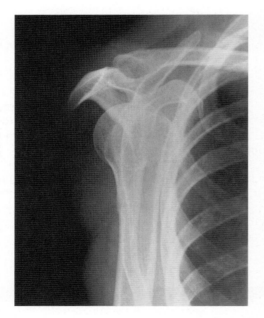
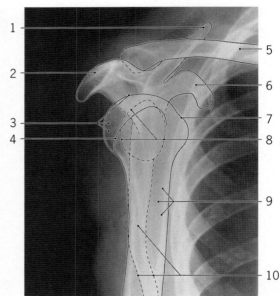

Scapula, oblique X-ray

1: Superior margin of scapula
2: Acromion
3: Head of humerus
4: Greater tubercle

5: Clavicle
6: Coracoid process
7: Lesser tubercle
8: Glenoid cavity

9: Surgical neck of humerus
10: Scapula from edge

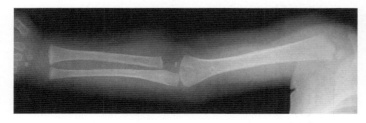
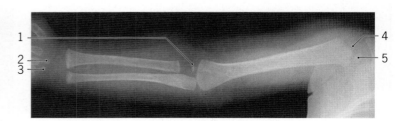

Shoulder and arm, a-p X-ray, child one year

1: Capitulum (ossification center)
2: Capitate bone (ossification center)

3: Hamate bone (ossification center)
4: Greater tubercle (ossification center)

5: Humeral head (ossification center)

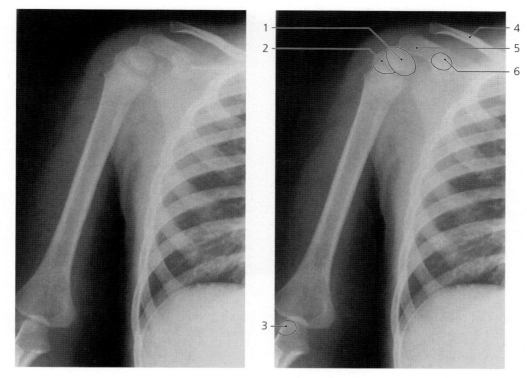

Shoulder and arm, a-p X-ray, child 5 years

1: **Humeral head (ossification center)**
2: **Greater tubercle (ossification center)**

3: **Capitulum (ossification center)**
4: **Clavicle**

5: **Acromion**
6: **Coracoid process (ossification center)**

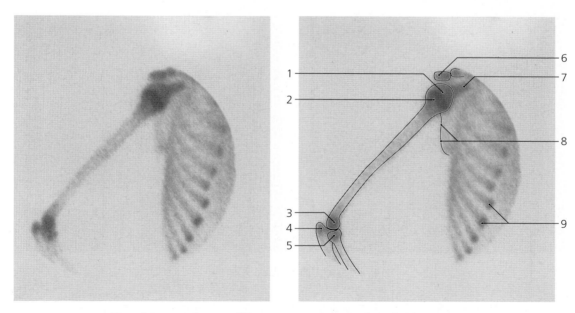

Shoulder and arm, ^{99m} Tc-MDP, scintigraphy, child 12 years

1: **Humeral head**
2: **Growth plate of proximal epiphysis of humerus**
3: **Trochlea and capitulum**

4: **Olecranon**
5: **Head of radius**
6: **Acromion**
7: **Coracoid process**

8: **Lateral margin of scapula**
9: **Osteochondral transition of ribs**

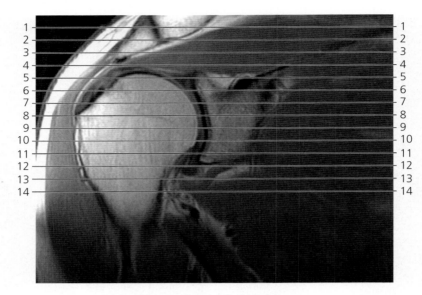

Scout view of shoulder

Lines #1–14 indicate planes of sectioning in the following axial MR series. Arrows ←, → and ↔ in the figure legends indicate that a structure can be seen in a preceding or following section or both. Interpretation of the scout image can be found in the coronal series, page 63, image #9.

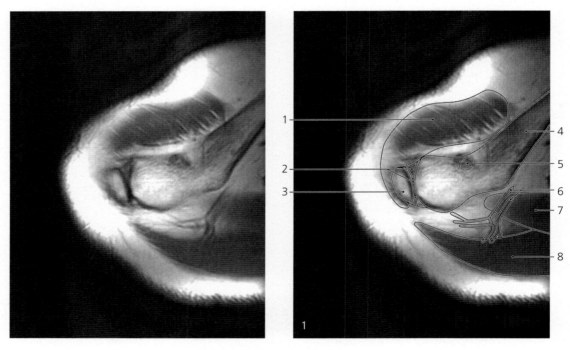

Shoulder, axial MR

1: Deltoideus →

2: Acromioclavicular joint with articular disc →

3: Acromion →

4: Clavicle →

5: Coracoclavicular (trapezoid) ligament (attachment) →

6: Suprascapular artery and vein →

7: Supraspinatus →

8: Trapezius →

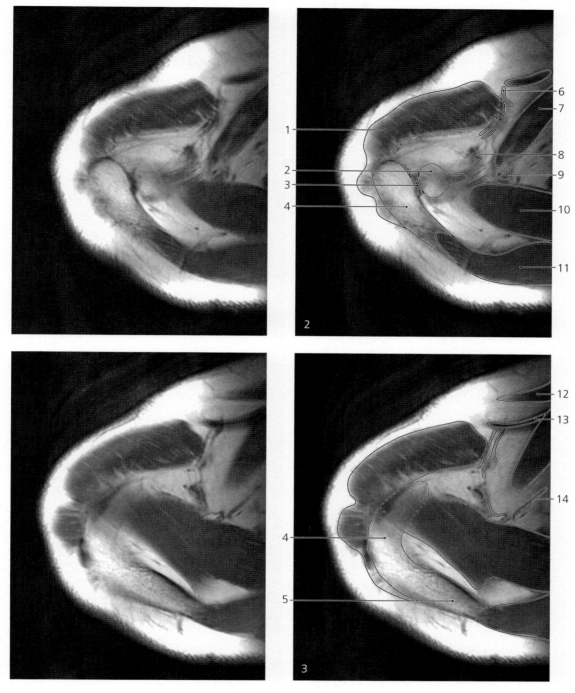

Shoulder, axial MR

Scout view on page 52

1: Deltoideus ↔
2: Clavicle (acromial extremity) ←
3: Acromioclavicular joint ←
4: Acromion ↔
5: Spine of scapula →

6: Thoracoacromial artery/vein
7: Subclavius muscle
8: Coracoclavicular (trapezoid) ligament ↔
9: Coracoclavicular (conoid) ligament →
10: Supraspinatus ↔

11: Trapezius ↔
12: Pectoralis major →
13: Cephalic vein →
14: Suprascapular artery/vein ←

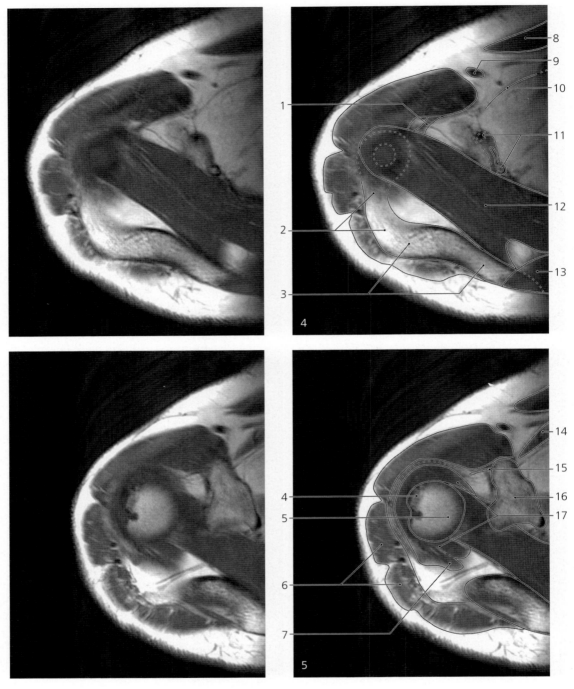

Shoulder, axial MR

Scout view on page 52

1: Coracoacromial ligament →
2: Acromion ←
3: Spine of scapula ↔
4: Greater tubercle of humerus →
5: Head of humerus →
6: Deltoideus ↔

7: Infraspinatus →
8: Pectoralis major ↔
9: Cephalic vein ↔
10: Clavipectoral fascia
11: Trapezoid and conoid ligament
   (attachment on coracoid process) ←
12: Supraspinatus ↔

13: Trapezius ↔
14: Pectoralis minor →
15: Coracoacromial ligament (attachment)
   ←
16: Coracoid process →
17: Articular capsule/rotator cuff →

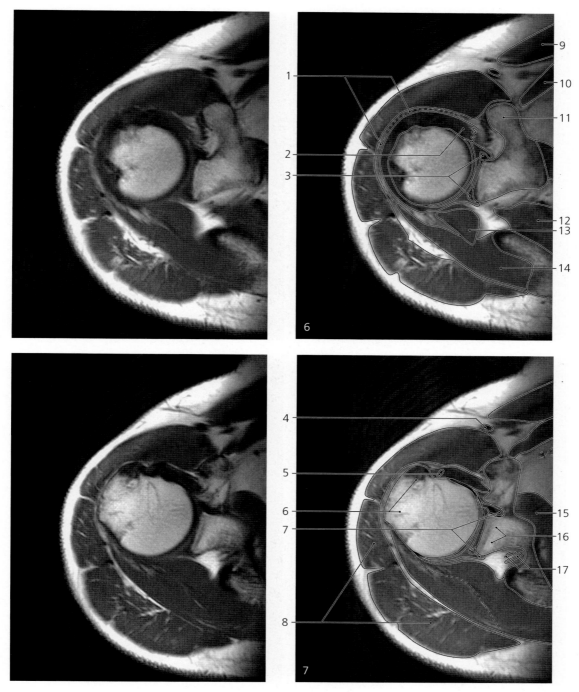

Shoulder, axial MR

Scout view on page 52

1: Subdeltoid bursa
2: Coracohumeral ligament
3: Glenoid labrum →
4: Cephalic vein ↔
5: Biceps brachii, long head →

6: Greater tubercle of humerus ↔
7: Reflection of articular capsule →
8: Deltoideus ↔
9: Pectoralis major ↔
10: Pectoralis minor ↔
11: Coracoid process ←

12: Supraspinatus →
13: Infraspinatus ↔
14: Teres minor →
15: Subscapularis →
16: Neck of scapula →
17: Suprascapular artery and vein →

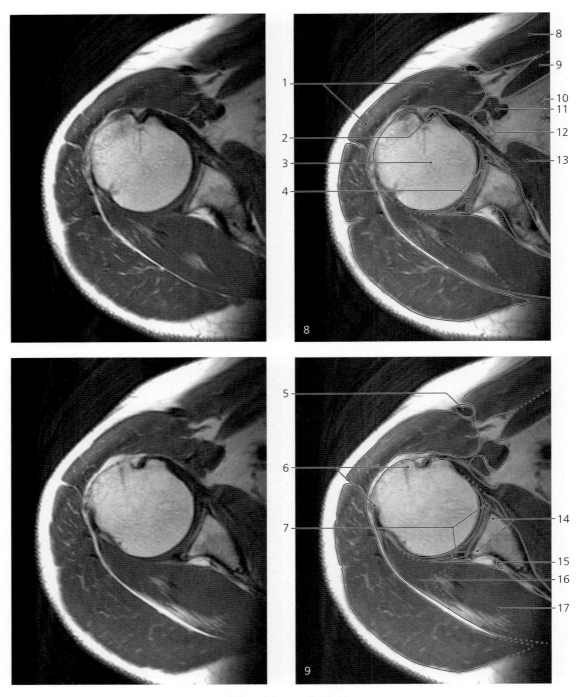

Shoulder, axial MR

Scout view on page 52

1: Deltoideus ↔
2: Biceps brachii, long head in intertubercular sulcus ↔
3: Head of humerus ↔
4: Glenoid cavity ↔
5: Cephalic vein ↔
6: Greater tubercle of humerus ↔
7: Glenoid labrum ↔
8: Pectoralis major ↔
9: Pectoralis minor ↔
10: Lymph node
11: Biceps brachii, short head →
12: Coracobrachialis →
13: Subscapularis ↔
14: Neck of scapula ↔
15: Suprascapular artery and vein
16: Teres minor ↔
17: Infraspinatus ↔

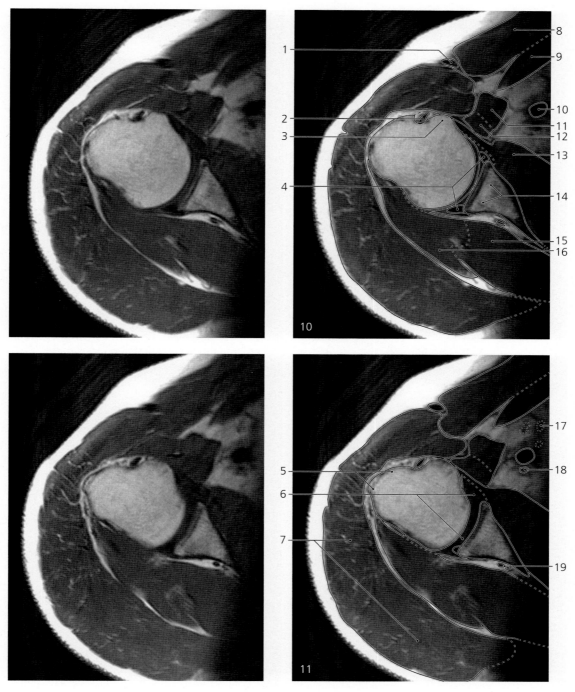

Shoulder, axial MR

Scout view on page 52
1: Cephalic vein ↔
2: Biceps brachii, long head ↔
3: Lesser tubercle of humerus →
4: Glenoid labrum ←
5: Greater tubercle of humerus ↔
6: Articular capsule, lower recess →

7: Deltoideus ↔
8: Pectoralis major ↔
9: Pectoralis minor ↔
10: Axillary artery →
11: Biceps brachii, short head ↔
12: Coracobrachialis ↔
13: Subscapularis ↔

14: Neck of scapula ↔
15: Infraspinatus ↔
16: Teres minor ↔
17: Lymph node →
18: Posterior cord of brachial plexus
19: Suprascapular artery and vein ←

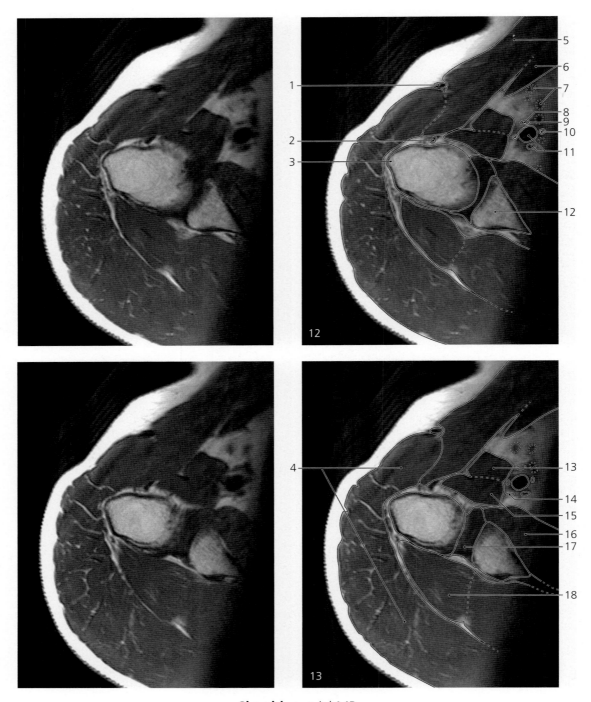

Shoulder, axial MR

Scout view on page 52
1: Cephalic vein ↔
2: Biceps brachii, long head ↔
3: Greater tubercle of humerus ←
4: Deltoideus ↔
5: Pectoralis major ↔
6: Pectoralis minor ↔

7: Lymph nodes ↔
8: Median nerve →
9: Musculocutaneous nerve →
10: Ulnar nerve →
11: Axillary artery and radial nerve →
12: Neck of scapula ←
13: Biceps brachii, short head ↔

14: Axillary nerve →
15: Coracobrachialis ↔
16: Subscapularis ↔
17: Articular capsule, lower recess ↔
18: Teres minor ↔

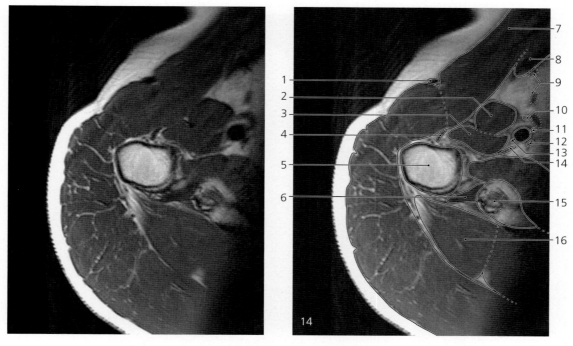

Shoulder, axial MR

Scout view on page 52
1: Cephalic vein ←
2: Biceps brachii, short head ←
3: Coracobrachialis ←
4: Biceps brachii, long head ←
5: Surgical neck of humerus

6: Articular capsule, lower recess ←
7: Pectoralis major ←
8: Pectoralis minor ←
9: Lymph nodes ←
10: Median nerve ←
11: Ulnar nerve ←

12: Radial nerve ←
13: Musculocutaneous nerve ←
14: Axillary nerve ←
15: Triceps brachii, long head (origin)
16: Teres minor ←

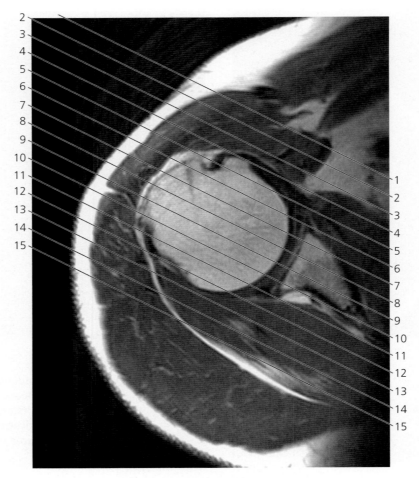

Scout view of shoulder

Lines #1–15 indicate planes of sectioning in the following MR series. The planes are approximately parallel to the scapular blade ("oblique coronal"). Interpretation of the scout image can be found in the axial series, page 56, image #9.

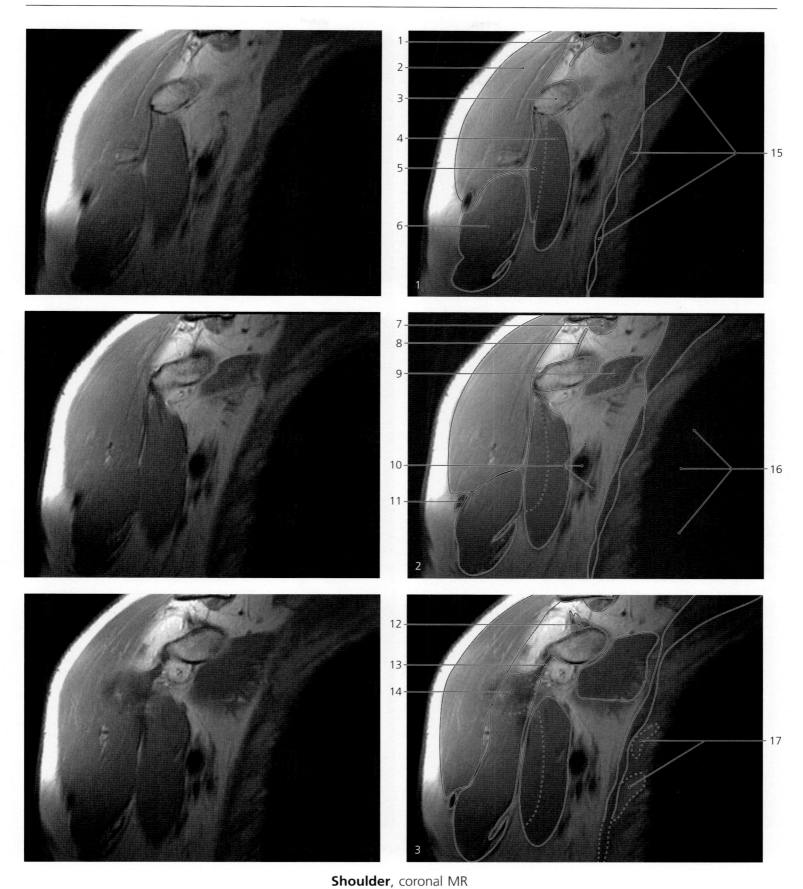

Shoulder, coronal MR

Scout view on page 60

1: Clavicle →
2: Deltoideus →
3: Coracoid process →
4: Coracobrachialis →
5: Biceps brachii, short head →
6: Pectoralis major →
7: Subclavius muscle →

8: Coracoclavicular (trapezoid) ligament
9: Subscapularis →
10: Vessels, lymph nodes and nerves in axillary fossa →
11: Cephalic vein →
12: Coracoclavicular (coronoid) ligament →
13: Coracoacromial ligament →

14: Head of humerus →
15: Serratus anterior →
16: Lung
17: Ribs

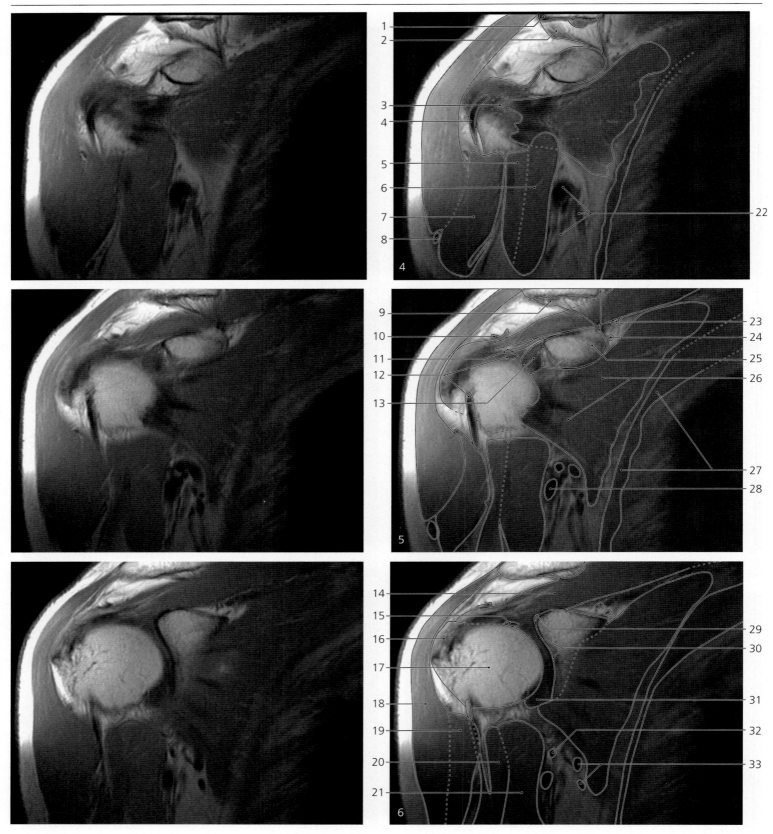

Shoulder, coronal MR

Scout view on page 60

1: Clavicle ↔
2: Coracoclavicular (coronoid) ligament ←
3: Lesser tubercle of humerus
4: Biceps brachii, long head →
5: Biceps brachii, short head ↔
6: Coracobrachialis ↔
7: Pectoralis major ↔
8: Cephalic vein ←
9: Coracoclavicular (coronoid) ligament ←
10: Coracoacromial ligament ↔
11: Coracohumeral ligament

12: Biceps brachii, long head ↔
13: Articular capsule, lower recess →
14: Supraspinatus →
15: Biceps brachii, long head ↔
16: Greater tubercle of humerus →
17: Head of humerus ↔
18: Deltoideus ↔
19: Pectoralis major ↔
20: Biceps brachii, short head →
21: Coracobrachialis ↔
22: Vessels, lymph nodes and nerves in axillary fossa ↔
23: Suprascapular artery →

24: Suprascapular nerve →
25: Coracoid process (root) ←
26: Subscapularis ↔
27: Serratus anterior ↔
28: Axillary artery →
29: Glenoid labrum →
30: Glenoid fossa →
31: Articular capsule, lower recess →
32: Posterior circumflex humeral artery →
33: Circumflex scapular artery and vein →

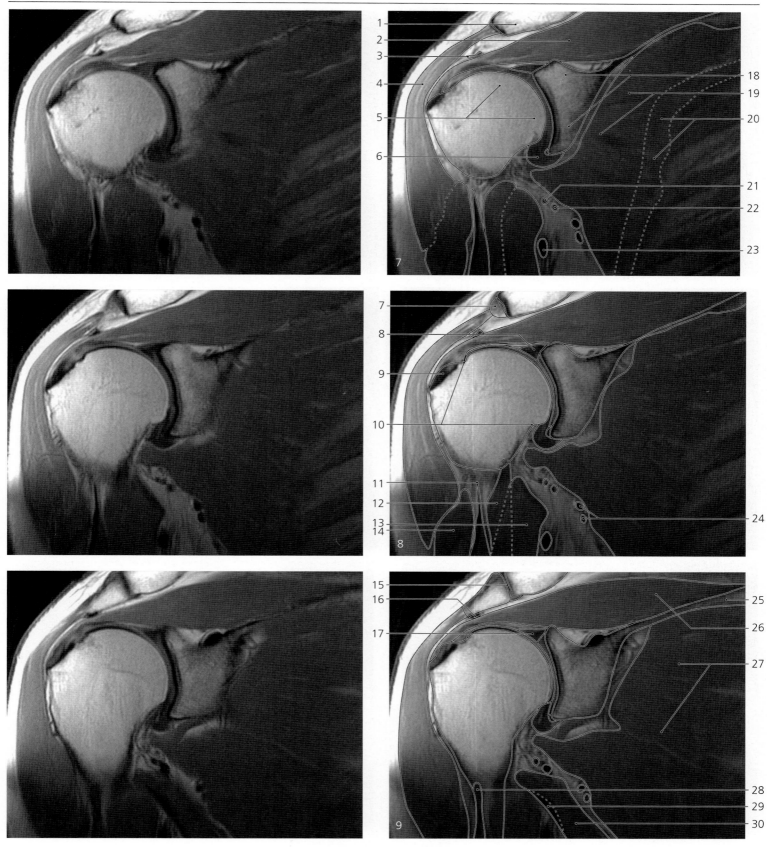

Shoulder, coronal MR

Scout view on page 60

1: Clavicle ←
2: Supraspinatus ↔
3: Coracoacromial ligament ↔
4: Deltoideus ↔
5: Head of humerus ↔
6: Articular capsule, lower recess ↔
7: Acromion →
8: Glenoid labrum ↔
9: Greater tubercle of humerus ↔
10: Anatomical neck of humerus

11: Biceps brachii, long head ←
12: Latissimus dorsi and teres major (insertion) →
13: Coracobrachialis ↔
14: Pectoralis major ↔
15: Acromioclavicular joint
16: Coracoacromial ligament (attachment) ←
17: Glenoid labrum ↔
18: Neck of scapula →
19: Subscapularis ↔
20: Serratus anterior ←
21: Posterior circumflex humeral artery ↔

22: Axillary nerve →
23: Axillary artery ←
24: Circumflex scapular artery and vein ↔
25: Spine of scapula →
26: Supraspinatus ↔
27: Subscapularis ↔
28: Pectoralis major (insertion) ←
29: Latissimus dorsi (tendon) →
30: Teres major →

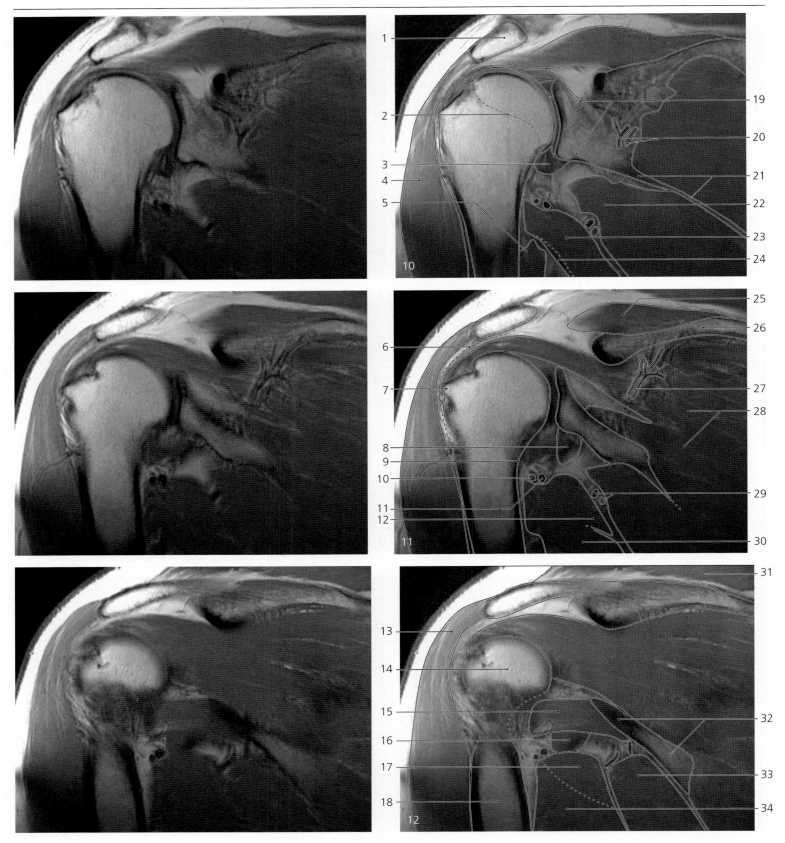

Shoulder, coronal MR

Scout view on page 60

1: Acromion ←
2: Epiphysial line
3: Articular capsule, lower recess ←
4: Deltoideus ↔
5: Coracobrachialis (insertion) ←
6: Subacromial and subdeltoid bursa
7: Greater tubercle of humerus ←
8: Triceps brachii, long head (origin) →
9: Surgical neck of humerus
10: Axillary nerve ↔
11: Posterior circumflex humeral artery ↔

12: Teres major ↔
13: Deltoideus ↔
14: Head of humerus ←
15: Teres minor →
16: Triceps brachii, long head ↔
17: Teres major ←
18: Shaft of humerus
19: Neck of scapula ←
20: Branches of #29
21: Blade of scapula
22: Subscapularis →
23: Teres major ↔

24: Latissimus dorsi (tendon) ↔
25: Supraspinatus ←
26: Spine of scapula ↔
27: Branches of #29
28: Infraspinatus →
29: Circumflex scapular artery and vein ↔
30: Latissimus dorsi ↔
31: Trapezius →
32: Lateral margin of scapula
33: Teres minor →
34: Latissimus dorsi →

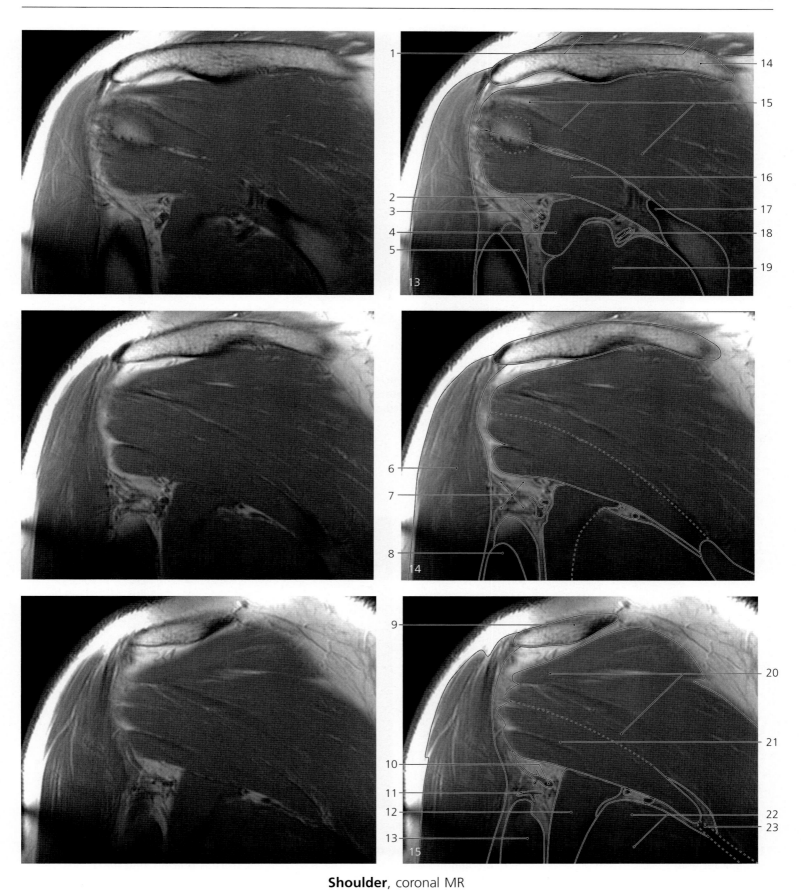

Shoulder, coronal MR

Scout view on page 60

1: Trapezius ←
2: Posterior circumflex humeral artery ↔
3: Axillary nerve ↔
4: Triceps brachii, long head ↔
5: Triceps brachii, lateral head →
6: Deltoideus ←
7: "Quadrangular space"

8: Shaft of humerus ←
9: Spine of scapula ←
10: Posterior circumflex humeral artery ←
11: Axillary nerve ←
12: Triceps brachii, long head ←
13: Triceps brachii, lateral head ←
14: Spine of scapula →
15: Infraspinatus →
16: Teres minor ↔

17: Lateral margin of scapula
18: Circumflex scapular artery and vein ↔
19: Latissimus dorsi ↔
20: Infraspinatus ←
21: Teres minor ←
22: Latissimus dorsi ←
23: Lateral margin of scapula ←

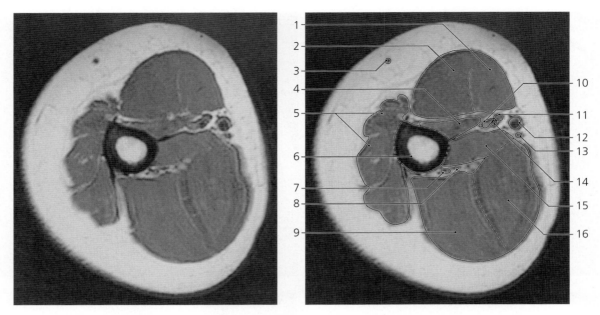

Arm, upper third, axial MR

1: Biceps brachii, short head
2: Biceps brachii, long head
3: Cephalic vein
4: Coracobrachialis
5: Deltoid muscle
6: Shaft of humerus

7: Radial nerve
8: Profunda brachii artery
9: Triceps brachii, lateral head
10: Median and musculocutaneus nerve
11: Brachial vein
12: Basilic vein

13: Ulnar nerve
14: Brachial artery
15: Triceps brachii, medial head
16: Triceps brachii, long head

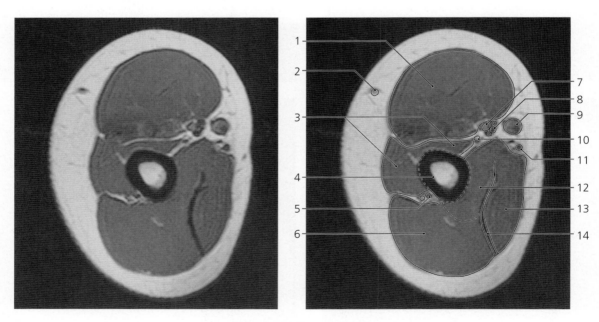

Arm, middle, axial MR

1: Biceps brachii
2: Cephalic vein
3: Brachialis muscle
4: Shaft of humerus
5: Radial nerve and profunda brachii artery

6: Triceps brachii, lateral head
7: Median nerve
8: Brachial artery and veins
9: Basilic veins
10: Musculocutaneous nerve
11: Ulnar nerve

12: Triceps brachii, medial head
13: Triceps brachii, long head
14: Internal aponeurosis of triceps brachii

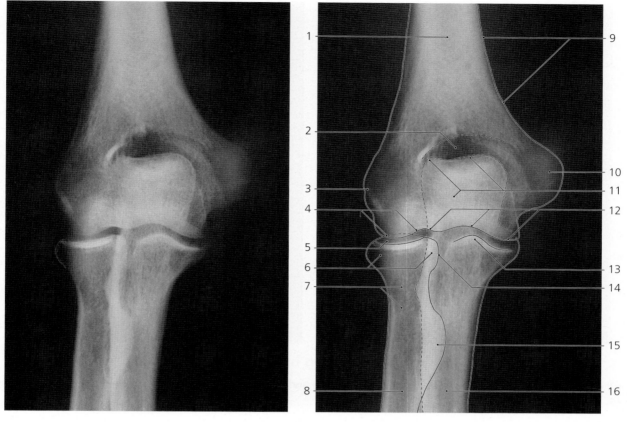

Elbow, a-p X-ray

1: Shaft of humerus
2: Olecranon fossa, and coronoid fossa (superimposed)
3: Lateral epicondyle
4: Capitulum
5: Humeroradial joint

6: Head of radius
7: Neck of radius
8: Shaft of radius
9: Medial supracondylar ridge
10: Medial epicondyle
11: Olecranon

12: Trochlea
13: Coronoid process
14: Articular circumference of radius
15: Radial tuberosity
16: Shaft of ulna

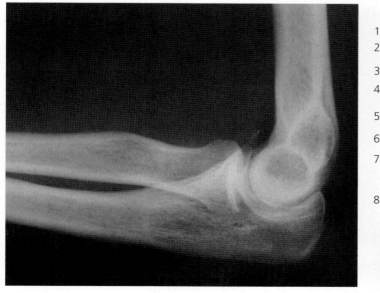
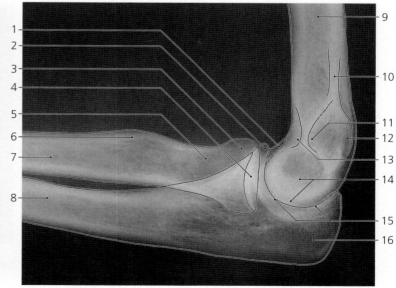

Elbow, lateral X-ray

1: Capitulum
2: Coronoid process
3: Head of radius
4: Articular fovea of radius
5: Neck of radius
6: Radial tuberosity

7: Shaft of radius
8: Shaft of ulna
9: Shaft of humerus
10: Medial supracondylar ridge
11: Olecranon fossa
12: Medial epicondyle

13: Coronoid fossa
14: Trochlea
15: Humero-ulnar joint
16: Olecranon

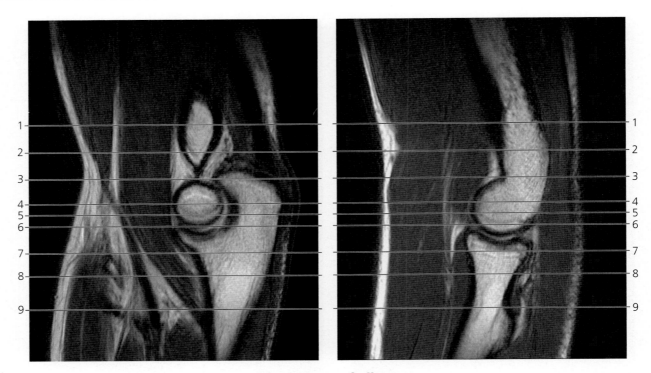

Scout views of elbow

Lines #1–9 indicate planes of sectioning in the following axial MR series. Interpretation of the scout images can be found in the sagittal series, page 73–74, image #1 and #3.

Note that the radial artery in this series has branched off from the brachial artery before reaching the cubital fossa. The frequency of this variation is about 15%. The artery termed "brachial artery" below might as well be termed "ulnar artery". However, it takes up the position of the brachial artery.

The forearm is pronated.

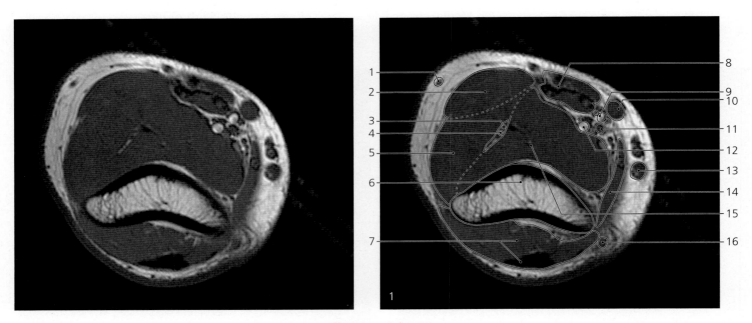

Elbow, axial MR

1: Cephalic vein →
2: Brachioradialis →
3: Radial nerve, superficial branch →
4: Radial nerve, deep branch →
5: Extensor carpi radialis longus →
6: Humerus →
7: Triceps brachii, muscle and tendon →

8: Biceps brachii →
9: Radial artery (high division) with comitant veins →
10: Median cubital vein →
11: Median nerve →
12: Brachial artery with comitant veins →
13: Basilic vein →

14: Pronator teres (humeral head) →
15: Brachialis muscle →
16: Ulnar nerve →

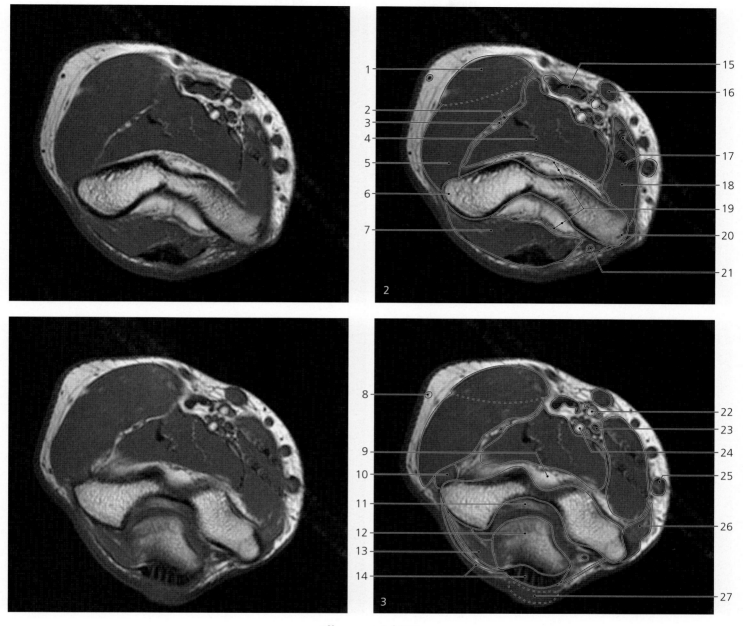

Elbow, axial MR

Scout view on page 68
1: Brachioradialis ↔
2: Radial nerve, superficial branch ↔
3: Radial nerve, deep branch ↔
4: Brachialis muscle ↔
5: Extensor carpi radialis longus ↔
6: Lateral epicondyle of humerus ↔
7: Triceps brachii ↔
8: Cephalic vein ←
9: Coronoid fossa with subsynovial fat

10: Extensor carpi radialis brevis →
11: Olecranon fossa
12: Olecranon →
13: Anconeus →
14: Triceps brachii, insertion ←
15: Biceps brachii ↔
16: Median cubital vein ↔
17: Flow artefacts from arteries
18: Pronator teres (humeral head) ↔
19: Articular capsule and subsynovial fat

20: Medial epicondyle of humerus
21: Ulnar nerve ↔
22: Radial artery with comitant veins ↔
23: Median nerve ↔
24: Brachial artery with comitant veins ↔
25: Basilic vein ↔
26: Flexor carpi radialis →
27: Olecranon bursa →

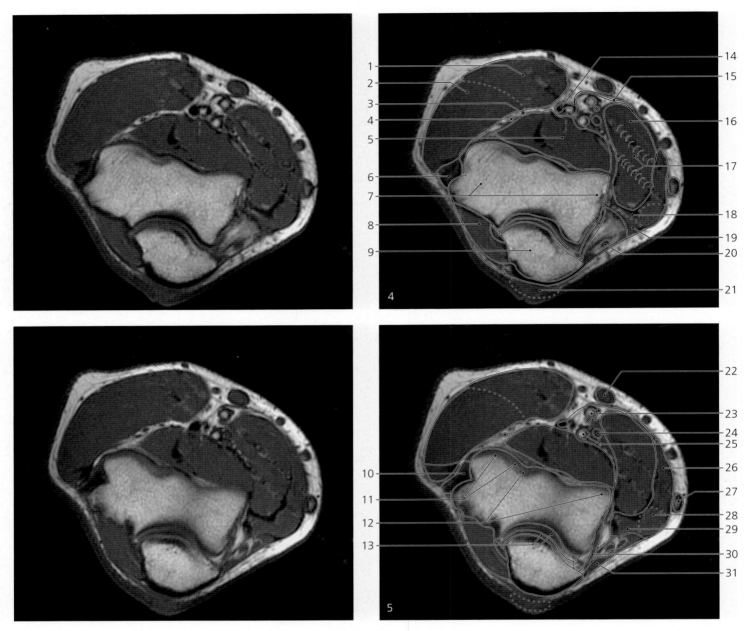

Elbow, axial MR

Scout view on page 68

1: Brachioradialis ↔
2: Extensor carpi radialis longus ↔
3: Radial nerve, superficial branch ↔
4: Radial nerve, deep branch ↔
5: Brachialis muscle ↔
6: Extensor carpi radialis brevis ↔
7: Condyle of humerus
8: Anconeus ↔
9: Olecranon ↔
10: Extensor digitorum and extensor carpi ulnaris (humeral head), common origin →

11: Capitulum of humerus →
12: Trochlea of humerus →
13: Articular cartilage
14: Biceps brachii, tendon ↔
15: Biceps brachii, aponeurosis →
16: Pronator teres ↔
17: Flow artefacts from arteries
18: Flexor digitorum superficialis (humeral head) →
19: Flexor carpi ulnaris (humeral head) →
20: Ulnar nerve ↔
21: Olecranon bursa ←
22: Median cubital vein ↔

23: Radial artery with comitant veins ↔
24: Median nerve ↔
25: Brachial artery ↔
26: Flexor carpi radialis ↔
27: Basilic vein ↔
28: Palmaris longus →
29: Flexor digitorum superficialis ↔
30: Ulnar collateral ligament ←
31: Flexor carpi ulnaris (ulnar head) →

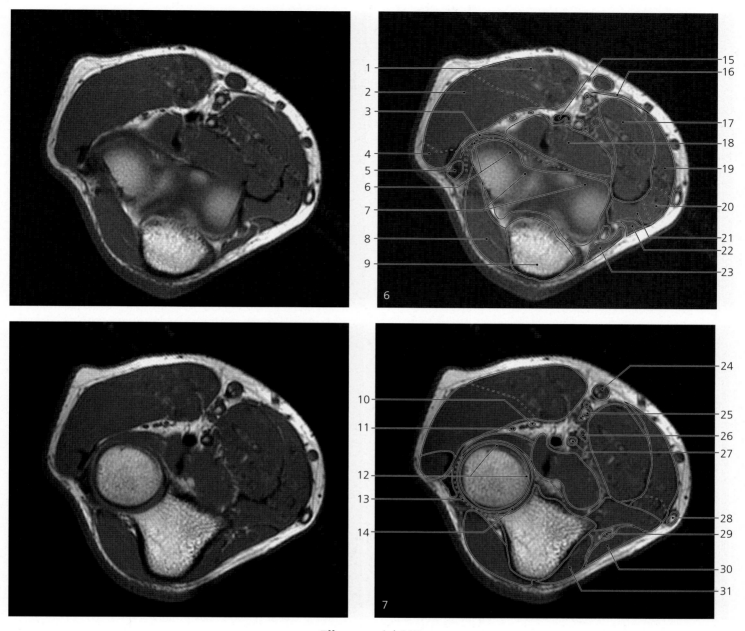

Elbow, axial MR

Scout view on page 68
 1: Brachioradialis ↔
 2: Extensor carpi radialis longus ↔
 3: Supinator, humeral head →
 4: Extensor carpi radialis brevis ↔
 5: Extensor digitorum and extensor
    carpi ulnaris ↔
 6: Capitulum and radial collateral
    ligament ←
 7: Trochlea of humerus ←
 8: Anconeus ↔
 9: Olecranon ↔
10: Radial nerve, superficial branch ↔

11: Radial nerve, deep branch ↔
12: Articular circumference of head of
    radius
13: Anular ligament
14: Proximal radio-ulnar joint
15: Biceps brachii, tendon ↔
16: Biceps brachii, aponeurosis ←
17: Pronator teres ↔
18: Brachialis muscle ↔
19: Flexor carpi radialis ↔
20: Palmaris longus ↔
21: Flexor digitorum superficialis
    (humeral head) ↔

22: Flexor carpi ulnaris (humeral head) ↔
23: Flexor carpi ulnaris (ulnar head) →
24: Median cubital vein ↔
25: Radial artery with comitant veins ↔
26: Median nerve ↔
27: Brachial artery ↔
28: Basilic vein ↔
29: Ulnar nerve ↔
30: Flexor carpi ulnaris (humeral and
    ulnar head fused) ↔
31: Flexor digitorum profundus →

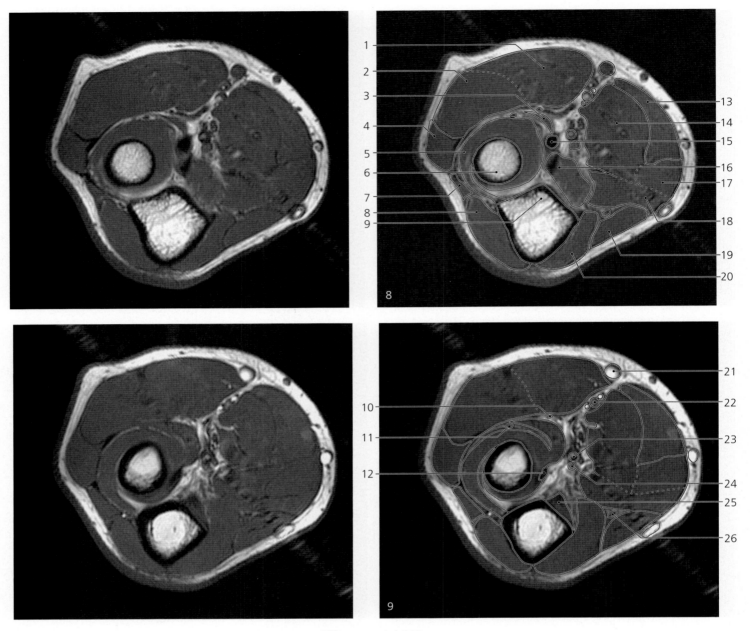

Elbow, axial MR

Scout view on page 68
1: Brachioradialis ↔
2: Extensor carpi radialis longus ↔
3: Supinator, humeral head ↔
4: Extensor carpi radialis brevis ↔
5: Supinator, ulnar head ↔
6: Neck of radius →
7: Extensor digitorum and extensor carpi ulnaris ↔
8: Anconeus ↔

9: Coronoid process →
10: Radial nerve, superficial branch ←
11: Radial nerve, deep branch ←
12: Biceps brachii, tendon ←
13: Flexor carpi radialis ↔
14: Pronator teres ↔
15: Biceps brachii, tendon ↔
16: Brachialis muscle ↔
17: Palmaris longus ↔
18: Flexor digitorum superficialis ↔

19: Flexor carpi ulnaris ↔
20: Flexor digitorum profundus ↔
21: Median cubital vein ←
22: Radial artery with comitant veins ←
23: Brachial artery ←
24: Median nerve ←
25: Brachialis muscle, insertion ←
26: Ulnar nerve ←

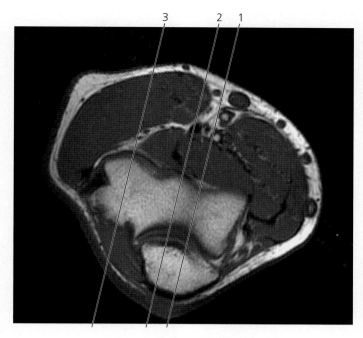

Scout view of elbow

Lines #1–3 indicate planes of sectioning in the following sagittal MR series. Interpretation of the scout image can be found in the axial series, page 70, image #5.

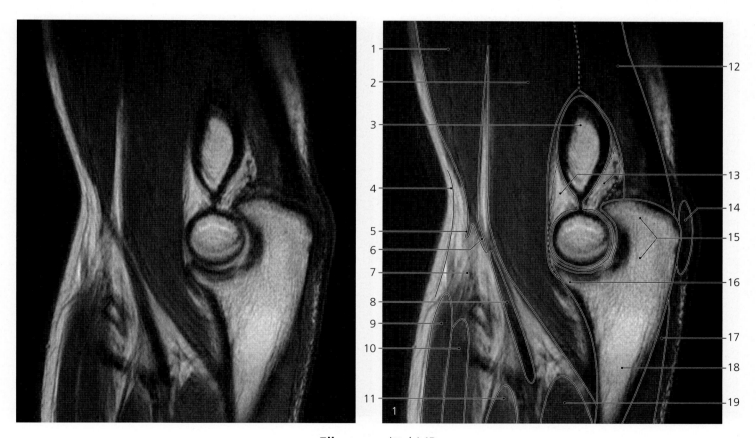

Elbow, sagittal MR

1: Biceps brachii →
2: Brachialis muscle →
3: Humerus shaft →
4: Cubital fascia
5: Biceps brachii, aponeurosis
6: Biceps tendon →
7: Cubital fossa →
8: Brachial artery

9: Flexor carpi radialis
10: Pronator teres
11: Flexor digitorum superficialis
12: Triceps brachii →
13: Coronoid fossa and olecranon fossa
    with subsynovial fat →
14: Olecranon bursa
15: Olecranon →

16: Coronoid process →
17: Anconeus →
18: Ulna, shaft →
19: Flexor digitorum profundus

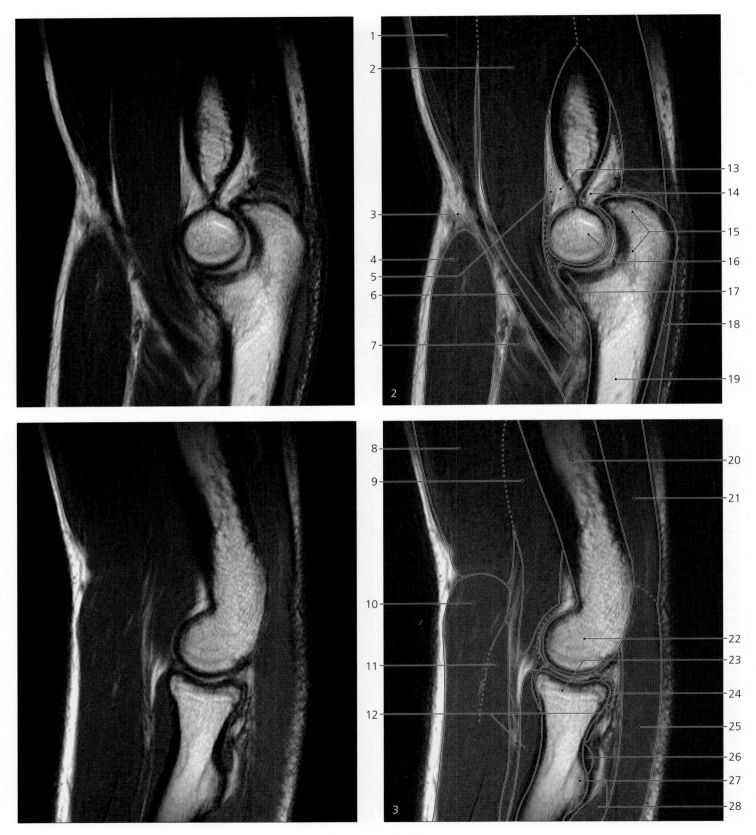

Elbow, sagittal MR

Scout view on page 73

1: Biceps brachii ↔
2: Brachialis muscle ↔
3: Cubital fossa ←
4: Brachioradialis ←
5: Articular capsule ↔
6: Biceps brachii, tendon ←
7: Supinator →
8: Biceps brachii ←
9: Brachialis muscle ←
10: Brachioradialis ←

11: Extensor carpi radialis longus
12: Supinator ←
13: Coronoid fossa with
    subsynovial fat ←
14: Olecranon fossa with
    subsynovial fat ←
15: Olecranon ←
16: Trochlea of humerus
17: Coronoid process ←
18: Anconeus ↔
19: Ulna, shaft ←

20: Humerus, shaft ←
21: Triceps brachii ←
22: Capitulum of humerus
23: Head of radius
24: Anular ligament
25: Anconeus ←
26: Biceps brachii (insertion)
27: Radial tuberosity
28: Extensor digitorum

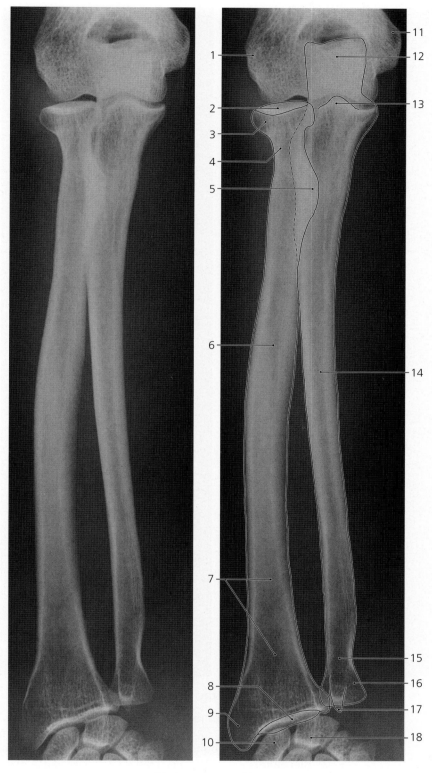

Forearm, a-p X-ray

1: Lateral epicondyle
2: Articular fovea of radius
3: Head of radius
4: Neck of radius
5: Tuberosity of radius
6: Shaft of radius
7: Distal end of radius

8: Carpal articular surface of radius
9: Styloid process of radius
10: Scaphoid bone
11: Medial epicondyle
12: Olecranon
13: Coronoid process
14: Shaft of ulna

15: Neck of ulna
16: Head of ulna
17: Styloid process of ulna
18: Lunate bone

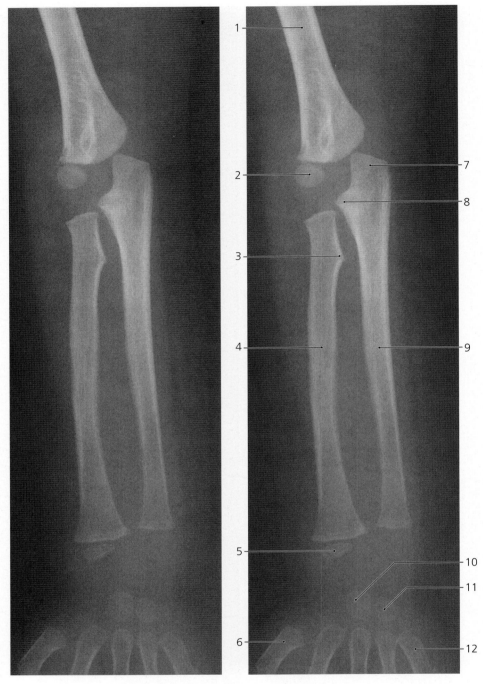

Forearm, a-p X-ray, child 2 years

1: Diaphysis of humerus
2: Capitulum (ossification
   center)
3: Tuberosity of radius
4: Diaphysis of radius

5: Distal epiphysis of radius (ossification
   center)
6: First metacarpal bone
7: Olecranon
8: Coronoid process of ulna

9: Diaphysis of ulna
10: Capitate bone (ossification center)
11: Hamate bone (ossification center)
12: Fifth metacarpal bone

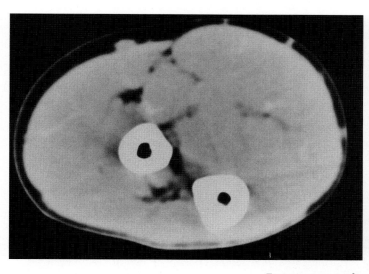
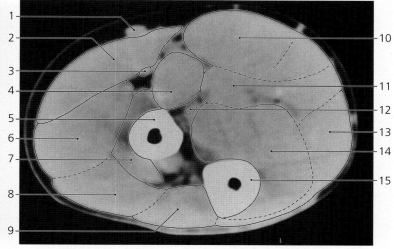

Forearm, supinated, middle, axial CT

1: Subcutaneous vein
2: Brachioradialis
3: Radial artery
4: Pronator teres
5: Radius
6: Extensor carpi radialis longus, and brevis
7: Supinator
8: Extensor digitorum
9: Extensor carpi ulnaris
10: Flexor carpi radialis, and palmaris longus
11: Flexor digitorum superficialis
12: Median nerve
13: Flexor carpi ulnaris
14: Flexor digitorum profundus
15: Ulna

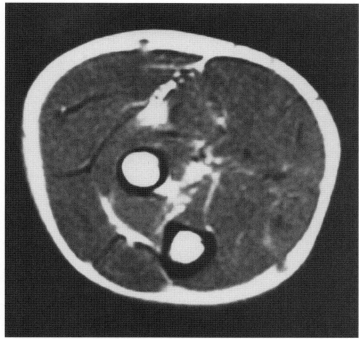
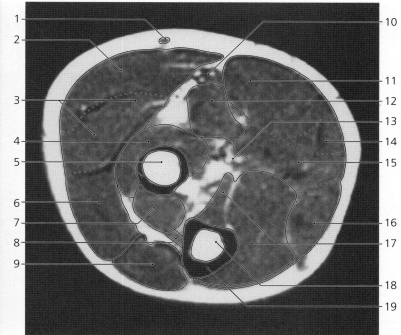

Forearm, pronated, middle, axial MR

1: Cephalic vein
2: Brachioradialis
3: Extensor carpi radialis longus and brevis
4: Supinator
5: Shaft of radius
6: Extensor digitorum
7: Abductor pollicis longus
8: Extensor pollicis brevis
9: Extensor carpi ulnaris
10: Radial artery and veins
11: Flexor carpi radialis
12: Pronator teres
13: Ulnar artery and veins
14: Palmaris longus
15: Flexor digitorum superficialis
16: Flexor carpi ulnaris
17: Flexor digitorum profundus
18: Shaft of ulna (bone marrow)
19: Compact bone

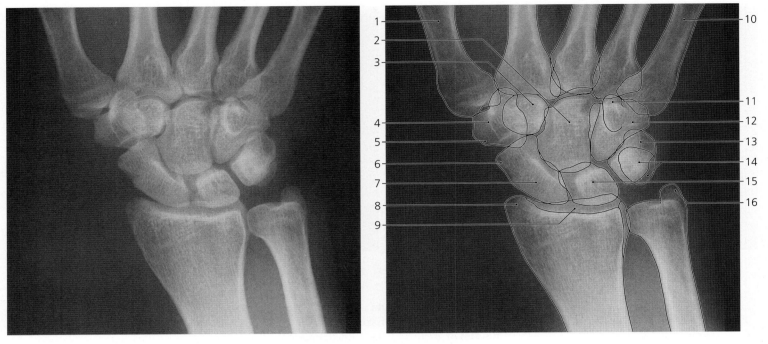

Wrist, dorso-volar X-ray

1: First metacarpal bone
2: Capitate bone
3: Trapezoid bone
4: Trapezium
5: Tubercle of trapezium
6: Tubercle of scaphoid bone

7: Scaphoid (navicular) bone
8: Styloid process of radius
9: Carpal articular surface of radius
10: Fifth metacarpal bone
11: Hook of hamate bone
12: Hamate bone

13: Triquetrum bone
14: Pisiform bone
15: Lunate bone
16: Styloid process of ulna

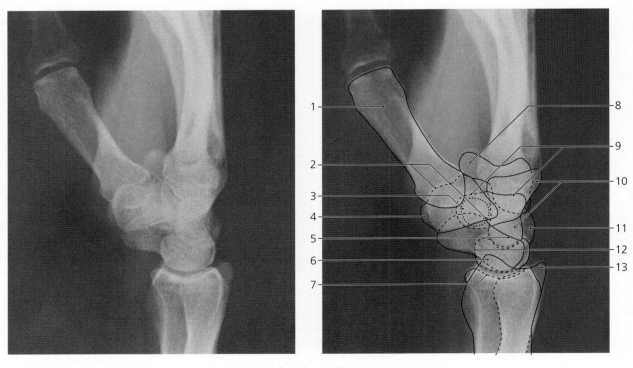

Wrist, lateral X-ray

1: First metacarpal bone
2: Trapezium
3: Pisiform bone
4: Tubercle of trapezium
5: Scaphoid bone

6: Styloid process of radius
7: Carpal articular surface of radius
8: Hook of hamate bone
9: Trapezoid bone
10: Capitate bone

11: Triquetrum bone
12: Lunate bone
13: Styloid process of ulna

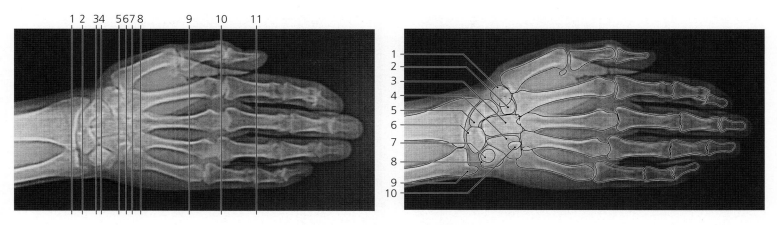

Scout view of wrist and hand

Lines # 1-11 indicate position of sections (1.5 mm thick) in the following CT series. Arrows ←, →, and ↔ in the legends indicate that a structure can be seen on a previous or following section, or both.

1: Trapezium
2: Trapezoid bone
3: Capitate bone
4: Hamate bone

5: Scaphoid bone
6: Lunate bone
7: Pisiform bone
8: Triquetrum bone

9: Styloid process of ulna
10: Hook of hamate bone

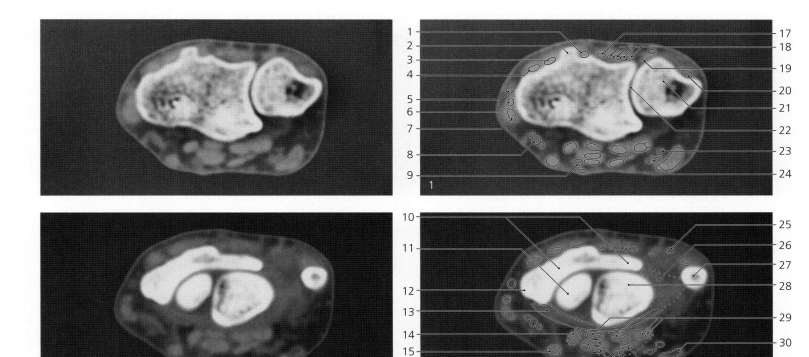

Wrist, axial CT

1: Extensor pollicis longus (tendon) →
2: Dorsal tubercle of radius
3: Extensor carpi radialis brevis (tendon) →
4: Extensor carpi radialis longus (tendon) →
5: Cephalic vein →
6: Extensor pollicis brevis (tendon) →
7: Abductor pollicis longus (tendon) →
8: Radial artery and veins →
9: Median nerve →
10: Distal edge of radius

11: Scaphoid bone →
12: Styloid process of radius
13: Joint capsule with palmar radiocarpal ligament
14: Flexor pollicis longus (tendon) ↔
15: Flexor carpi radialis (tendon) ↔
16: Palmaris longus (tendon) ↔
17: Extensor indicis (tendon) →
18: Extensor digitorum (tendons) →
19: Extensor digiti minimi (tendon) →
20: Extensor carpi ulnaris (tendon) →
21: Head of ulna

22: Distal radio-ulnar joint
23: Ulnar nerve →
24: Ulnar artery and veins →
25: Basilic vein ↔
26: Articular disc
27: Styloid process of ulna
28: Lunate bone →
29: Flexor digitorum profundus (tendons) ↔
30: Flexor carpi ulnaris (tendon) ↔
31: Flexor digitorum superficialis (tendons) ↔

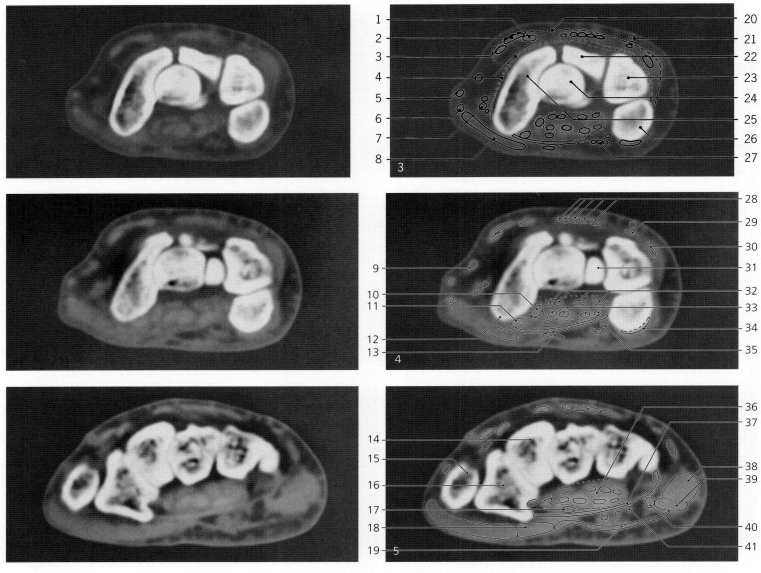

Wrist, axial CT

Scout view on page 79

 1: **Extensor carpi radialis brevis (tendon)** ↔
 2: **Extensor pollicis longus (tendon)** ↔
 3: **Extensor carpi radialis longus (tendon)** ↔
 4: **Articular capsule**
 5: **Extensor pollicis brevis (tendon)** ↔
 6: **Abductor pollicis longus (tendon)** ↔
 7: **Radial artery and veins** ↔
 8: **Abductor pollicis brevis** →
 9: **Cephalic vein** ↔
10: **Flexor pollicis longus (tendon)** ↔
11: **Flexor carpi radialis (tendon)** ↔
12: **Tubercle of scaphoid bone**
13: **Palmaris longus (tendon)** ←

14: **Trapezoid bone** →
15: **Base of first metacarpal bone**
16: **Trapezium** →
17: **Median nerve** ↔
18: **Flexor pollicis brevis** →
19: **Palmar aponeurosis** →
20: **Extensor retinacle**
21: **Basilic vein** ↔
22: **Lunate bone** ←
23: **Triquetrum bone** →
24: **Capitate bone** →
25: **Scaphoid bone** ↔
26: **Pisiform bone** →
27: **Ulnar artery and veins** ↔
28: **Extensor indicis and digitorum (tendons)** ↔

29: **Extensor digiti minimi (tendon)** ↔
30: **Extensor carpi ulnaris (tendon)** ↔
31: **Hamate bone** →
32: **Flexor digitorum profundus (tendons)** ↔
33: **Flexor digitorum superficialis (tendons)** ↔
34: **Flexor carpi ulnaris (insertion)** ←
35: **Ulnar nerve** ↔
36: **Common synovial sheath of digital flexors** ↔
37: **Flexor retinacle** ↔
38: **Abductor digiti minimi** →
39: **Flexor digiti minimi** →
40: **Pisometacarpeal ligament** →
41: **Pisohamate ligament**

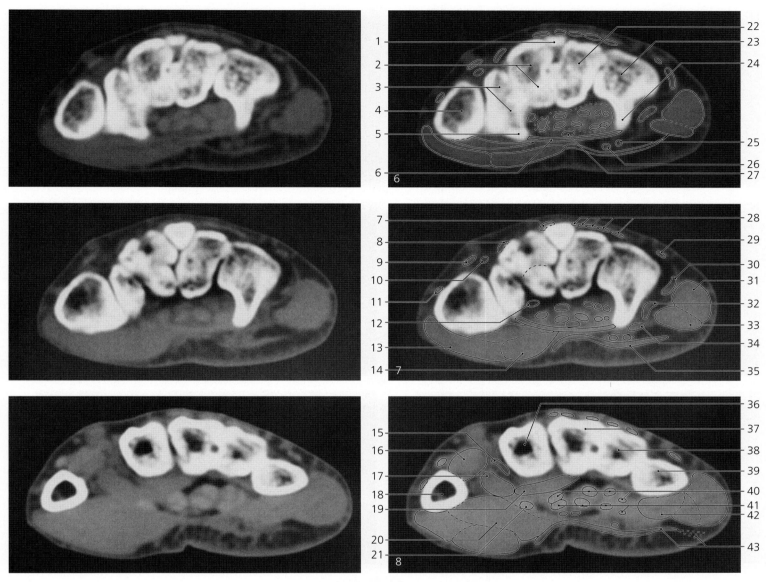

Wrist, axial CT

Scout view on page 79

1: Styloid process of third metacarpal bone
2: Trapezoid bone ←
3: Trapezium ←
4: Base of first metacarpal bone ↔
5: Tubercle of trapezium ←
6: Flexor retinacle ↔
7: Extensor carpi radialis brevis (insertion) ←
8: Extensor carpi radialis longus (insertion) ←
9: Extensor pollicis longus (tendon) ↔
10: Radial artery ↔
11: Extensor pollicis brevis (tendon) ↔
12: Flexor carpi radialis (tendon) ←
13: Abductor pollicis brevis ↔

14: Flexor pollicis brevis ↔
15: Radial artery (turning into deep palmar arch) ←
16: First dorsal interosseus muscle →
17: Flexor pollicis brevis, deep head
18: Shaft of first metacarpal bone ↔
19: Adductor pollicis →
20: Opponens pollicis ←
21: Flexor pollicis longus (tendon) ↔
22: Capitate bone ↔
23: Hamate bone ↔
24: Hook of hamate bone
25: Ulnar nerve ↔
26: Ulnar artery ↔
27: Median nerve ↔
28: Extensor indicis and digitorum (tendons) ↔

29: Extensor digiti minimi (tendon) ↔
30: Extensor carpi ulnaris (tendon) ←
31: Abductor digiti minimi ↔
32: Pisometacarpeal ligament ←
33: Flexor digiti minimi ↔
34: Palmar carpometacarpeal ligament
35: Palmar aponeurosis ↔
36: Base of second metacarpal bone →
37: Base of third metacarpal bone →
38: Base of fourth metacarpal bone
39: Base of fifth metacarpal bone
40: Flexor digitorum profundus (tendons) ↔
41: Flexor digitorum superficialis (tendons) ↔
42: Opponens digiti minimi ←
43: Palmaris brevis

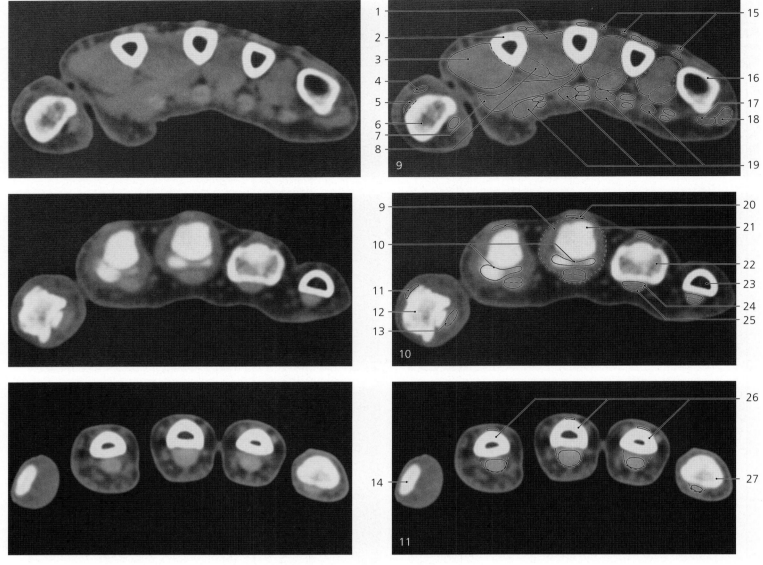

Metacarpus and fingers, axial CT

Scout view on page 79

1: Second dorsal interosseus muscle ←
2: Shaft of second metacarpal bone ←
3: First dorsal interosseus muscle ←
4: Extensor pollicis longus (tendon) ↔
5: Extensor pollicis brevis (insertion) ←
6: Proximal phalanx of thumb
7: Adductor pollicis ←
8: First palmar interosseus muscle
9: Joint capsule of third carpometacarpeal joint

10: Fibrocartilaginous plates of palmar ligament
11: Extensor pollicis longus (insertion) ←
12: Distal phalanx of thumb
13: Flexor pollicis longus (tendon) ←
14: Tuberosity of distal phalanx
15: Veins
16: Head of fifth metacarpal bone
17: Flexor digiti minimi ←
18: Abductor digiti minimi ←
19: Lumbrical muscles

20: Extensor digitorum (tendon) ↔
21: Head of third metacarpal bone
22: Base of proximal phalanx of fourth finger
23: Shaft of proximal phalanx of fifth finger
24: Flexor digitorum profundus ↔
25: Flexor digitorum superficialis ↔
26: Shafts of proximal phalanges of second, third and fourth finger
27: Base of middle phalanx of fifth finger

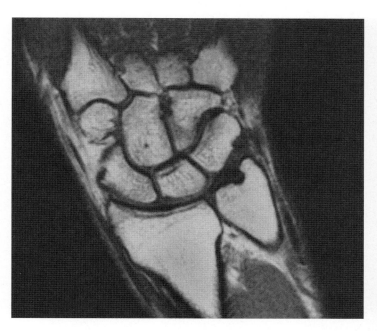

Wrist, coronal MR

1: Interossei muscles
2: Base of fourth metacarpal bone
3: Base of third metacarpal bone
4: Base of second metacarpal bone
5: Interosseous ligaments
6: Trapezoid bone
7: Capitate bone
8: Scaphoid bone
9: Styloid process of radius
10: Base of fifth metacarpal bone
11: Hamate bone
12: Triquetrum bone
13: Styloid process of ulna
14: Articular disc
15: Head of ulna
16: Distal radio-ulnar joint
17: Lunate bone
18: Radiocarpal joint

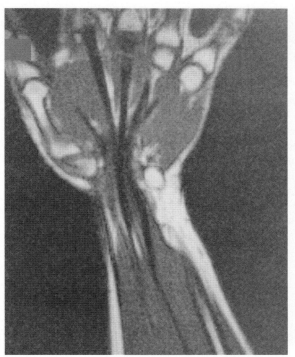
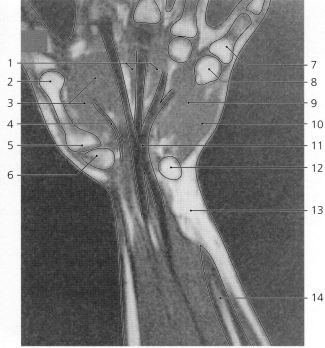

Wrist, carpal tunnel, coronal MR

1: Lumbricals
2: Head of first metacarpal bone
3: Flexor pollicis brevis, and adductor pollicis
4: Flexor pollicis longus (tendon)
5: Base of first metacarpal bone
6: Trapezium
7: Proximal phalanx of fifth finger
8: Head of fifth metacarpal bone
9: Flexor digiti minimi
10: Abductor digiti minimi
11: Long flexor tendons in canalis carpi
12: Pisiform bone
13: Subcutaneous fat
14: Shaft of ulna

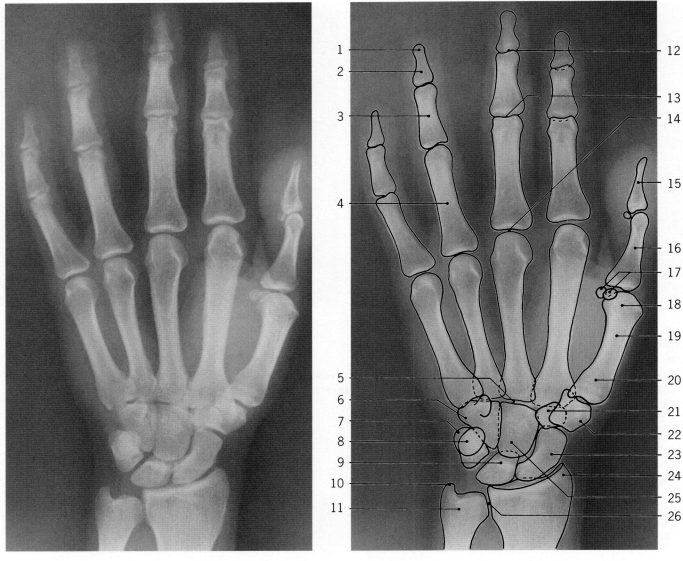

Hand, left, dorso-volar X-ray

1: Tuberosity of distal phalanx
2: Distal phalanx
3: Middle phalanx
4: Proximal phalanx
5: Carpometacarpeal joint
6: Hamate bone
7: Triquetrum bone
8: Pisiform bone
9: Lunate bone

10: Styloid process of ulna
11: Head of ulna
12: Distal interphalangeal joint "DIP"
13: Proximal interphalangeal joint "PIP"
14: Metacarpophalangeal joint "MCP"
15: Distal phalanx of thumb
16: Proximal phalanx of thumb
17: Sesamoid bones
18: Head of first metacarpal bone

19: Shaft of first metacarpal bone
20: Base of first metacarpal bone
21: Trapezoid bone
22: Trapezium
23: Scaphoid bone
24: Styloid process of radius
25: Capitate bone
26: Distal radio-ulnar joint

Skeletal age of hand

The skeletal development of the hand of boys and girls is displayed on the following pages 85–92

The skeletal (bone) age of each hand (left) is given according to Greulich and Pyle (1) (upper line), and according to the 20 bone scoring system of Tanner et al. (2) followed by the 10 to 90 centile interval of variation (lower line).

(1) W.W. Greulich and S.J. Pyle: Radiographic atlas of skeletal development of the hand and wrist. Stanford University Press 1959.

(2) J.M. Tanner, R.H. Whitehouse, N. Cameron, W.A. Marshall, M.J.R. Healy and H. Goldstein: Assessment of skeletal maturity and prediction of adult height (TW2 method). Academic Press 1983.

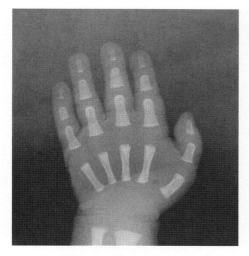

Boy, newborn 0 years

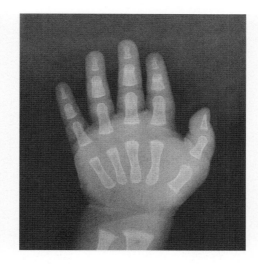

Boy, ½ year

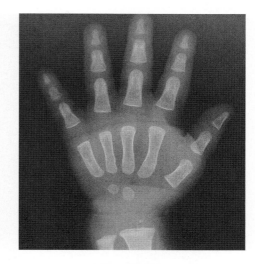

Boy, 1 year

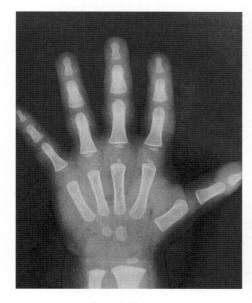

Boy, 1 ½ year
1 $\frac{7}{12}$ year (1–2$\frac{5}{12}$)

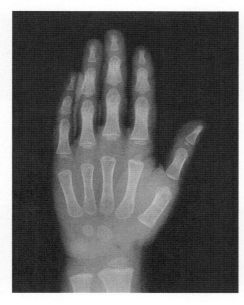

Boy, 2 years
2 years (1 $\frac{5}{12}$–2 $\frac{9}{12}$)

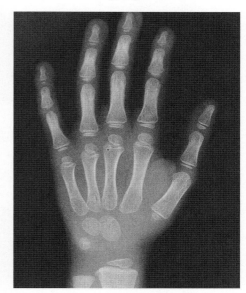

Boy, 3 years
3 $\frac{6}{12}$ years (2 $\frac{8}{12}$–4 $\frac{7}{12}$)

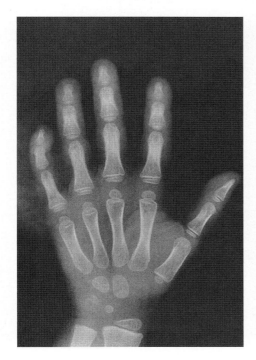

Boy, 4 years
4 years (3 $\frac{1}{12}$–5 $\frac{4}{12}$)

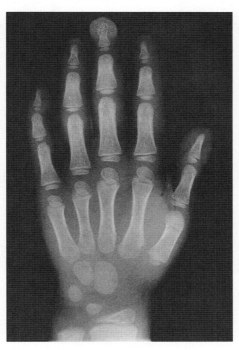

Boy, 5 years
4 $\frac{7}{12}$ years (3 $\frac{6}{12}$–5 $\frac{11}{12}$)

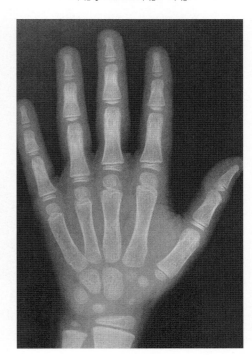

Boy, 6 years
7 years (5 $\frac{10}{12}$–8 $\frac{6}{12}$)

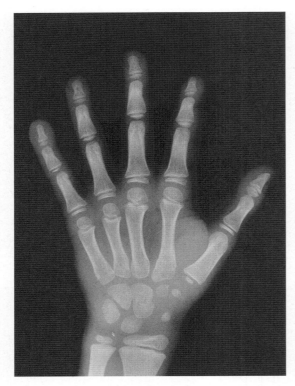

Boy, 7 years
7 9/12 years (6 6/12–9 4/12)

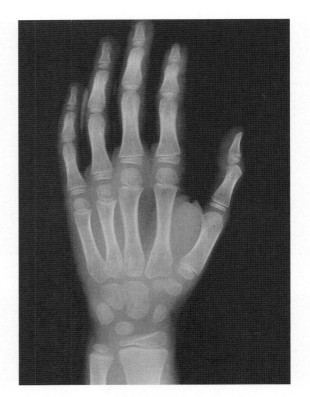

Boy, 8 years
8 2/12 years (6 10/12–9 8/12)

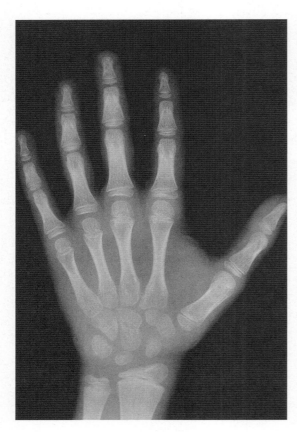

Boy, 9 years
9 years (7 7/12–10 5/12)

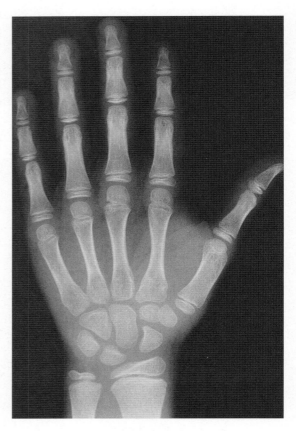

Boy, 10 years
10 6/12 years (9 1/12–11 11/12)

Explanation of age figures is given on page 84

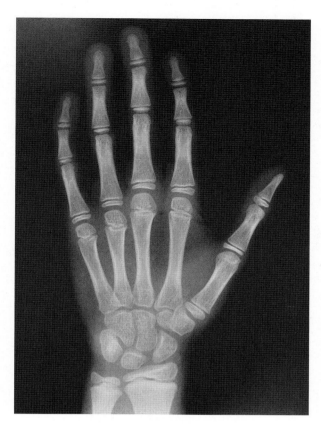

Boy, 11 years
11 2/12 years (9 9/12–12 6/12)

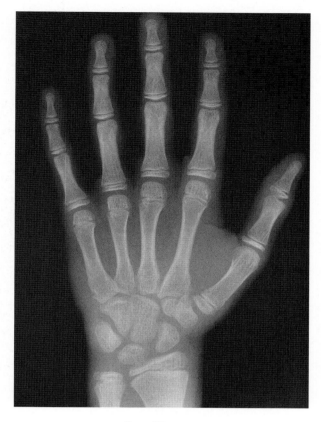

Boy, 12 years
11 10/12 years (10 5/12–13 1/12)

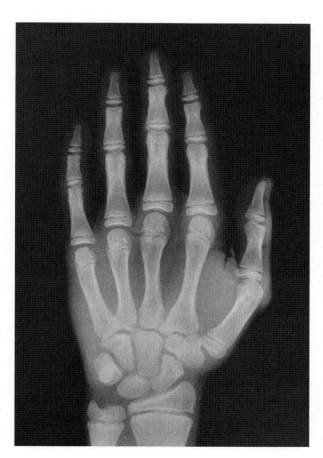

Boy, 13 years
13 5/12 years (12–14 9/12)

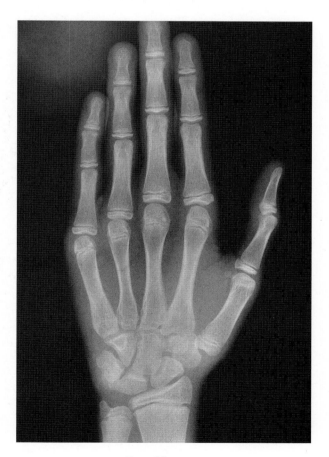

Boy, 14 years
13 10/12 years (12 6/12–15 1/12)

Explanation of age figures is given on page 84

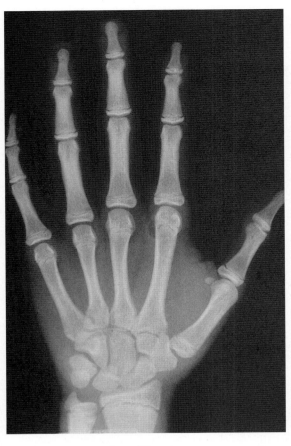

Boy, 15 years
15 $\frac{1}{12}$ years (13 $\frac{9}{12}$–16 $\frac{6}{12}$)

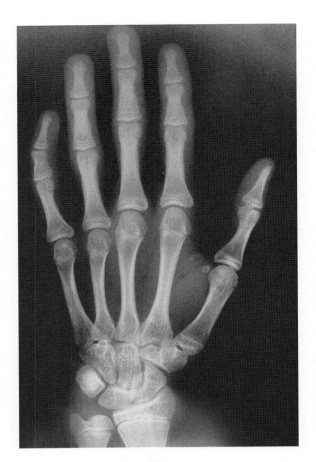

Boy, 16 years
15 $\frac{8}{12}$ years (14 $\frac{5}{12}$–17 $\frac{1}{12}$)

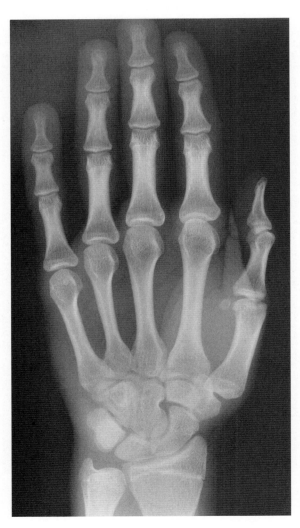

Boy, 17 years
17 years (15 $\frac{7}{12}$–18 $\frac{5}{12}$)

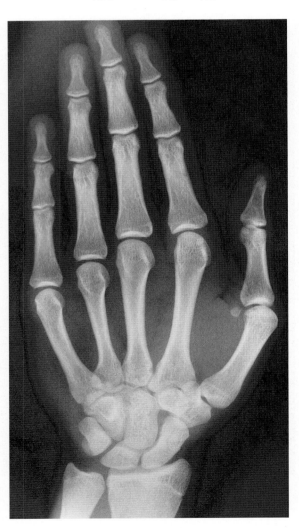

Boy, 18 years
18 years (16 $\frac{6}{12}$–19 $\frac{4}{12}$)

Explanation of age figures is given on page 84

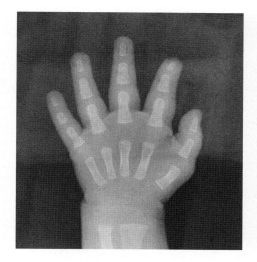

Girl, newborn 0 years

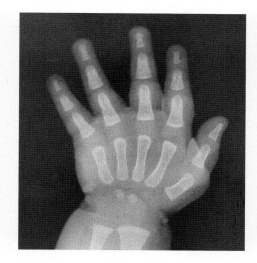

Girl, ½ year

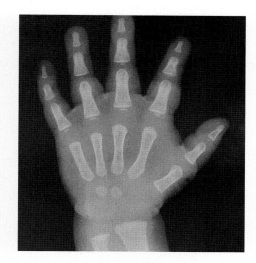

Girl, 1 year

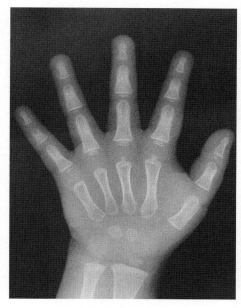

Girl, 1 ½year
1 ⁵/₁₂ year (1–2)

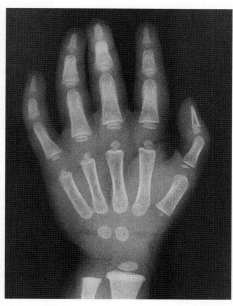

Girl, 2 years
1 ¹⁰/₁₂ years (1 ³/₁₂–2 ⁶/₁₂)

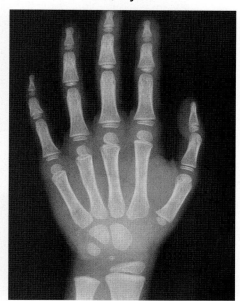

Girl, 3 years
3 ⁹/₁₂ years (2 ¹⁰/₁₂–5)

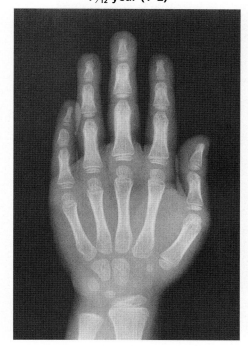

Girl, 4 years
4 ³/₁₂ years (3 ⁵/₁₂–5 ⁶/₁₂)

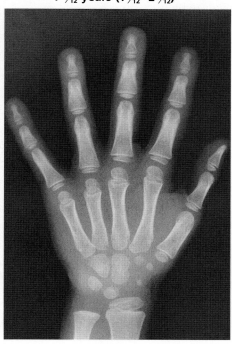

Girl, 5 years
5 ⁷/₁₂ years (4 ⁶/₁₂–7)

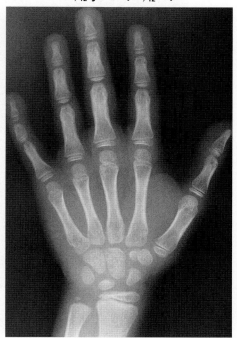

Girl, 6 years
6 ⁸/₁₂ years (5 ⁶/₁₂–8 ²/₁₂)

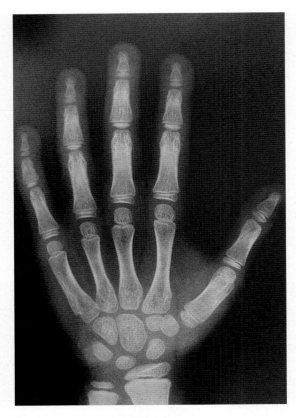

Girl, 7 years
7 $\frac{2}{12}$ years (6 $\frac{1}{12}$–8 $\frac{7}{12}$)

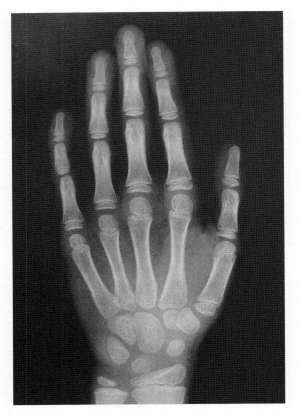

Girl, 8 years
7 $\frac{11}{12}$ years (6 $\frac{10}{11}$–9 $\frac{1}{12}$)

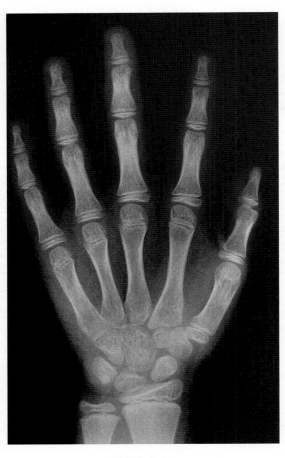

Girl, 9 years
9 $\frac{6}{12}$ years (8 $\frac{6}{12}$–10 $\frac{7}{12}$)

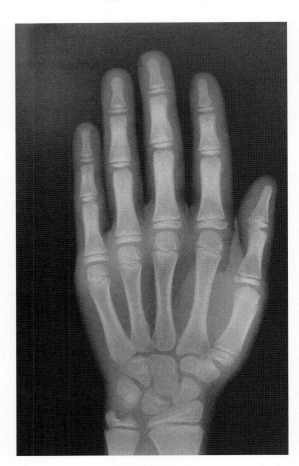

Girl, 10 years
9 $\frac{11}{12}$ years (8 $\frac{10}{12}$–11)

Explanation of age figures is given on page 84

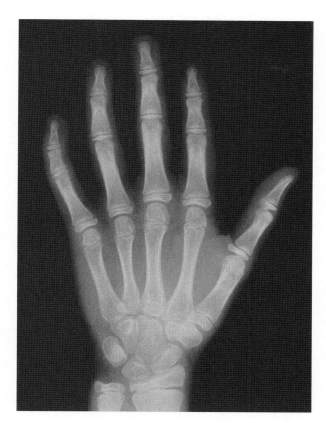

Girl, 11 years
10 ⁶⁄₁₂ years (9 ³⁄₁₂–11 ⁷⁄₁₂)

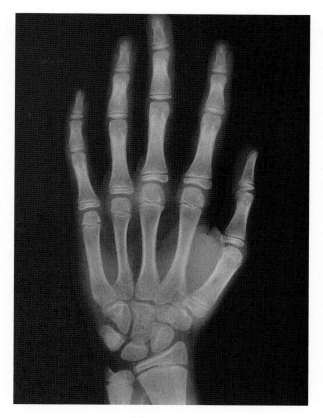

Girl, 12 years
11 ³⁄₁₂ years (10–12 ⁴⁄₁₂)

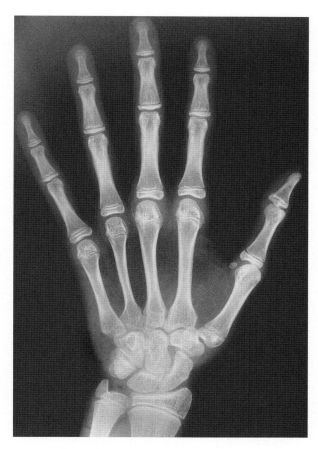

Girl, 13 years
12 ⁵⁄₁₂ years (11 ³⁄₁₂–13 ⁵⁄₁₂)

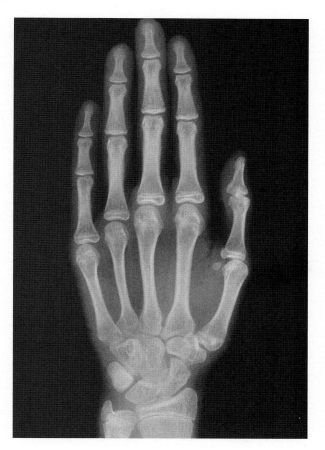

Girl, 14 years
13 ¹⁄₁₂ years (11 ¹⁰⁄₁₂–14 ⁴⁄₁₂)

Explanation of age figures is given on page 84

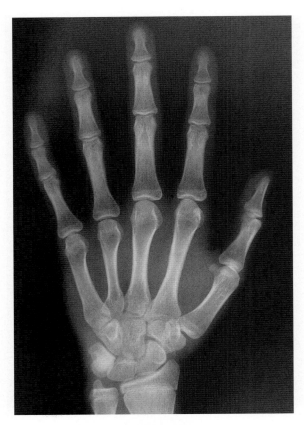

Girl, 15 years
14 ⁵⁄₁₂ years (13–15 ⁷⁄₁₂)

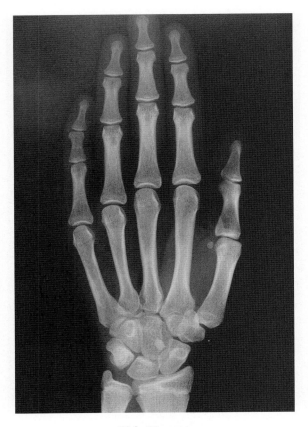

Girl, 16 years
15 ¹¹⁄₁₂ years (14 ⁷⁄₁₂–17 ⁷⁄₁₂)

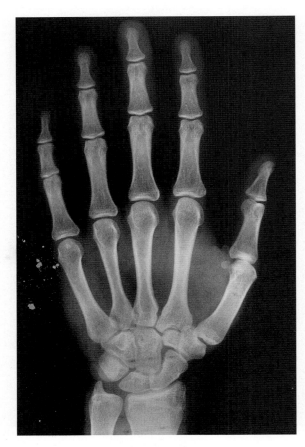

Girl, 17 years

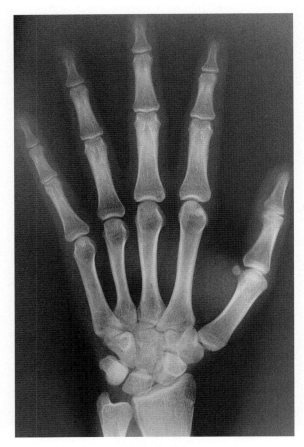

Girl, 18 years

Explanation of age figures is given on page 84

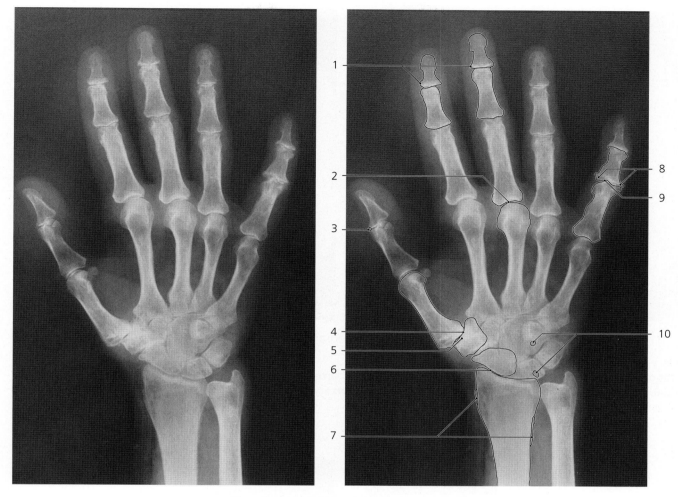

Hand, senescent, dorso-volar X-ray

1: Osteophytes
2: Subluxation of metacarpophalangeal joint
3: Soft tissue calcification

4: First carpometacarpeal joint (narrowed)
5: Subchondral sclerosis (sign of arthrosis)
6: Radiocarpal joint (narrowed)

7: Periosteal calcifications
8: Osteophytes
9: Interphalangeal joint (arthrosis)
10: Cysts in carpal bones

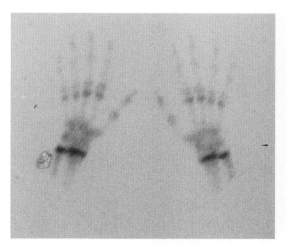
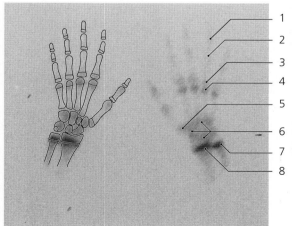

Hand, dorso-volar, ^{99m}Tc-MDP, scintigraphy, child 12 years

1: Growth plate of distal phalanx IV
2: Growth plate of middle phalanx IV
3: Growth plate proximal phalanx IV

4: Growth plate of fourth metacarpal bone
5: Growth plate first metacarpal bone
6: Carpal bones

7: Growth plate of distal epiphysis of ulna
8: Growth plate of distal epiphysis of radius

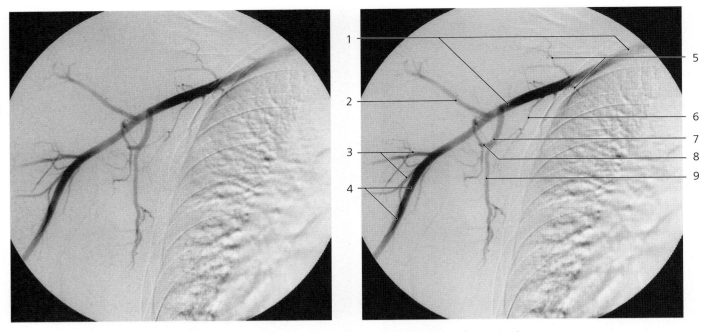

Shoulder, a-p X-ray, arteriography (digital subtraction)

1: Axillary artery
2: Posterior circumflex humeral artery
3: Profunda brachii artery

4: Brachial artery
5: Thoraco-acromial artery
6: Lateral thoracic artery

7: Subscapular artery
8: Circumflex scapular artery
9: Thoracodorsal artery

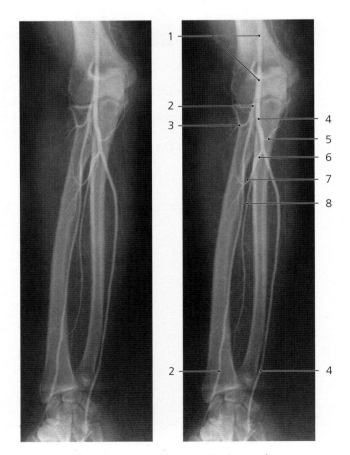

Forearm, a-p X-ray, arteriography

1: Brachial artery
2: Radial artery
3: Recurrent radial artery

4: Ulnar artery
5: Recurrent ulnar artery
6: Common interosseous artery

7: Posterior interosseous artery
8: Anterior interosseous artery

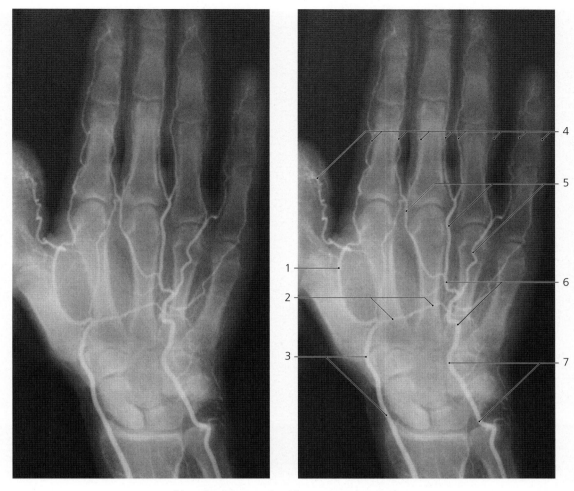

Hand, dorso-volar X-ray, arteriography

1: **Arteria princeps pollicis**
2: **Deep palmar arch**
3: **Radial artery**

4: **Proper palmar digital arteries**
5: **Common palmar digital arteries**
6: **Superficial palmar arch (incomplete)**

7: **Ulnar artery**

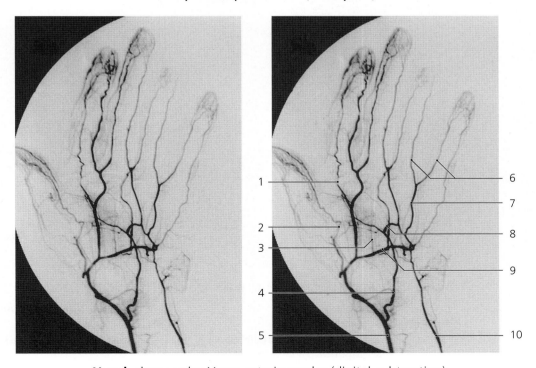

Hand, dorso-volar X-ray, arteriography (digital subtraction)
Radial dominance

1: **Radialis indicis artery**
2: **Princeps pollicis artery**
3: **Metacarpeal artery**

4: **Superficial palmar branch of radial artery**
5: **Radial artery**
6: **Proper palmar digital arteries**

7: **Common palmar digital artery**
8: **Superficial palmar arch**
9: **Deep palmar arch**
10: **Ulnar artery**

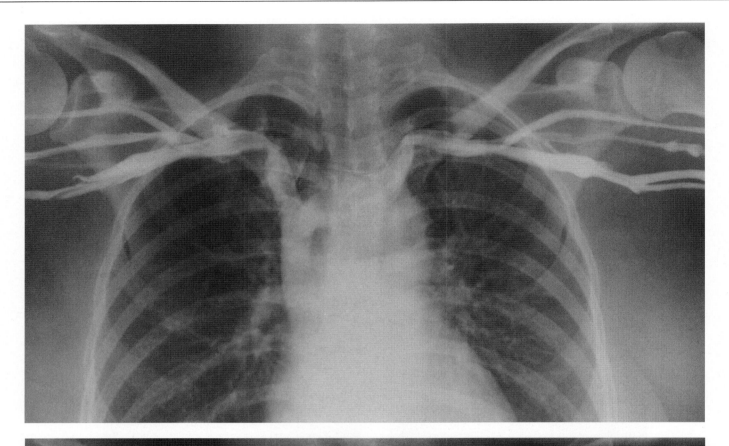

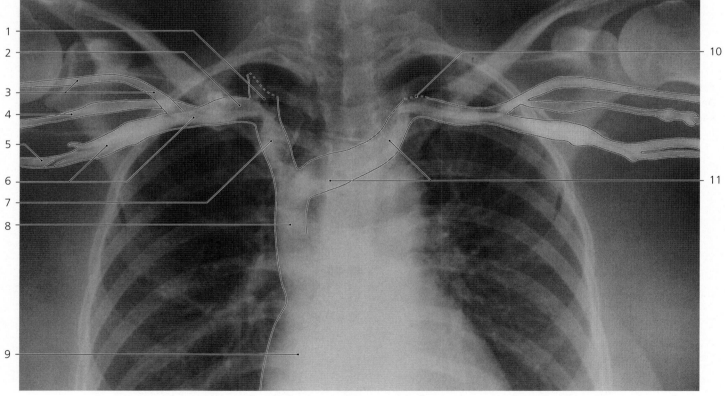

Shoulder, a-p X-ray, phlebography

1: Right internal jugular vein
   (termination)
2: Subclavian vein
3: Cephalic vein
4: Brachial vein

5: Basilic vein
6: Axillary vein
7: Right brachiocephalic vein
8: Superior caval vein
9: Right atrium

10: Left internal jugular vein
    (termination)
11: Left brachiocephalic vein

Lower Limb

Pelvis

Hip and thigh

Knee

Leg

Ankle and foot

Arteries and veins

Lymphatics

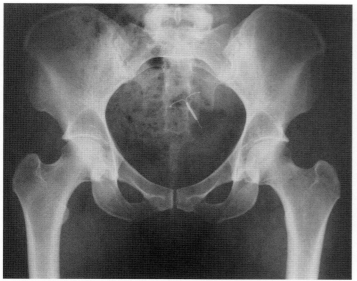
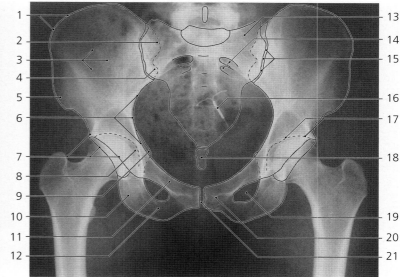

Pelvis, female, a-p X-ray, tilted

1: Iliac crest
2: Posterior superior iliac spine
3: Wing of ilium
4: Posterior inferior iliac spine
5: Anterior superior iliac spine
6: Arcuate line of ilium
7: Acetabular rim
8: Acetabular fossa
9: Ischial spine
10: Ischial tuberosity
11: Superior ramus of pubis
12: Inferior ramus of pubis
13: Ala of sacrum
14: Pelvic sacral foramina
15: Sacro-iliac joint
16: Intrauterine contraceptive device (IUD)
17: Lunate surface of acetabulum
18: Coccyx
19: Obturator foramen
20: Body of pubis
21: Pubic symphysis

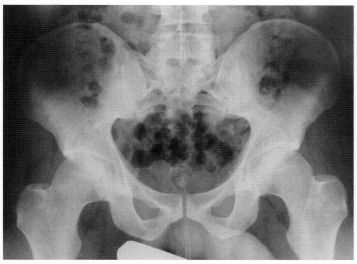
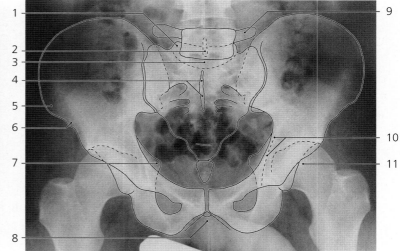

Pelvis, male, a-p X-ray, tilted

1: Zygapophysial (facet) joint L V-S I
2: Spinous process of L V
3: Promontory
4: Median sacral crest
5: Anterior superior iliac spine
6: Anterior inferior iliac spine
7: Ischial spine
8: Subpubic angle
9: Transverse process of L V
10: Ilio-ischial line (radiology term)
11: Femoral head

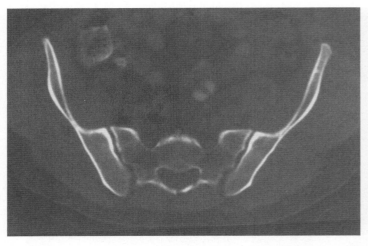

Sacro-iliac joints, axial CT (bone settings)

1: Sacro-iliac joint
2: Interosseous sacro-iliac ligament
3: Sacral canal
4: Ala of ilium
5: Ala of sacrum

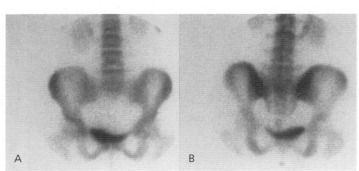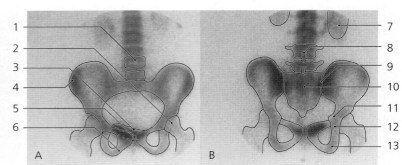

Pelvis, ^{99m} Tc-MDP scintigraphy

A: Anterior view. B: Posterior view

1: Body of fourth lumbar vertebra
2: Femoral head
3: Urinary bladder
4: Tubercle of ilium
5: Pubic symphysis
6: Inferior ramus of pubis
7: Right kidney
8: Spinous process L IV
9: Sacro-iliac joint
10: Sacrum
11: Ischial spine
12: Body of ischium
13: Ischial tuberosity

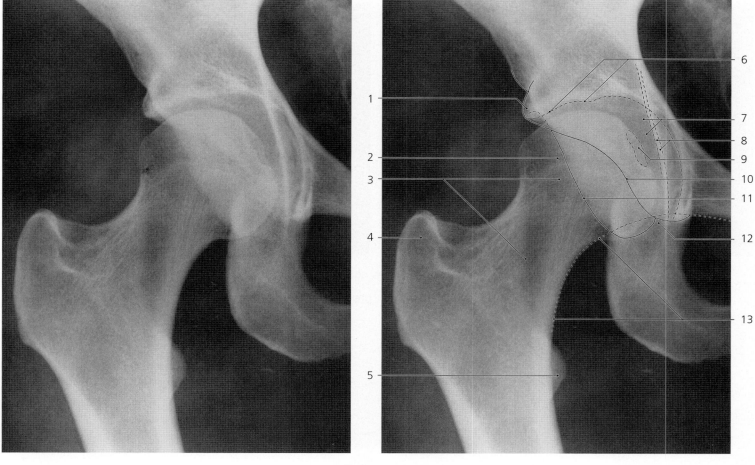

Hip, a-p X-ray

1: Acetabular rim	6: Lunate surface	11: Acetabular rim (posterior)
2: Femoral head	7: Acetabular fossa	12: Acetabular notch
3: Femoral neck	8: Ilio-ischial line (radiology term)	13: Shenton's line (radiology term)
4: Greater trochanter	9: Fovea of femoral head	
5: Lesser trochanter	10: Acetabular rim (anterior lip)	

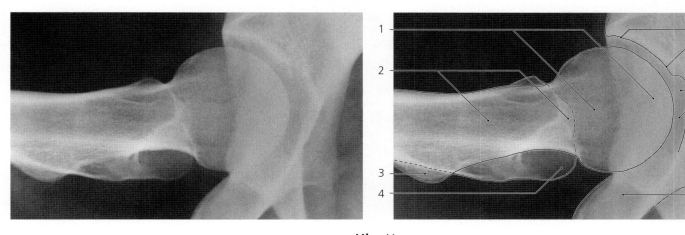

Hip, X-ray

Lauenstein projection (flexed abduced, outward rotated hip joint)

1: Femoral head	4: Greater trochanter	7: Ischial spine
2: Femoral neck	5: Lunate surface of acetabulum	8: Body of ischium
3: Lesser trochanter	6: Acetabular fossa	

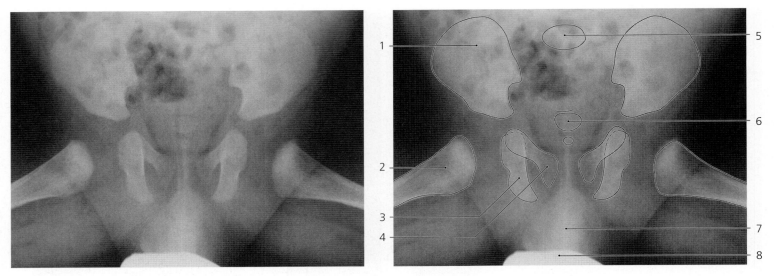

Pelvis, a-p X-ray, child 3 months

Lauenstein projection

1: Ilium
2: Metaphysis of femur
3: Ischium

4: Pubis
5: Sacral vertebra I
6: Sacral vertebra V

7: Penis
8: Gonadal lead shield

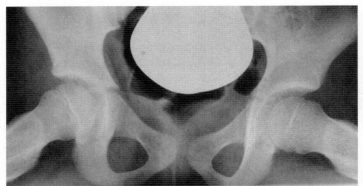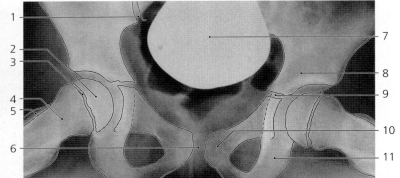

Pelvis, X-ray, child 7 years

Lauenstein projection

1: Sacro-iliac joint
2: Femoral head (epiphysis)
3: Epiphyseal growth plate
4: Femoral neck

5: Greater trochanter
6: Pubic symphysis
7: Gonadal lead shield
8: Body of ilium

9: Synchondrosis of acetabulum
10: Body of pubis
11: Body of ischium

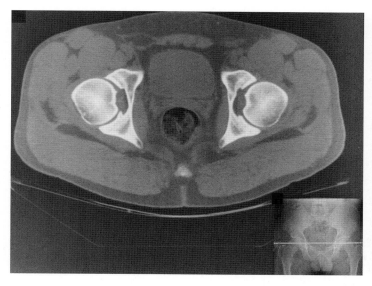

Hip, axial CT

1: Acetabular fossa
2: Femoral head

3: Fovea of femoral head
4: Ischial spine

5: Lunate surface of acetabulum

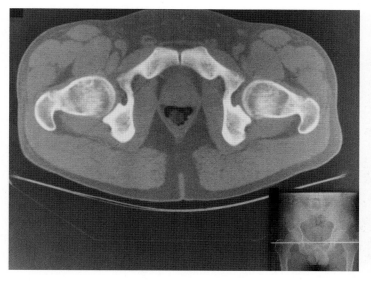
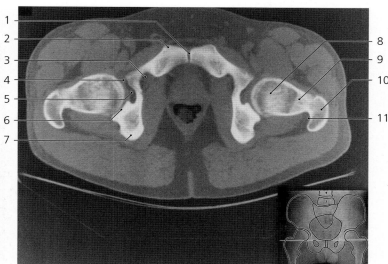

Hip, axial CT

1: Pubic symphysis
2: Pubic tubercle
3: Obturator canal
4: Acetabular notch

5: Acetabular fossa
6: Lunate surface
7: Body of ischium
8: Femoral head

9: Femoral neck
10: Greater trochanter
11: Trochanteric fossa

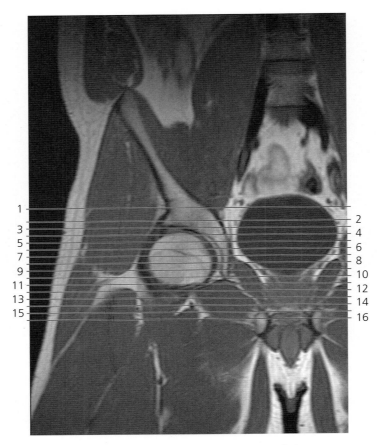

Scout view of hip and male pelvis

Lines #1–16 indicate planes of sectioning in the following axial MR series. Arrows ←, → and ↔ in the figure legends indicate that a structure can be seen in a preceding or following section or both. Interpretation of the scout image can be found in the coronal series, page 114, image #2.

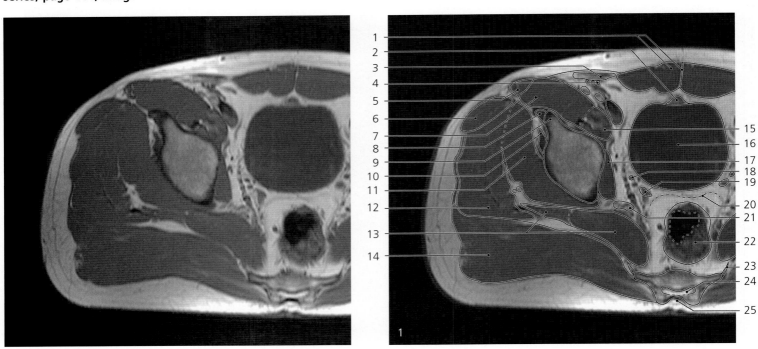

Hip and male pelvis, axial MR

1: Rectus abdominis and linea alba →
2: Median umbilical ligament
3: Spermatic cord in inguinal canal →
4: Inferior epigastric artery and veins →
5: Sartorius →
6: Tensor fasciae latae →
7: Iliacus →
8: Rectus femoris, straight head →
9: Anterior inferior iliac spine

10: Rectus femoris, reflected head
11: Gluteus minimus →
12: Gluteus medius →
13: Piriformis and gemellus superior→
14: Gluteus maximus →
15: Psoas major →
16: Urinary bladder →
17: Obturator internus →
18: Ureter →

19: Ductus (vas) deferens →
20: Recto-vesical pouch →
21: Sciatic nerve →
22: Rectum with feces and gas →
23: Sacrotuberous and sacrospinous
    ligaments →
24: Sacral canal
25: Sacral hiatus

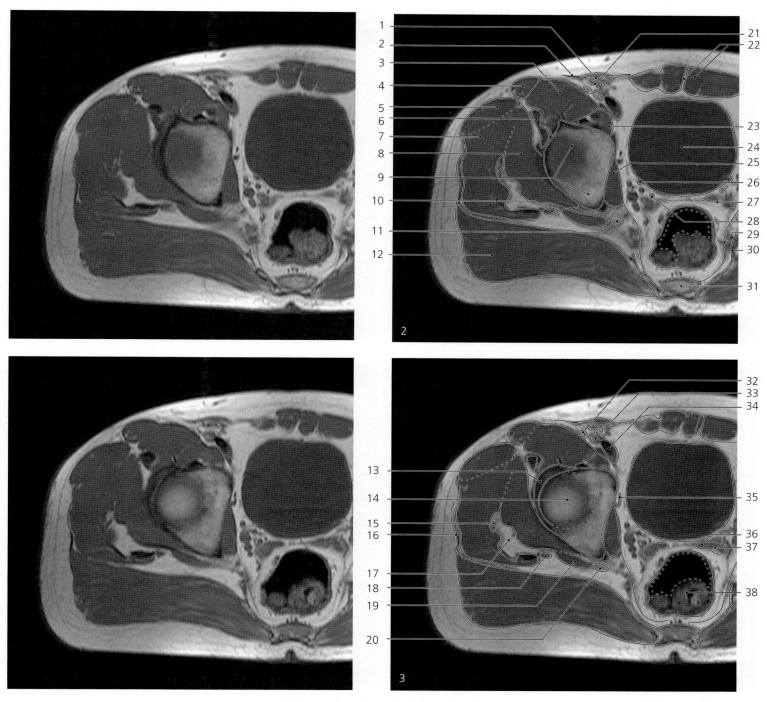

Hip and male pelvis, axial MR

Scout view on page 104

 1: Spermatic cord in inguinal canal ↔
 2: Fascia lata →
 3: Iliacus ↔
 4: Sartorius ↔
 5: Tensor fasciae latae ↔
 6: Rectus femoris ↔
 7: Gluteus medius ↔
 8: Gluteus minimus ↔
 9: Body of ilium ↔
10: Piriformis (tendon) ↔
11: Sciatic nerve ↔
12: Gluteus maximus ↔
13: Articular capsule →

14: Head of femus →
15: Superior gluteal artery ←
16: Iliotibial tract ↔
17: Intergluteal space ↔
18: Piriformis (tendon) ↔
19: Gemellus superior ↔
20: Sciatic nerve ↔
21: Inferior epigastric artery and veins ↔
22: Rectus abdominis and linea alba ↔
23: Psoas major ↔
24: Urinary bladder ↔
25: Obturator internus ↔
26: Ureter (termination in bladder) ←
27: Recto-vesical pouch ←

28: Ductus (vas) deferens ←
29: Levator ani →
30: Sacrotuberous and sacrospinous
    ligaments ↔
31: Coccyx →
32: Femoral nerve ←
33: External iliac artery ↔
34: External iliac vein ↔
35: Obturator artery and nerve →
36: Ampulla of ductus (vas) deferens
37: Seminal vesicle (gland) →
38: Rectum with feces and gas ↔

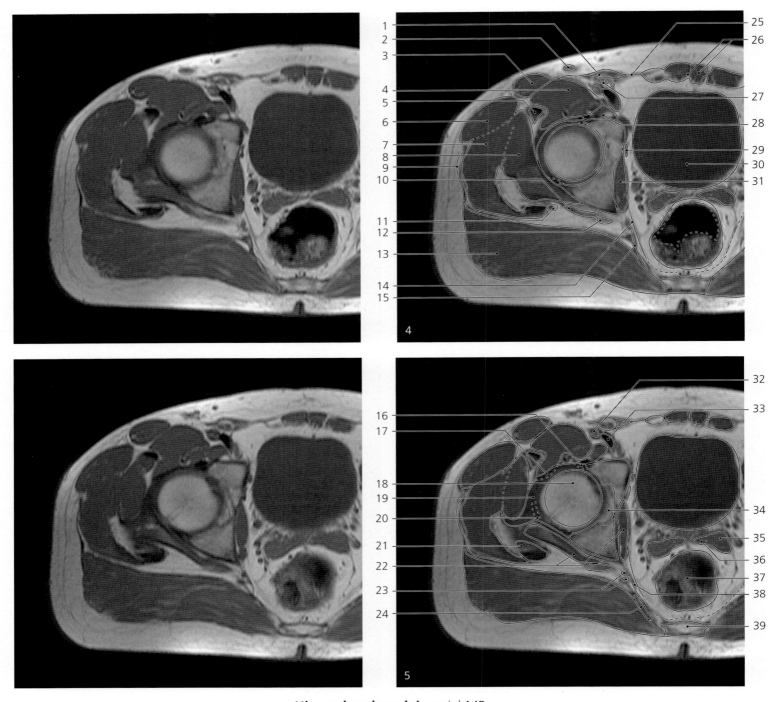

Hip and male pelvis, axial MR

Scout view on page 104
1: Spermatic cord in inguinal canal ↔
2: Superficial inguinal lymph node
3: Sartorius ↔
4: Iliacus ↔
5: Rectus femoris ↔
6: Tensor fasciae latae ↔
7: Gluteus medius ↔
8: Gluteus minimus ↔
9: Iliotibial tract ↔
10: Gemellus superior ←
11: Piriformis (tendon) ←
12: Sciatic nerve ↔
13: Gluteus maximus ↔
14: Levator ani ↔

15: Sacrotuberous and sacrospinous
    ligaments ↔
16: Acetabular labrum →
17: Iliofemoral ligament →
18: Head of femur ↔
19: Articular capsule ↔
20: Ischiofemoral ligament →
21: Greater trochanter (with insertion of
    gluteus medius and piriformis) →
22: Obturator internus ↔
23: Inferior gluteal artery and vein →
24: Sacrotuberous ligament ↔
25: External oblique (aponeurosis) →
26: Rectus abdominis and linea alba ↔
27: Inferior epigastric artery and veins ←

28: Psoas major ↔
29: Obturator artery and nerve ↔
30: Urinary bladder ↔
31: Obturator internus ↔
32: External iliac artery ←
33: External iliac vein ←
34: Acetabular fossa →
35: Seminal vesicle (gland) ↔
36: Ampulla of ductus (vas) deferens ↔
37: Rectum with feces ↔
38: Sacrospinous ligament ↔
39: Coccyx ↔

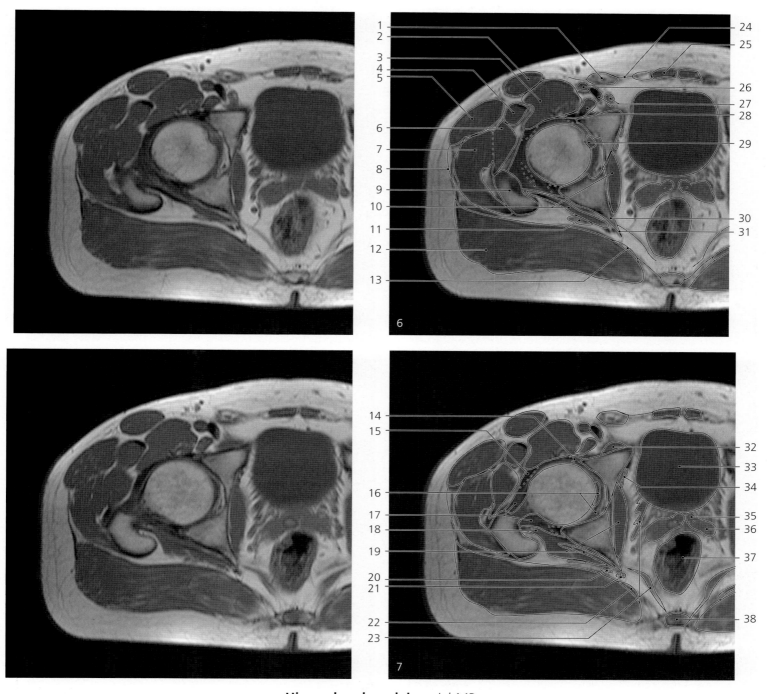

Hip and male pelvis, axial MR

Scout view on page 104
1: Spermatic cord ↔
2: Sartorius ↔
3: Iliacus ↔
4: Rectus femoris ↔
5: Tensor fasciae latae ↔
6: Gluteus minimus ↔
7: Gluteus medius ↔
8: Iliotibial tract ↔
9: Greater trochanter ↔
10: Obturator internus ↔
11: Sciatic nerve ↔
12: Gluteus maximus ↔
13: Sacrotuberous ligament ↔
14: Acetabular labrum ↔
15: Iliofemoral ligament ↔
16: Ligament of head of femur in pulvinar acetabuli
17: Articular capsule ↔
18: Gemellus inferior
19: Obturator internus ↔
20: Inferior gluteal artery and vein ↔
21: Internal pudendal artery and nerve →
22: Sacrotuberous ligament ↔
23: Levator ani ↔
24: External oblique (aponeurosis) ←
25: Rectus abdominis ↔
26: Femoral artery →
27: Femoral vein and deep inguinal lymph node
28: Psoas major ↔
29: Ligament of head of femur (attaching in fovea of head)
30: Ischial spine
31: Sacrospinous ligament ←
32: Pectineus →
33: Urinary bladder ↔
34: Obturator artery and nerve ↔
35: Ampulla of ductus (vas) deferens ←
36: Seminal vesicle (gland) ↔
37: Rectum with feces ↔
38: Coccyx ↔

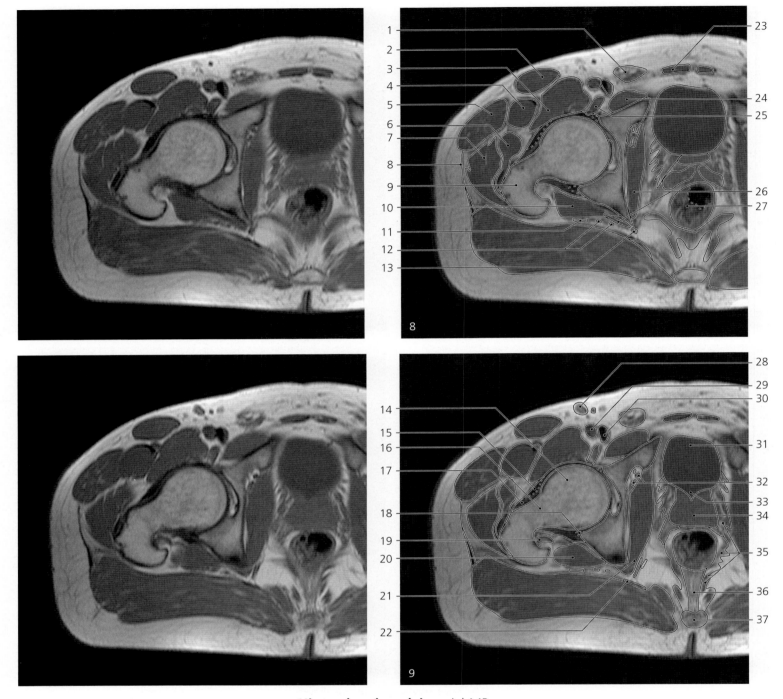

Hip and male pelvis, axial MR

Scout view on page 104

1: Spermatic cord ↔
2: Sartorius ↔
3: Iliacus ↔
4: Rectus femoris ↔
5: Tensor fasciae latae ↔
6: Gluteus minimus ↔
7: Gluteus medius ↔
8: Iliotibial tract ↔
9: Greater trochanter ↔
10: Gemellus inferior and quadratus femoris
11: Sciatic nerve ↔
12: Inferior gluteal artery and vein ↔

13: Internal pudendal artery and pudendal nerve ↔
14: Head of femur ↔
15: Iliofemoral ligament ↔
16: Neck of femur →
17: Articular capsule ↔
18: Acetabular labrum ←
19: Obturator externus (insertion) →
20: Quadratus femoris →
21: Obturator internus ↔
22: Sacrotuberous ligament ↔
23: Rectus abdominis ↔
24: Pectineus muscle ↔
25: Psoas major ↔

26: Obturator internus ↔
27: Rectum ↔
28: Superficial inguinal lymph node
29: Femoral artery ↔
30: Femoral vein ↔
31: Urinary bladder ↔
32: Obturator artery, vein and nerve in obturator canal ↔
33: Internal urethral orifice
34: Prostate →
35: Levator ani ↔
36: Anococcygeal ligament
37: Coccyx ↔

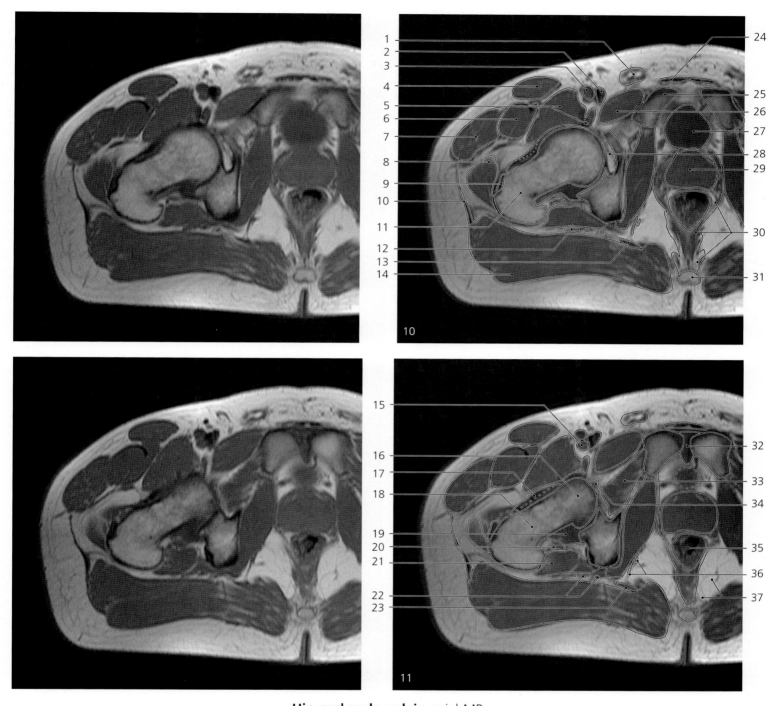

Hip and male pelvis, axial MR

Scout view on page 104

1: Spermatic cord ↔
2: Femoral vein ↔
3: Femoral artery ↔
4: Sartorius ↔
5: Iliopsoas →
6: Rectus femoris ↔
7: Tensor fasciae latae ↔
8: Gluteus medius ↔
9: Gluteus minimus (insertion) ←
10: Iliotibial tract ↔
11: Greater trochanter ↔
12: Sciatic nerve ↔

13: Sacrotuberous ligament ↔
14: Gluteus maximus ↔
15: Deep femoral artery →
16: Head of femur ←
17: Iliofemoral ligament ↔
18: Neck of femur ↔
19: Articular capsule ↔
20: Obturator externus (tendon) ↔
21: Quadratus femoris ↔
22: Inferior gluteal artery and vein ↔
23: Sacrotuberous ligament ↔
24: Rectus abdominis (tendon) ↔
25: Pubic tubercle

26: Pectineus ↔
27: Urinary bladder (fundus) ←
28: Acetabular fossa ←
29: Prostate ↔
30: Levator ani ↔
31: Coccyx ↔
32: Pubic symphysis →
33: Obturator externus ↔
34: Pubofemoral ligament
35: Rectum ↔
36: Internal pudendal artery and pudendal nerve ←
37: Ischio-anal fossa →

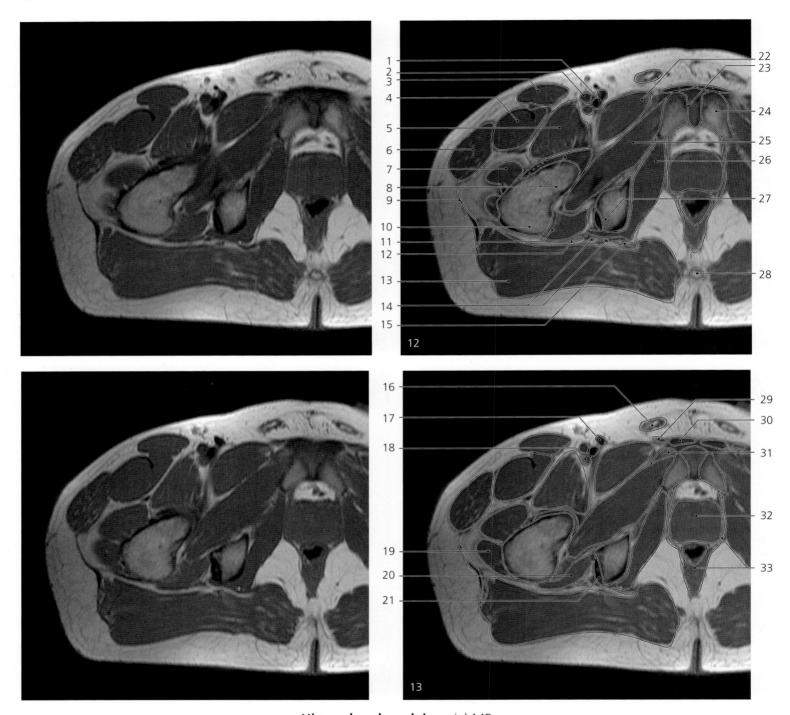

Hip and male pelvis, axial MR

Scout view on page 104

1: Femoral vein ↔
2: Femoral artery ↔
3: Sartorius ↔
4: Rectus femoris ↔
5: Iliopsoas ↔
6: Tensor fasciae latae ↔
7: Vastus intermedius →
8: Neck of femur ← and articular capsule ↔
9: Iliotibial tract ↔
10: Greater trochanter ←

11: Quadratus femoris ←
12: Sciatic nerve ↔
13: Gluteus maximus ↔
14: Inferior gluteal artery and vein ←
15: Sacrotuberous ligament ↔
16: Spermatic cord ↔
17: Great saphenous vein →
18: Deep femoral artery ↔
19: Vastus lateralis →
20: Adductor magnus →
21: Hamstring muscles (origin) →
22: Pectineus ↔

23: Pubic symphysis ↔
24: Body of pubic
25: Obturator externus ↔
26: Obturator internus ↔
27: Ischial tuberosity →
28: Coccyx ←
29: Adductor longus →
30: Gracilis →
31: Adductor brevis →
32: Prostate ↔
33: Levator ani ↔

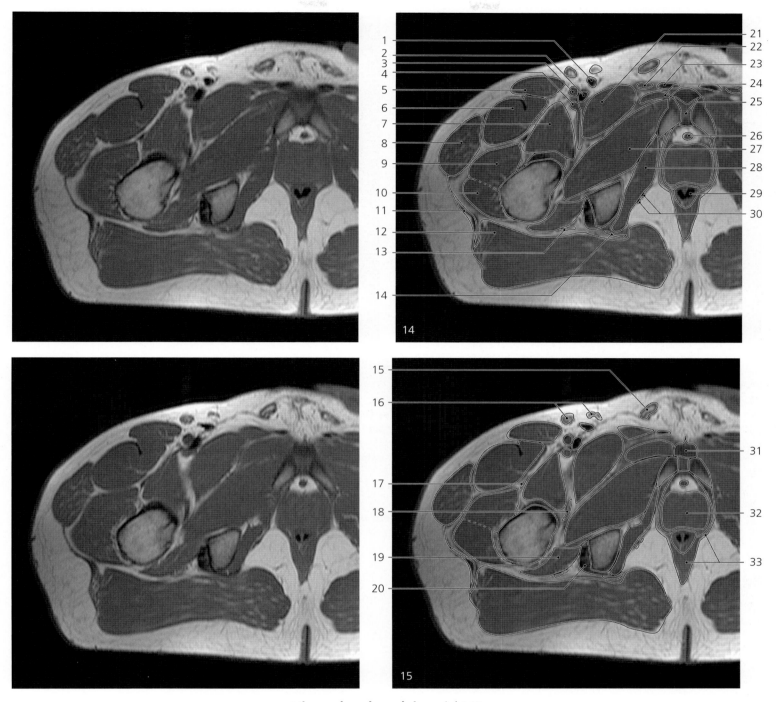

Hip and male pelvis, axial MR

Scout view on page 104
1: Great saphenous vein ↔
2: Femoral vein ↔
3: Femoral artery ↔
4: Deep femoral artery ↔
5: Sartorius ↔
6: Rectus femoris ↔
7: Iliopsoas ↔
8: Tensor fasciae latae ↔
9: Vastus intermedius ↔
10: Vastus lateralis ↔
11: Iliotibial tract ↔

12: Gluteus maximus ↔
13: Sciatic nerve ↔
14: Sacrotuberous ligament ↔
15: Spermatic cord ↔
16: Superficial inguinal lymph nodes
17: Lateral circumflex artery of femur →
18: Medial circumflex artery of femur →
19: Adductor magnus ↔
20: Hamstring muscles (origin) ↔
21: Pectineus ↔
22: Adductor longus ↔
23: Gracilis ↔

24: Adductor brevis ↔
25: Pubic symphysis ↔
26: Dorsal vein of penis →
27: Obturator externus ↔
28: Obturator internus ↔
29: Rectum ←
30: Internal pudendal artery and pudendal nerve ↔
31: Fundiform ligament of penis
32: Prostate ↔
33: Levator ani (puborectalis) ↔

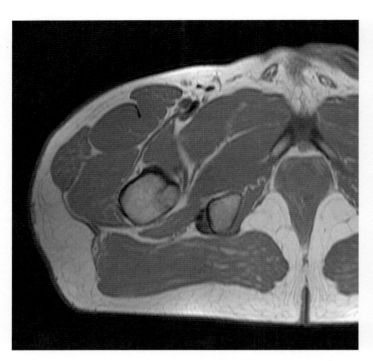
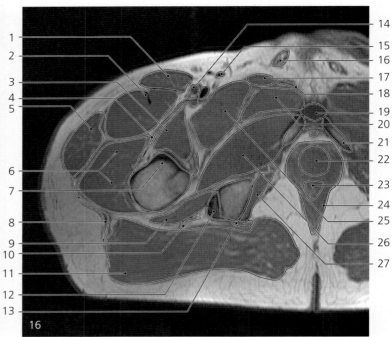

Hip and male pelvis, axial MR

Scout view on page 104

1: Sartorius ←
2: Rectus femoris ←
3: Iliopsoas ←
4: Lateral circumflex artery of femur ←
5: Tensor fasciae latae ←
6: Vastus intermedius and lateralis ←
7: Lesser trochanter
8: Iliotibial tract ←
9: Adductor magnus ←

10: Sciatic nerve ←
11: Gluteus maximus ←
12: Hamstring muscles (origin) ←
13: Sacrotuberous ligament ←
14: Femoral artery ←
15: Great saphenous vein ←
16: Spermatic cord ←
17: Adductor longus ←
18: Gracilis ←
19: Fundiform ligament of penis ←

20: Adductor brevis ←
21: Inferior pubic ramus
22: Prostate ←
23: Anal canal
24: Levator ani ←
25: Pectineus ←
26: Obturator externus ←
27: Obturator internus ←

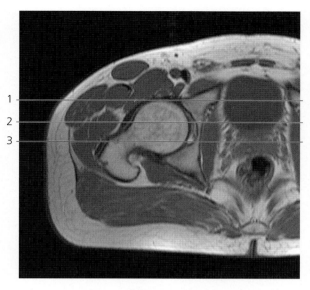

Scout view of hip and male pelvis

Lines #1–3 indicate planes of sectioning in the following coronal MR series. Interpretation of the scout image can be found in the axial series, page 108, image #8.

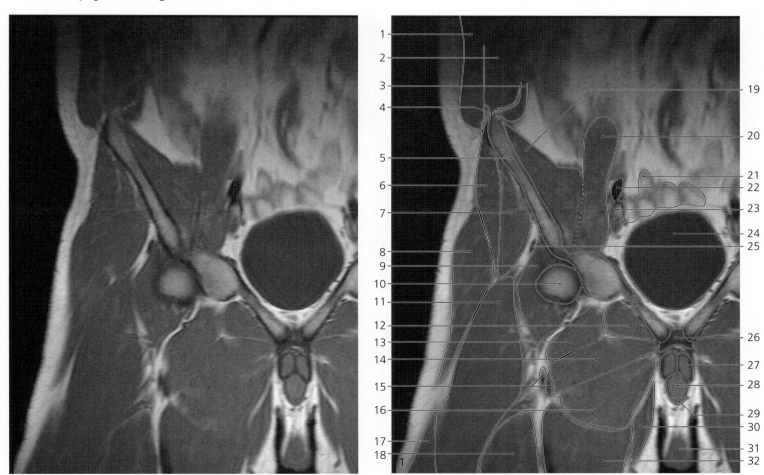

Hip and male pelvis, coronal MR

Scout view above
1: External oblique →
2: Internal oblique →
3: Transversus abdominis →
4: Iliac crest →
5: Ala of ilium →
6: Gluteus medius →
7: Gluteus minimus →
8: Tensor fasciae latae →
9: Iliopsoas →
10: Head of femur →

11: Vastus intermedius →
12: Obturator externus →
13: Pectineus →
14: Adductor brevis →
15: Deep femoral artery and vein →
16: Adductor longus →
17: Vastus lateralis →
18: Rectus femoris
19: Iliacus →
20: Psoas major →
21: Sigmoid colon →

22: External iliac artery →
23: External iliac vein →
24: Urinary bladder →
25: Rectus femoris (reflected head)
26: Pubic symphysis
27: Corpus cavernosum penis →
28: Corpus spongiosum penis →
29: Bulbocavernosus muscle →
30: Gracilis →
31: Testis in scrotum
32: Adductor magnus →

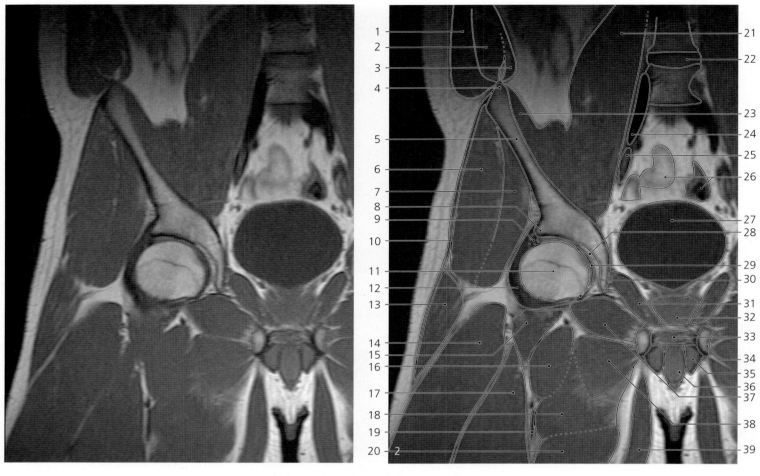

Hip and male pelvis, coronal MR

Scout view on page 113
1: External oblique ↔
2: Internal oblique ↔
3: Transversus abdominis ↔
4: Iliac crest ↔
5: Ala of ilium ↔
6: Gluteus medius ↔
7: Gluteus minimus ↔
8: Acetabular rim ↔
9: Acetabular labrum ↔
10: Iliotibial tract ↔
11: Head of femur ↔
12: Articular capsule ↔
13: Tensor fasciae latae ↔

14: Vastus lateralis ↔
15: Iliopsoas ↔
16: Pectineus ↔
17: Vastus intermedius ↔
18: Adductor longus ←
19: Deep femoral artery ←
20: Adductor magnus ↔
21: Psoas major ↔
22: Intervertebral disc
23: Iliacus ↔
24: External iliac artery ↔
25: External iliac vein ↔
26: Sigmoid colon ←
27: Urinary bladder ↔

28: Acetabular fossa →
29: Ligament of head of femur
30: Transverse acetabular ligament →
31: Obturator internus →
32: Prostate →
33: Urogenital diaphragm →
34: Inferior pubic ramus →
35: Crus of penis →
36: Corpus spongiusum penis ↔
37: Obturator externus ↔
38: Adductor brevis ↔
39: Gracilis ↔

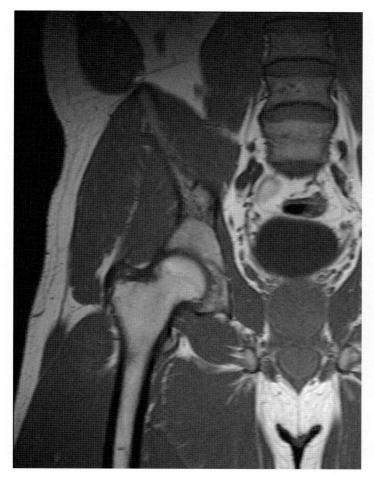
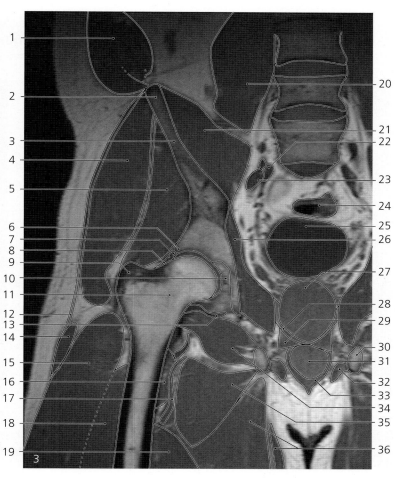

Hip and male pelvis, coronal MR

Scout view on page 113

1: External oblique, internal oblique and transversus abdominis ←
2: Iliac crest ←
3: Ala of ilium ←
4: Gluteus medius ←
5: Gluteus minimus ←
6: Acetabular rim ←
7: Acetabular labrum ←
8: Articular capsule ←
9: Greater trochanter
10: Acetabular fossa ←
11: Femoral neck

12: Iliotibial tract ←
13: Transverse acetabular ligament ←
14: Tensor fasciae latae ←
15: Vastus lateralis ←
16: Pectineus ←
17: Perforating artery from deep femoral artery
18: Vastus intermedius ←
19: Vastus medialis
20: Psoas major ←
21: Iliacus ←
22: External and internal iliac arteries ←
23: External iliac vein ←

24: Rectum
25: Urinary bladder ←
26: Obturator internus ←
27: Prostate ←
28: Levator ani
29: Urogenital diaphragm ←
30: Inferior pubic ramus ←
31: Bulb of penis
32: Ischiocavernosus muscle
33: Bulbospongiosus muscle ←
34: Obturator externus ←
35: Adductor brevis ←
36: Adductor magnus and gracilis ←

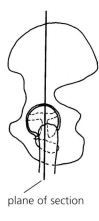

plane of section

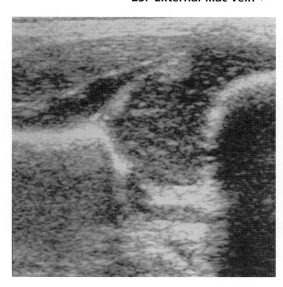
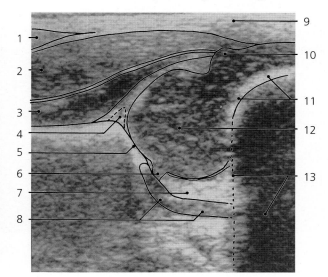

Hip, child, 3 months, coronal US

Plane of section shown on drawing

1: Tensor fasciae latae
2: Gluteus medius
3: Gluteus minimus
4: Acetabular labrum
5: Lunate surface

6: Ligament of head of femur
7: Acetabular fat pad
8: Triradiate cartilage
9: Subcutaneous fat
10: Greater trochanter

11: Ossification deep in femoral neck and shaft
12: Head of femur
13: Acoustic shadow

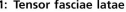

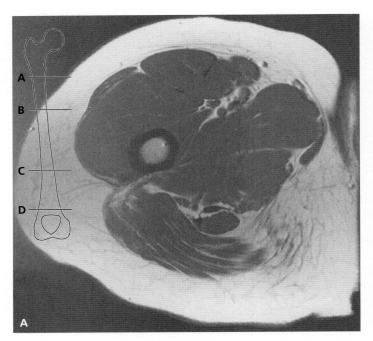

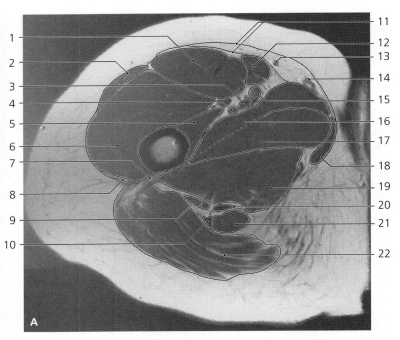

Thigh, axial MR

1: Rectus femoris →
2: Tensor fasciae latae
3: Femoral artery →
4: Deep artery of thigh
5: Vastus medialis →
6: Vastus lateralis →
7: Insertion of gluteus maximus in gluteal tuberosity
8: Insertion of gluteus maximus in iliotibial tract

9: Sciatic nerve →
10: Biceps femoris (long head) →
11: Fascia lata, deep and superficial layer of femoral triangle
12: Sartorius →
13: Accessory saphenous vein →
14: Great saphenous vein →
15: Femoral vein →
16: Adductor longus →
17: Adductor brevis

18: Gracilis →
19: Adductor magnus →
20: Semimembranosus →
21: Semitendinosus →
22: Gluteus maximus

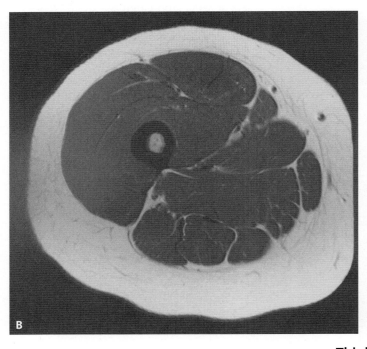

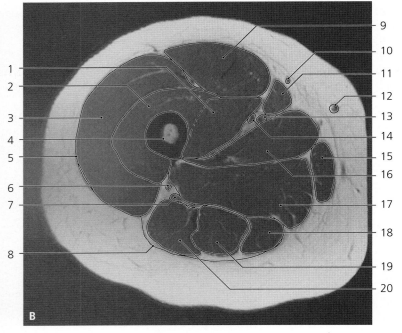

Thigh, axial MR

1: Vastus medialis ↔
2: Vastus intermedius →
3: Vastus lateralis ↔
4: Shaft of femur
5: Iliotibial tract ↔
6: Branches of perforant arteries of thigh

7: Sciatic nerve ↔
8: Fascia lata →
9: Rectus femoris ↔
10: Accessory saphenous vein ↔
11: Sartorius ↔
12: Great saphenous vein ↔
13: Femoral artery ↔

14: Femoral vein ↔
15: Gracilis ↔
16: Adductor longus ←
17: Adductor magnus ↔
18: Semimembranosus →
19: Semitendinosus ↔
20: Biceps femoris (long head) ↔

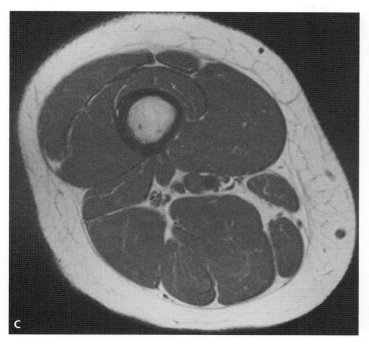

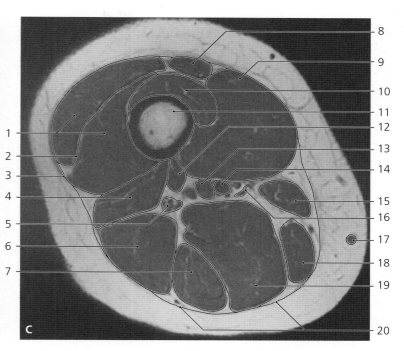

Thigh, axial MR

1: **Vastus lateralis** ↔
2: **Internal aponeurosis of vastus lateralis**
3: **Iliotibial tract** ↔
4: **Biceps femoris (short head)**
5: **Sciatic nerve** ←
6: **Biceps femoris (long head)** ↔
7: **Semitendinosus** ↔
8: **Rectus femoris** ↔

9: **Vastus medialis** ↔
10: **Vastus intermedius** ↔
11: **Shaft of femur**
12: **Adductor magnus** ↔
13: **Femoral/popliteal vein in adductor hiatus** ↔
14: **Femoral/popliteal artery in adductor hiatus** ↔
15: **Sartorius** ↔

16: **Adductor magnus (tendon)** ↔
17: **Great saphenous vein** ↔
18: **Gracilis** ↔
19: **Semimembranosus** ↔
20: **Fascia lata** ↔

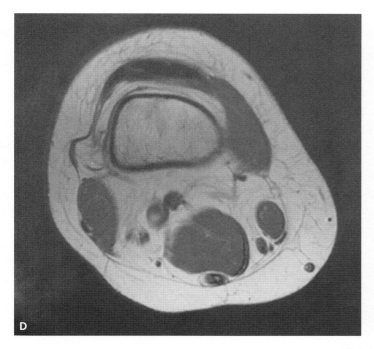

Thigh, axial MR

1: **Vastus lateralis** ←
2: **Suprapatellar bursa**
3: **Iliotibial tract** ←
4: **Popliteal artery** ←
5: **Popliteal vein** ←
6: **Tendon of long head of biceps femoris** ←

7: **Belly of short head of biceps femoris** ←
8: **Common peroneal nerve**
9: **Tibial nerve**
10: **Fascia lata** ←
11: **Rectus femoris** ←
12: **Vastus intermedius** ←

13: **Vastus medialis** ←
14: **Adductor magnus** ←
15: **Sartorius** ←
16: **Gracilis** ←
17: **Semimembranosus** ←
18: **Semitendinosus** ←

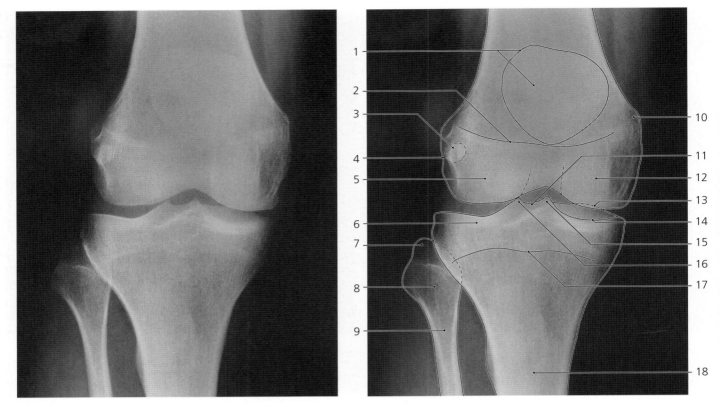

Knee, a-p X-ray

1: Patella
2: Epiphyseal scar
3: Fabella
4: Insertion of popliteus tendon
5: Lateral condyle of femur
6: Lateral condyle of tibia
7: Apex of fibula

8: Head of fibula
9: Neck of fibula
10: Adductor tubercle
11: Intercondylar eminence
12: Medial condyle of femur
13: Medial condyle of tibia (anterior margin)

14: Medial condyle of tibia (posterior margin)
15: Medial intercondylar tubercle
16: Lateral intercondylar tubercle
17: Epiphyseal scar
18: Body of tibia

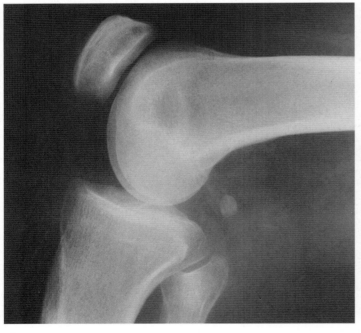

Knee, flexed, lateral X-ray

1: Base of patella
2: Articular surface of patella
3: Apex of patella
4: Femoral condyles
5: Superior articular surface of tibia

6: Tibial tuberosity
7: Patellar surface of femur
8: Shaft of femur
9: Intercondylar fossa (bottom)
10: Intercondylar eminence

11: Fabella
12: Tibiofibular joint
13: Apex of fibula
14: Head of fibula

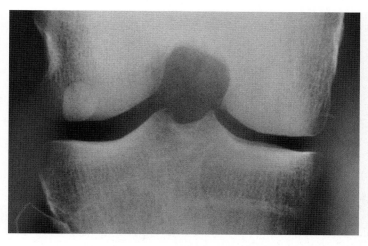
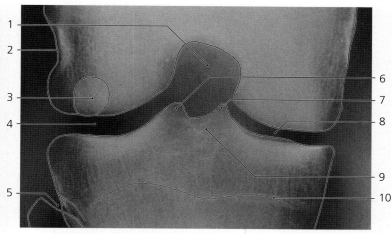

Knee, half flexed, tilted X-ray ("intercondylar notch projection")

1: Intercondylar fossa
2: Insertion of popliteus tendon
3: Fabella
4: Lateral femurotibial joint

5: Tibiofibular joint
6: Lateral intercondylar tubercle
7: Medial intercondylar tubercle
8: Medial femurotibial joint

9: Intercondylar eminence
10: Epiphyseal scar

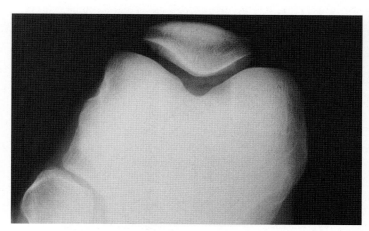
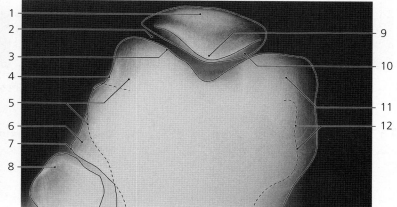

Knee, flexed, axial X-ray

"Sunrise" or "skyview" of patella

1: Patella
2: Femuropatellar joint
3: Articular surface of femur
4: Site of insertion of popliteus muscle

5: Lateral condyle of femur
6: Lateral condyle of tibia
7: Tibiofibular joint
8: Apex of fibula

9: Apex of patella
10: Articular surface of patella
11: Medial condyle of femur
12: Medial condyle of tibia

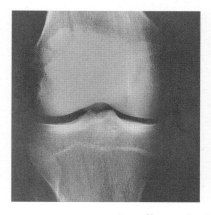
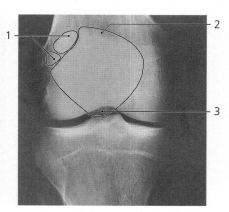

Patella variation (2%), a-p X-ray

Patella partita (tripartita)

1: Unfused ossification centers

2: Basis of patella

3: Apex of patella

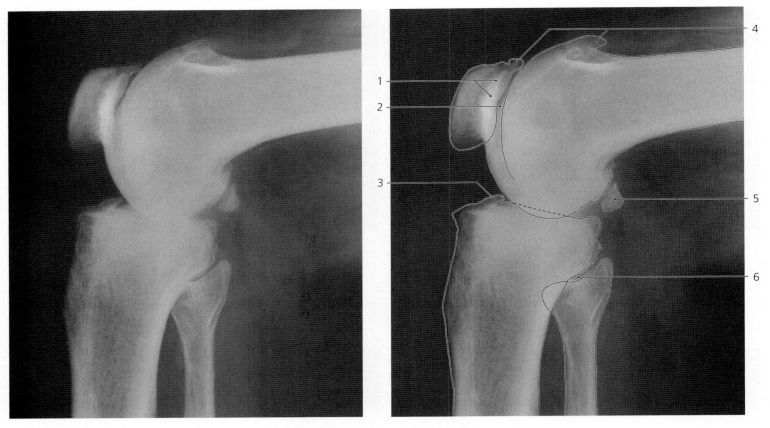

Knee, flexed, lateral X-ray, old age

With signs of arthrosis

1: Subchondral sclerosis of patella
2: Femuropatellar joint (narrow)

3: Osteophytes in anterior intercondylar area
4: Osteophytes

5: Fabella
6: Tibiofibular joint

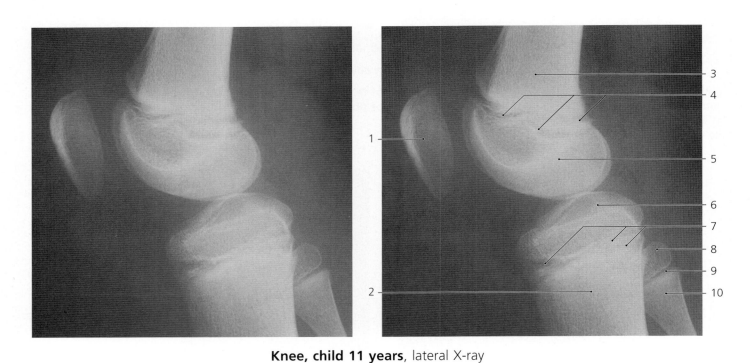

Knee, child 11 years, lateral X-ray

1: Patella
2: Metaphysis of tibia
3: Metaphysis of femur
4: Growth plate

5: Epiphysis of femur
6: Epiphysis of tibia
7: Growth plate
8: Epiphysis of fibula

9: Growth plate
10: Metaphysis of fibula

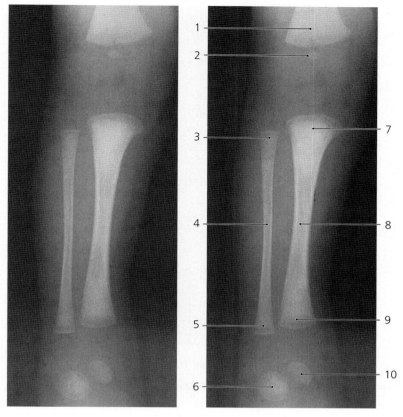

Knee and leg, newborn, a-p X-ray

1: Distal metaphysis of femur
2: Epiphysis of femur (ossification center, Béclard)
3: Proximal metaphysis of fibula

4: Diaphysis of fibula
5: Distal metaphysis of fibula
6: Calcaneus (ossification center)
7: Proximal metaphysis of tibia

8: Diaphysis of tibia
9: Distal metaphysis of tibia
10: Talus (ossification center)

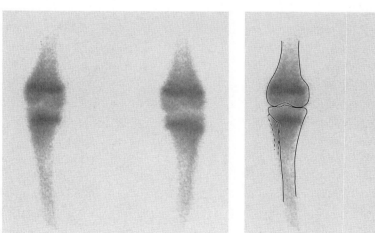
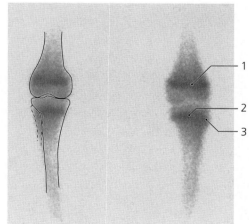

Knee, ^{99m}Tc-MDP, a-p scintigraphy, child 12 years

1: Growth plate of distal epiphysis of femur

2: Growth plate of proximal epiphysis of tibia

3: Growth plate of proximal epiphysis of fibula

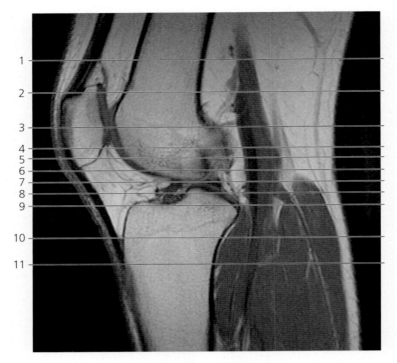

Scout view of knee

Lines #1–11 indicate position of sections in the following axial MR series. Interpretation of the scout image can be found in the sagittal series, page 132, image # 8.

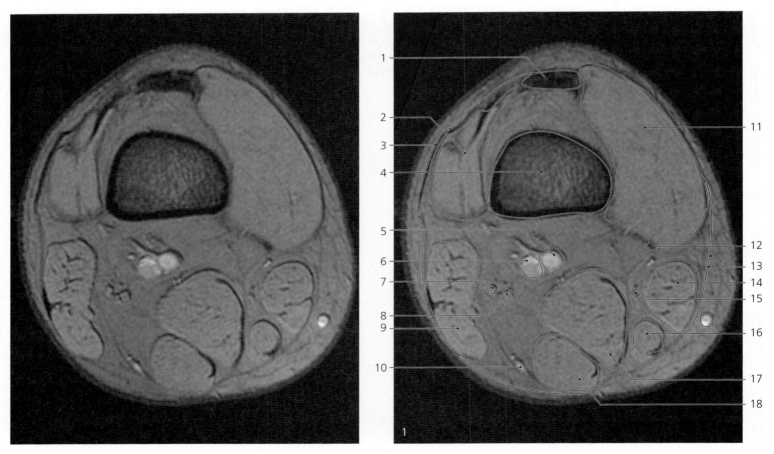

Knee, axial MR

1: Quadriceps tendon
2: Vastus lateralis →
3: Iliotibial tract →
4: Femur (shaft)
5: Popliteal artery →
6: Popliteal vein →
7: Common peroneal nerve →
8: Tibial nerve →
9: Biceps femoris →
10: Small saphenous vein →
11: Vastus medialis →
12: Adductor magnus (tendon) →
13: Fascia lata →
14: Sartorius →
15: Saphenous nerve →
16: Gracilis →
17: Semimembranosus →
18: Semitendinosus →

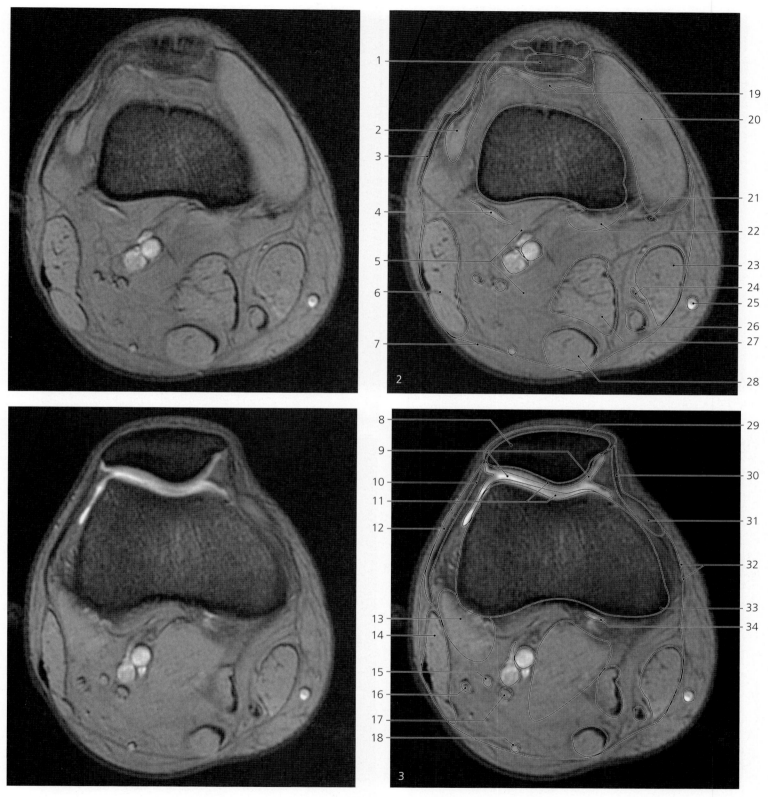

Knee, axial MR

Scout view on page 122

1: Patella (basis) →
2: Vastus lateralis ↔
3: Iliotibial tract ↔
4: Plantaris →
5: Popliteal fossa →
6: Biceps femoris →
7: Popliteal fascia →
8: Patella →
9: Patellofemoral joint cavity (with synovia)
10: Lateral retinaculum patellae →

11: Articular cartilage of patella and femur
12: Iliotibial tract ↔
13: Plantaris muscle →
14: Biceps femoris ↔
15: Lymph node
16: Common peroneal nerve ↔
17: Tibial nerve ↔
18: Small saphenous vein ↔
19: Suprapatellar bursa
20: Vastus medialis ←
21: Adductor magnus (tendon) ←
22: Gastrocnemius (medial head) →

23: Sartorius ↔
24: Saphenous nerve ←
25: Great saphenous vein ↔
26: Gracilis ↔
27: Semimembranosus ↔
28: Semitendinosus ↔
29: Quadriceps femoris (tendon)
30: Medial patellofemoral ligament
31: Vastus medialis ←
32: Fascia lata ↔
33: Adductor tubercle (adductor magnus insertion)
34: Bursa

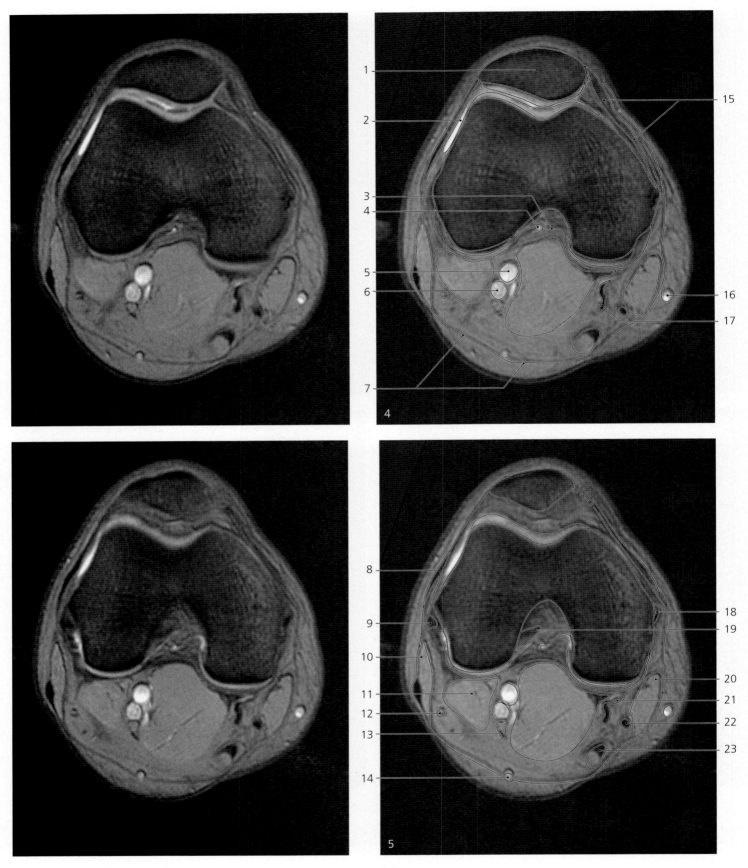

Knee, axial MR

Scout view on page 122

1: Patella ↔
2: Synovia in joint cavity
3: Posterior joint capsule
4: Median articular artery
5: Popliteal artery ↔
6: Popliteal vein ↔
7: Popliteal fascia ↔
8: Iliotibial tract ↔

9: Fibular (lateral) collateral ligament →
10: Biceps femoris ↔
11: Plantaris and gastrocnemius (lateral head)
12: Common peroneal nerve ←
13: Tibial nerve ↔
14: Small saphenous vein ↔
15: Medial patellofemoral ligament ↔
16: Great saphenous vein ↔

17: Semimembranosus (tendon) ↔
18: Tibial (medial) collateral ligament →
19: Anterior cruciate ligament →
20: Sartorius ↔
21: Semimembranosus (tendon) ↔
22: Gracilis ↔
23: Semitendinosus ↔

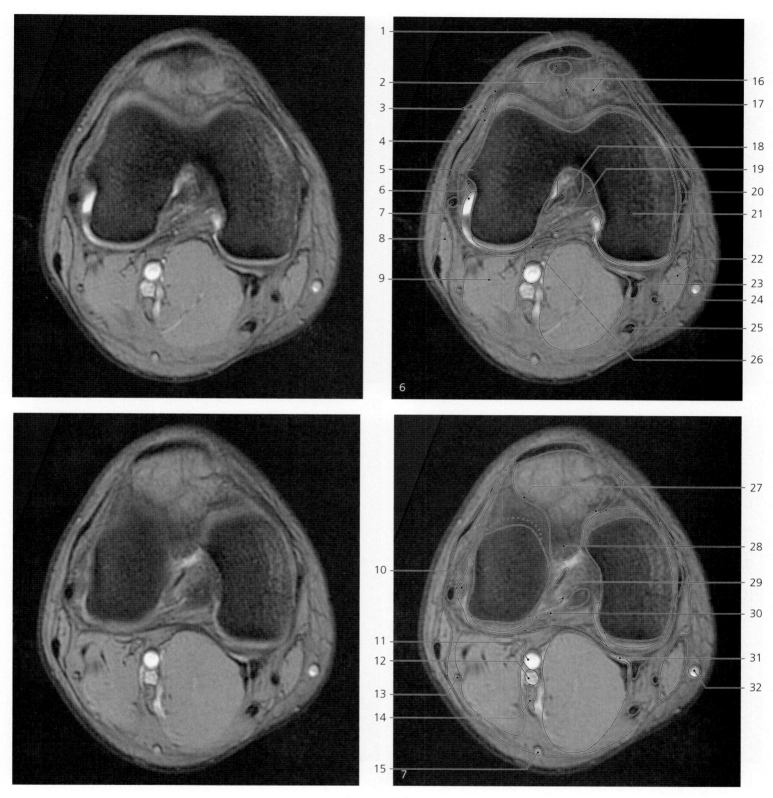

Knee, axial MR

Scout view on page 122
1: Patellar ligament →
2: Apex of patella
3: Lateral patellar retinacula →
4: Iliotibial tract ↔
5: Lateral epicondyle of femur
6: Popliteus tendon (insertion) and synovia →
7: Fibular (lateral) collateral ligament ↔
8: Biceps femoris ↔
9: Gastrocnemius (lateral head) ↔
10: Popliteus (tendon) ↔

11: Popliteal artery ↔
12: Popliteal vein ↔
13: Common peroneal nerve ↔
14: Tibial nerve ↔
15: Small saphenous vein ↔
16: Infrapatellar fat pad (Hoffa) ↔
17: Medial patellar retinacula →
18: Anterior cruciate ligament ↔
19: Posterior cruciate ligament →
20: Tibial (medial) collateral ligament ↔
21: Medial condyle of femur ↔
22: Sartorius ↔

23: Semimembranosus (tendon) ↔
24: Gracilis (tendon) ↔
25: Semitendinosus (tendon) ↔
26: Oblique popliteal ligament →
27: Alar fold
28: Infrapateller band
29: Anterior meniscofemoral ligament (Humphrey)
30: Posterior meniscofemoral ligament (Wrisberg)
31: Synovial bursa
32: Great saphenous vein ↔

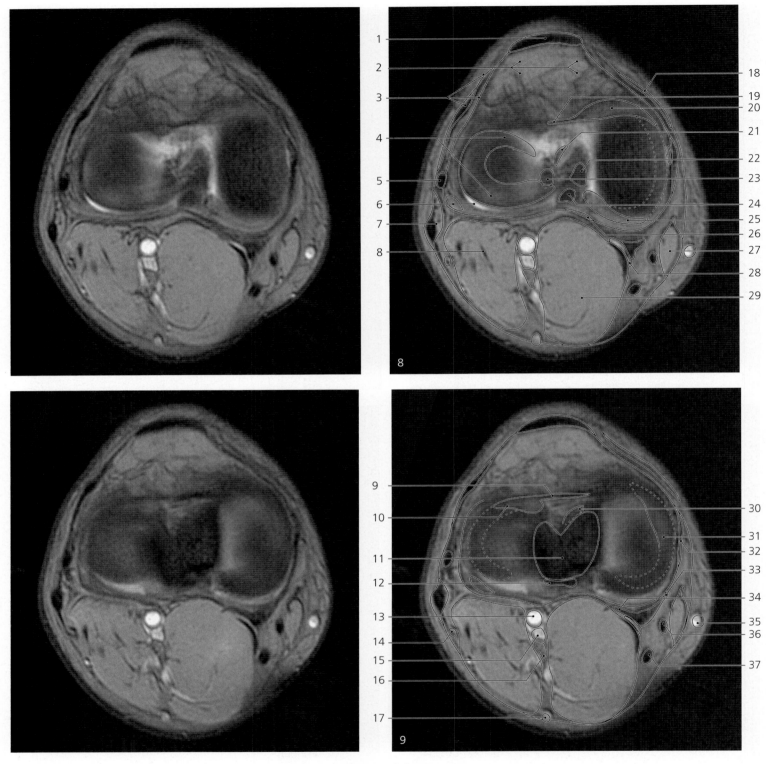

Knee, axial MR

Scout view on page 122

1: Patellar ligament ↔
2: Infrapatellar fat pad (Hoffa) ↔
3: Iliotibial tract and lateral patellar retinacula ↔
4: Lateral meniscus
5: Fibular (lateral) collateral ligament ↔
6: Popliteus tendon and synovial recess ←
7: Biceps femoris ←
8: Gastrocnemius (lateral head) ↔
9: Transverse ligament ←
10: Lateral meniscus (anterior horn)
11: Intercondylar eminence

12: Posterior cruciate ligament ←
13: Popliteal artery ↔
14: Common peroneal nerve ↔
15: Popliteal vein ↔
16: Tibial nerve ↔
17: Small saphenous vein ↔
18: Medial patellar retinacula ←
19: Transverse ligament →
20: Medial meniscus (anterior horn)
21: Anterior cruciate ligament ←
22: Medial tubercle of intercondylar eminence
23: Lateral tubercle of intercondylar eminence

24: Posterior cruciate ligament ←
25: Medial meniscus (posterior horn)
26: Oblique popliteal ligament ←
27: Sartorius ↔
28: Synovial bursa ←
29: Gastrocnemius (medial head) ←
30: Anterior cruciate ligament ←
31: Medial meniscus
32: Tibial (medial) collateral ligament ←
33: Semimembranosus (horizontal crus)
34: Semimembranosus (oblique crus)
35: Great saphenous vein ↔
36: Gracilis (tendon) ↔
37: Semitendinosus (tendon) ↔

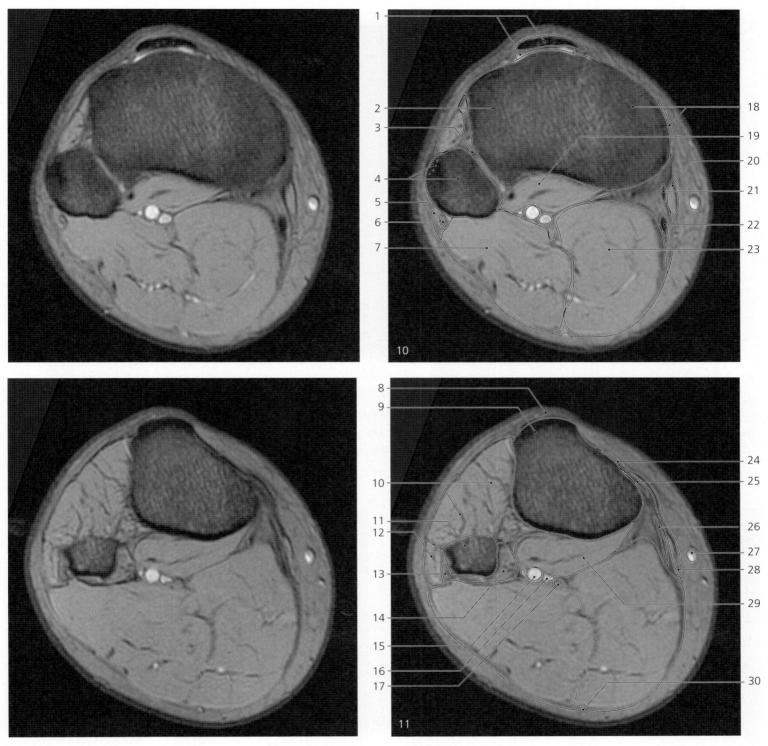

Knee, axial MR

Scout view on page 122

1: Patellar ligament with subtendinous bursa ←
2: Lateral condyle of tibia
3: Superior tibiofibular joint
4: Head of fibula with insertion of fibular collateral ligament
5: Peroneus longus
6: Common peroneal nerve ←
7: Gastrocnemius (lateral head) ←
8: Patellar ligament (insertion) ←
9: Tibial tuberosity

10: Tibialis anterior and extensor digitorum longus
11: Neck of fibula
12: Peroneus longus
13: Common peroneal nerve
14: Soleus
15: Popliteal artery ←
16: Popliteal vein ←
17: Tibial nerve ←
18: Medial condyle of tibia and tibial collateral ligament (insertion)
19: Popliteus ←

20: Sartorius ←
21: Gracilis (tendon) ←
22: Semitendinosus (tendon) ←
23: Gastrocnemius (medial head) ←
24: Pes anserinus (sartorius)
25: Pes anserinus (gracilis)
26: Pes anserinus (semitendinosus)
27: Great saphenous vein ←
28: Sartorius ←
29: Popliteus ←
30: Small saphenous vein ←

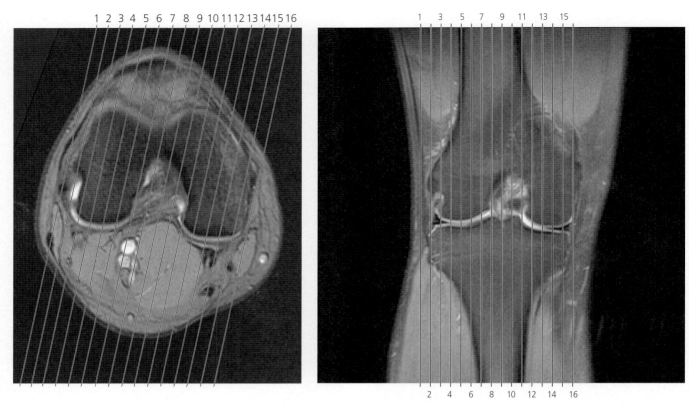

Scout views of knee

Lines #1–16 indicate position of sections in the following sagittal MR series. Interpretation of the scout images can be found in the axial series, page 125, image #6 and in the coronal series, page 140, image #5.

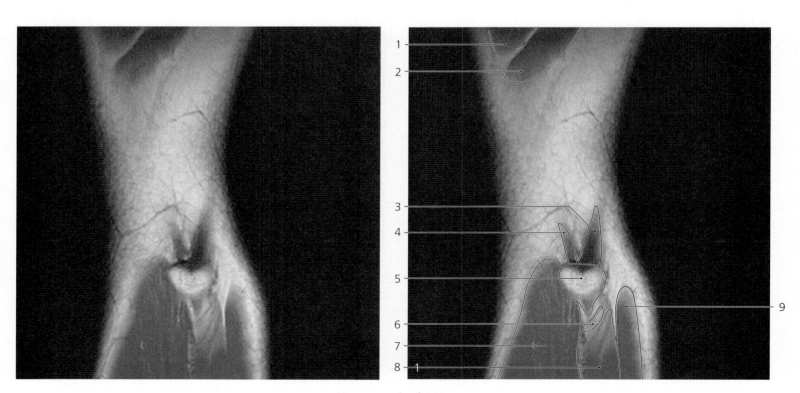

Knee, sagittal MR

1: Vastus lateralis →
2: Vastus intermedius →
3: Biceps femoris (insertion) →

4: Fibular (lateral) collateral ligament
   (fibular attachment) →
5: Head of fibula →
6: Common peroneal nerve →

7: Tibialis anterior →
8: Peroneus longus →
9: Gastrocnemius (lateral head) →

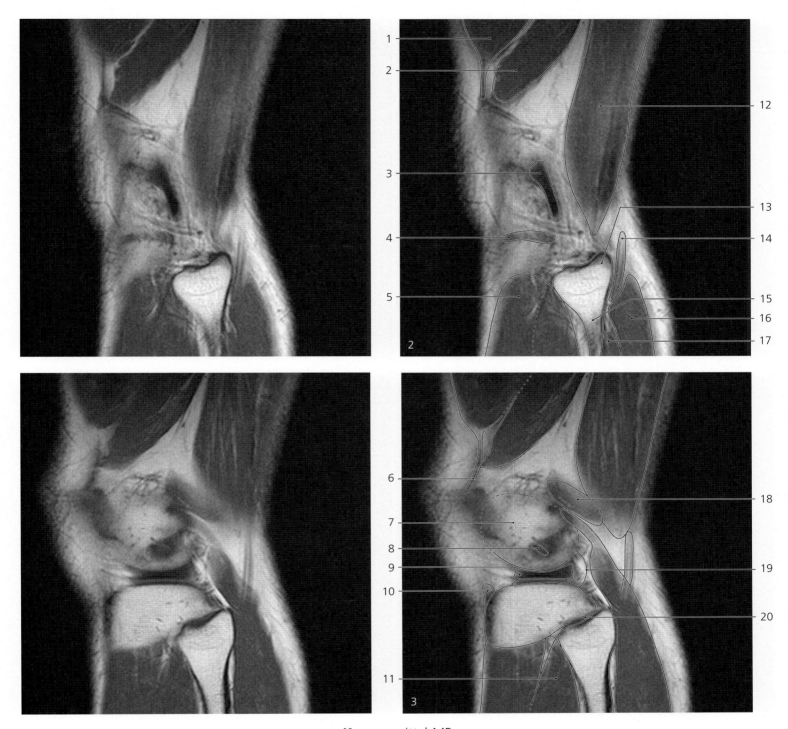

Knee, sagittal MR

Scout view on page 128

1: Vastus lateralis ↔
2: Vastus intermedius ↔
3: Fibular collateral ligament
   (femoral attachment) ←
4: Rim of lateral tibial condyle →
5: Tibialis anterior ↔
6: Lateral patellar retinaculum →

7: Lateral femoral condyle →
8: Popliteus tendon (insertion) →
9: Lateral meniscus →
10: Lateral patellar retinaculum
    (insertion)
11: Extensor digitorum longus →
12: Biceps femoris ↔
13: Apex of fibula

14: Common peroneal nerve ↔
15: Neck of fibula →
16: Gastrocnemius (lateral head) ↔
17: Peroneus longus ←
18: Plantaris →
19: Articular capsule →
20: Superior tibiofibular joint →

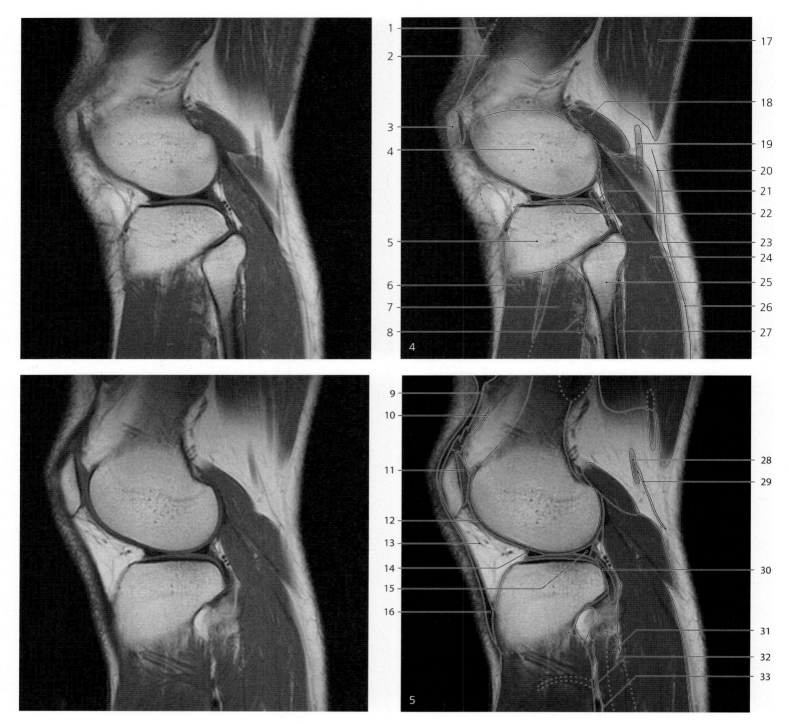

Knee, sagittal MR

Scout view on page 128

1: Vastus lateralis ←
2: Vastus intermedius ←
3: Patella →
4: Lateral femoral condyle ↔
5: Lateral tibial condyle ↔
6: Tibialis anterior ←
7: Extensor digitorum longus ←
8: Anterior tibial vessels
9: Quadriceps (tendon) →
10: Suprapatellar bursa →
11: Articular cartilage of patella
12: Articular cartilage of lateral femoral condyle

13: Infrapatellar fat pad (Hoffa) →
14: Lateral meniscus (anterior horn) ↔
15: Lateral meniscus (posterior horn) ↔
16: Patellar ligament →
17: Biceps femoris ↔
18: Plantaris ↔
19: Common peroneal nerve ←
20: Popliteal fascia →
21: Popliteus (tendon, sliding over lateral meniscus) ↔
22: Articular cartilage of lateral tibial condyle
23: Superior tibiofibular joint ←
24: Gastrocnemius (lateral head) ↔

25: Neck of fibula ←
26: Deep fascia of leg
27: Soleus →
28: Tibial nerve →
29: Medial sural cutaneous nerve
30: Popliteus (tendon) ↔
31: Soleus →
32: Interosseus membrane
33: Tibialis posterior →

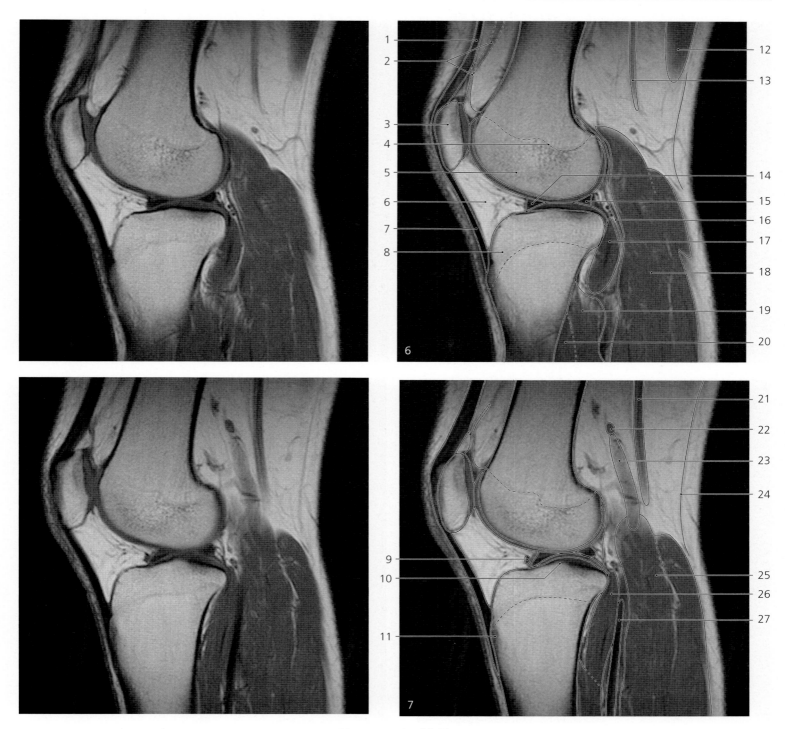

Knee, sagittal MR

Scout view on page 128

1: Quadriceps (tendon) ↔
2: Suprapatellar bursa and
   articular muscle ↔
3: Patella ↔
4: Epiphysial line →
5: Lateral condyle of femur ↔
6: Infrapatellar fat pad (Hoffa) ↔
7: Patellar ligament ↔
8: Lateral condyle of tibia ←

9: Transverse ligament of knee →
10: Intercondylar eminence →
11: Tibial tuberosity →
12: Biceps femoris ←
13: Tibial nerve ↔
14: Lateral meniscus (anterior horn) ↔
15: Lateral meniscus (posterior horn) ↔
16: Articular capsule
17: Popliteus ↔
18: Gastrocnemius (lateral head) ↔

19: Soleus ↔
20: Tibialis posterior
21: Tibial nerve ↔
22: Lymph node
23: Popliteal artery →
24: Popliteal fascia ↔
25: Plantaris ←
26: Popliteus ↔
27: Popliteal artery →

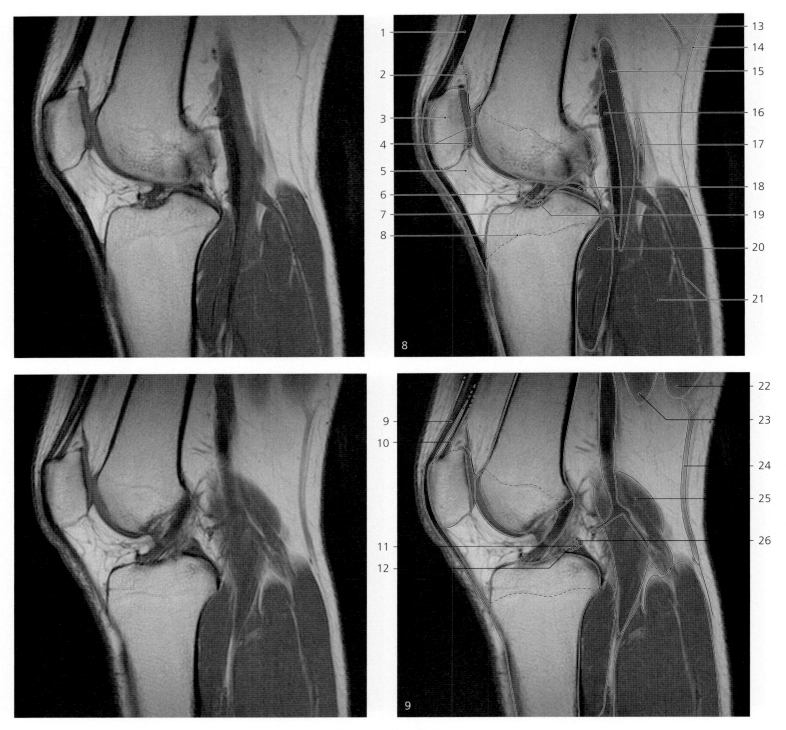

Knee, sagittal MR

Scout view on page 128
1: Quadriceps tendon ↔
2: Suprapatellar bursa ↔
3: Patella ↔
4: Articular cartilage
5: Infrapatellar fat pad (Hoffa) ↔
6: Transverse ligament of knee ↔
7: Anterior cruciate ligament →
8: Epiphysial line ↔
9: Rectus femoris (tendon) ↔
10: Quadriceps (tendon) ↔
11: Lateral meniscus (posterior horn, attachment) ←

12: Anterior meniscofemoral ligament (Humphrey) →
13: Small saphenous vein →
14: Popliteal fascia ↔
15: Popliteal vein ↔
16: Popliteal artery ↔
17: Tibial nerve ←
18: Lateral meniscus (posterior horn) ↔
19: Lateral meniscus (anterior horn, insertion)
20: Popliteus ↔
21: Gastrocnemius (lateral head with nutrient vessels) ↔

22: Semitendinosus →
23: Semimembranosus →
24: Small saphenous vein (in popliteal fascia) ←
25: Gastrocnemius (medial head) ↔
26: Posterior meniscofemoral ligament (Wrisberg)

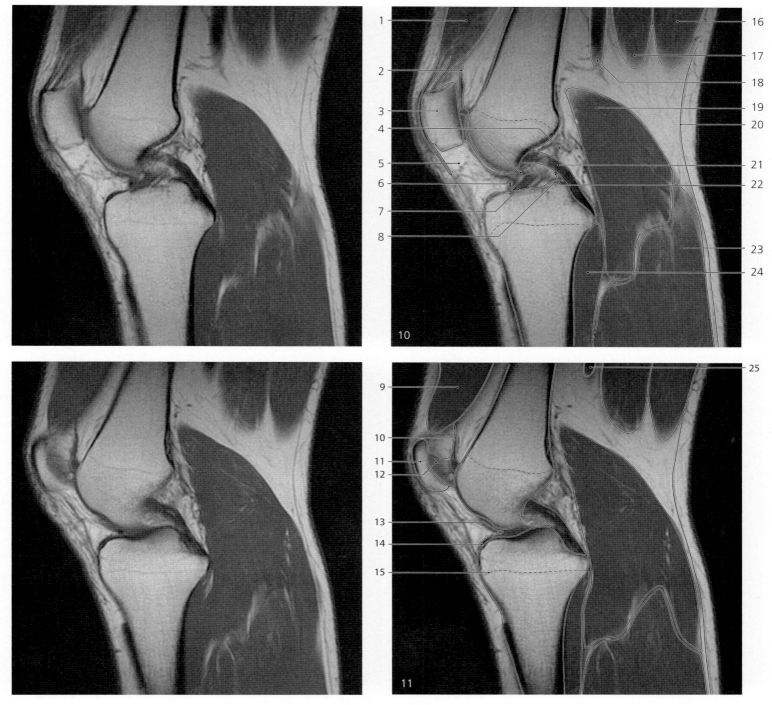

Knee, sagittal MR

Scout view on page 128

1: Quadriceps femoris ↔
2: Suprapatellar bursa ↔
3: Patella ↔
4: Intercondylar fossa
5: Infrapatellar fat pad (Hoffa) ↔
6: Transverse ligament of knee ↔
7: Anterior cruciate ligament ←
8: Intercondylar eminence →
9: Quadriceps femoris ↔

10: Suprapatellar bursa ↔
11: Patella ←
12: Wall of suprapatellar bursa in imaging plane
13: Transverse ligament of knee ←
14: Medial meniscus (anterior horn, attachment) →
15: Epiphysial line ↔
16: Semitendinosus ↔
17: Semimembranosus ↔

18: Popliteal artery and vein ↔
19: Gastrocnemius (lateral head) ↔
20: Popliteal fascia ↔
21: Posterior cruciate ligament →
22: Anterior meniscofemoral ligament (Humphrey) ←
23: Gastrocnemius (lateral head) ↔
24: Popliteus ↔
25: Popliteal artery and vein ←

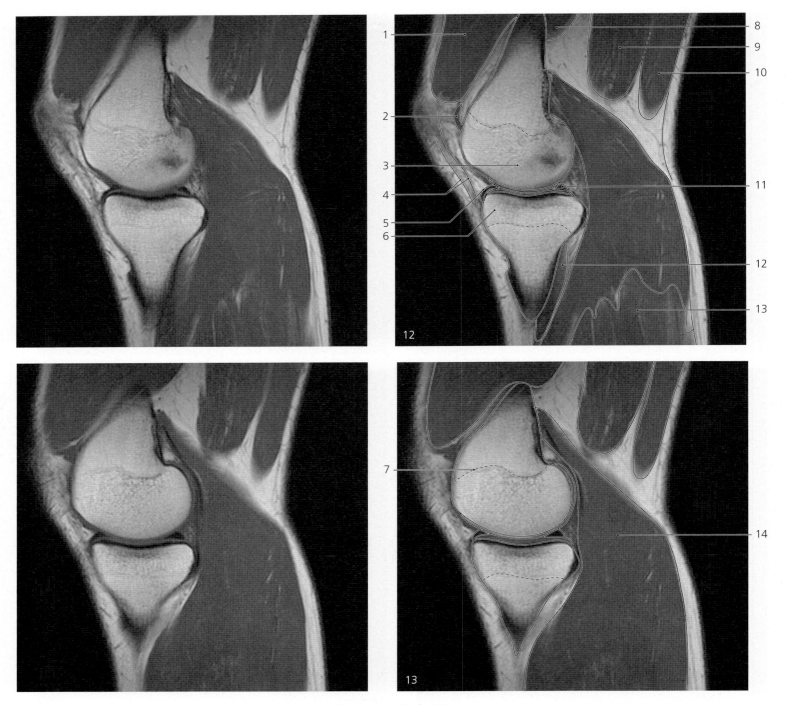

Knee, sagittal MR

Scout view on page 128

1: Quadriceps femoris ↔
2: Suprapatella bursa ←
3: Medial condyle of femur →
4: Medial patellar retinaculum
5: Medial meniscus (anterior horn) and anterior meniscotibial ligament ↔
6: Medial condyle of tibia →
7: Epiphysial line ↔
8: Vastus medialis ↔
9: Semimembranosus ↔
10: Semitendinosus ↔
11: Medial meniscus (posterior horn) ←
12: Popliteus ←
13: Gastrocnemius (lateral head) ←
14: Gastrocnemius (medial head) →

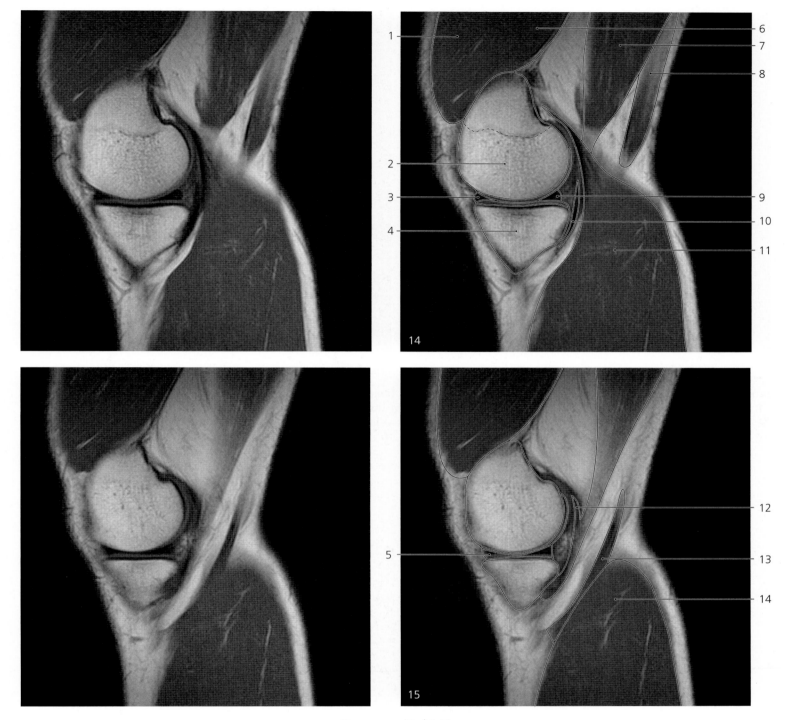

Knee, sagittal MR

Scout view on page 128
1: Quadriceps femoris ↔
2: Medial condyle of femur ↔
3: Medial meniscus (anterior horn) ↔
4: Medial condyle of tibia
5: Medial meniscus ↔

6: Vastus medialis ↔
7: Semimembranosus ↔
8: Semitendinosus ↔
9: Medial meniscus (posterior horn) ↔
10: Semimembranosus (vertical crus) →
11: Gastrocnemius (medial head) ↔

12: Semimembranosus (oblique crus/
    oblique popliteal ligament)
13: Semitendinosus ↔
14: Gastrocnemius (medial head) ↔

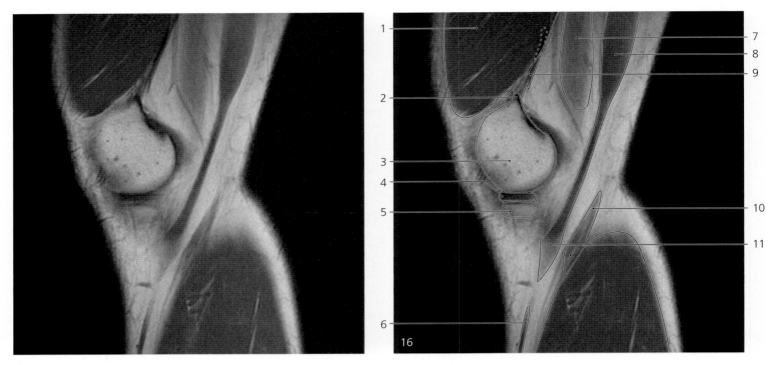

Knee, sagittal MR

Scout view on page 128

1: Quadriceps femoris ←
2: Adductor tubercle
3: Medial condyle of femur ←
4: Medial meniscus (medial rim) ←
5: Medial condyle of tibia (rim) ←
6: Great saphenous vein
7: Sartorius
8: Gracilis
9: Adductor magnus (tendon)
10: Semitendinosus ←
11: Pes anserinus

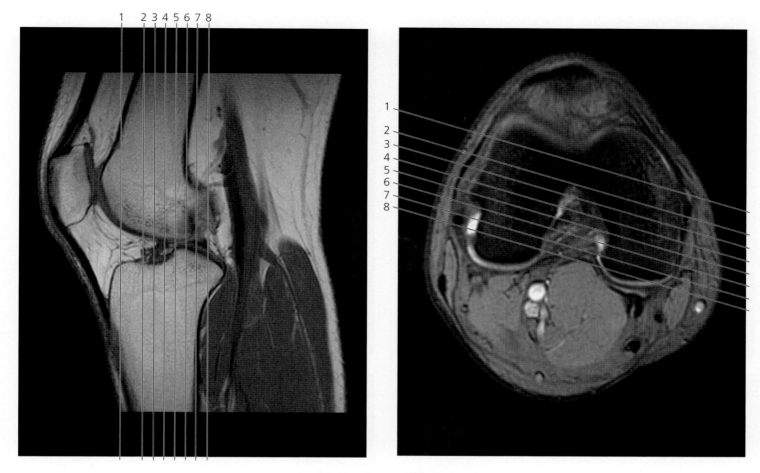

Scout views of knee

Lines #1–8 indicate position of sections in the following coronal MR series. Interpretation of the scout images can be found in the sagittal series, page 132, image #8 and in the axial series, page 125, image #6.

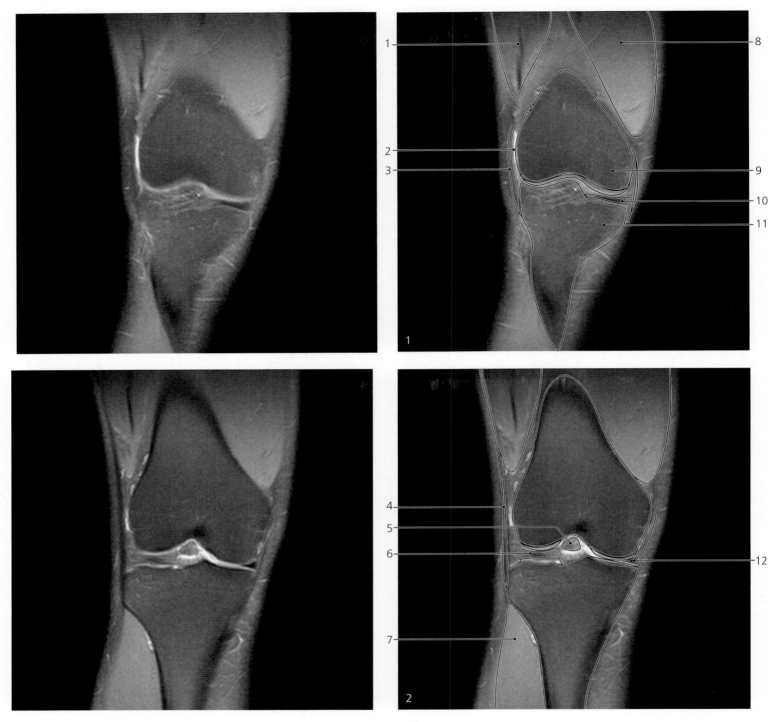

Knee, coronal MR

Scout view on page 137
1: Vastus lateralis →
2: Synovia in joint cavity
3: Articular capsule
4: Iliotibial tract →

5: Infrapatellar synovial fold
6: Lateral meniscus (anterior horn) →
7: Tibialis anterior →
8: Vastus medialis →
9: Medial condyle of femur →

10: Medial meniscus (anterior horn) →
11: Medial condyle of tibia →
12: Medial meniscus →

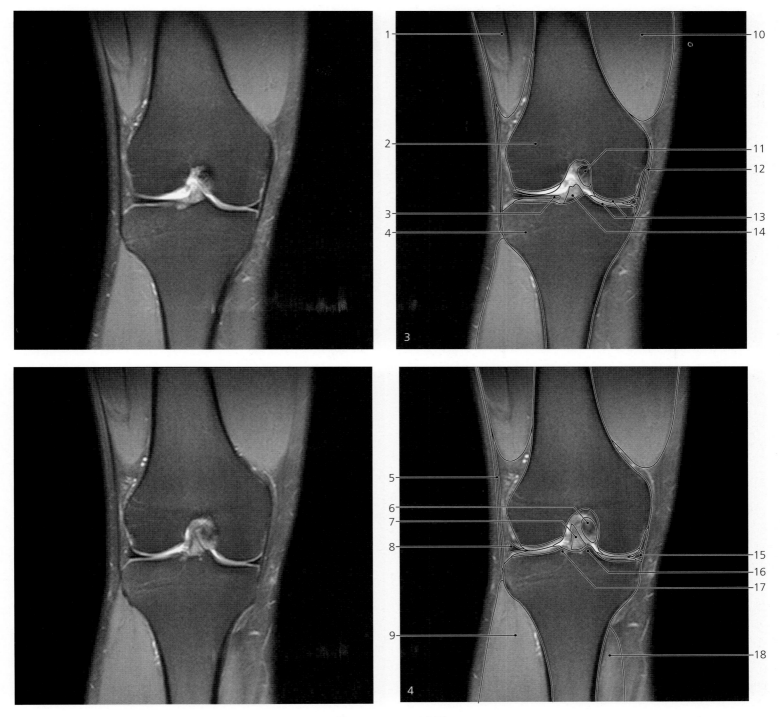

Knee, coronal MR

Scout view on page 137
1: Vastus lateralis ↔
2: Lateral condyle of femur ↔
3: Lateral meniscus (anterior horn) ↔
4: Lateral condyle of tibia ↔
5: Iliotibial tract ↔
6: Posterior cruciate ligament ↔

7: Anterior cruciate ligament →
8: Lateral meniscus ↔
9: Tibialis anterior ↔
10: Vastus medialis ↔
11: Posterior cruciate ligament →
12: Tibial (medial) collateral ligament →
13: Articular cartilage of femur and tibia

14: Anterior cruciate ligament ↔
15: Medial meniscus ↔
16: Intercondular eminence (medial tubercle)
17: Intercondular eminence (lateral tubercle)
18: Gastrocnemius (medial head) →

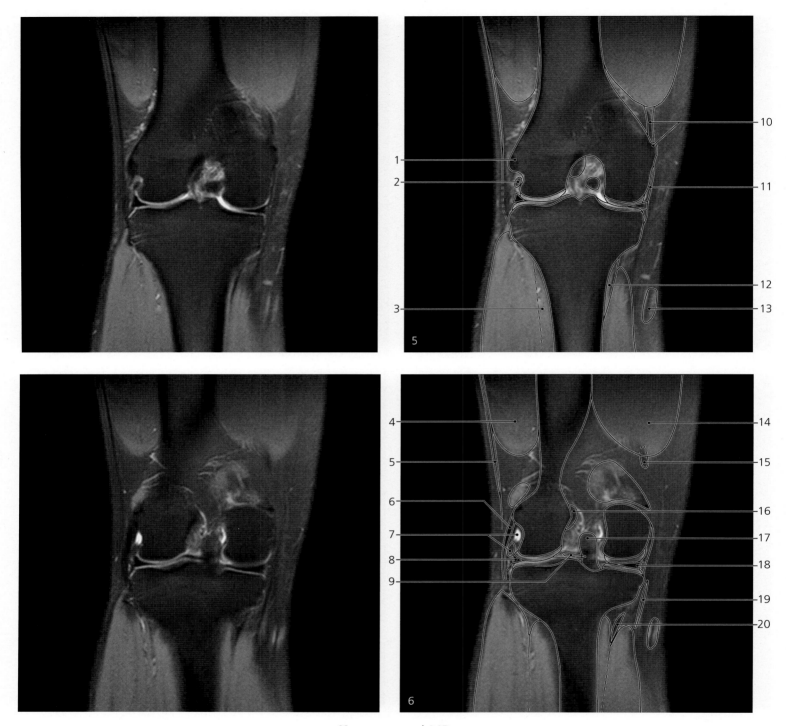

Knee, coronal MR

Scout view on page 137
1: Lateral epicondyle of femur
2: Popliteus (tendon) →
3: Extensor digitorum longus
4: Vastus lateralis ↔
5: Iliotibial tract ↔
6: Fibular (lateral) collateral ligament →
7: Popliteus (tendon) and synovial
   recess →

8: Lateral meniscus ↔
9: Anterior meniscofemoral ligament
   (Humphrey)
10: Adductor magnus (insertion on
    adductor tubercle) →
11: Tibial (medial) collateral ligament ←
12: Popliteus muscle ↔
13: Great saphenous vein →
14: Vastus medialis ↔

15: Adductor magnus (tendon) ↔
16: Anterior cruciate ligament ↔
17: Posterior cruciate ligament ↔
18: Medial meniscus ↔
19: Sartorius (tendon) →
20: Semimembranosus (vertical crus)

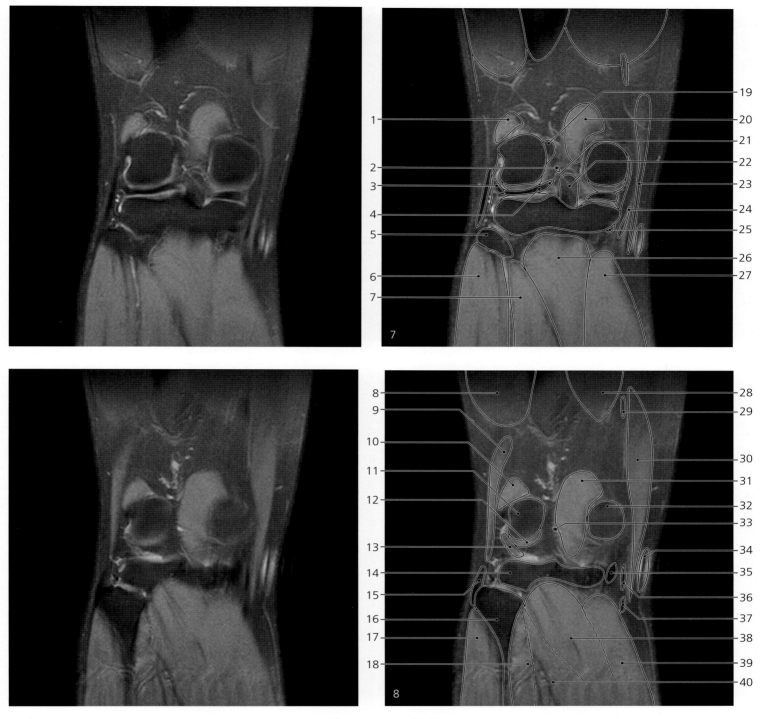

Knee, coronal MR

Scout view on page 137
1: Gastrocnemius, lateral head →
2: Middle genicular artery →
3: Popliteus (tendon, sliding over lateral meniscus) ↔
4: Lateral meniscus (posterior horn) ←
5: Head of fibula →
6: Tibialis anterior ↔
7: Tibialis posterior ↔
8: Vastus lateralis ↔
9: Biceps femoris
10: Gastrocnemius (lateral head) ←
11: Lateral femoral condyle ←
12: Articular cartilage
13: Popliteus (tendon) ←

14: Lateral condyle of tibia ←
15: Fibular collateral ligament (attachment) ←
16: Head of fibula ←
17: Tibialis anterior ←
18: Tibialis posterior ←
19: Anterior cruciate ligament ←
20: Gastrocnemius (medial head) ←
21: Posterior meniscofemoral ligament (Wrisberg)
22: Posterior cruciate ligament ←
23: Gracilis →
24: Sartorius →
25: Semimembranosus (horizontal crus)
26: Popliteus ↔

27: Gastrocnemius (medial head) ↔
28: Vastus medialis ←
29: Adductor magnus (tendon)
30: Gracilis ←
31: Gastrocnemius (medial head) ←
32: Medial condyle of femur ←
33: Middle genicular artery ←
34: Great saphenous vein ←
35: Semimembranosus (tendon) ←
36: Sartorius ←
37: Semitendinosus
38: Popliteus ←
39: Gastrocnemius (medial head) ←
40: Soleus

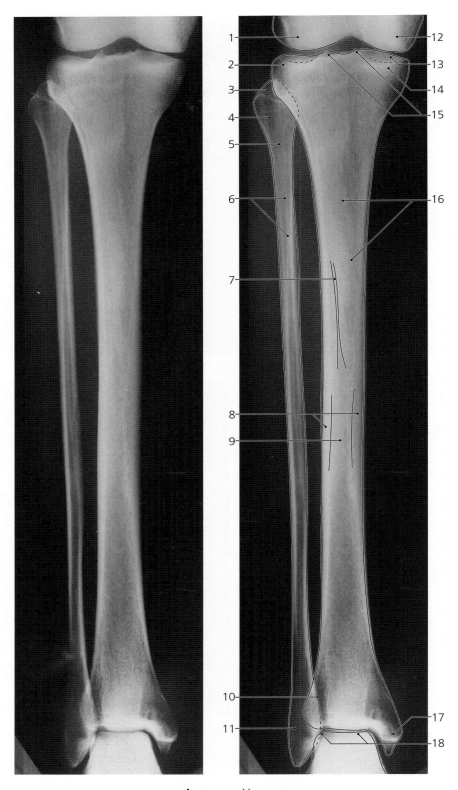

Leg, a-p X-ray

1: Lateral condyle of femur	7: Nutrient canal	13: Superior articular surface of tibia
2: Lateral condyle of tibia	8: Compact bone of tibial shaft	14: Medial condyle of tibia
3: Apex of fibula	9: Medullary cavity of tibia	15: Medial and lateral tubercle
4: Head of fibula	10: Fibular notch of tibia (syndesmosis)	16: Shaft of tibia
5: Neck of fibula	11: Lateral malleolus	17: Medial malleolus
6: Shaft of fibula	12: Medial condyle of femur	18: Trochlea of talus

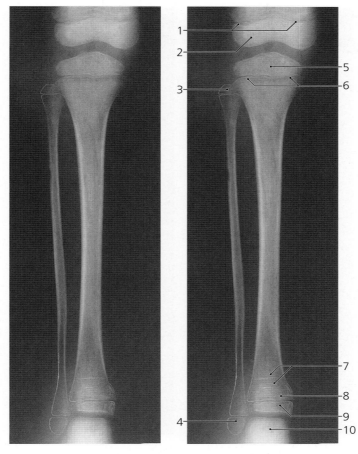

Leg, child 6 years, a-p X-ray

1: Growth plate
2: Distal epiphysis of femur
3: Proximal epiphysis of fibula
4: Distal epiphysis of fibula

5: Proximal epiphysis of tibia
6: Growth plate
7: Harris lines (signs of temporary growth arrest)

8: Growth plate
9: Distal epiphysis of tibia
10: Talus

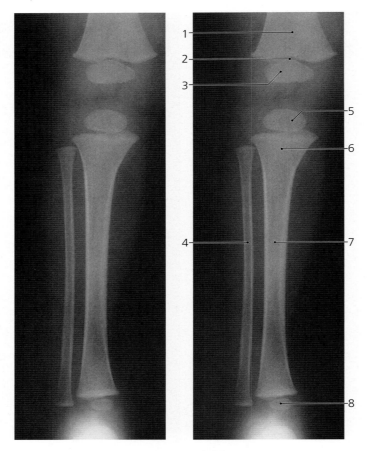

Leg, a-p X-ray, child 1 year

1: Metaphysis of femur	4: Diaphysis of fibula	7: Diaphysis of tibia
2: Growth plate	5: Proximal epiphysis of tibia	8: Distal epiphysis of tibia
3: Distal epiphysis of femur	6: Metaphysis of tibia	

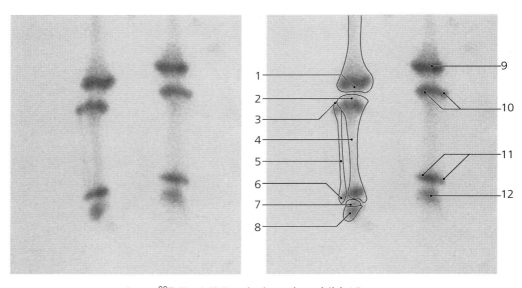

Leg, ^{99m} Tc- MDP, scintigraphy, child 12 years

1: Distal epiphysis of femur	7: Talus	11: Distal growth plates of tibia and fibula
2: Proximal epiphysis of tibia	8: Calcaneus	12: Tarsal bones
3: Proximal epiphysis of fibula	9: Distal growth plate of femur	
4: Diaphysis of tibia	10: Proximal growth plates of tibia and fibula	
5: Diaphysis of fibula		
6: Distal epiphysis of fibula		

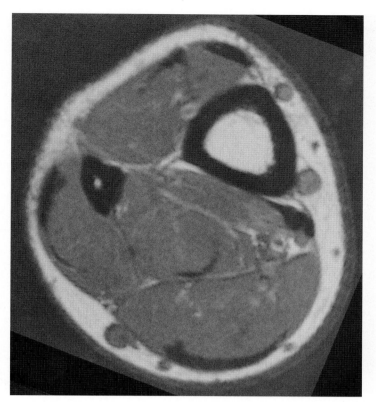

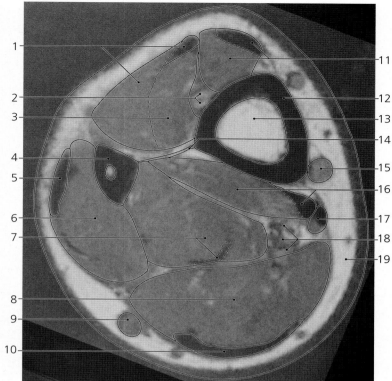

Leg, middle, axial MR

1: Extensor digitorum longus with tendon
2: Anterior tibial artery, and deep peroneal nerve
3: Extensor hallucis longus
4: Fibula
5: Peroneus longus (tendon)
6: Peroneus brevis
7: Flexor hallucis longus with tendon
8: Soleus
9: Small saphenous vein
10: Gastrocnemius (tendon)
11: Tibialis anterior (with tendon)
12: Compact bone of tibia
13: Bone marrow (yellow)
14: Interosseus membrane
15: Great saphenous vein
16: Tibialis posterior (with tendon)
17: Flexor digitorum longus (with tendon)
18: Posterior tibial artery, tibial nerve, and veins
19: Subcutaneous fat

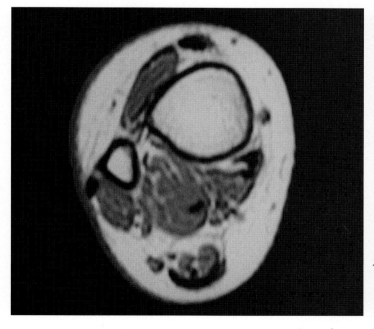

Leg, lower fourth, axial MR

1: Tibialis anterior
2: Extensor hallucis longus
3: Extensor digitorum longus
4: Tibia
5: Interosseus membrane
6: Fibula
7: Flexor hallucis longus (with tendon)
8: Peroneus longus (tendon)
9: Peroneus brevis
10: Small saphenous vein and sural nerve
11: Anterior tibial artery
12: Great saphenous vein
13: Tibialis posterior
14: Flexor digitorum longus
15: Posterior tibial veins
16: Posterior tibial artery
17: Tibial nerve
18: Soleus
19: Calcaneal tendon (Achilles)

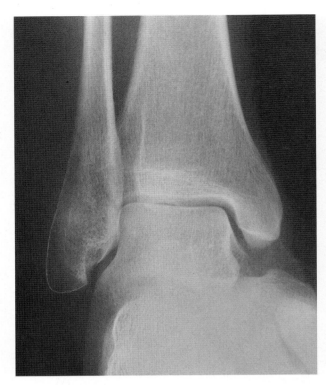

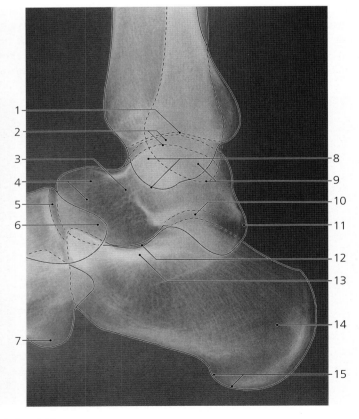

Ankle, a-p X-ray

1: Fibula
2: Tibiofibular syndesmosis
3: Lateral malleolus

4: Trochlea of talus
5: Lateral process of talus
6: Calcaneus

7: Tibia
8: Medial malleolus
9: Talocrural joint

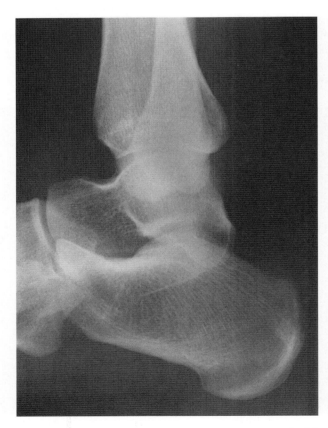

Ankle, lateral X-ray

1: Inferior articular surface of tibia
2: Trochlea of talus
3: Neck of talus
4: Head of talus
5: Talonavicular joint

6: Tuberosity of navicular bone
7: Tuberosity of cuboid bone
8: Medial malleolus
9: Lateral malleolus
10: Subtalar joint

11: Posterior process of talus
12: Middle talocalcanean joint
13: Sustentaculum tali
14: Tuber calcanei
15: Calcaneal tuberosity

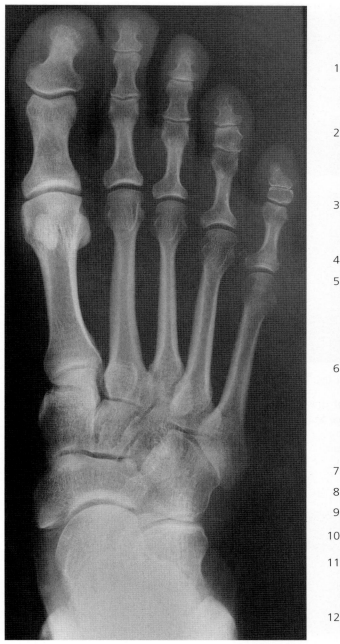
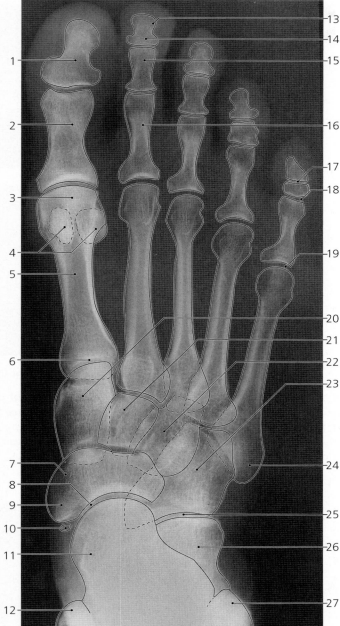

Foot, dorso-plantar X-ray

1: Distal phalanx of great toe
2: Proximal phalanx of great toe
3: Head of first metatarsal bone
4: Sesamoid bones
5: Shaft of first metatarsal bone
6: Base of first metatarsal bone
7: Navicular bone
8: Talonavicular joint
9: Tuberosity of navicular bone
10: Sesamoid bone in tendon of flexor
    digitorum longus

11: Head of talus
12: Medial malleolus
13: Tuberosity of distal phalanx
14: Distal phalanx
15: Middle phalanx
16: Proximal phalanx
17: Distal interphalangeal joint ("DIP")
18: Proximal interphalangeal joint ("PIP")
19: Metatarsophalangeal joint ("MTP")
20: Medial cuneiform bone
21: Intermediate cuneiform bone

22: Lateral cuneiform bone
23: Cuboid bone
24: Tuberosity of fifth metatarsal
25: Calcaneocuboideal joint
26: Calcaneus
27: Lateral malleolus

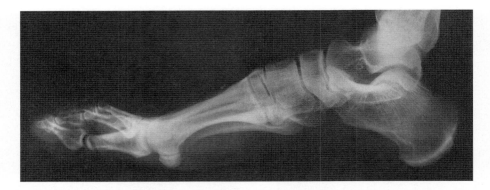

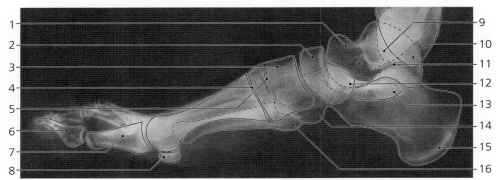

Foot, lateral X-ray

1: Head of talus
2: Navicular bone
3: Medial cuneiform bone
4: First tarsometatarseal joint
5: Second and third tarsometatarseal joints

6: Distal phalanx of great toe
7: Proximal phalanx of great toe
8: Sesamoid bones
9: Lateral malleolus
10: Medial malleolus
11: Subtalar joint

12: Tuberosity of navicular bone
13: Sustentaculum tali
14: Tuberosity of cuboid bone
15: Tuber calcanei
16: Tuberosity of fifth metatarseal

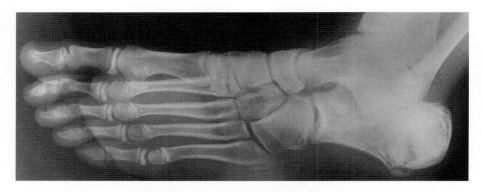

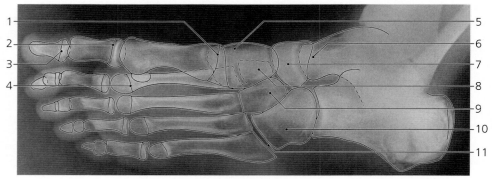

Foot, oblique X-ray

1: Growth plate of first metatarseal
2: Growth plate of proximal phalanx of great toe
3: Growth plate of distal phalanx of great toe

4: Growth plate of second metatarsal bone
5: Medial cuneiform bone
6: Head of talus
7: Navicular bone

8: Intermediate cuneiform bone
9: Lateral cuneiform bone
10: Cuboid bone
11: Fifth tarsometatarseal joint

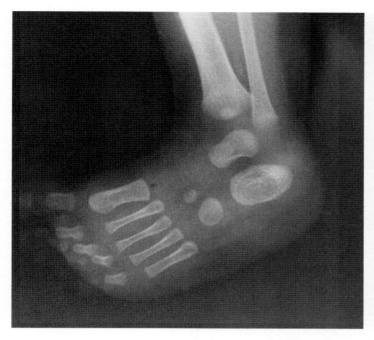
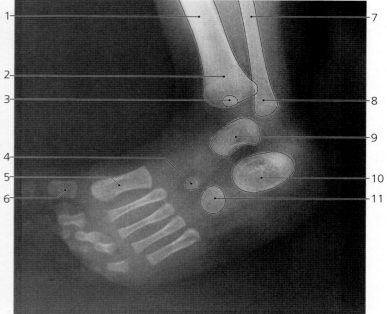

Foot, oblique X-ray, child 3 months

1: Diaphysis of tibia
2: Distal metaphysis of tibia
3: Distal epiphysis of tibia (ossification center)
4: Lateral cuneiform bone (ossification center)
5: Diaphysis of first metatarsal bone
6: Diaphysis of proximal phalanx of great toe
7: Diaphysis of fibula
8: Distal metaphysis of fibula
9: Talus (ossification center)
10: Calcaneus (ossification center)
11: Cuboid bone (ossification center)

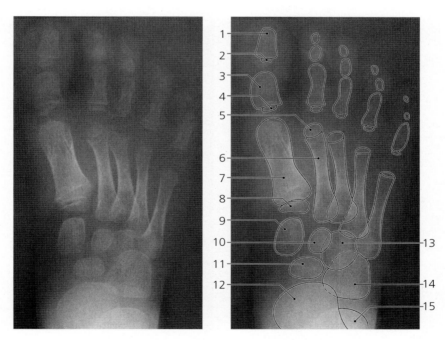

Foot, dorso-plantar X-ray, child 5 years

1: Diaphysis of distal phalanx
2: Epiphysis of distal phalanx
3: Diaphysis of proximal phalanx
4: Epiphysis of proximal phalanx
5: Epiphysis of second metatarsal bone
6: Diaphysis of second metatarsal bone
7: Diaphysis of first metatarsal bone
8: Epiphysis of first metatarsal bone
9: Medial cuneiforme bone
10: Intermediate cuneiforme bone
11: Navicular bone
12: Head of talus
13: Lateral cuneiforme bone
14: Cuboid bone
15: Calcaneus

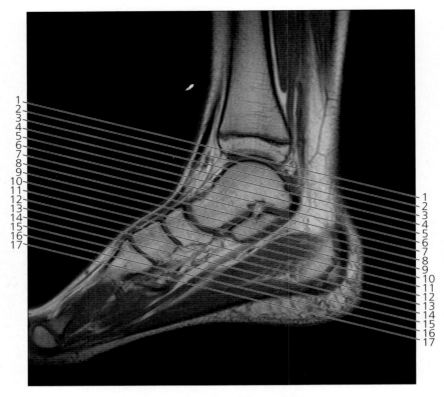

Scout view of ankle and foot

Lines #1–17 indicate position of sections in the following axial MR series. Interpretation of the scout image can be found in the sagittal series, page 167, image #8.

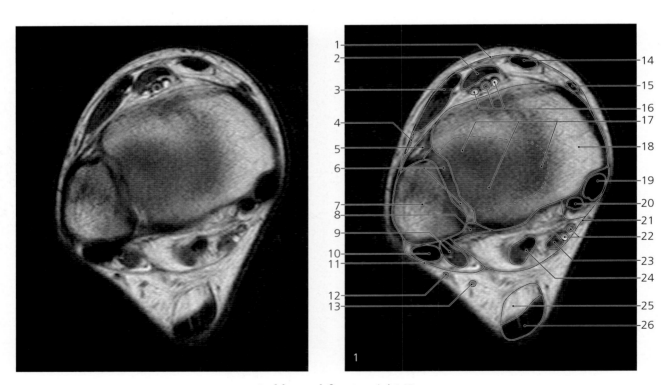

Ankle and foot, axial MR

1: Superior extensor retinaculum/ fascia cruris →
2: Extensor hallucis longus →
3: Extensor digitorum longus →
4: Peroneus tertius →
5: Anterior tibiofibular ligament →
6: Syndesmosis →
7: Lateral malleolus →
8: Posterior tibiofibular ligament →

9: Peroneus brevis →
10: Peroneus longus →
11: Superior peroneal retinaculum →
12: Small saphenous vein →
13: Sural nerve →
14: Tibialis anterior →
15: Great saphenous vein →
16: Dorsalis pedis artery and veins →
17: Articular cartilage of talocrural joint

18: Medial malleolus →
19: Tibialis posterior →
20: Flexor digitorum longus →
21: Flexor retinaculum →
22: Posterior tibial artery and vein →
23: Tibial nerve →
24: Flexor hallucis longus →
25: Karger's fat pad →
26: Calcaneal tendon (Achilles) →

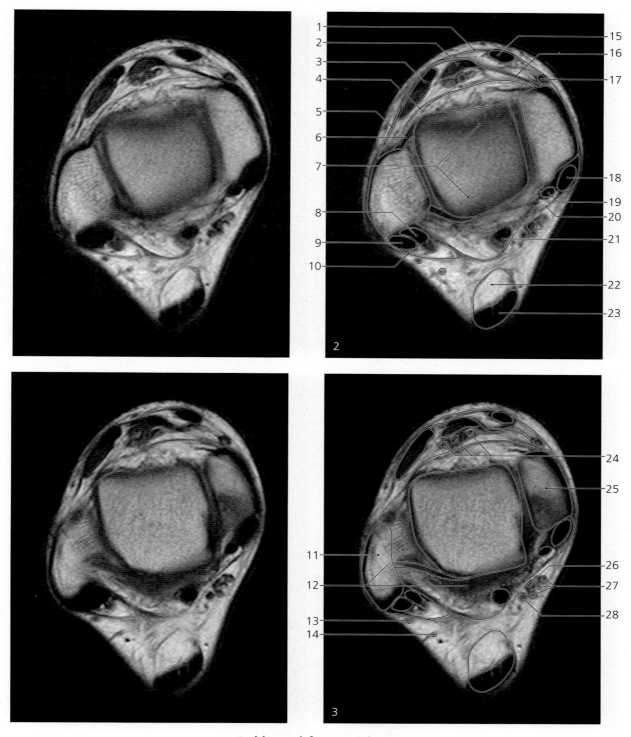

Ankle and foot, axial MR

Scout view on page 150

 1: **Superior extensor retinaculum/ fascia cruris** ↔
 2: **Extensor hallucis longus** ↔
 3: **Extensor digitorum longus** ↔
 4: **Anterior articular capsule** →
 5: **Peroneus tertius** ↔
 6: **Anterior tibiofibular ligament (lower edge)** ←
 7: **Trochlea tali** →
 8: **Peroneus brevis (muscle and tendon)** ↔

 9: **Peroneus longus** ↔
10: **Superior peroneal retinaculum** ↔
11: **Lateral malleolus** ↔
12: **Posterior articular capsule and syndesmosis tibiofibulare**
13: **Small saphenous vein** ↔
14: **Sural nerve** ↔
15: **Tibialis anterior** ↔
16: **Inferior extensor retinaculum** →
17: **Great saphenous vein** ↔
18: **Tibialis posterior** ↔
19: **Flexor digitorum longus** ↔

20: **Flexor retinaculum** ↔
21: **Flexor hallucis longus (muscle and tendon)** ↔
22: **Karger's fat pad** ↔
23: **Calcaneal tendon (Achilles)** ↔
24: **Dorsalis pedis artery and veins** ↔
25: **Medial malleolus** ↔
26: **Medial plantar nerve** ↔
27: **Posterior tibial artery and veins** ↔
28: **Lateral plantar nerve** ↔

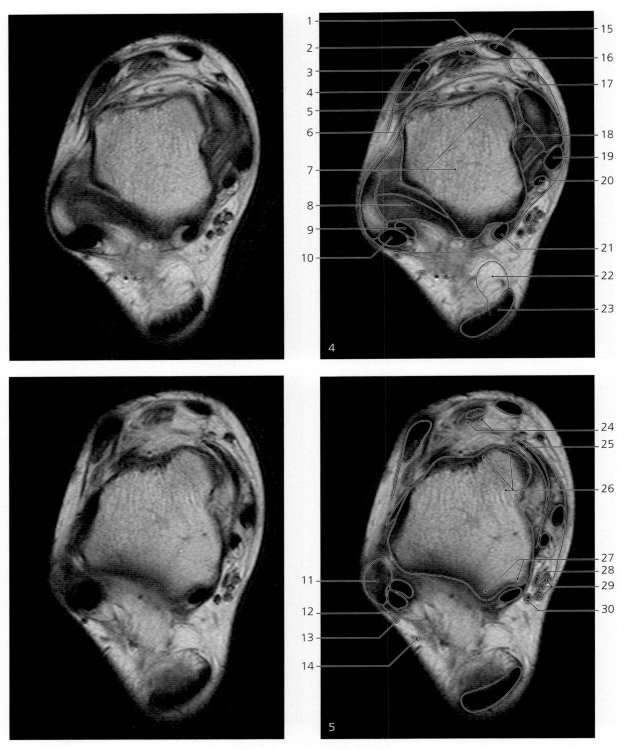

Ankle and foot, axial MR

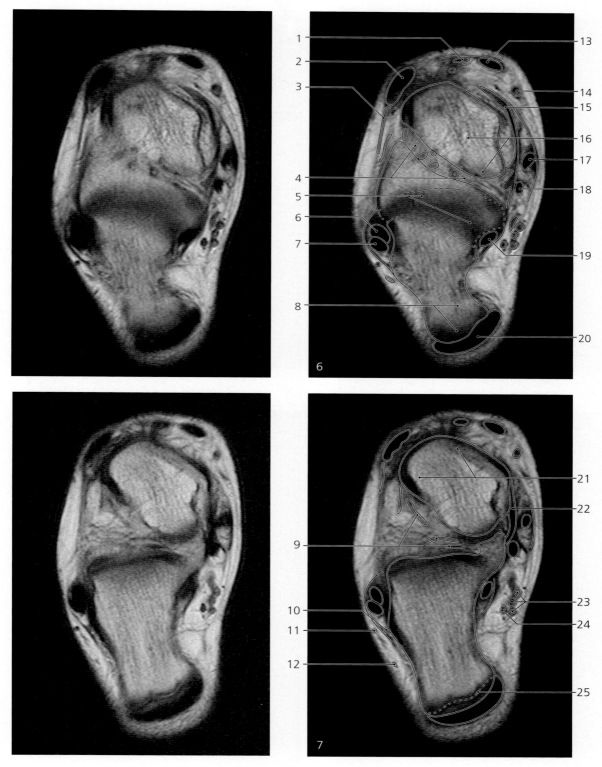

Ankle and foot, axial MR

Scout view on page 150

1: Extensor hallucis longus ↔
2: Extensor digitorum longus ↔
3: Peroneus tertius ↔
4: Tarsal sinus with talocalcanean ligaments →
5: Subtalar joint, posterior chamber (articular cartilage)
6: Peroneus brevis ↔
7: Peroneus longus ↔

8: Tuber calcanei
9: Talocalcanean ligaments in tarsal sinus ↔
10: Calcaneofibular ligament ←
11: Small saphenous vein ↔
12: Sural nerve ↔
13: Tibialis anterior ↔
14: Great saphenous vein →
15: Deltoid ligament ↔
16: Neck of talus ←

17: Tibialis posterior ↔
18: Flexor digitorum longus ↔
19: Flexor hallucis longus ↔
20: Calcanean tendon (Achilles) ↔
21: Head of talus →
22: Deltoid ligament ←
23: Posterior tibial artery and veins ←
24: Lateral plantar nerve ↔
25: Apophysial cartilage disc →

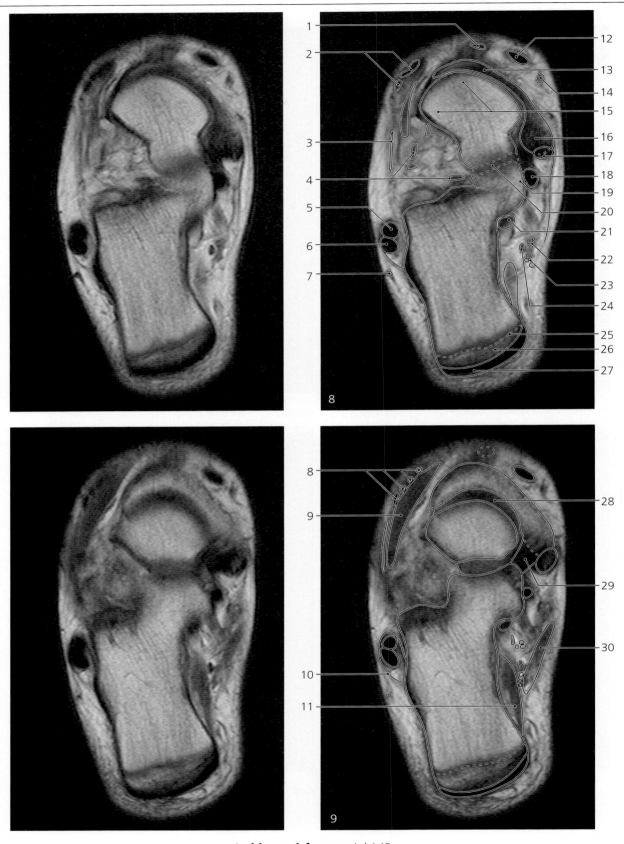

Ankle and foot, axial MR

Scout view on page 150

1: **Extensor hallucis longus** ↔
2: **Extensor digitorum longus** ↔
3: **Peroneus tertius** ↔
4: **Talocalcanean ligaments in tarsal sinus** ←
5: **Peroneus brevis** ↔
6: **Peroneus longus** ↔
7: **Small saphenous vein** ↔
8: **Extensor digitorum longus** ↔
9: **Extensor digitorum brevis** ↔
10: **Inferior peroneal retinaculum** ↔

11: **Quadratus plantae** →
12: **Tibialis anterior** ↔
13: **Navicular bone** →
14: **Great saphenous vein** ←
15: **Head of talus** ↔
16: **Tuberosity of navicular** →
17: **Tibialis posterior (insertion)** ↔
18: **Flexor digitorum longus** ↔
19: **Sustentaculum tali** →
20: **Calcaneonavicular joint (anterior chamber of subtalar joint)**

21: **Flexor hallucis longus** ↔
22: **Medial plantar artery and veins** ↔
23: **Lateral plantar artery and veins** ↔
24: **Lateral plantar nerve** ↔
25: **Apophysial disc** ↔
26: **Calcanean tuberosity** →
27: **Calcanean (Achilles) tendon** ↔
28: **Talonavicular joint** ←
29: **Plantar calcaneonavicular (spring) ligament** →
30: **Abductor hallucis** →

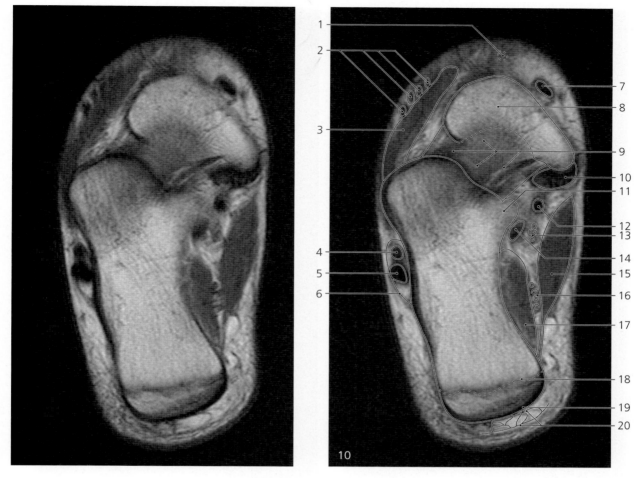

Ankle and foot, axial MR

Scout view on page 150

1: Extensor hallucis longus ↔
2: Extensor digitorum longus →
3: Extensor digitorum brevis ↔
4: Peroneus brevis ↔
5: Peroneus longus ↔
6: Inferior peroneal retinaculum ↔
7: Tibialis anterior ↔

8: Navicular bone ↔
9: Plantar calcaneonavicular (spring)
   ligament ←
10: Sesamoid bone (tibialis externum)
    and tibialis posterior (insertion)
11: Sustentaculum tali ←
12: Flexor digitorum longus ↔
13: Medial plantar artery and veins ↔

14: Flexor hallucis longus ↔
15: Abductor hallucis ↔
16: Lateral plantar artery and veins ↔
17: Quadratus plantae ↔
18: Apophysial disc ↔
19: Calcanean tuberosity ↔
20: Retinacula cutis (skin ligaments) ↔

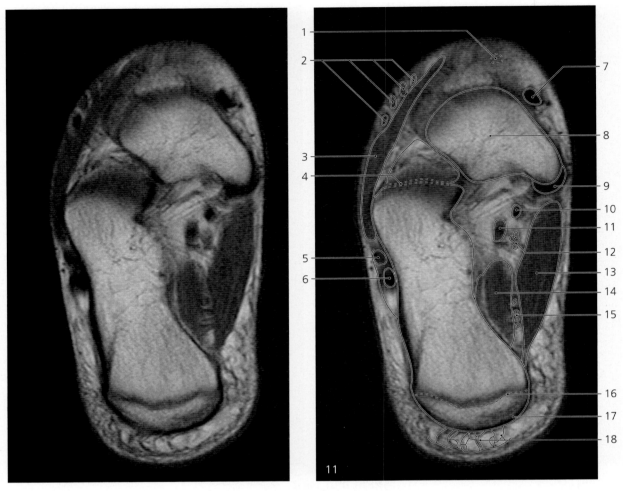

Ankle and foot, axial MR

Scout view on page 150
1: Extensor hallucis longus ↔
2: Extensor digitorum longus ↔
3: Extensor digitorum brevis ↔
4: Calcaneocuboid joint
5: Peroneus brevis ↔
6: Peroneus longus ↔

7: Tibialis anterior ↔
8: Navicular bone ↔
9: Tibialis posterior (insertion) ←
10: Flexor digitorum longus ↔
11: Flexor hallucis longus ↔
12: Medial plantar artery and veins ↔
13: Abductor hallucis ↔

14: Quadratus plantae ↔
15: Lateral plantar artery and veins ↔
16: Apophysial disc ↔
17: Calcanean tuberosity ↔
18: Retinacula cutis (skin ligaments) ↔

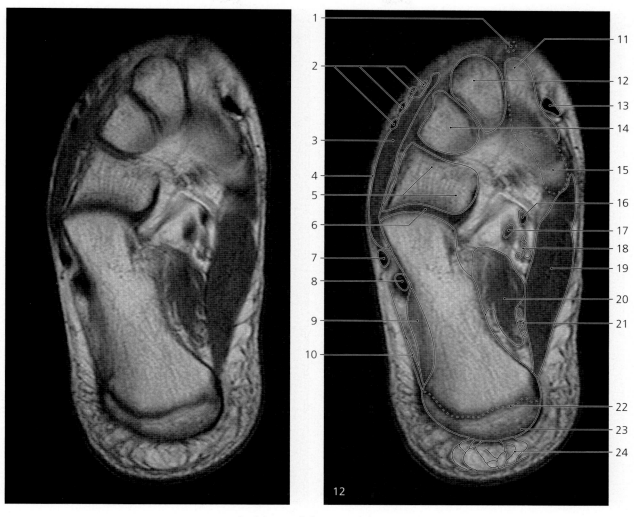

Ankle and foot, axial MR

Scout view on page 150
1: Extensor hallucis longus ↔
2: Extensor digitorum longus ↔
3: Extensor digitorum brevis ↔
4: Peroneus tertius ↔
5: Cuboid bone ↔
6: Calcaneocuboid joint ↔
7: Peroneus brevis ↔
8: Peroneus longus ↔

9: Flexor digitorum brevis →
10: Abductor digiti minimi →
11: Medial cuneiform bone →
12: Intermediate cuneiform bone →
13: Tibialis anterior ↔
14: Lateral cuneiform bone →
15: Navicular bone ←
16: Flexor digitorum longus ↔
17: Flexor hallucis longus ↔

18: Medial plantar artery and veins ↔
19: Abductor hallucis ↔
20: Quadratus plantae ↔
21: Lateral plantar artery and veins ↔
22: Apophysial disc ↔
23: Calcanean tuberosity ←
24: Retinacula cutis (skin ligaments) ↔

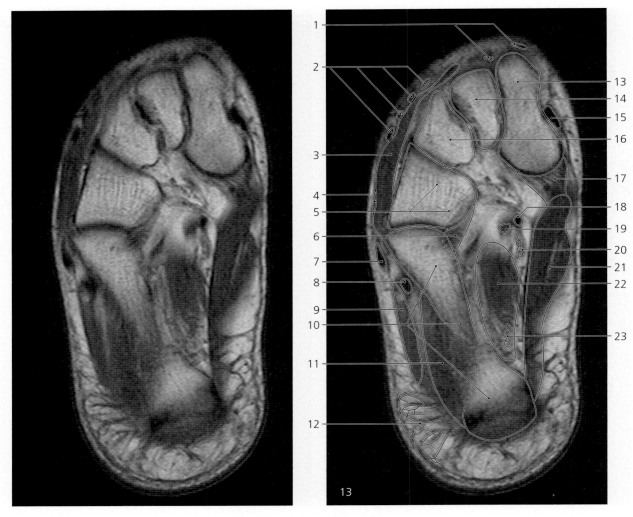

Ankle and foot, axial MR

Scout view on page 150
1: Extensor hallucis longus ↔, dorsalis pedis artery and deep peroneal nerve →
2: Extensor digitorum longus ↔
3: Extensor digitorum brevis ↔
4: Peroneus tertius ↔
5: Cuboid bone ↔
6: Short plantar ligament →
7: Peroneus brevis ↔

8: Peroneus longus ↔
9: Abductor digiti minimi ↔
10: Calcaneus ↔
11: Flexor digitorum brevis ↔
12: Retinacula cutis (skin ligaments) ↔
13: Medial cuneiform bone ↔
14: Intermediate cuneiform bone ↔
15: Tibialis anterior ↔
16: Lateral cuneiform bone ↔

17: Medial plantar cuneonavicular ligament
18: Flexor digitorum longus ↔
19: Flexor hallucis longus ↔
20: Medial plantar artery and veins ↔
21: Abductor hallucis ↔
22: Quadratus plantae ↔
23: Lateral plantar artery and veins ↔

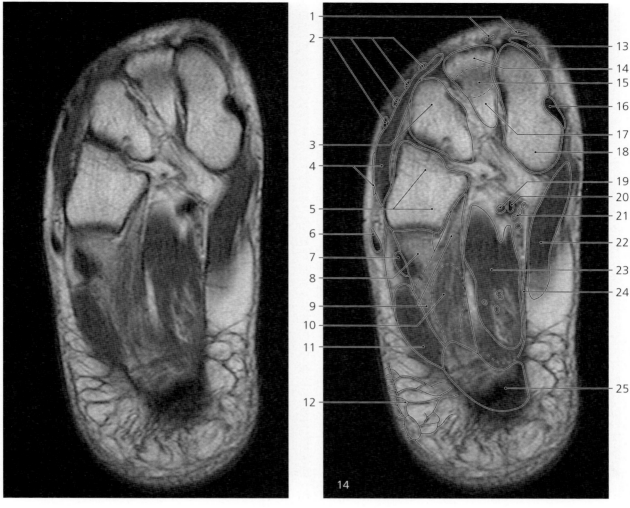

Ankle and foot, axial MR

Scout view on page 150

1: Extensor hallucis longus, dorsalis pedis artery and deep peroneal nerve ↔
2: Extensor digitorum longus ↔
3: Intermediate cuneiform bone ↔
4: Extensor digitorum brevis and peroneus tertius ↔
5: Cuboid bone ↔
6: Peroneus brevis ↔
7: Peroneus longus ↔

8: Short plantar ligament ←
9: Long plantar ligament →
10: Flexor digitorum brevis (superimposed on #9)
11: Abductor digiti minimi ↔
12: Retinacula cutis (skin ligaments) ↔
13: Edge of base of 1st metatarsal bone →
14: 2nd metatarsal bone →
15: 2nd tarsometatarsal joint
16: Tibialis anterior (insertion) ↔

17: Intermediate cuneiform bone ←
18: Medial cuneiform bone ↔
19: Flexor hallucis longus ↔
20: Flexor digitorum longus ↔
21: Medial plantar artery and veins ↔
22: Abductor hallucis ↔
23: Quadratus plantae ↔
24: Intermuscular septum from plantar aponeurosis →
25: Calcaneus ←

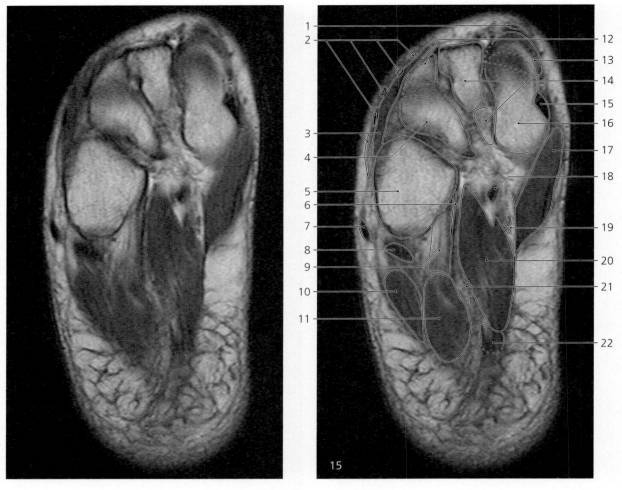

Ankle and foot, axial MR

Scout view on page 150
1: Extensor hallucis longus ↔
2: Extensor digitorum longus ↔
3: Extensor digitorum brevis and
   peroneus tertius ↔
4: Lateral cuneiform bone ↔
5: Cuboid bone ↔
6: Intermuscular septum from plantar
   aponeurosis ←

7: Peroneus brevis ↔
8: Peroneus longus ↔
9: Long plantar ligament ←
10: Abductor digiti minimi ↔
11: Flexor digitorum brevis ↔
12: 3rd metatarsal bone →
13: 1st metatarsal bone ↔
14: 2nd metatarsal and intermediate
    cuneiform bone ↔

15: Tibialis anterior (insertion) ←
16: Medial cuneiform bone ↔
17: Abductor hallucis ↔
18: Flexor hallucis longus and flexor
    digitorum longus (crossing) ↔
19: Medial plantar artery and veins ←
20: Quadratus plantae ↔
21: Lateral plantar artery and veins ←
22: Plantar aponeurosis ↔

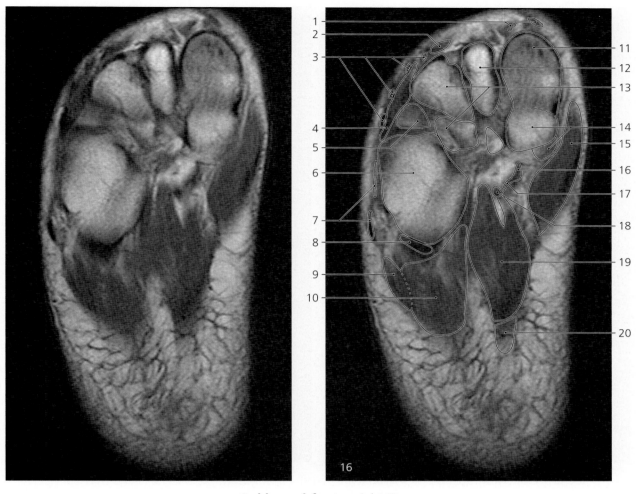

Ankle and foot, axial MR

Scout view on page 150

1: Extensor hallucis longus, dorsalis pedis artery and deep peroneal nerve ↔

2: Extensor hallucis brevis →

3: Extensor digitorum longus ↔

4: Extensor digitorum brevis ↔

5: 5th metatarsal bone (basis)

6: Cuboid bone ↔

7: Peroneus brevis and peroneus tertius ↔

8: Peroneus longus ↔

9: Abductor digiti minimi ↔

10: Flexor digitorum brevis ↔

11: 1st metatarsal bone ↔

12: 2nd metatarsal bone ↔

13: 3rd metatarsal bone ↔ and lateral cuneiform bone ←

14: Medial cuneiform bone ← and flexor hallucis brevis →

15: Abductor hallucis ↔

16: Flexor hallucis longus ↔

17: Intertendinous bridge

18: Flexor digitorum longus ↔

19: Quadratus plantae ↔

20: Plantar aponeurosis ↔

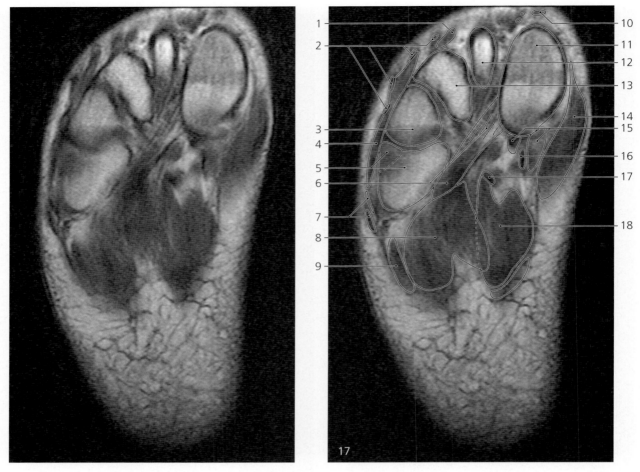

Ankle and foot, axial MR

Scout view on page 150
1: Extensor hallucis brevis ←
2: Extensor digitorum longus ←
3: 4th metatarsal bone
4: Extensor digitorum brevis ←
5: Cuboid bone and 5th metatarsal
   bone ←

6: Peroneus longus (insertion) ←
7: Peroneus brevis and
   peroneus tertius ←
8: Flexor digitorum brevis ←
9: Abductor digiti minimi ←
10: Extensor hallucis longus ←
11: 1st metatarsal bone ←

12: 2nd metatarsal bone ←
13: 3rd metatarsal bone ←
14: Abductor hallucis ←
15: Flexor hallucis brevis ←
16: Flexor hallucis longus ←
17: Flexor digitorum longus ←
18: Quadratus plantae ←

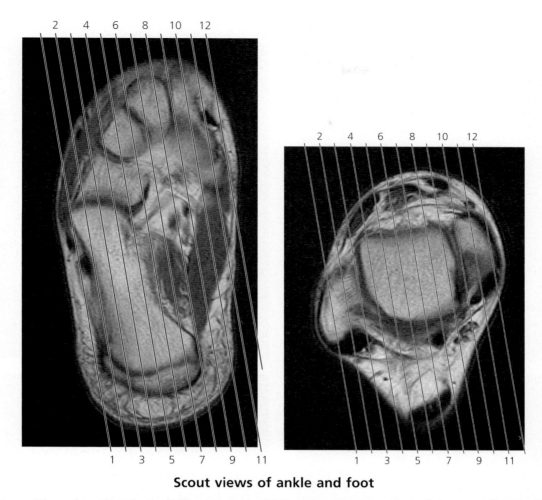

Scout views of ankle and foot

Lines #1–12 indicate position of sections in the following sagittal MR series. Interpretation of the scout images can be found in the axial series, page 157, image #12 and page 151, image #3.

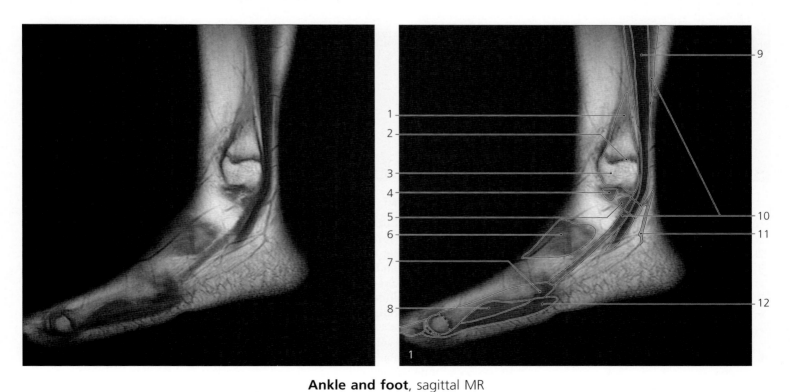

Ankle and foot, sagittal MR

1: Fibula →
2: Epiphysial line →
3: Lateral malleolus →
4: Joint capsule with anterior talofibular ligament →

5: Peroneal retinaculum →
6: Inferior extensor retinaculum and extensor digitorum brevis →
7: Tuberosity of 5th metacarpal bone
8: Flexor digiti minimi brevis →

9: Peroneus longus →
10: Peroneus brevis →
11: Small saphenous vein →
12: Abductor digiti minimi →

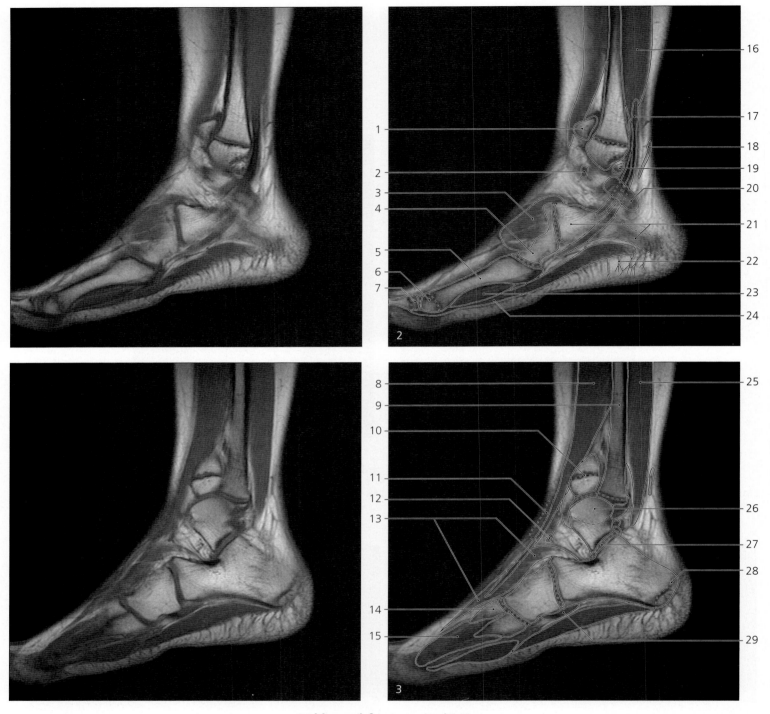

Ankle and foot, sagittal MR

Scout view on page 163
 1: Tibia →
 2: Anterior talofibular ligament ↔
 3: Extensor digitorum brevis →
 4: Cuboid bone →
 5: 5th metatarsal bone ←
 6: Epiphysis of 5th metatarsal bone
 7: Epiphysis of proximal phalanx of
    5th toe
 8: Extensor digitorum longus →
 9: Fibula ←

10: Epiphysial line of tibia →
11: Inferior extensor retinaculum ↔
12: Anterior talofibular ligament ↔
13: Extensor digitorum brevis ↔
14: 4th metatarsal bone (base) →
15: Interosseous muscles →
16: Flexor hallucis longus →
17: Peroneus longus ↔
18: Small saphenous vein ↔
19: Posterior talofibular ligament →
20: Peroneal retinaculum ←

21: Calcaneus →
22: Retinacula cutis (skin ligaments) →
23: Flexor digiti minimi brevis ←
24: Abductor digiti minimi ↔
25: Flexor hallucis longus →
26: Trochlea tali
    (lateral articular surface) →
27: Subtalar joint (posterior chamber) →
28: Apophysial line →
29: Peroneus longus ↔

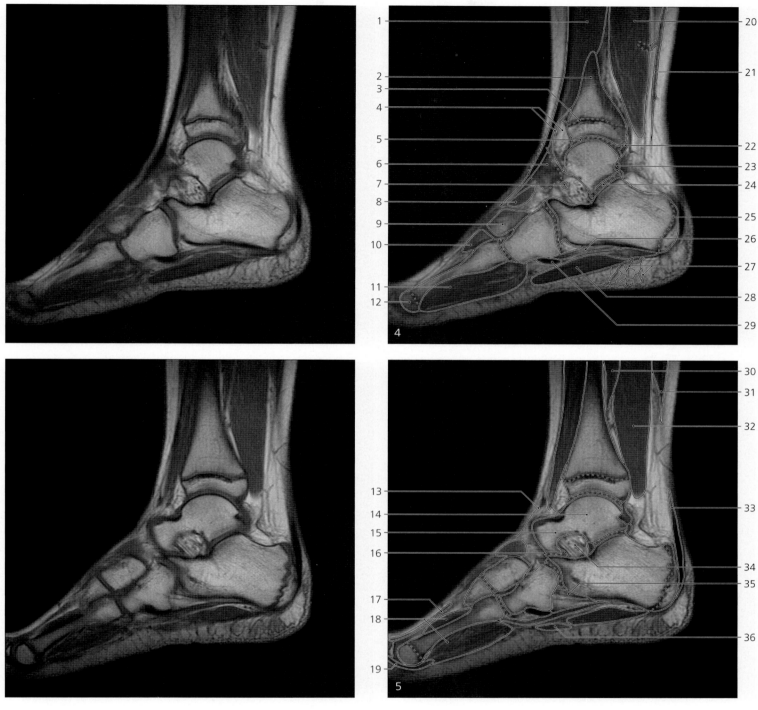

Ankle and foot, sagittal MR

Scout view on page 163

 1: Extensor digitorum longus ↔
 2: Tibia ↔
 3: Epiphysial line ↔
 4: Joint capsule and subsynovial fat pad →
 5: Talocrural joint →
 6: Inferior extensor retinaculum ↔
 7: Anterior talofibular ligament ←
 8: Extensor digitorum brevis ↔
 9: Lateral cuneiform bone →
10: 3rd metatarsal bone (base) →
11: Interosseous muscles ↔
12: 4th metatarsal bone (epiphysis) →

13: Inferior extensor retinaculum ↔
14: Trochlea of talus ↔
15: Neck of talus →
16: Subtalar joint (anterior chamber) ↔
17: Extensor digitorum longus ↔
18: Interosseous muscles ↔
19: Flexor tendons to 4th toe
20: Flexor hallucis longus ↔
21: Small saphenous vein ←
22: Joint capsule →
23: Posterior talofibular ligament (attachment) ←
24: Subtalar joint (posterior chamber) ↔
25: Apophysial line ↔

26: Long plantar ligament →
27: Retinacula cutis (skin ligaments) ↔
28: Abductor digiti minimi ↔
29: Peroneus longus ↔
30: Flexor digitorum longus →
31: Soleus →
32: Flexor hallucis longus ↔
33: Calcaneal tendon (Achilles) →
34: Tarsal sinus with talocalcanean ligaments →
35: Short plantar ligament →
36: Flexor digitorum brevis →

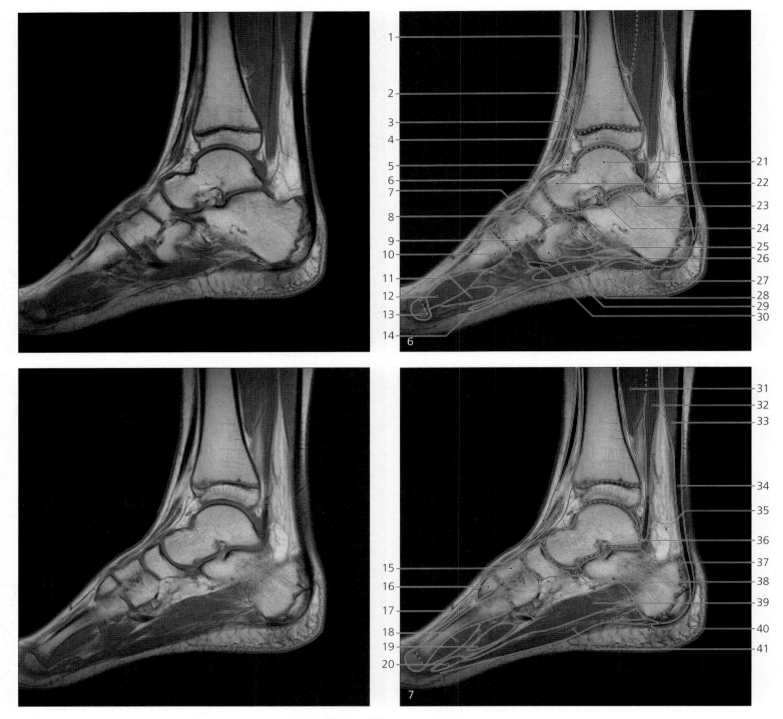

Ankle and foot, sagittal MR

Scout view on page 163
1: Tibialis anterior →
2: Extensor hallucis longus →
3: Extensor digitorum longus ↔
4: Epiphysis of tibia ↔
5: Joint capsule with subsynovial fat pad ↔
6: Inferior extensor retinaculum ↔
7: Extensor hallucis brevis ←
8: Navicular bone →
9: Lateral cuneiform bone ←
10: 3rd metatarsal ←
11: Adductor hallucis (oblique head) →
12: Interosseous muscles ↔
13: 4th metatarsal bone (epiphysis) ←

14: Flexor tendons
15: Intermediate cuneiform bone →
16: 2nd metatarsal bone (base) →
17: Extensor tendons
18: Interosseous muscles ↔
19: Adductor hallucis (oblique head) ↔
20: Adductor hallucis (transverse head)
21: Trochlea of talus ↔
22: Head of talus →
23: Subtalar joint (posterior chamber) ↔
24: Tarsal sinus ↔
25: Subtalar joint (anterior chamber) ↔
26: Short plantar ligament ←
27: Abductor digiti minimi ←
28: Flexor digitorum brevis ↔

29: Cuboid bone ←
30: Peroneus longus ↔
31: Flexor digitorum longus ↔
32: Flexor hallucis longus ↔
33: Soleus ↔
34: Calcaneal tendon (Achilles) ↔
35: Kager's fat pad ←
36: Posterior process of talus
37: Apophysial line ↔
38: Plantar calcaneonavicular (spring) ligament →
39: Quadratus plantae →
40: Plantar aponeurosis →
41: Flexor digitorum brevis ↔

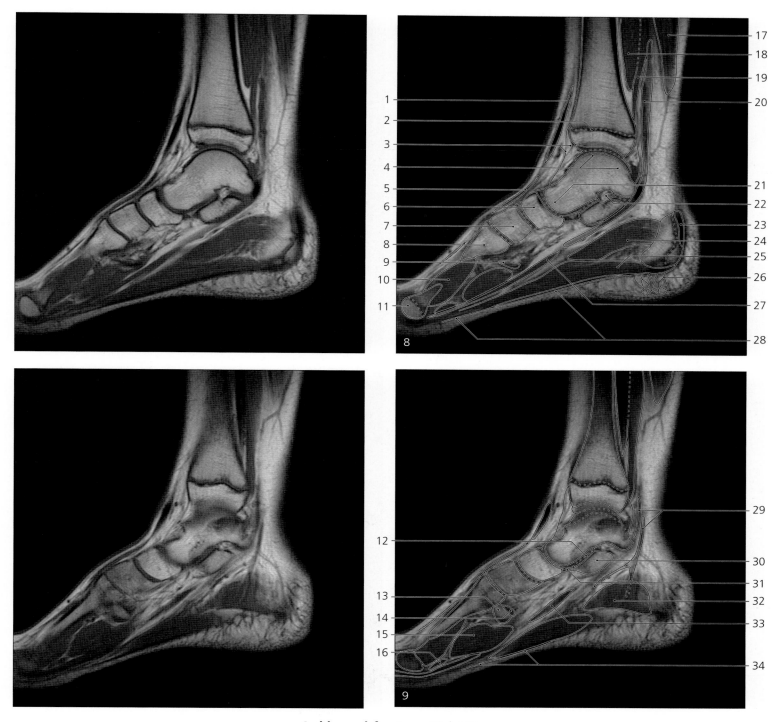

Ankle and foot, sagittal MR

Scout view on page 163

1: Tibialis anterior ↔
2: Epiphysial line ↔
3: Joint capsule and subsynovial fat pad ←
4: Trochlea of talus ↔
5: Extensor hallucis longus ↔
6: Navicular bone ↔
7: Intermediate cuneiform bone ↔
8: 2nd metatarsal bone ↔
9: Peroneus longus ↔
10: Interosseous muscles ↔
11: 3rd metatarsal bone (epiphysis) ←

12: Subtalar joint (anterior chamber) ←
13: 1st metatarsal bone (base) →
14: Peroneus longus (insertion) ←
15: Adductor hallucis ↔
16: Flexor tendons to 2nd toe
17: Soleus ←
18: Tibialis posterior →
19: Flexor digitorum longus ↔
20: Flexor hallucis longus ↔
21: Head of talus ↔
22: Tarsal sinus ←
23: Calcaneal tendon (Achilles), insertion ←

24: Quadratus plantae ←
25: Flexor digitorum brevis ←
26: Retinacula cutis (skin ligaments) ↔
27: Flexor digitorum longus ↔
28: Plantar aponeurosis ↔
29: Posterior tibial artery and vein →
30: Sustentaculum tali
31: Plantar calcaneonavicular (spring) ligament ←
32: Abductor hallucis →
33: Flexor digitorum longus and flexor hallucis longus (crossing) ↔
34: Plantar aponeurosis ↔

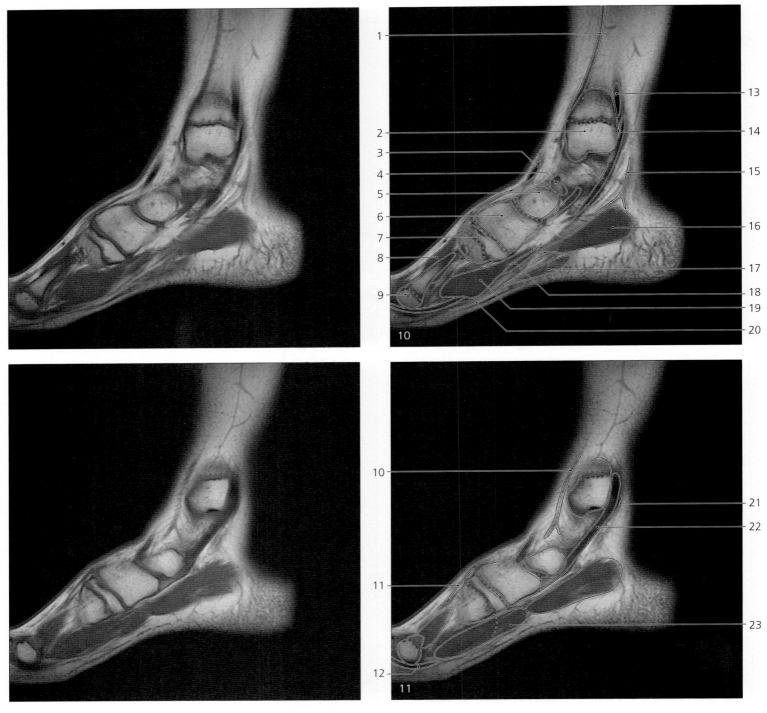

Ankle and foot, sagittal MR

Scout view on page 163

1: Great saphenous vein →
2: Medial malleolus →
3: Tibialis anterior ↔
4: Head of talus ←
5: Navicular bone ↔
6: Medial cuneiform bone →
7: 1st metatarsal bone (epiphysis) ↔

8: Interosseous muscles ←
9: 2nd metatarsal bone (epiphysis) ↔
10: Great saphenous vein ↔
11: Extensor hallucis longus ↔
12: Flexor tendons to 2nd toe
13: Tibialis posterior ↔
14: Flexor digitorum longus ←
15: Posterior tibial vessel

16: Abductor hallucis ↔
17: Flexor digitorum brevis ←
18: Flexor hallucis longus ↔
19: Adductor hallucis ↔
20: Plantar aponeurosis ←
21: Flexor retinaculum
22: Tibialis posterior ↔
23: Flexor hallucis brevis (lateral head)

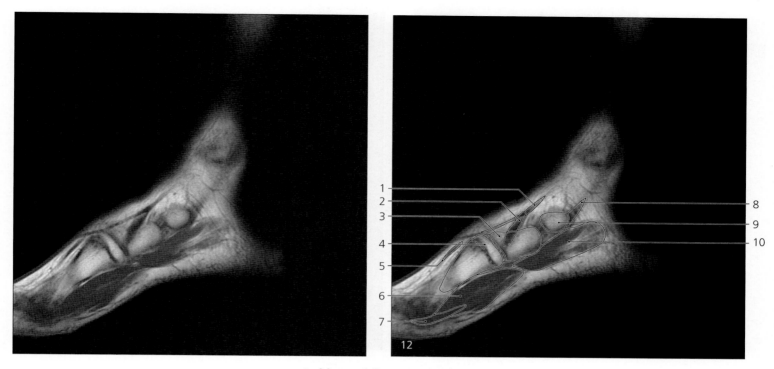

Ankle and foot, sagittal MR

Scout view on page 163
1: Great saphenous vein ←
2: Tibialis anterior (insertion) ←
3: Medial cuneiform bone ←

4: 1st metatarsal bone (epiphysis) ←
5: Extensor hallucis longus ←
6: Adductor hallucis and
   flexor hallucis brevis ←

7: Flexor hallucis longus ←
8: Tibialis posterior (insertion) ←
9: Tuberosity of navicular bone ←
10: Abductor hallucis ←

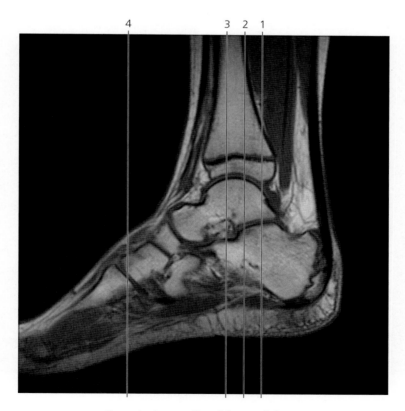

Scout view of ankle and foot

Lines #1–4 indicate position of sections in the following coronal MR series. Interpretation of the scout image can be found in the sagittal series, page 166, image #6.

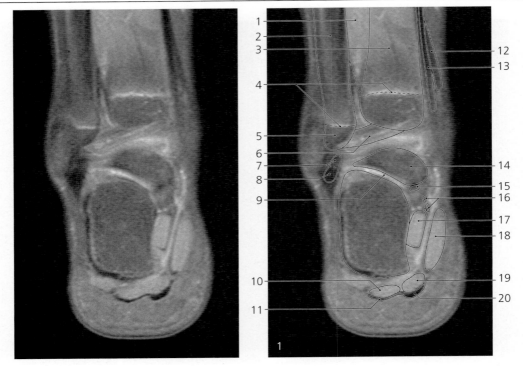

Ankle, coronal MR

Scout view on page 169

1: Flexor hallucis longus ←
2: Fibula ←
3: Tibia ←
4: Epiphysial lines ←
5: Lateral malleolus ←
6: Posterior tibiofibular ligament

7: Peroneus brevis ←
8: Peroneus longus ←
9: Subtalar joint (posterior chamber)
10: Abductor digiti minimi ←
11: Plantar aponeurosis (lateral band)
12: Tibialis posterior ←
13: Flexor digitorum longus ←

14: Posterior process of talus
15: Flexor hallucis longus ←
16: Medial and lateral plantar vessels and nerves ←
17: Quadratus plantae ←
18: Abductor hallucis ←
19: Flexor digitorum brevis ←
20: Plantar aponeurosis (medial band) ←

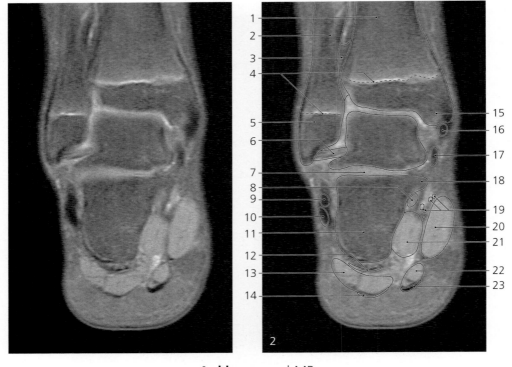

Ankle, coronal MR

Scout view on page 169

1: Tibia ↔
2: Fibula ↔
3: Syndesmosis
4: Epiphysial lines ↔
5: Lateral malleolus ↔
6: Posterior talofibular ligament
7: Tarsal sinus ←

8: Flexor hallucis longus ↔
9: Peroneus brevis ↔
10: Peroneus longus ↔
11: Calcaneus
12: Long plantar ligament ↔
13: Abductor digiti minimi ↔
14: Plantar aponeurosis (lateral band) ↔
15: Medial malleolus ←

16: Tibialis posterior ↔
17: Flexor digitorum longus ↔
18: Sustentaculum tali ←
19: Medial and lateral plantar vessels and nerves ↔
20: Abductor hallucis ↔
21: Quadratus plantae ↔
22: Flexor digitorum brevis ↔
23: Plantar aponeurosis (medial band) ↔

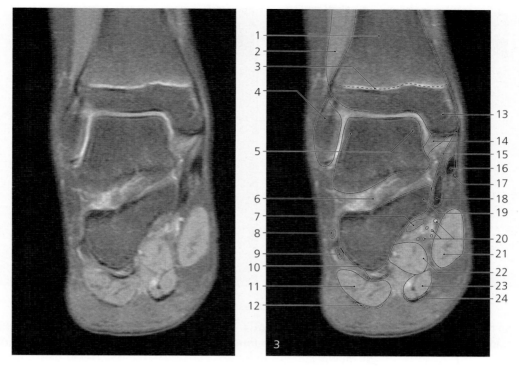

Ankle, coronal MR

Scout view on page 169
1: Tibia →
2: Extensor digitorum longus/ peroneus
   tertius
3: Epiphysial line →
4: Lateral malleolus →
5: Trochlea of talus →
6: Tarsal sinus →
7: Flexor hallucis longus →
8: Peroneus brevis →

9: Peroneus longus →
10: Long plantar ligament →
11: Abductor digiti minimi →
12: Plantar aponeurosis (lateral band) →
13: Medial malleolus →
14: Tibiotalar ligament (part of deltoid
    ligament)
15: Tibiocalcanean ligament (part of
    deltoid ligament)
16: Tibialis posterior →

17: Flexor retinaculum
18: Flexor digitorum longus →
19: Sustentaculum tali →
20: Medial and lateral plantar vessels and
    nerves →
21: Abductor hallucis →
22: Quadratus plantae →
23: Flexor digitorum brevis →
24: Plantar aponeurosis (medial band) →

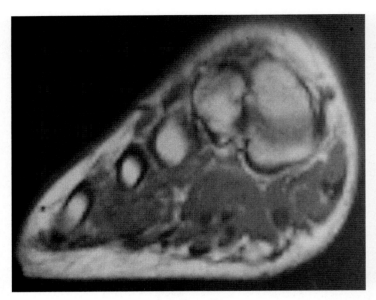
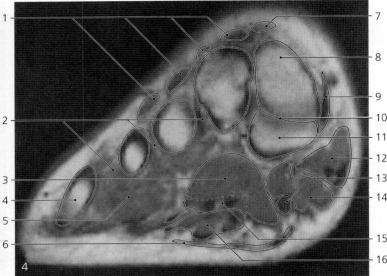

Metatarsus, cross-section MR

Scout view on page 169

1: Extensor digitorum longus, and
   brevis (tendons)
2: Interossei muscles
3: Adductor hallucis, oblique head
4: Fifth metatarsal bone
5: Flexor digiti minimi

6: Plantar aponeurosis
7: Extensor hallucis longus (tendon)
8: Medial cuneiform bone
9: Tibialis anterior (insertion)
10: First tarsometatarsal joint
11: First metatarsal bone
12: Abductor hallucis

13: Flexor hallucis longus (tendon)
14: Flexor hallucis brevis
15: Flexor digitorum longus, and
    lumbricals
16: Flexor digitorum brevis

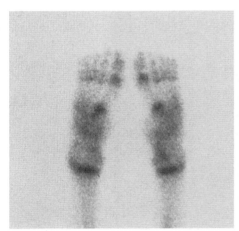
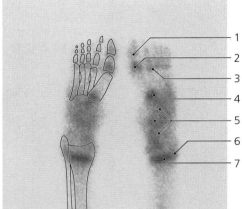

Foot, ^{99m} Tc-MDP, scintigraphy, child 14 years

1: Growth plate of distal phalanx of
   hallux
2: Growth plate of proximal phalanx of
   hallux

3: Growth plate of second metatarsal
   bone
4: Growth plate of first metatarsal bone
5: Tarsal bones

6: Growth plate of distal epiphysis of
   fibula
7: Growth plate of distal epiphysis of
   tibia

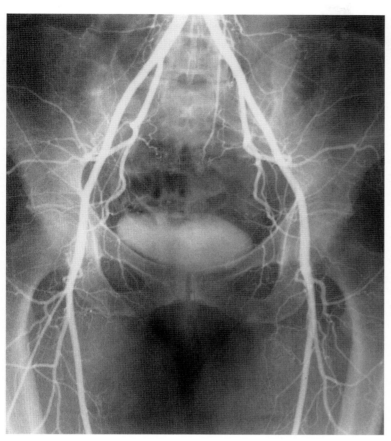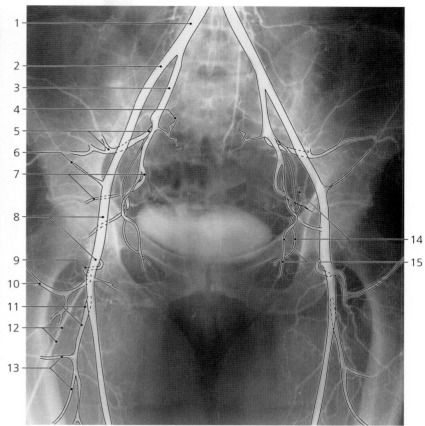

Iliac and femoral arteries, a-p X-ray, arteriography

1: Common iliac artery
2: External iliac artery
3: Internal iliac artery
4: Lateral sacral artery
5: Superior gluteal artery
6: Deep circumflex iliac artery
7: Inferior gluteal artery
8: Femoral artery
9: Medial circumflex femoral artery
10: Lateral circumflex femoral artery
11: Profunda femoris artery
12: Catheter
13: Perforating arteries
14: Internal pudendal artery
15: Obturator artery

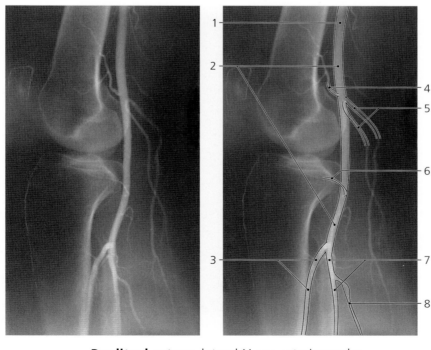

Popliteal artery, lateral X-ray, arteriography

1: Femoral artery
2: Popliteal artery
3: Anterior tibial artery
4: Superior genicular artery
5: Muscular branches to gastrocnemius
6: Inferior genicular artery
7: Posterior tibial artery
8: Muscular branch (Peroneal artery not visible)

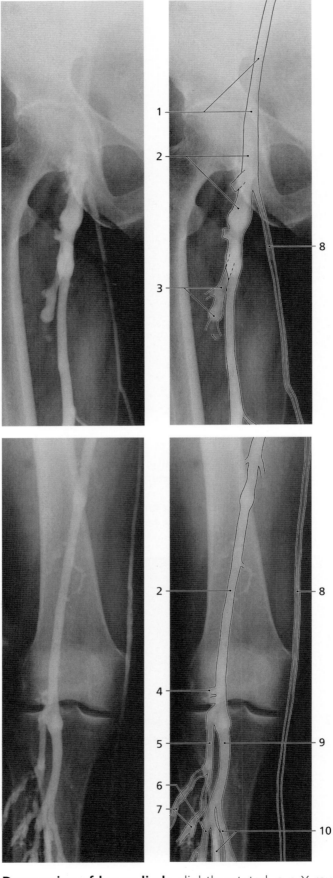

Deep veins of lower limb, slightly rotated, a-p X-ray

1: External iliac vein
2: Femoral vein
3: Deep femoral vein
4: Sural/Small saphenous vein

5: Accessory popliteal vein
6: Peroneal vein
7: Anterior tibial veins
8: Great saphenous vein

9: Popliteal vein
10: Posterior tibial veins

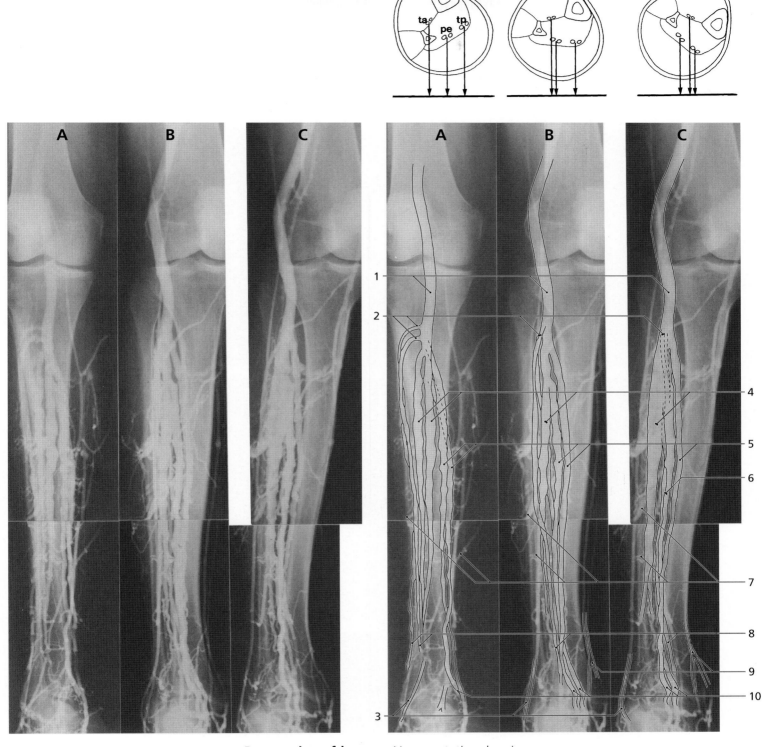

Deep veins of leg, a-p X-ray, rotational series

A: Outward rotation. B: Medium inward
rotation. C: Max. inward rotation
  1: Popliteal vein
  2: Anterior tibial veins
  3: Small saphenous vein

  4: Peroneal veins
  5: Posterior tibial veins
  6: Peroneal and anterior tibial veins
     superpositioned
  7: Perforant veins

  8: Anterior tibial veins
  9: Great saphenous vein
10: Posterior tibial veins behind medial
     malleolus

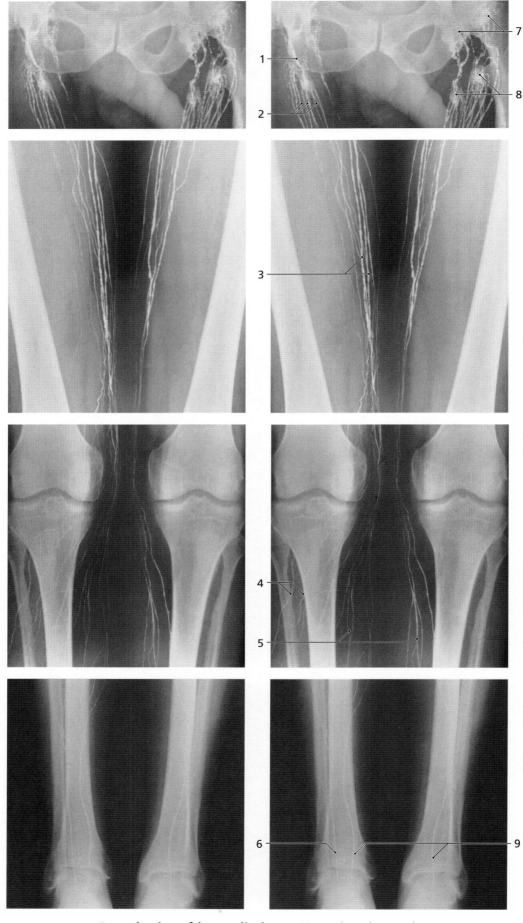

Lymphatics of lower limb, a-p X-ray, lymphography

Contrast infused in lymphatic vessel
of first interdigital space

1: Efferent lymphatic vessel
2: Afferent lymphatic vessels
3: Superficial lymphatics along great
    saphenous vein on thigh

4: Superficial lymphatics coursing
    lateral on lower leg
5: Superficial lymphatics coursing along
    great saphenous vein on lower leg
6: Lateral lymphatic on front of wrist

7: Superficial inguinal lymph nodes (prox. group)
8: Superficial inguinal lymph nodes (distal group)
9: Medial lymphatic along great saphenous vein at wrist

Spine

Cervical spine
Thoracic spine
Lumbar spine

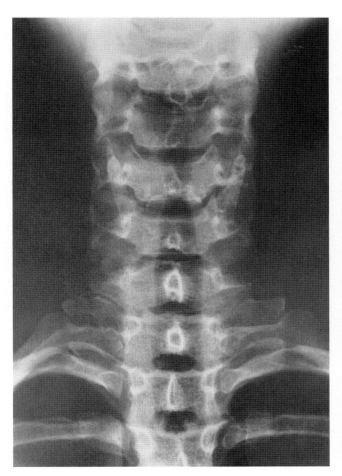
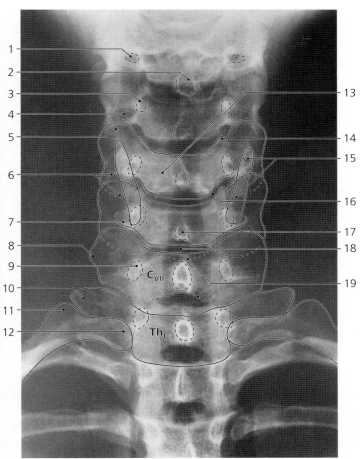

Cervical spine, a-p X-ray

1: Foramen transversarium of C III
2: Spinous process of C III
3: Pedicle of vertebral arch
4: Foramen transversarium of C IV
5: Superior articular process of C V
6: Inferior articular process of C V
7: Anterior tubercle of C VI

8: Transverse process of C VII
9: Pedicle of C VII
10: Transverse process of Th I
11: Tubercle of first rib
12: Head of first rib
13: Body of vertebra C V
14: Uncus (lip) of C V

15: Lamina of thyroid cartilage (calcified)
16: Uncovertebral joint (Luschka)
17: Spinous process of C VI
18: Intervertebral disc C VI – C VII
19: Lamina of vertebral arch C VII

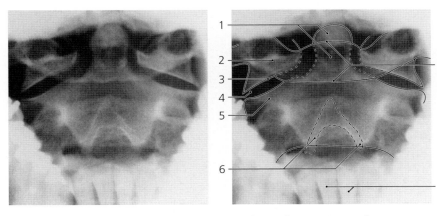

Atlas and axis, a-p X-ray, through open mouth

1: Dens axis
2: Lateral mass of atlas
3: Inferior articular facet of atlas

4: Lateral atlanto-axial joint
5: Superior articular process of axis
6: Spinous process of axis (bifid)

7: Anterior and posterior arch of atlas
8: Lower incisor teeth

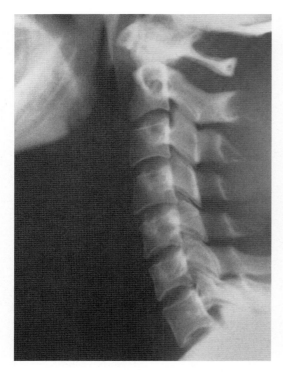
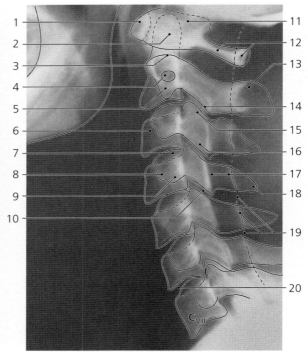

Cervical spine, lateral X-ray

1: Anterior arch of atlas
2: Dens axis
3: Superior articular facet of axis
4: Foramen transversarium of axis
5: Transverse process of axis
6: Body of C III
7: Uncus of C IV
8: Anterior tubercle of transverse process

9: Posterior tubercle of transverse process
10: Zygapophysial (facet) joint C IV – C V
11: Lateral mass of atlas
12: Posterior arch of atlas
13: Spinous process of axis
14: Inferior articular process of axis
15: Superior articular process of C III
16: Inferior articular process of C III

17: Lamina of vertebral arch C IV
18: Spinous process of C IV
19: Posterior wall of vertebral canal
20: Intervertebral disc C VI – C VII

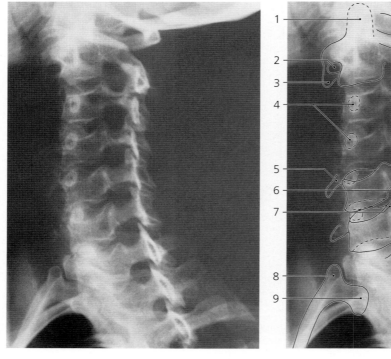
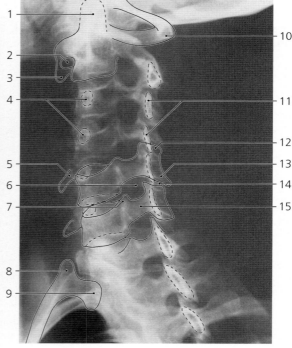

Cervical spine, oblique X-ray

1: Dens axis
2: Foramen transversarium of axis
3: Transverse process of axis
4: Pedicles of vertebral arches C III and C IV
5: Transverse process of C V

6: Intervertebral foramen for sixth cervical spinal nerve
7: Uncus (lip) of vertebral body
8: Tubercle of first rib
9: Head of first rib
10: Posterior arch of atlas

11: Laminae of vertebral arches C III and C IV
12: Superior articular process C V
13: Inferior articular process C V
14: Zygapophysial (facet) joint C V – C VI
15: Pedicle of vertebral arch C VI

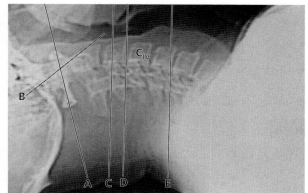
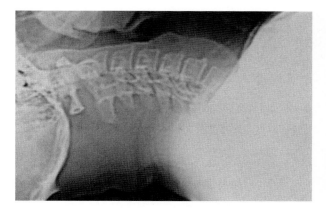

Scout view

Lines A to E indicate position of following sections

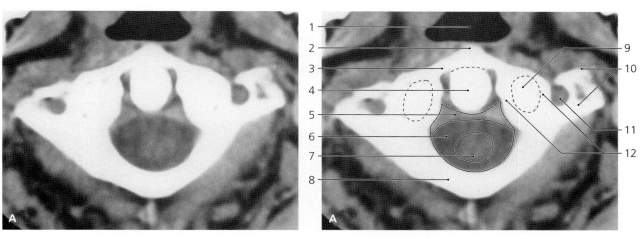

Atlas and axis, axial CT

Position of section A indicated on scout view

1: Pharynx, nasal part
2: Anterior tubercle of atlas
3: Anterior arch of atlas
4: Dens axis
5: Transverse ligament of atlas
6: Subarachnoid space
7: Spinal cord
8: Posterior arch of atlas
9: Occipital condyle
10: Transverse process of atlas
11: Foramen transversarium of atlas
12: Lateral mass of atlas

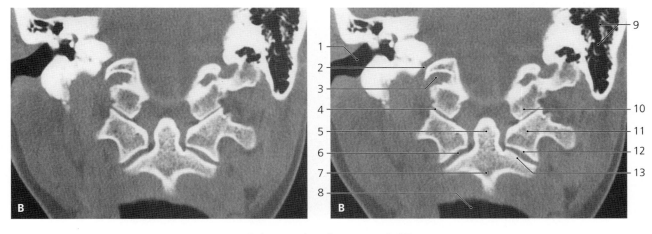

Atlas and axis, coronal CT

Position of section B indicated on scout view

1: External acoustic meatus
2: Jugular foramen
3: Hypoglossal canal
4: Atlanto-occipital joint
5: Dens axis
6: Lateral atlanto-axial joint
7: Body of axis
8: Pharynx
9: Mastoid process
10: Occipital condyle
11: Lateral mass of atlas
12: Inferior articular facet of atlas
13: Superior articular facet of axis

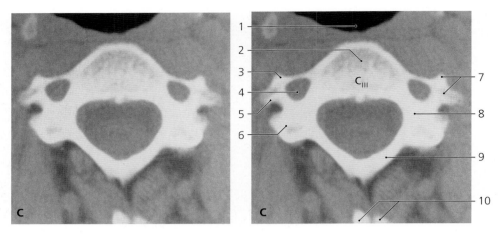

Cervical spine, axial CT

Position of section C indicated on scout
view page 181
  1: Pharynx
  2: Body of vertebra

3: Anterior tubercle
4: Foramen transversarium
5: Posterior tubercle
6: Superior articular process

7: Transverse process
8: Pedicle of vertebral arch
9: Lamina of vertebral arch
10: Spinous process of axis

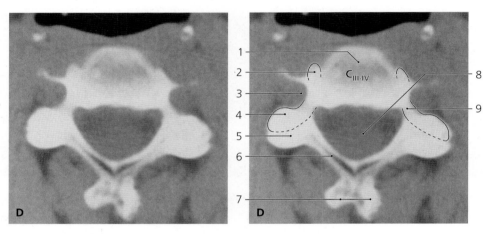

Cervical spine, axial CT

Position of section D indicated on scout
view page 181
  1: Intervertebral disc
  2: Uncus (lip) of body of C IV

3: Groove for spinal nerve
4: Superior articular process of C IV
5: Inferior articular process of C III
6: Lamina of vertebral arch C III

7: Spinous process of C III (bifid)
8: Vertebral canal
9: Pedicle of vertebral arch C IV

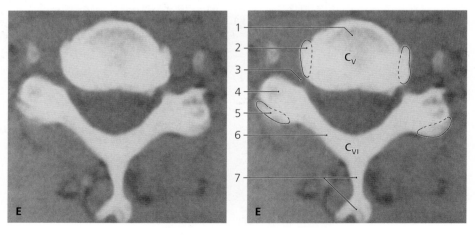

Cervical spine, axial CT

Position of section E indicated on scout
view page 181
  1: Body of vertebra
  2: Uncus (lip) of body of C VI

3: Intervertebral foramen for sixth
   cervical spinal nerve
4: Superior articular process of C VI
5: Inferior articular process of C VI

6: Lamina of vertebral arch
7: Spinous process

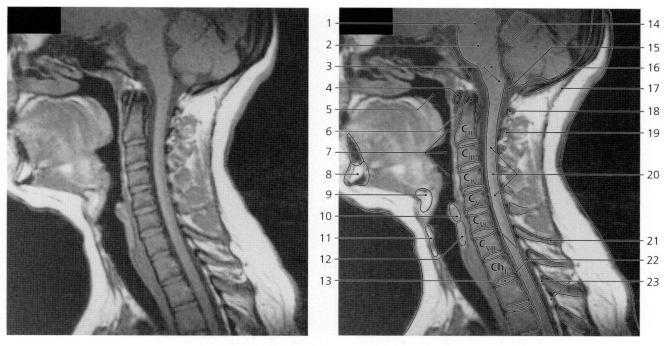

Cervical spine, median MR

1: Mesencephalon
2: Pons
3: Medulla oblongata
4: Anterior arch of atlas
5: Nasal part of pharynx
6: Dens axis
7: Oral part of pharynx
8: Mandible

9: Body of hyoid bone
10: Arythenoid cartilage
11: Thyroid cartilage
12: Lamina of cricoid cartilage
13: Intervertebral disc Th I – Th II
14: Fourth ventricle
15: Cerebello-medullary cistern
16: Squamous part of occipital bone

17: Lig. nuchae
18: Posterior arch of atlas
19: Lamina of vertebral arch C II
20: Spinal cord
21: Spinous process of C VII
22: Subarachnoid space
23: Fat in epidural space

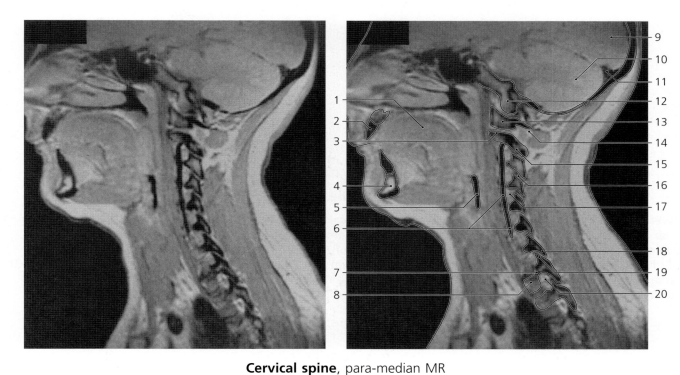

Cervical spine, para-median MR

1: Tongue
2: Upper incisive tooth
3: Superior articular facet of axis
4: Mandible
5: Piriform fossa
6: Vertebral artery
7: Pedicle of vertebral arch Th I
8: Body of vertebra Th I

9: Occipital lobe
10: Cerebellum
11: Transverse sinus
12: Occipital condyle
13: Lateral mass of atlas
14: Posterior arch of atlas
15: Inferior articular process of axis
16: Zygapophysial (facet) joint C III – C IV

17: Intervertebral foramen with fifth
    cervical spinal nerve, vessels and fat
18: Inferior articular process of C VII
19: Superior articular process of Th I
20: Intervertebral foramen of first
    thoracic spinal nerve

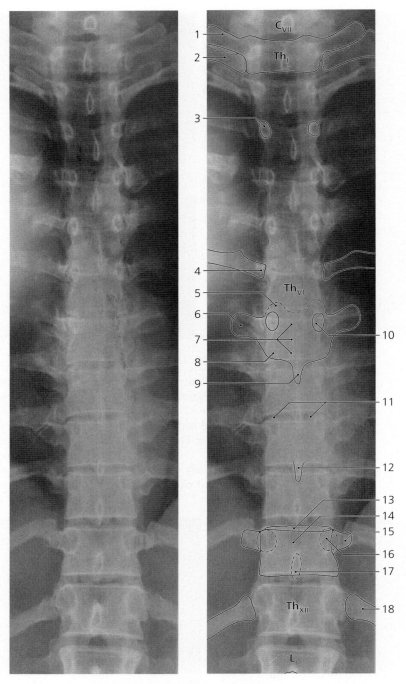

Thoracic spine, a-p X-ray

1: Transverse process
2: First rib
3: Pedicle of vertebral arch Th III
4: Head of sixth rib
5: Superior articular process of Th VII
6: Transverse process of Th VII

7: Lamina of vertebral arch Th VII
8: Inferior articular process of Th VII
9: Spinous process of Th VII
10: Pedicle of vertebral arch Th VII
11: Intervertebral disc Th VIII – Th IX
12: Spinous process of Th IX

13: End plate of vertebral body of Th XI
14: Body of vertebra Th XI
15: Transverse process of Th XI
16: Pedicle of vertebral arch Th XI
17: Spinous process of Th XI
18: 12th rib

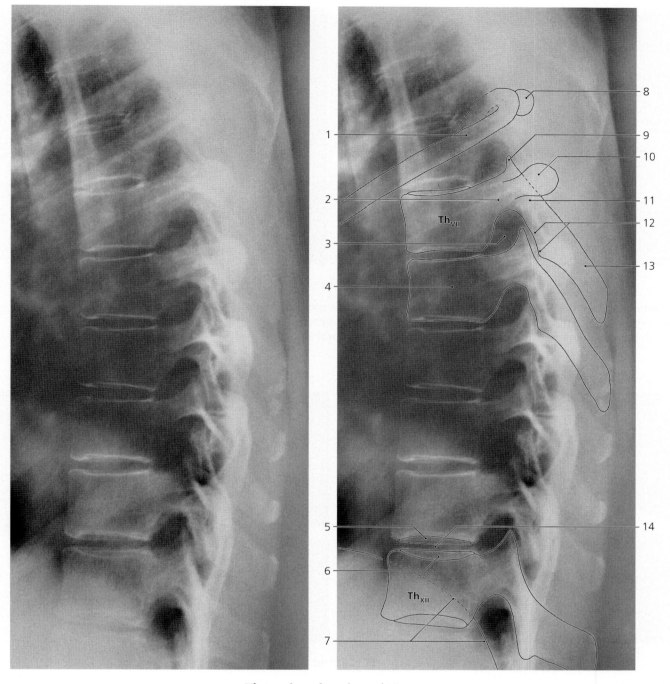

Thoracic spine, lateral X-ray

1: 6th rib
2: Pedicle of vertebral arch
3: Intervertebral foramen
4: Body of vertebra
5: Lower end plate of Th XI

6: Upper end plate of Th XII
7: Diaphragm
8: Transverse process of Th VI
9: Superior articular process
10: Transverse process

11: Lamina of vertebral arch
12: Inferior articular process
13: Spinous process
14: Intervertebral disc Th XI – Th XII

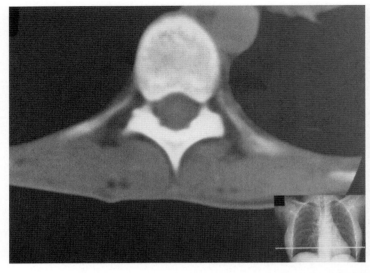

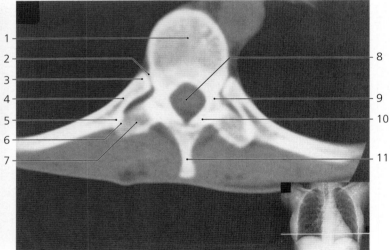

Thoracic spine, axial CT

Level of intervertebral disc Th X – Th XI
1: Intervertebral disc Th X – Th XI
2: Intervertebral foramen

3: Superior articular process Th XI
4: Inferior articular process Th X
5: Lamina of vertebral arch

6: Spinous process of Th X
7: Thoracic aorta

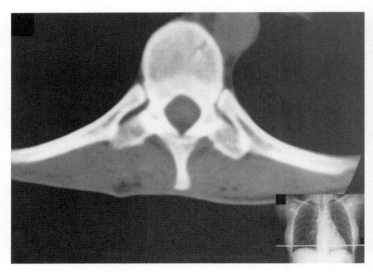

Thoracic spine, axial CT

Level of vertebral body Th XI
1: Body of vertebra Th XI
2: Costovertebral joint
3: Head of 11th rib

4: Neck of 11th rib
5: Tubercle of 11th rib
6: Costotransverse joint
7: Transverse process Th XI

8: Vertebral foramen
9: Pedicle of vertebral arch
10: Lamina of vertebral arch
11: Spinous process of Th XI

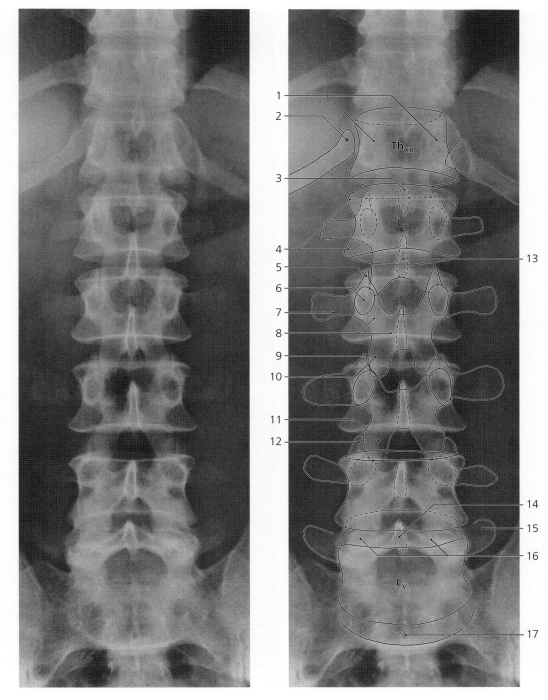

Lumbar spine, a-p X-ray

1: Body of vertebra Th XII
2: Head of 12th rib
3: Spinous process of Th XII
4: Upper and lower ambitus eminens of L I
5: Superior articular process of L II

6: Pedicle of vertebral arch L II
7: Transverse process L II
8: Lamina of vertebral arch L II
9: Zygapophysial (facet) joint L II – L III
10: Inferior articular process of L II
11: Inferior articular process of L III

12: Superior articular process of L IV
13: Spinous process of L I
14: Spinous process of L V
15: Transverse process of L V
16: Intervertebral disc L IV – L V
17: Base of sacrum

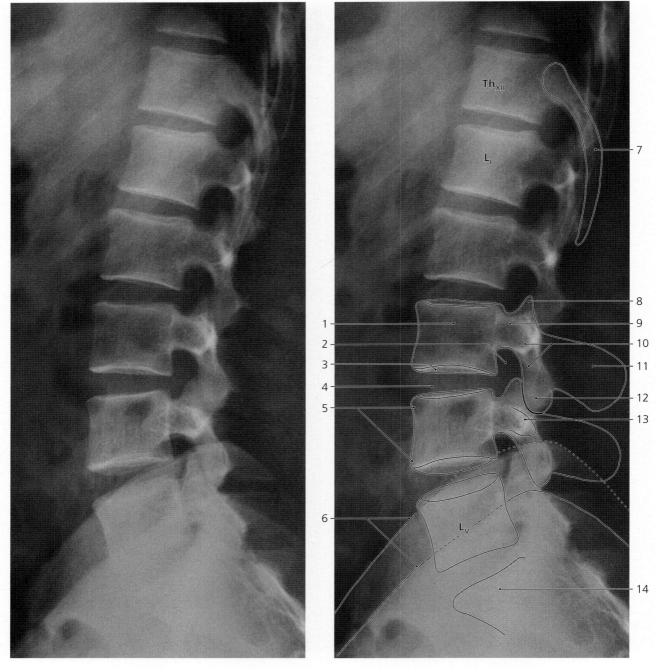

Lumbar spine, lateral X-ray

1: Body of vertebra
2: Intervertebral foramen
3: Lower end plate of L III
4: Intervertebral disc L III – L IV
5: Upper and lower ambitus eminens

6: Iliac crests
7: 12th rib
8: Superior articular process
9: Pedicle of vertebral arch
10: Lamina of vertebral arch

11: Spinous process
12: Inferior articular process
13: Transverse (costal) process
14: Sacrum

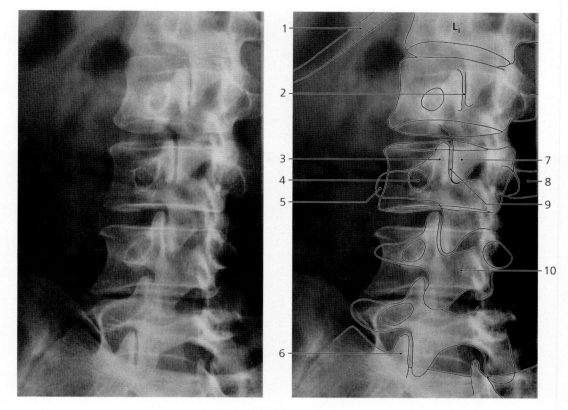

Lumbar spine, oblique X-ray

The "Scottie dog" projection
1: 12th rib
2: Zygapophysial (facet) joint L I – L II
3: Superior articular process of L III

4: Pedicle of vertebral arch L III (eye of "Scottie dog")
5: Transverse process of L III (snout of "Scottie dog")
6: Superior articular process of sacrum

7: Inferior articular process of L II
8: Transverse process of L III
9: Zygapophysial (facet) joint L II – L III
10: Lamina of vertebral arch L IV

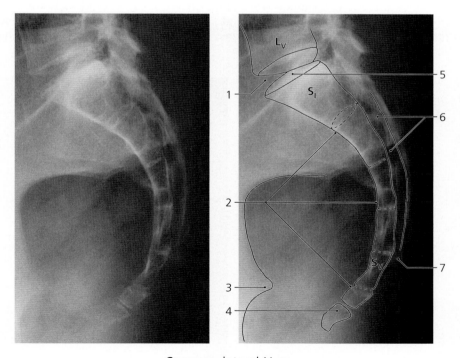

Sacrum, lateral X-ray

1: Intervertebral disc L V – S I
2: Pelvic surface of sacrum
3: Ischial spine

4: Coccyx
5: Base of sacrum
6: Sacral canal

7: Sacral hiatus

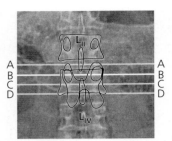

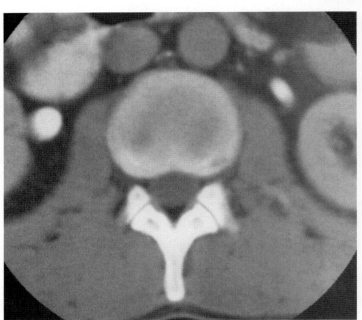

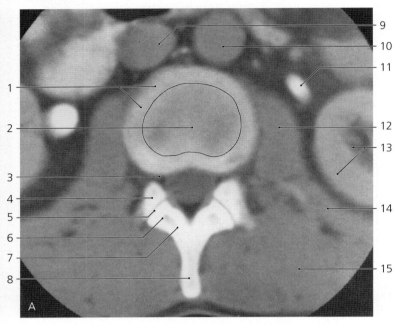

Lumbar spine, axial CT

Level of section A indicated on scout view above

1: Anulus fibrosus of intervertebral disc
2: Nucleus pulposus
3: Intervertebral foramen for spinal nerve L II

4: Superior articular process of L III
5: Zygapophysial (facet) joint
6: Inferior articular process of L II
7: Lamina of vertebral arch
8: Spinous process of L II
9: Inferior caval vein
10: Abdominal aorta

11: Left ureter/pelvis (with contrast medium)
12: Psoas major
13: Left kidney
14: Quadratus lumborum
15: Erector spinae

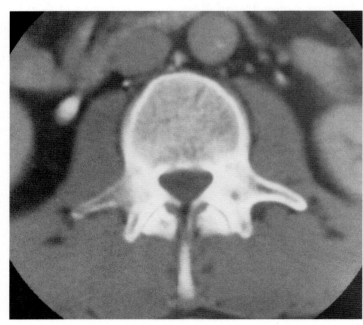

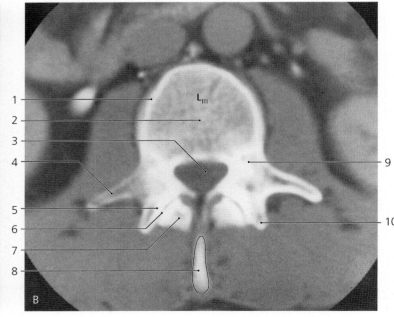

Lumbar spine, axial CT

Level of section B indicated on scout view above

1: Compact bone
2: Cancelleous bone

3: Vertebral foramen
4: Transverse (costal) process
5: Superior articular process
6: Zygapophysial (facet) joint L II – L III

7: Inferior articular process of L II
8: Spinous process of L III
9: Pedicle of vertebral arch
10: Mammillary process

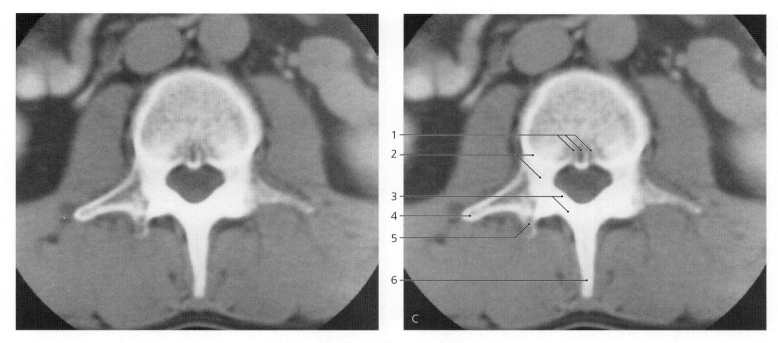

Lumbar spine, axial CT

Level of section C indicated on scout
view on previous page
 1: Basivertebral veins

2: Pedicle of vertebral arch
3: Lamina of vertebral arch
4: Transverse (costal) process

5: Accessory process
6: Spinous process

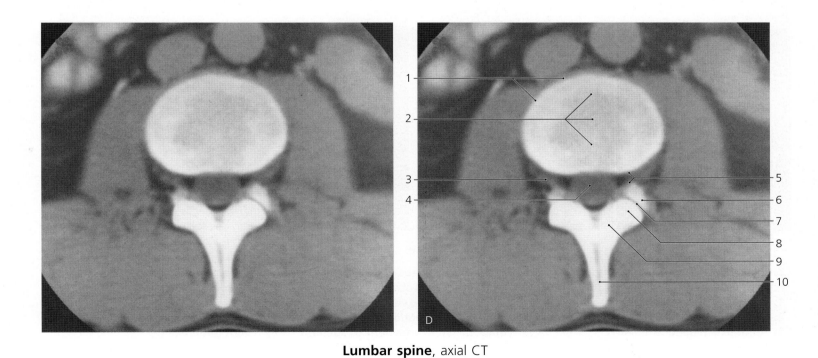

Lumbar spine, axial CT

Level of section D indicated on scout
view on previous page
 1: Ambitus eminens
 2: Lower "end plate" of vertebral body
    L III

3: Third lumbar spinal nerve with
   ganglion
4: Cauda equina
5: Intervertebral foramen
6: Superior articular process of L IV

7: Zygapophysial (facet) joint L III – L IV
8: Inferior articular process of L III
9: Lamina of vertebral arch
10: Spinous process of L III

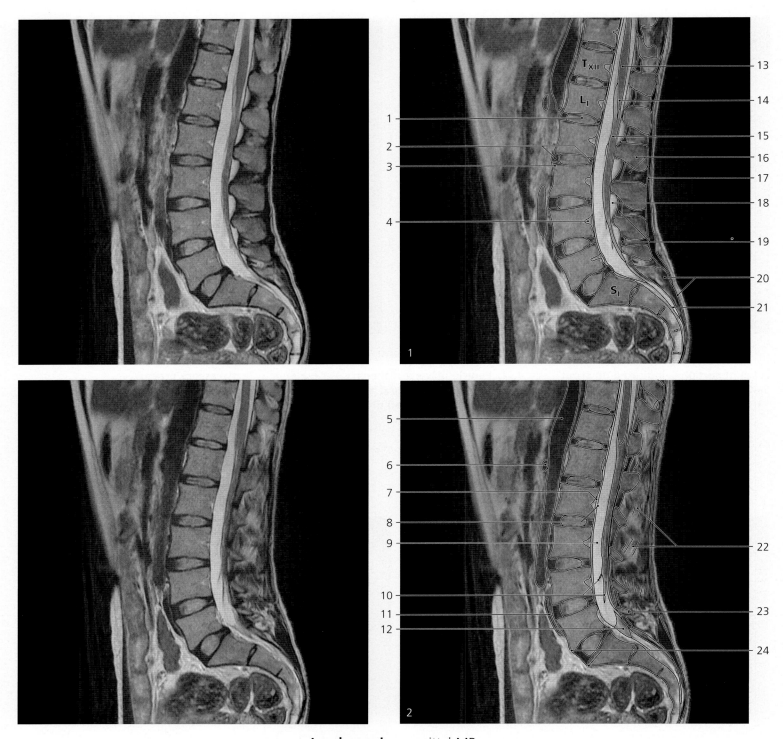

Lumbar spine, sagittal MR

Consecutive series of seven sagittal sections. No. 1 is median.

1: Nucleus pulposus L1/L2 →
2: Anulus fibrosus L2/L3→
3: Ambitus eminens →
4: Basivertebral vein (foramen)
5: Aorta →
6: Left renal vein →
7: Poaterior longitudinal ligament →
8: Dura mater

9: Subarachnoid space with liquor →
10: Rootles (fila radicularia)
11: Left common iliac vein →
12: Dural sac (termination)
13: Lumbosacral enlargement of spinal cord
14: Conus medullaris
15: Cauda equina →
16: Spinous process L2 and interspinal ligament

17: Supraspinous ligament
18: Fat in epidural space
19: Ligamenta flava
20: Median sacral crest
21: Filum terminale
22: Interspinous ligaments and muscles
23: Lamina of vertebral arch L5 →
24: Promontory →

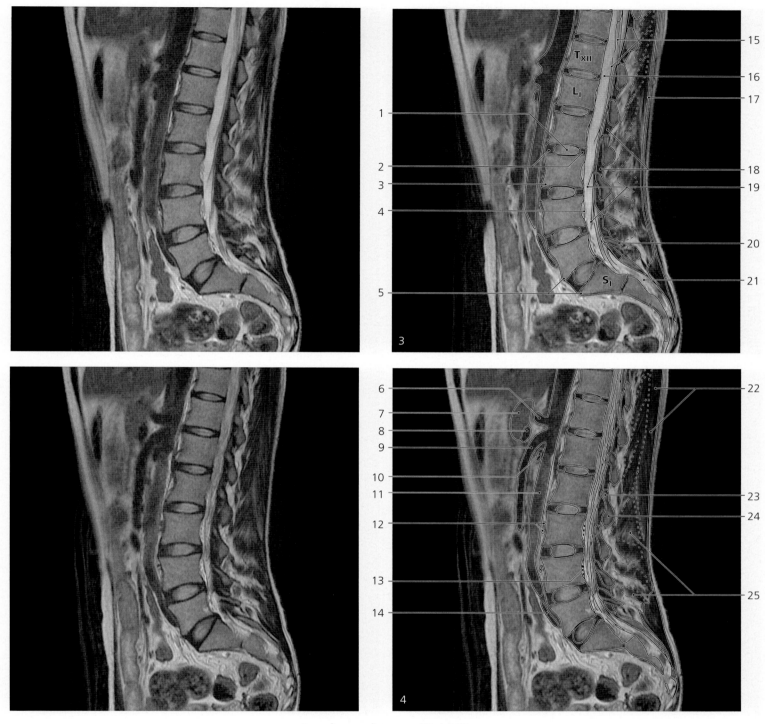

Lumbar spine, sagittal MR

1: Nucleus pulposus L2/L3 ↔
2: Anulus fibrosus ↔
3: Ambitus eminens ↔
4: Posterior longitudinal ligament ←
5: Promontory ↔
6: Celiac trunk →
7: Pancreas →
8: Portal vein →
9: Superior mesenteric artery →

10: Left renal vein ↔
11: Aorta ↔
12: Lumbar artery and vein →
13: Epidural space with internal vertebral venous plexus
14: Left common iliac vein ↔
15: Cauda equina ←
16: Subarachnaoid space with liquor ←
17: Thoracolumbar fascia →

18: Ligamanta flava ↔
19: Rootlets (fila radicularia) ↔
20: Lamina of vertebral arch L5
21: Sacral canal ←
22: Erector spinae →
23: Lamina of vertebral arch L2
24: Inferior articular process of L2
25: Rotator and multifidi muscles

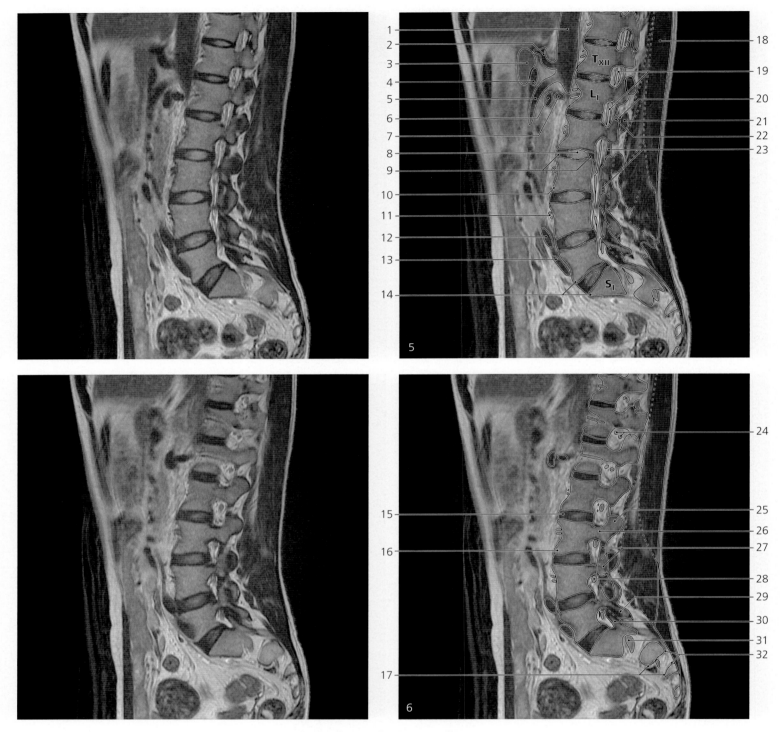

Lumbar spine, sagittal MR

1: Aorta ←
2: Celiac trunk ←
3: Pancreas ←
4: Portal vein ←
5: Superior mesenteric artery ←
6: Left renal vein ←
7: Left renal artery →
8: Nucleus pulposus L2/L3 ←
9: Anulus fibrosus
10: Ambitus eminens ↔
11: Lumbar artery and vein ↔
12: Right common iliac artery →

13: Left common iliac vein
14: Promontory ←
15: Intervertebral disc L2/L3
16: Ambitus eminens ↔
17: Anterior sacral foramen S2/S3
18: Erector spinae ↔
19: Rootlets (fila radicularia) ←
20: Zygapophysial joint L1/L2
21: Inferior articular process L1
22: Superior articular process L2 ↔
23: Ligamanta flava ←

24: Ventral and dorsal rot of spinal nerve T12 in intervertebral foramen
25: Superior articular process L3
26: Pediculus of vertebral arch L3
27: Inferior articular process of L3
28: Spinal nerve and ganglion L4
29: Inferior articular process L5 →
30: Superior articular process S1 →
31: Spinal ganglion S1
32: Posterior sacral foramen S2/S3

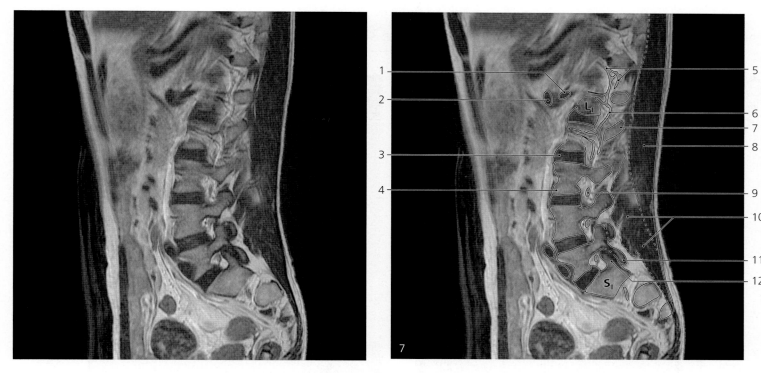

Lumbar spine, sagittal MR

1: Left renal artery ←
2: Left renal vein ←
3: Intervertebral disc L2/L3 ←
4: Ambitus eminens ←

5: External vertebral venous plexus
6: Intervertebral vein
7: Superior articular process L2
8: Erector spinae ←

9: Spinal nerve L3
10: Multifidi muscles ←
11: Inferior articular process L5 ←
12: Superior articular process S1 ←

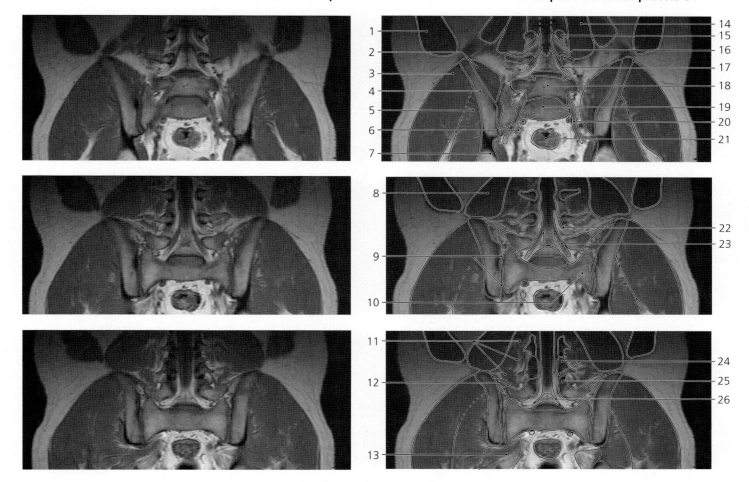

Lumbar spine coronal MR

Three sections, anterior to posterior
1: Abdominal wall muscles
2: Iliacus
3: Gluteus medius
4: Ala of ilium
5: Gluteus minimus
6: Internal iliac artery and vein
7: Ischium
8: Quadrarus lumborum

9: Sacroiliac joint
10: Ala of sacrum
11: Transversospinal (multifidi) muscles
12: Iliolumbar ligament
13: Piriformis
14: Psoas major
15: Pedicle of 3rd lumbar vertebra
16: Pedicle of 4th lumbar vertebra
17: 4th lumbar spinal nerve root

18: 5th lumbar vertebra (body)
19: Intervertebral disc L5/S1
20: Lumbosacral trunk
21: Rectum
22: 4th lumbar spinal nerve root
23: 5th lumbar spinal nerve root
24: Superior and inferior articular process
25: Articular processes of L5
26: 1st sacral spinal nerve root

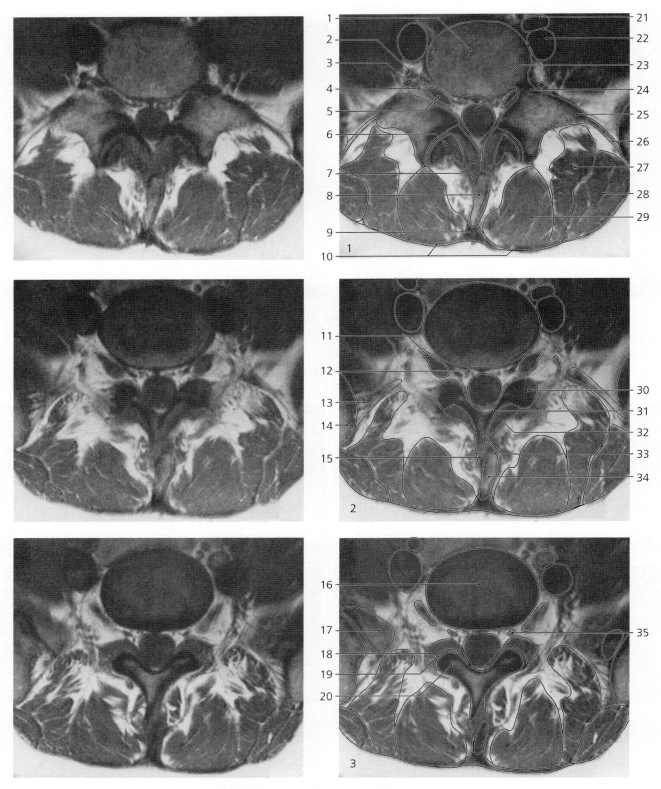

Lumbar spine, L5/S1, tilted axial MR

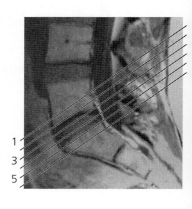

1: Body of lumbar vertebra L5
2: Branch from spinal nerve L4 to lumbosacral trunk
3: Iliolumbar artery
4: Motor root of spinal nerve L5
5: Spinal ganglion L5
6: Inferior articular process of L4
7: Lig. flavum
8: Spinous process of L4
9: Supraspinal ligament
10: Thoracolumbar fascia
11: Spinal nerve L5
12: Epidural space with fat and vessels
13: Iliolumbar ligament

14: Iliac crest
15: Interspinal muscle and ligament
16: Intervertebral disc L5/S1
17: Ala of sacrum
18: Superior articular process of S1
19: Zygapophysial joint L5/S1
20: Inferior articular process of L5
21: Common iliac artery
22: Common iliac vein
23: Cauda equina in dural sac
24: Pedicle of vertebra L5
25: Transverse process of L5
26: Iliolumbar ligament
27: Longissimus muscle

28: Iliocostalis muscle
29: Multifidus
30: Base of inferior articular process of L5
31: Lamina of vertebral arch L5
32: Lig. flavum
33: Spinous process of L5
34: Spinous process of L4
35: Spinal artery/vein

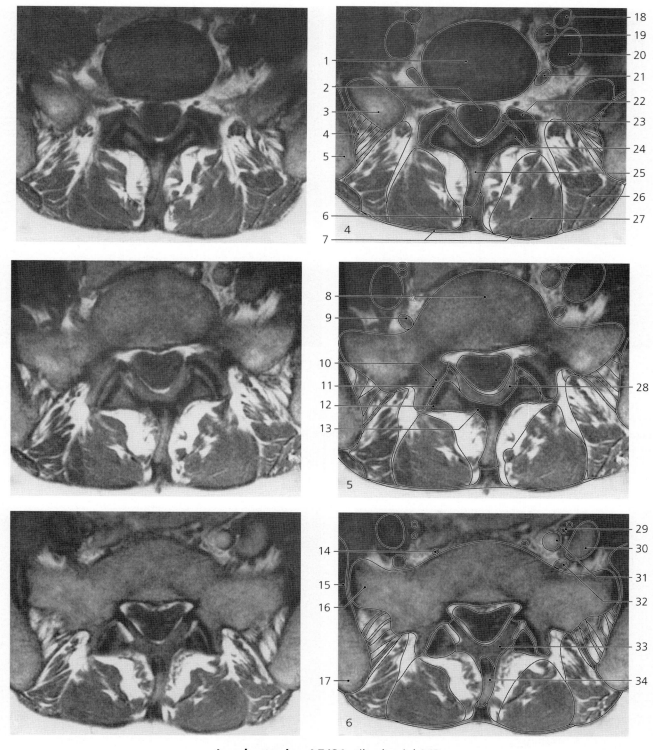

Lumbar spine L5/S1, tilted axial MR

Scout view on previous page

1: Intervertebral disc L5/S1
2: Cauda equina in dural sac
3: Ala of sacrum
4: Interosseous sacroiliac ligament
5: Iliac bone
6: Supraspinal ligament
7: Thoracolumbar fascia
8: Body of vertebra S1
9: Lumbosacral trunk
10: Superior articular process of S1
11: Zygapophysial joint L5/S1
12: Inferior articular process of L5

13: Lamina of vertebral arch L5
14: Lateral sacral artery
15: Sacroiliac joint
16: Ala of sacrum
17: Posterior superior iliac spine
18: External iliac artery
19: Internal iliac artery
20: Common iliac vein
21: Lumbosacral trunk
22: Superior articular process of S1
23: Lig. flavum
24: Inferior articular process of L5

25: Spinous process of L5
26: Longissimus muscle
27: Multifidus muscle
28: Lig. flavum
29: Internal iliac artery branches
30: External iliac vein
31: Internal iliac vein
32: Lumbosacral trunk
33: Lig. flavum
34: Spinous process of L5

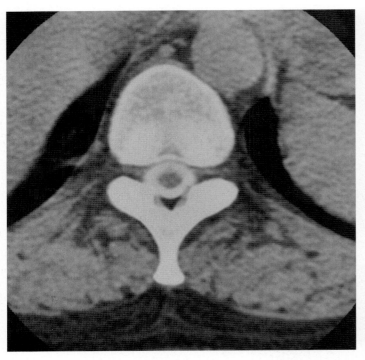

Thoracic spine, axial CT, myelography

1: Body of thoracic vertebra Th 11 (lower end)
2: Intervertebral foramen
3: Lig. flavum
4: Lamina of vertebral arch

5: Spinous process
6: Aorta
7: Spinal cord
8: Subarachnoid space with contrast agent

9: Spinal nerve and ganglion in dural pouch
10: Epidural space with fat

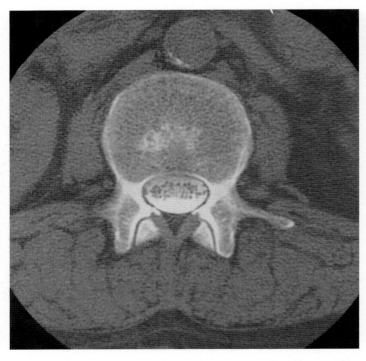

Lumbar spine, axial CT, myelography

1: Body of vertebra L3
2: Epidural space
3: Cauda equina
4: Subarachnoid space with contrast agent

5: Lig. flavum
6: Aorta (with calcification)
7: Psoas major
8: Pedicle of vertebral arch
9: Transverse process of vertebra

10: Superior articular process of L3
11: Mamillary process
12: Zygapophysial joint L2/L3
13: Inferior articular process of L2

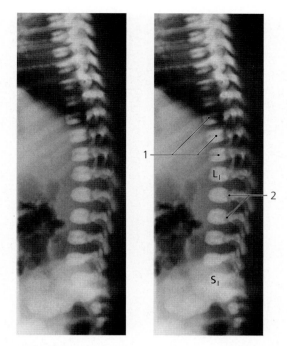

Thoracolumbar spine, lateral X-ray, newborn

1: **Yet incomplete fusion of ossification centers in vertebral body**

2: **Synchondrosis between arch and body of vertebra (neurocentral synchondrosis)**

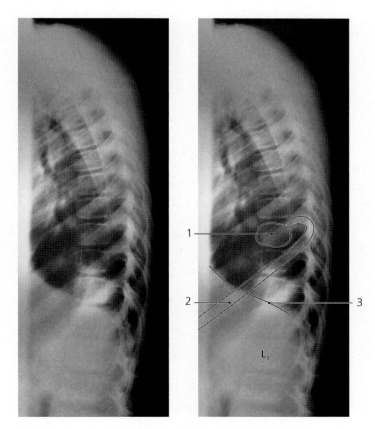

Thoracolumbar spine, lateral X-ray, child 12 years

1: **Body of vertebra Th IX. Annular ossification center of end plate has not yet appeared.**

2: **Ninth rib**

3: **Diaphragm**

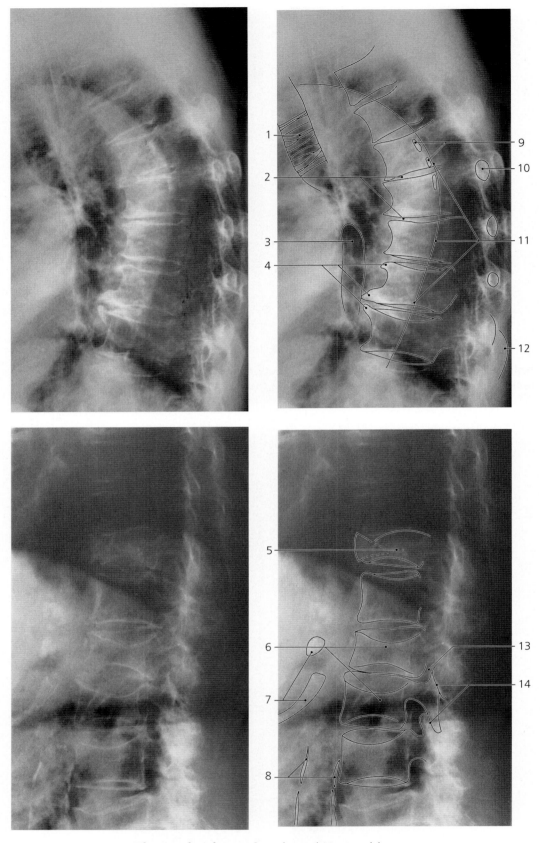

Thoracolumbar spine, lateral X-ray, old age

1: Trachea with calcified cartilages
2: Intervertebral disc (reduced thickness)
3: Esophagus with air
4: Osteophytes
5: Collapsed body of vertebra
6: Vertebral bodies with central
   compression/fracture

7: Calcified costal cartilage
8: Abdominal aorta (calcified)
9: Calcifications in thoracic aorta
10: Transverse process (tip)
11: Thoracic aorta (posterior wall),
    elongated
12: Rib

13: Intervertebral foramen (narrowed)
14: Zygapophysial (facet) joints with
    subchondral sclerosis (sign of
    arthrosis)

Head

Skull
Ear
Orbita
Paranasal sinuses
Temporomandibular joint
Teeth
Salivary glands
Arteries

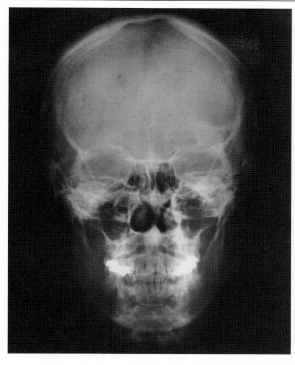

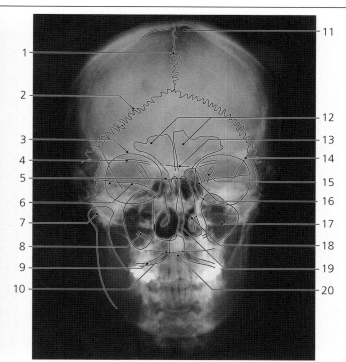

Skull, a-p X-ray

1: Sagittal suture
2: Lambdoid suture
3: Supra-orbital margin
4: Lesser wing of sphenoid bone
5: Hypophysial fossa
6: Crista pyramidis (upper edge of petrous bone)
7: Head of mandible
8: Atlanto-occipital joint

9: Lateral atlanto-axial joint
10: Squama occipitalis
11: Granular foveola
12: Frontal sinus
13: Jugum sphenoidale
14: Innominate line (radiology term) (tangential view of greater wing of sphenoid bone)

15: Superior orbital fissure
16: Ethmoidal air cells
17: Maxillary sinus
18: Inferior nasal concha
19: Nasal septum
20: Dens axis

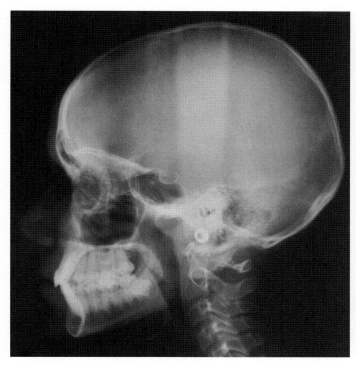

Skull, lateral X-ray

1: Coronal suture
2: Frontal bone
3: Outer table of calvaria
4: Diploë
5: Inner table of calvaria
6: Frontal sinus
7: Cribriform plate
8: Nasal bone
9: Ethmoidal air cells
10: Zygomatic process of maxilla
11: Maxillary sinus

12: Anterior nasal spine
13: Hard palate
14: Uvula
15: Mental protuberance
16: Angle of mandible
17: Parietal bone
18: Orbital plates of frontal bone
19: Greater wings of sphenoid bone
20: Jugum sphenoidale
21: Hypophysial fossa

22: Dorsum sellae
23: Sphenoidal sinus
24: Lambdoid suture
25: Occipitomastoid suture
26: Squamous part of occipital bone
27: Mastoid air cells
28: External acoustic meatus
29: Clivus
30: Mandibular neck
31: Anterior arch of atlas

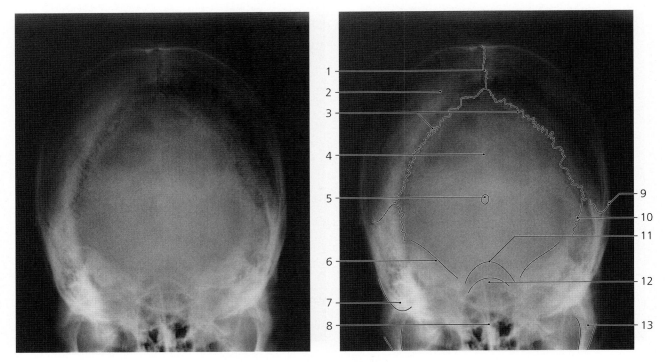

Skull, X-ray, Towne's projection

1: Sagittal suture
2: Parietal bone
3: Lambdoid suture
4: Squamous part of occipital bone
5: Pineal gland (calcified)

6: Petrous part of temporal bone
7: Mastoid process
8: Nasal septum
9: Squamosal suture
10: Occipitomastoid suture

11: Foramen magnum
12: Sphenoidal sinus
13: Mandibular neck

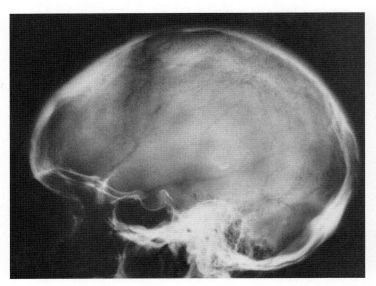
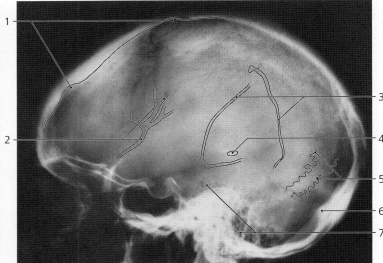

Skull, lateral X-ray, old age

1: Granular foveolae
2: Grooves for branches of middle
   meningeal artery

3: Diploic veins
4: Pineal gland (calcified)
5: Lambdoid suture

6: Internal occipital protuberance
7: Air cells in temporal bone

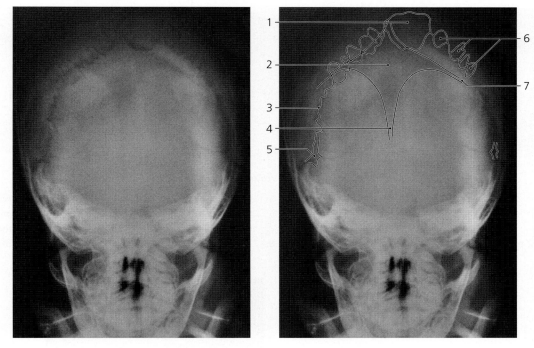

Skull, a-p, tilted X-ray, child 5 months

1: Interparietal bone (Inca bone)
2: Anterior fontanelle
3: Lambdoid suture

4: Sagittal suture
5: Mastoid fontanelle

6: Sutural (Wormian) bones in lambdoid suture
7: Coronal suture

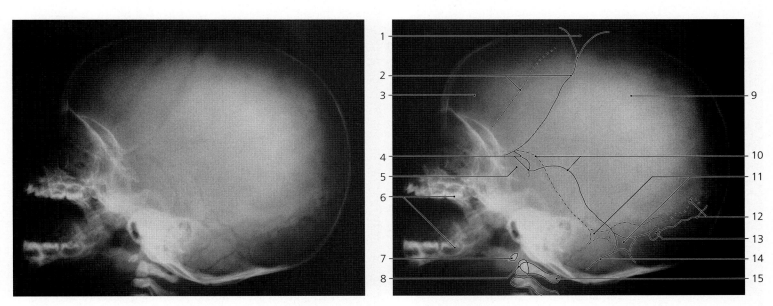

Skull, lateral X-ray, child 5 months

1: Anterior fontanelle
2: Coronal suture
3: Frontal bone
4: Pterion (sphenoidal fontanelle)
5: Greater wing of sphenoid bone

6: Deciduous teeth
7: Anterior arch of atlas
8: Dens axis
9: Parietal bone
10: Squamosal sutures

11: Mastoid fontanelles
12: Lambdoid suture
13: Sutural bone
14: Occipitomastoid suture
15: Posterior arch of atlas

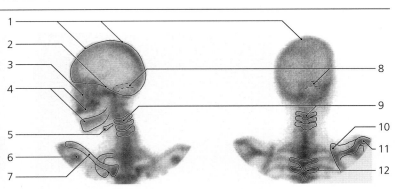

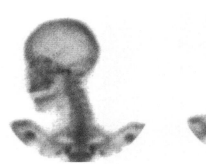
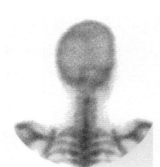

Skull, lateral and posterior view, ⁹⁹ᵐ Tc-MDP, scintigraphy

1:	Calvaria	5:	Hyoid bone	9:	Cervical vertebra
2:	Base of skull	6:	Coracoid process	10:	Superior angle of scapula
3:	Facial skeleton	7:	Clavicle	11:	Acromion
4:	Alveolar process of maxilla and alveolar part of mandible	8:	Transverse and sigmoid sinus	12:	Thoracic vertebra

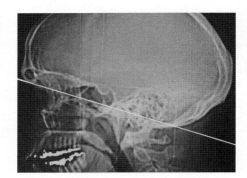

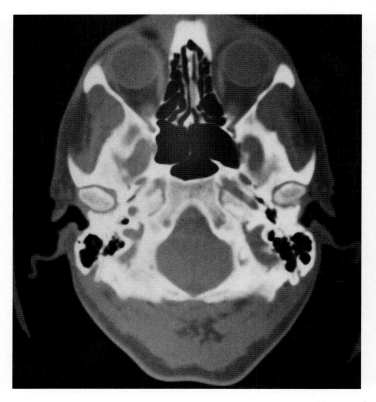
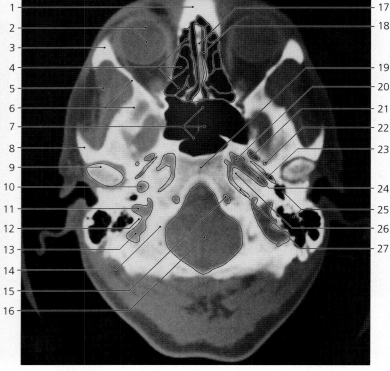

Base of skull, axial CT

1:	Nasal spine of frontal bone	10:	Carotid canal, first part	19:	Body of sphenoid bone
2:	Eyeball	11:	Jugular foramen, posterior to intrajugular process	20:	Foramen lacerum
3:	Frontal process of zygomatic bone	12:	Posterior border of jugular foramen	21:	Foramen ovale
4:	Ethmoidal air cells	13:	Sigmoid sinus	22:	Foramen spinosum
5:	Temporal fossa	14:	Lateral part of occipital bone	23:	Sphenopetrous fissure/ Eustachian tube
6:	Greater wing of sphenoid bone	15:	Hypoglossal canal	24:	Carotid canal, second part
7:	Sphenoidal sinus	16:	Foramen magnum	25:	Air cells in temporal bone
8:	Zygomatic process of temporal bone	17:	Nasal septum	26:	Apex of petrous bone
9:	Head of mandible	18:	Nasal cavity	27:	Petro-occipital fissure

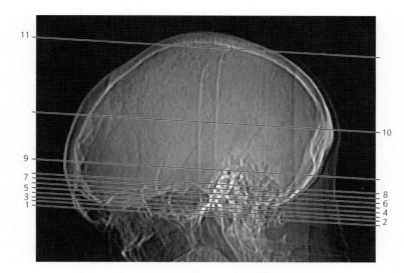

Scout view of skull

Lines #1–11 indicate position of sections in the following axial CT series displayed in bone settings. The corresponding series in brain settings is found on pages 245–7. This skull is highly pneumatized.

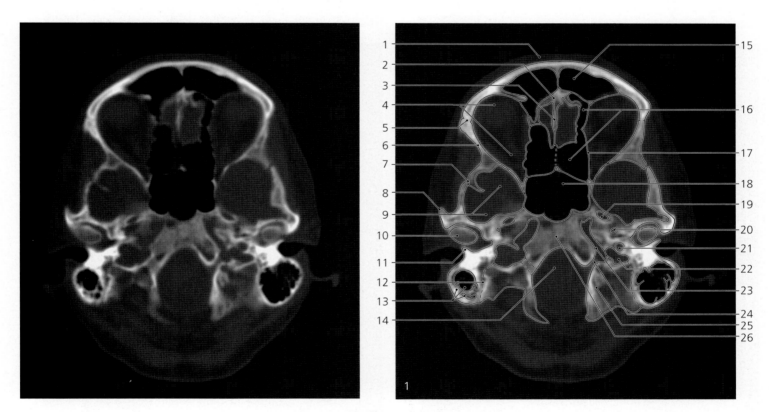

Skull, axial CT

1: Squamous part of frontal bone →
2: Frontal crest →
3: Crista galli →
4: Orbit →
5: Sphenofrontal suture →
6: Greater wing of sphenoidal bone →
7: Sphenosquamous suture →
8: Zygomatic process of temporal bone
9: Middle cranial fossa →

10: Head of mandible in mandibular fossa →
11: Tympanic part of temporal bone
12: Occipitomastoid suture →
13: Mastoid process (with air cells) →
14: Foramen magnum →
15: Frontal sinus →
16: Ethmoidal air cells →
17: Orbital plate (lamina papyracea)

18: Sphenoidal sinus →
19: Foramen ovale
20: Foramen spinosum
21: Carotid canal →
22: Jugular foramen →
23: Petrooccipital synchondrosis →
24: Hypoglossal canal →
25: Lateral part of occipital bone
26: Clivus (basilar part of occipital bone)

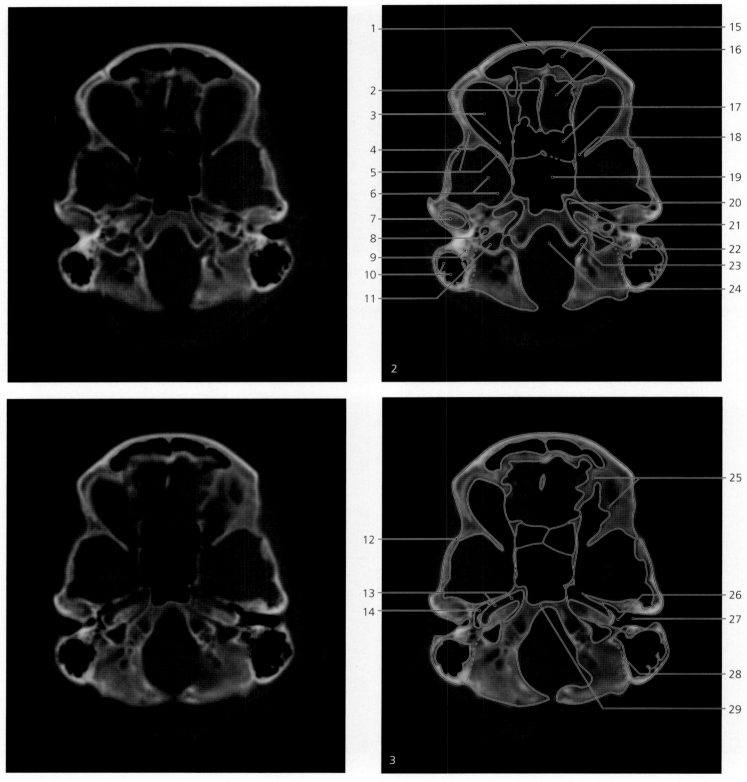

Skull, axial CT

Scout view on page 207

1: Squamous part of frontal bone ↔
2: Crista galli ↔
3: Orbit ←
4: Sphenosquamous suture ↔
5: Greater wing of sphenoidal bone ↔
6: Middle cranial fossa ↔
7: Head of mandible in mandibular fossa ←
8: Carotid canal ↔
9: Facial canal →
10: Mastoid process (with air cells) ↔
11: Jugular foramen ↔
12: Sphenosquamous suture ↔
13: Carotid canal (in petrous part of temporal bone) ↔
14: Musculotubal canal →
15: Frontal sinus ↔
16: Anterior cranial fossa ↔
17: Ethmoidal air cells ↔
18: Superior orbital fissure →
19: Sphenoidal sinus ↔
20: Foramen lacerum →
21: Sphenopetrous synchondrosis
22: Petrooccipital synchondrosis ↔
23: Hypoglossal canal ←
24: Foramen magnum ←
25: Orbital part of frontal bone →
26: Tympanic cavity →
27: External acoustic meatus →
28: Occipitomastoid suture ↔
29: Clivus (body of sphenoidal bone) ←

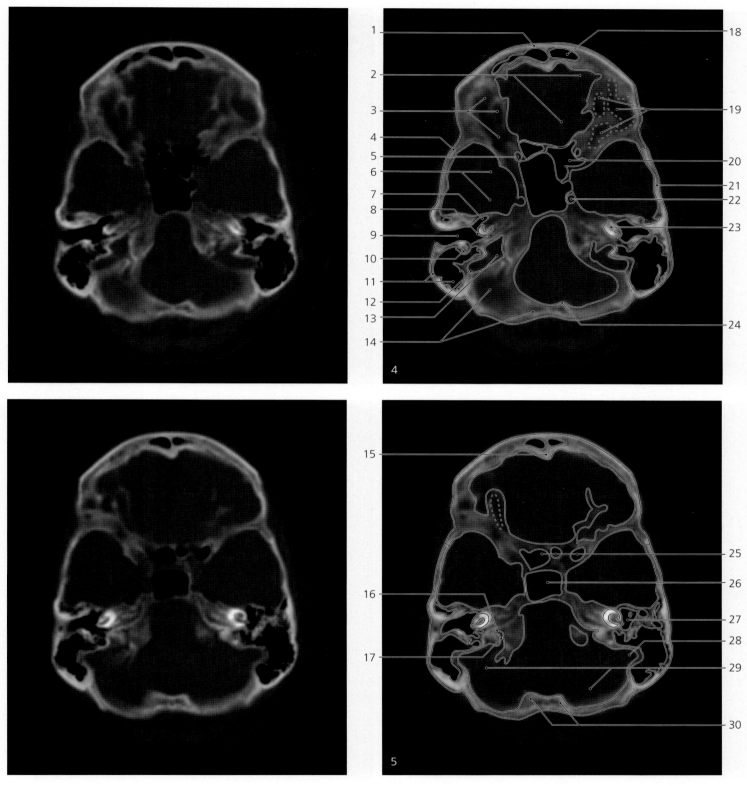

Skull, axial CT

Scout view on page 207
1: Squamous part of frontal bone ↔
2: Anterior cranial fossa ↔
3: Orbital part of frontal bone ←
4: Sphenosquamous suture ↔
5: Optic canal
6: Middle cranial fossa ↔
7: Musculotubal canal ←
8: Promontory (of middle ear)
9: External acoustic meatus ←
10: Facial canal ↔

11: Mastoid process (with air cells) ↔
12: Groove for sigmoid sinus →
13: Jugular foramen ←
14: Squamous part of occipital bone →
15: Frontal crest ↔
16: Cochlear canaliculus (for
    perilymphatic duct)
17: Grove for inferior petrosal sinus
18: Frontal sinus ↔
19: Impressions of cerebral gyri
20: Ethmoidal air cells ↔

21: Squamous part of temporal bone ↔
22: Carotid canal ←
23: Cochlea →
24: Internal occipital crest →
25: Ethmoidal air cells ←
26: Sphenoidal sinus ↔
27: Tympanic cavity ↔
28: Groove for sigmoid sinus ↔
29: Posterior cranial fossa →
30: Internal occipital protuberance →

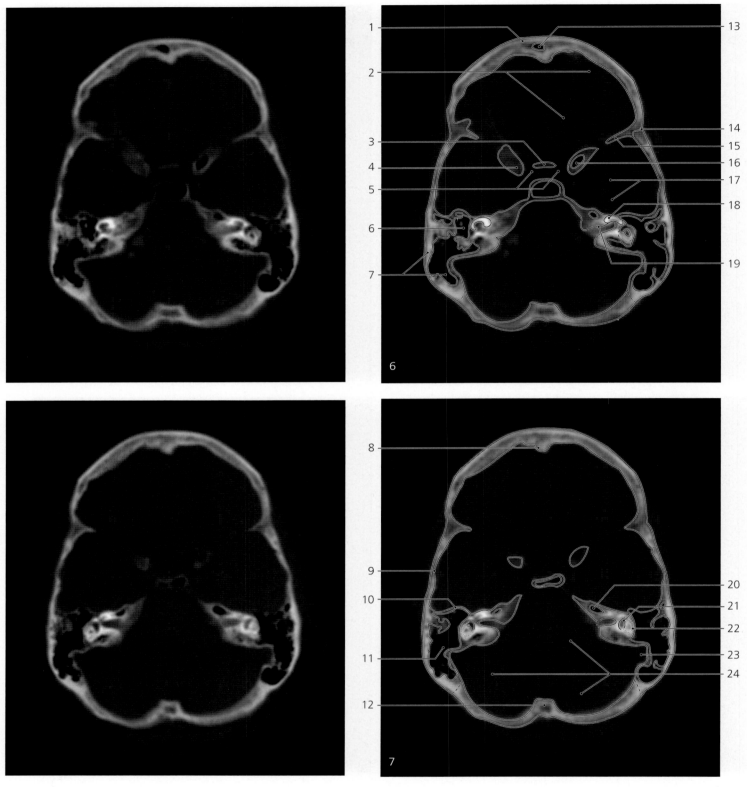

Skull, axial CT

Scout view on page 207

1: Squamous part of frontal bone ↔
2: Anterior cranial fossa ↔
3: Sella turcica (anterior rim)
4: Anterior clinoid process →
5: Hypophysial fossa
6: Tympanic cavity ↔
7: Mastoid process (with air cells) ↔
8: Frontal crest ↔

9: Squamous part of temporal bone ↔
10: Tegmen tympani →
11: Mastoid antrum →
12: Internal occipital crest ↔
13: Frontal sinus ←
14: Sphenofrontal suture
15: Lesser wing of sphenoidal bone →
16: Anterior clinoid process (with air cell) →

17: Middle cranial fossa ↔
18: Cochlea ←
19: Internal acoustic meatus →
20: Air cell in petrous bone
21: Vestibulum (of inner ear)
22: Lateral semicircular canal
23: Groove for sigmoid sinus ↔
24: Posterior cranial fossa ↔

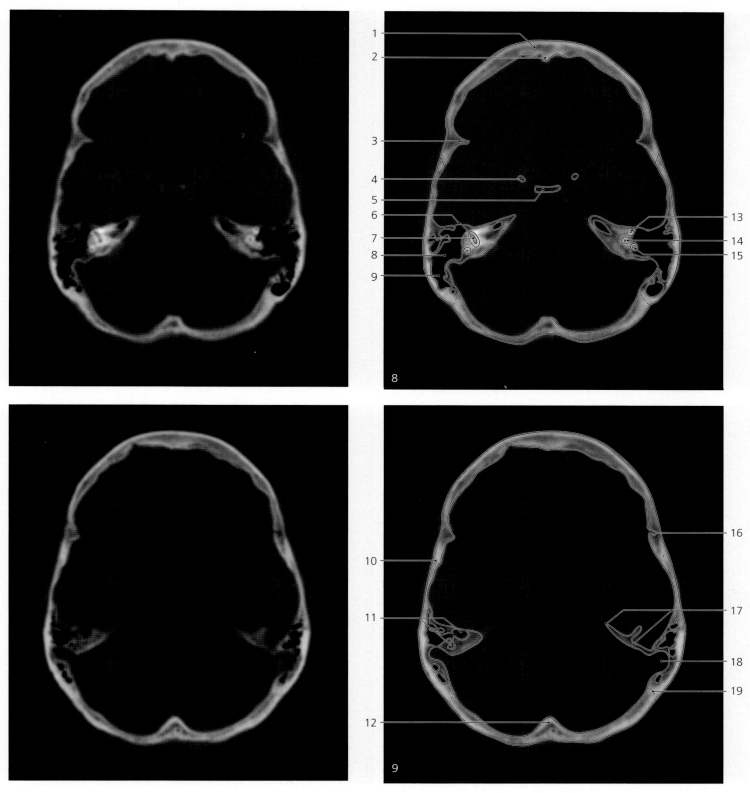

Skull, axial CT

Scout view on page 207

1: Squamous part of frontal bone ↔
2: Frontal crest ←
3: Lesser wing of sphenoidal bone ←
4: Anterior clinoid process ←
5: Dorsum sellae ←
6: Tegmen tympani ←
7: Anterior semicircular canal
8: Mastoid antrum ←

9: Mastoid process (with air cells) ←
10: Coronal suture →
11: Petrous part of temporal bone (with air cells) ←
12: Internal occipital crest ←
13: Anterior semicircular canal (ampullar limb)
14: Common limb of anterior and posterior semicircular canal

15: Posterior semicircular canal (ampullar limb)
16: Groove for middle meningeal artery →
17: Superior rim of petrous bone (crista pyramidis)
18: Groove for sigmoid sinus ←
19: Lambdoid suture ↔

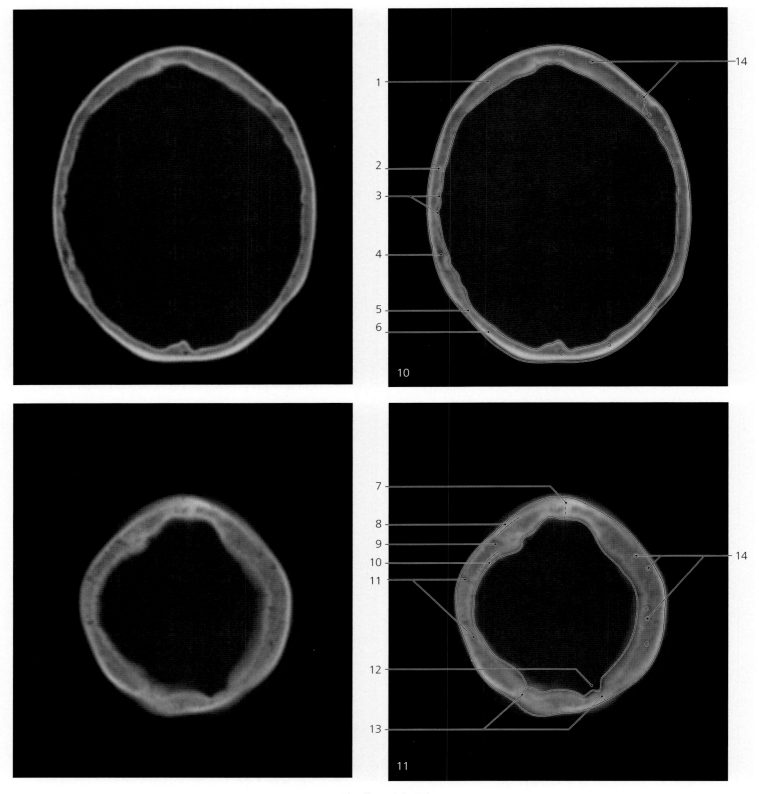

Skull, axial CT

Scout view on page 207

1: Frontal bone (squamous part) ←
2: Coronal suture ←
3: Grooves for branches of middle
    meningeal artery ←
4: Parietal bone →

5: Lambdoid suture ↔
6: Occipital bone (squamous part) ↔
7: Sagittal suture
8: External table of calvaria
9: Diploë
10: Internal table of calvaria

11: Parietal bone ←
12: Granular foveola
13: Lambdoid suture ←
14: Diploic veins

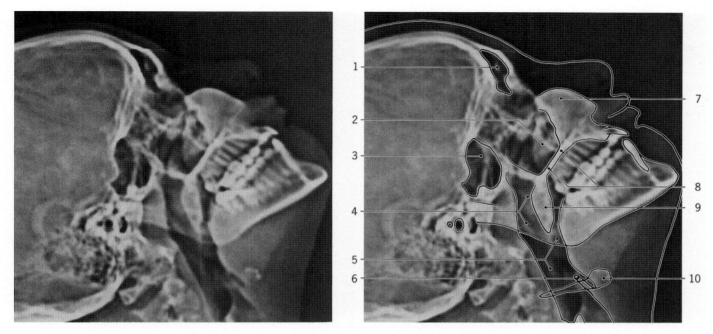

Scout view

1: Frontal sinus
2: Maxillary sinus
3: Sphenoidal sinus
4: Nasal part of pharynx

5: Oral part of pharynx
6: Epiglottis
7: Frontal process of maxilla
8: Hard palate

9: Soft palate
10: Hyoid bone

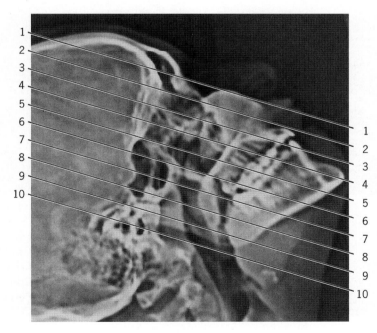

Scout view

Lines #1–10 indicate positions of sections in the following CT series.
Consecutive sections, 10 mm thick. Prone position with hyperextended neck.

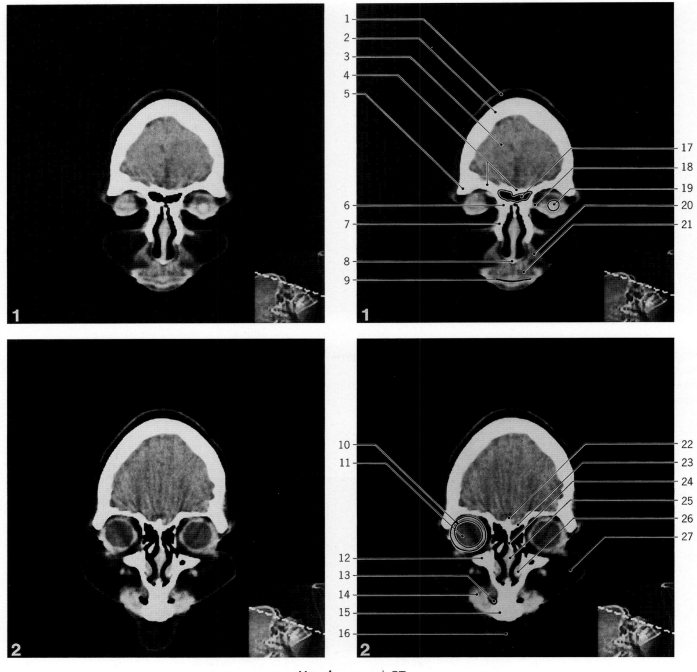

Head, coronal CT

Scout view on opposite page 213

1: Scalp
2: Squamous part of frontal bone
3: Frontal lobe
4: Orbital plate of frontal bone
5: Zygomatic process of frontal bone
6: Nasal spine of frontal bone
7: Frontal process of maxilla
8: Anterior nasal spine
9: Oral fissure
10: Sclera
11: Vitreous body
12: Body of maxilla
13: Air in vestibule of mouth
14: Orbicularis oris
15: Upper incisor teeth
16: Chin
17: Frontal sinus
18: Medial palpebral ligament
19: Lens
20: Levator labii superioris
21: Upper lip
22: Crista galli
23: Cribriform plate
24: Perpendicular plate of ethmoid bone
25: Cartilage of nasal septum
26: Inferior nasal concha
27: Cheek

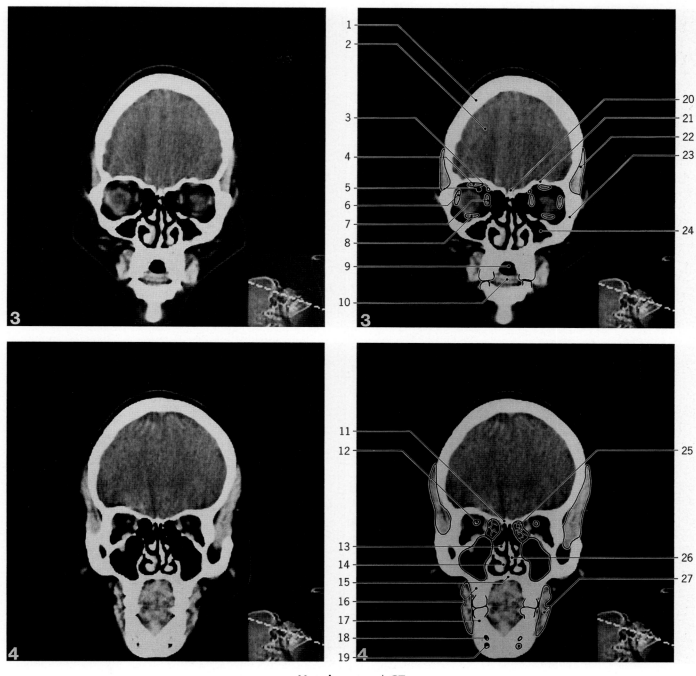

Head, coronal CT

Scout veiw on page 213

1: Squamous part of frontal bone
2: Frontal lobe
3: Obliquus superior
4: Rectus superior, and levator palpebrae
5: Ophthalmic artery, or superior orbital vein
6: Rectus lateralis
7: Rectus medialis
8: Rectus inferior
9: Air in oral cavity
10: Apex of tongue
11: Cribriform plate
12: Optic nerve
13: Middle nasal concha
14: Inferior nasal concha
15: Hard palate
16: Alveolar process of maxilla
17: Alveolar part of mandible
18: Mental foramen
19: Marrow cavity of mandible
20: Crista galli
21: Orbital plate of frontal bone
22: Temporalis muscle
23: Zygomatic bone
24: Maxillary sinus
25: Ethmoidal air cells
26: Nasal septum
27: Buccinator

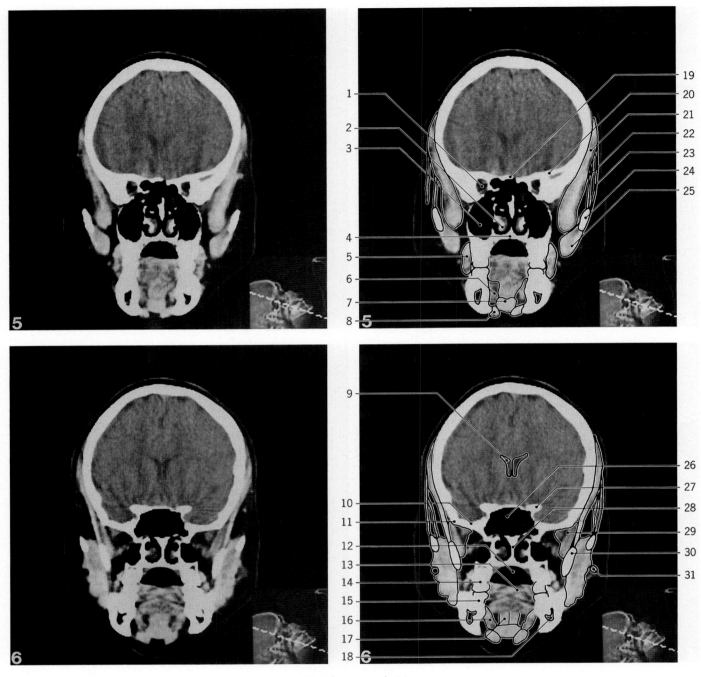

Head, coronal CT

Scout view on page 213
 1: Apex of orbita
 2: Inferior nasal concha
 3: Maxillary sinus
 4: Hard Palate
 5: Buccinator
 6: Sublingual region
 7: Geniohyoideus
 8: Digastricus, anterior belly
 9: Lateral ventricle
10: Greater wing of sphenoid bone

11: Infratemporal crest
12: Oral cavity
13: Tongue
14: Upper molar tooth
15: Lower molar tooth
16: Mylohyoideus
17: Genioglossus
18: Marrow cavity of mandible/
    mandibular canal
19: Jugum sphenoidale
20: Lesser wing of sphenoid bone

21: Temporalis muscle
22: Temporal fascia
23: Galea aponeurotica
24: Zygomatic arch
25: Masseter
26: Sphenoidal sinus
27: Anterior clinoid process
28: Vomer
29: Lateral pterygoid muscle
30: Coronoid process of mandible
31: Parotid duct

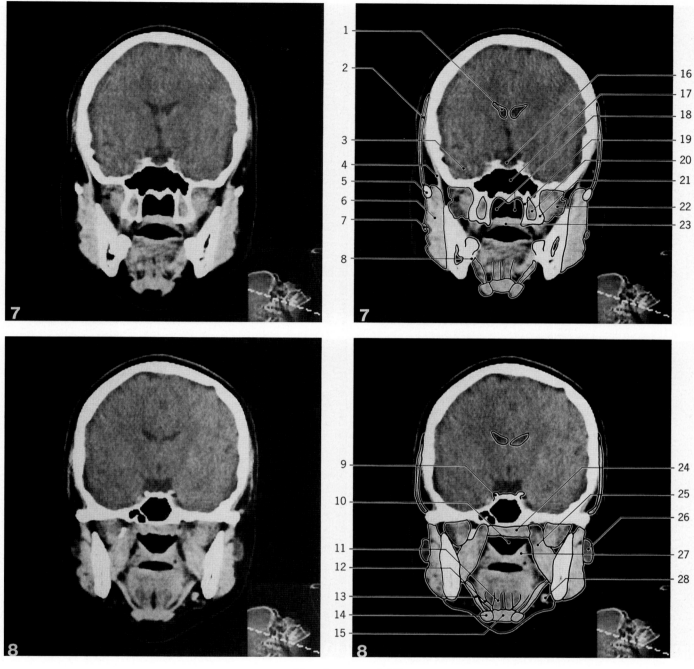

Head, coronal CT

Scout view on page 213
1: Lateral ventricle of brain
2: Galea aponeurotica
3: Temporal lobe
4: Temporalis (tendon)
5: Zygomatic arch
6: Masseter
7: Parotid duct
8: Mylohyoid line
9: Posterior clinoid process

10: Nasal part of pharynx
11: Genioglossus
12: Hyoglossus
13: Mylohyoideus
14: Digastricus, anterior belly
15: Geniohyoideus
16: Hypophyseal fossa
17: Sphenoidal sinus
18: Choanae
19: Medial pterygoid plate

20: Pterygoid fossa
21: Lateral pterygoid plate
22: Lateral pterygoid muscle
23: Soft palate
24: Longus capitis
25: Medial pterygoid muscle
26: Accessory parotid gland
27: Levator veli palatini
28: Submandibular lymph node

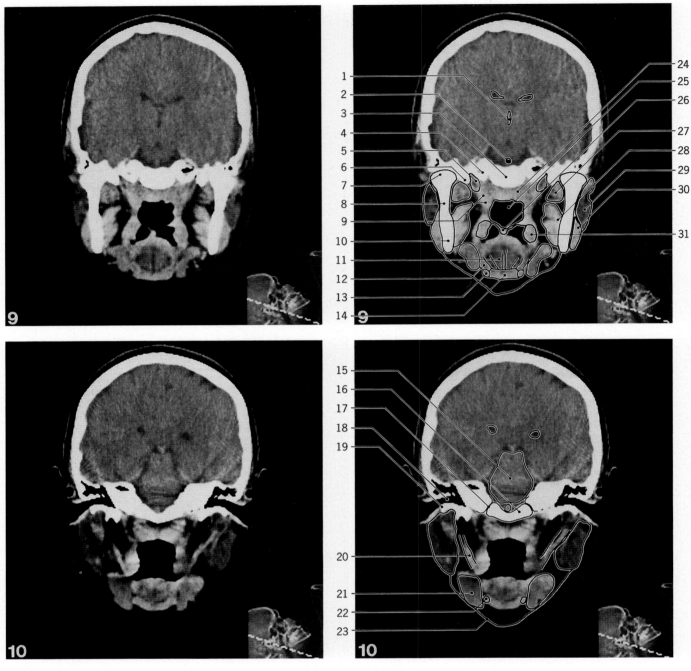

Head, coronal CT

Scout view on page 213

1: Third ventricle
2: Basilary artery
3: Body of sphenoid bone
4: Petrous part of temporal bone
5: Auditory tube
6: Spine of sphenoid bone
7: Head of mandible
8: Neck of mandible
9: Levator and tensor veli palatini
10: Angle of mandible

11: Genioglossus
12: Hyoglossus
13: Digastricus, anterior belly
14: Geniohyoideus
15: Brain stem
16: Basilar part of occipital bone
17: Petro-occipital fissure
18: External acoustic meatus
19: Tympanic part of temporal bone
20: Styloglossus
21: Submandibular gland

22: Digastricus (tendon)
23: Platysma
24: Longus capitis
25: Nasal part of pharynx
26: Uvula
27: Lateral pterygoid muscle
28: Medial pterygoid muscle
29: Parotid gland
30: Masseter
31: Palatine tonsil

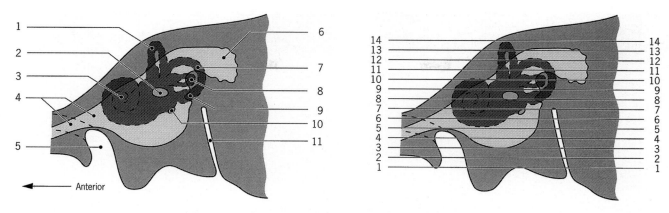

Petrous bone, CT series, diagrammatic scout view

Lines #1–14 indicate positions of sections in the following CT series. Consecutive sections, 3 mm thick

1: Anterior semicircular canal
2: Fenestra vestibuli
3: Cochlea
4: Auditory tube

5: Carotid canal
6: Mastoid antrum
7: Posterior semicircular canal
8: Lateral semicircular canal

9: Pyramidal process
10: Fenestra cochleae
11: Facial canal

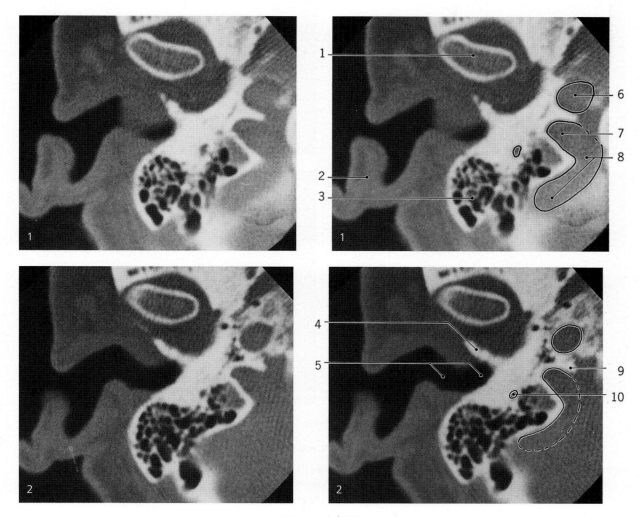

Ear, axial CT

Positions of sections are indicated above

1: Head of mandible
2: Auricle
3: Mastoid process with air cells
4: Tympanic part of temporal bone

5: External acoustic meatus
6: Carotid canal
7: Bulb of internal jugular vein
8: Sigmoid sinus

9: Intrajugular process
10: Facial canal

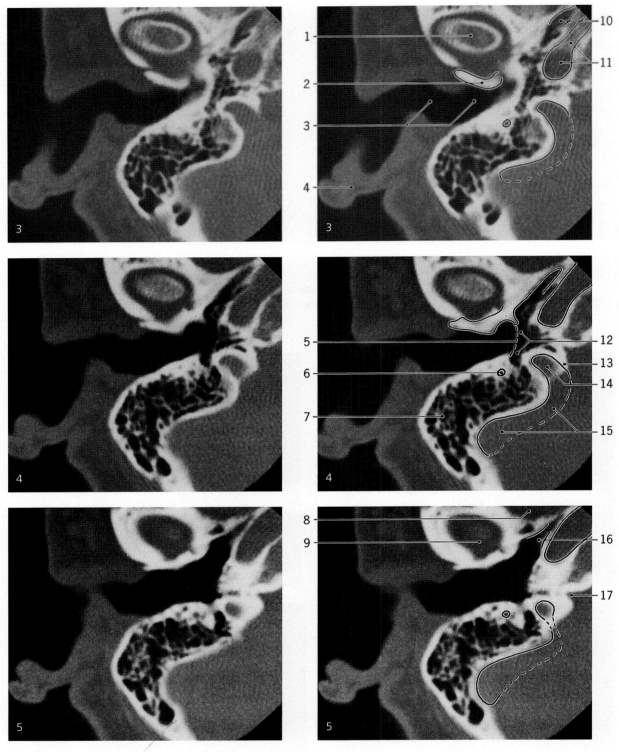

Ear, axial CT

Positions of section #3–5 are indicated on previous page

1: Head of mandible
2: Tympanic part (plate) of temporal bone
3: External acoustic meatus
4: Auricle
5: Tympanic membrane
6: Facial canal
7: Mastoid process with air cells
8: Middle cranial fossa
9: Articular disc of temporomandibular joint
10: Auditory tube
11: Carotid canal
12: Tympanic cavity
13: Intrajugular process
14: Bulb of internal jugular vein
15: Sigmoid sinus
16: Tympanic ostium of auditory tube
17: Aperture of cochlear canaliculus (perilymphatic duct)

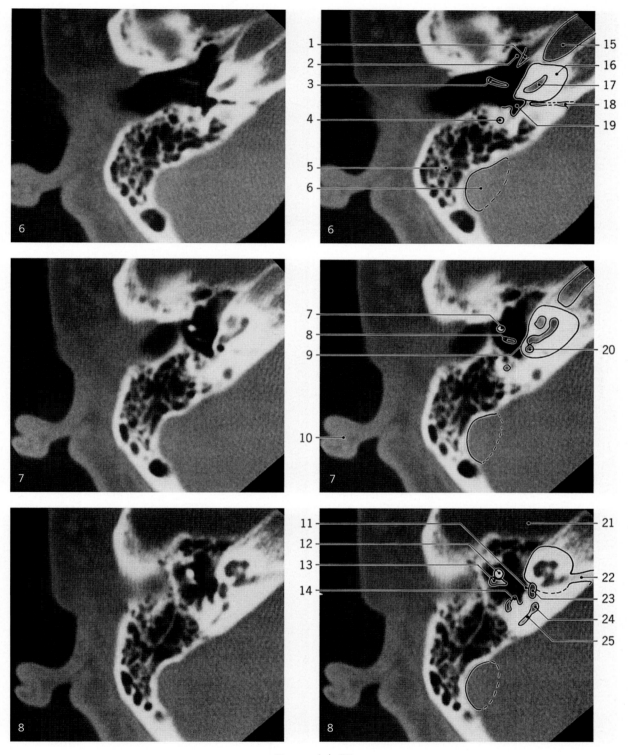

Ear, axial CT

Positions of section #6–8 are indicated on page 219

1: Tensor tympani muscle
2: Tympanic ostium of auditory tube
3: Manubrium of malleus
4: Facial canal
5: Air cells in mastoid process
6: Sigmoid sinus
7: Neck of malleus
8: Crus longum of incus
9: Promontory
10: Auricle

11: Base of stapes in fenestra vestibuli
12: Head of malleus
13: Body of incus
14: Pyramidal eminence
15: Carotid canal
16: Cochlea
17: Spiral canal
18: Canaliculus cochleae (perilymphatic duct)
19: Sinus tympani

20: Fenestra cochleae
21: Middle cranial fossa
22: Internal acoustic meatus
23: Vestibulum
24: Ampulla of posterior semicircular canal
25: Posterior semicircular canal

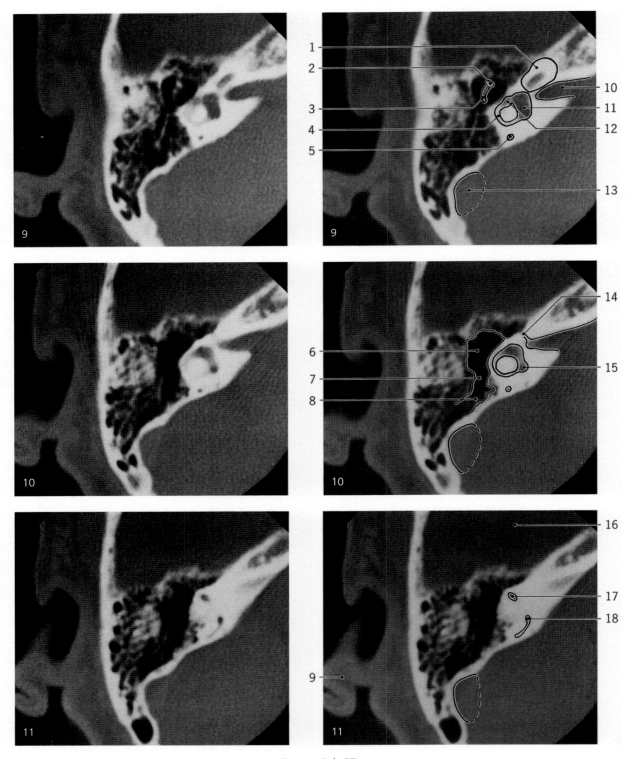

Ear, axial CT

Positions of section #9–11 are indicated on page 219

1: Cochlea
2: Head of malleus
3: Crus breve of incus
4: Lateral semicircular canal
5: Posterior semicircular canal
6: Epitympanic recess
7: Aditus ad antrum

8: Mastoid antrum
9: Auricle
10: Internal acoustic meatus
11: Vestibulum
12: Ampulla of lateral semicircular canal
13: Sigmoid sinus
14: Facial canal

15: Elliptical recess
16: Middle cranial fossa
17: Ampulla of anterior semicircular canal
18: Crus commune of ant. and post. semicircular canals

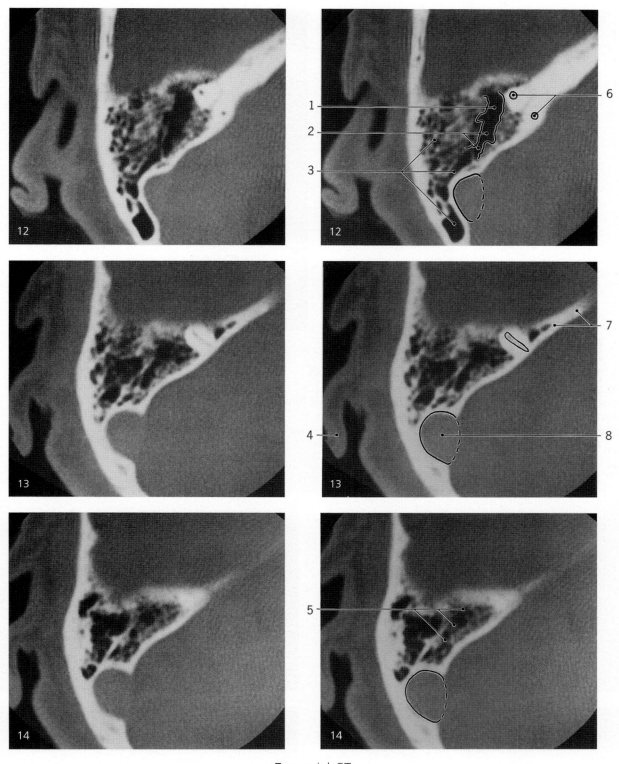

Ear, axial CT

Positions of section #12–14 are indicated on page 219

1: Epitympanic recess
2: Mastoid antrum
3: Air cells in mastoid process
4: Auricle
5: Tegmen tympani
6: Anterior semicircular canal
7: Superior margin of petrous bone
8: Sigmoid sinus

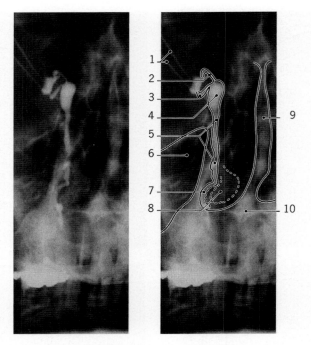

Lacrimal ducts, a-p X-ray, dacryography

1: Catheters inserted in puncta
   lacrimalia
2: Superior lacrimal canaliculus
3: Inferior lacrimal canaliculus
4: Lacrimal sac

5: Nasolacrimal duct
6: Maxillary sinus
7: Contrast medium flowing into nasal
   cavity
8: Inferior nasal concha

9: Nasal septum
10: Hard palate

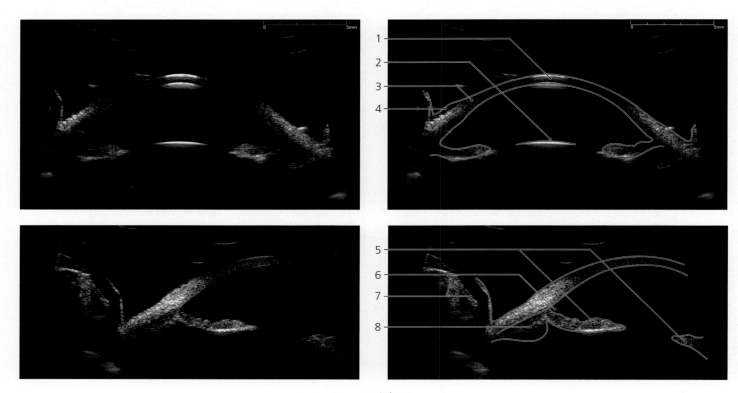

Eye, axial US

1: Cornea
2: Front of lens
3: Limbus of cornea

4: Conjunctiva
5: Iris
6: Irido-corneal angle

7: Lacrimal caruncle
8: Ciliary body

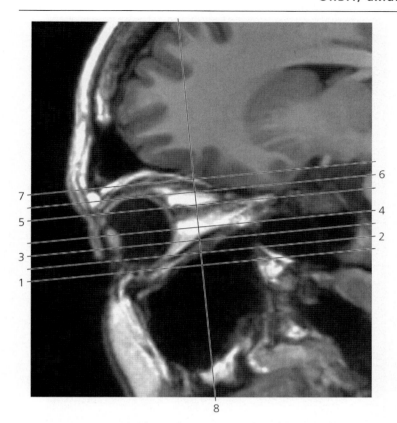

Scout view of orbita

Lines #1–7 indicate position of sections in the following axial MR series. Line #8 indicates the position of a coronal section. Note that bulbar structures do not correspond to the indicated planes in some of the images due to ocular movements during the period of examination.

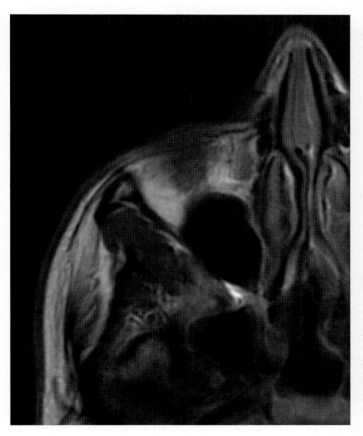

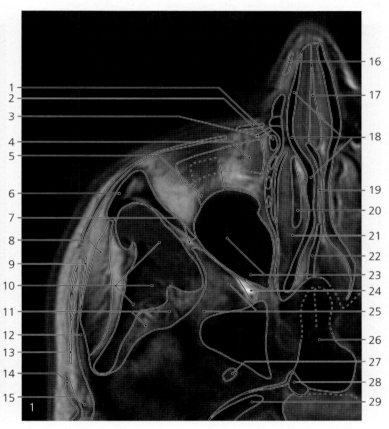

Orbita, axial MR

1: Lacrimal sac →
2: Levator labii superioris alaeque nasi
3: Orbicularis oculi (lacrimal part) →
4: Inferior oblique
5: Inferior rectus →
6: Zygomatic bone →
7: Inferior orbital fissure →
8: Masseter
9: Temporal fascia (superficial layer) →
10: Temporalis →

11: Pterygoid venous plexus
12: Zygomatic process of temporal bone
13: Temporo-parietal fascia →
14: Anterior auricular muscle →
15: Superficial temporal artery →
16: Nasal cartilage →
17: Nasal septum (cartilaginous part) →
18: Middle nasal meatus →
19: Ethmoidal bone (perpendicular plate) →
20: Middle nasal concha

21: Mucosa of middle nasal concha
22: Vomer →
23: Maxillary sinus →
24: Pterygopalatine fossa →
25: Greater wing of sphenoidal bone (with air cell) →
26: Sphenoidal sinus →
27: Foramen ovale
28: Foramen lacerum
29: Internal carotid artery (in carotid canal) →

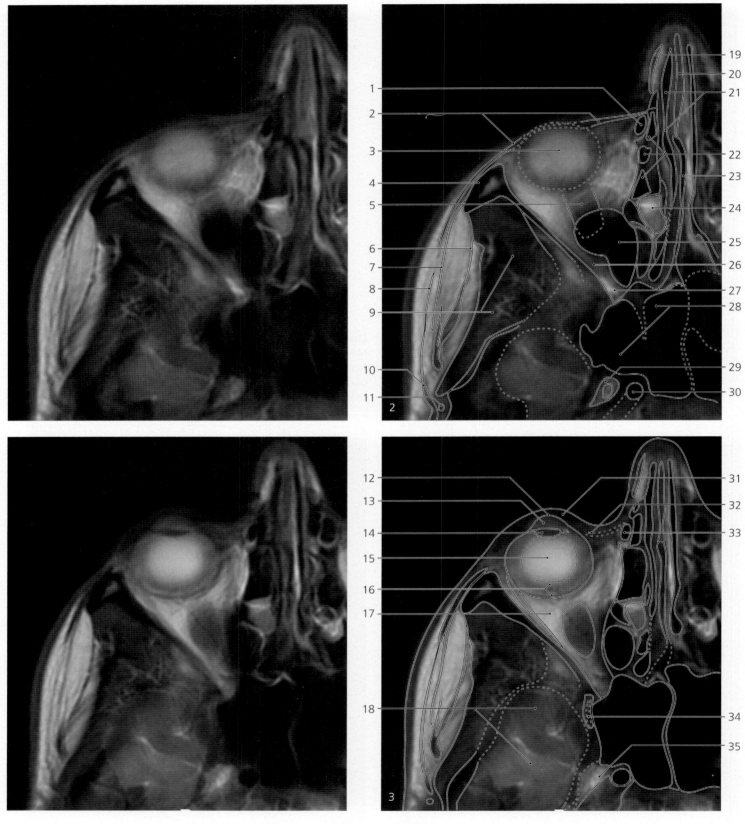

Orbita, axial MR

Scout view on page 225

1: Lacrimal sac ↔
2: Orbicularis oculi ↔
3: Eye ball →
4: Zygomatic bone ↔
5: Inferior rectus ↔
6: Temporal fascia (deep layer) →
7: Temporal fascia (superficial layer) ↔
8: Temporo-parietal fascia ↔
9: Temporalis ↔
10: Anterior auricular muscle ←
11: Superficial temporal artery ↔
12: Cornea →

13: Anterior eye chamber →
14: Lens ↔
15: Vitreous body →
16: Sclera, choroidea and retina tangentially cut
17: Retrobulbar fat ↔
18: Temporal lobe →
19: Nasal cartilage ←
20: Nasal septum (cartilaginous part) ←
21: Middle nasal meatus ←
22: Ethmoidal air cells ↔
23: Ethmoidal bone (perpendicular plate) ←
24: Air cell with fluid
25: Maxillary sinus ←

26: Inferior orbital fissure closed by fibromuscular tissue (Müller's muscle)
27: Pterygopalatine fossa ←
28: Sphenoidal sinus (extending into greater wing of sphenoidal bone) ↔
29: Trigeminal cave (Meckeli) →
30: Internal carotid artery ↔
31: Eyelid ↔
32: Medial palpebral ligament
33: Lacrimal sac in lacrimal fossa ↔
34: Maxillary nerve in foramen rotundum
35: Trigeminal cave with trigeminal ganglion ↔

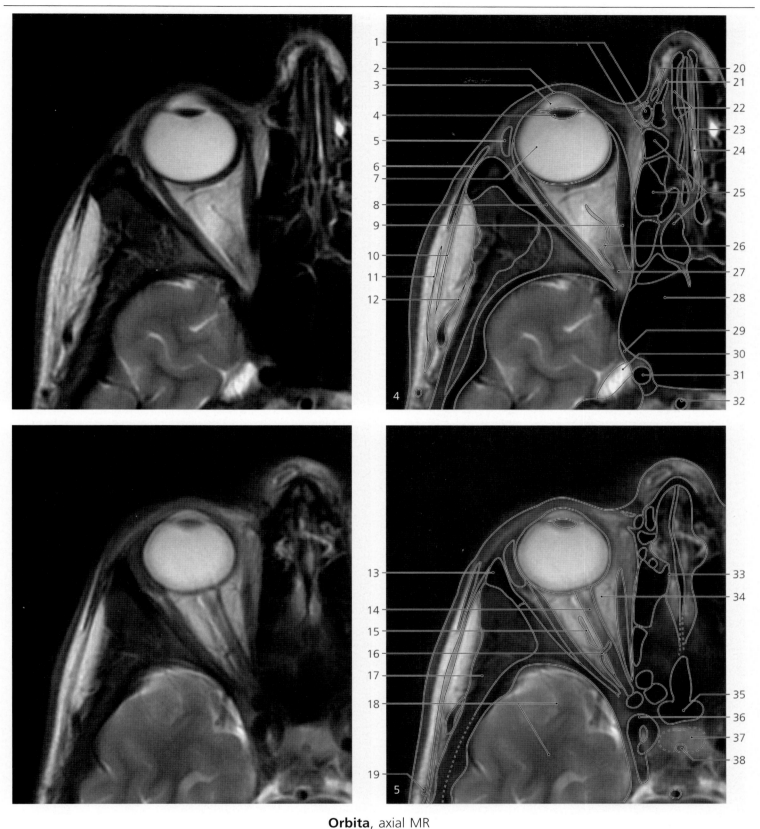

Orbita, axial MR

Scout view on page 225

1: Lacrimal sac and orbicularis oculi attaching on posterior lacrimal crest ↔
2: Cornea ↔
3: Anterior chamber of eye ↔
4: Lens ↔
5: Lacrimal gland →
6: Orbicularis oculi ↔
7: Vitreous body ↔
8: Rectus lateralis →
9: Rectus medialis →
10: Temporal fascia (superficial layer) ↔
11: Temporo-parietal fascia ↔
12: Temporal fascia (deep layer) ←

13: Zygomatic bone ←
14: Optic nerve →
15: Retrobulbar vein
16: Ophthalmic artery
17: Temporalis ↔
18: Temporal lobe ↔
19: Superficial temporal artery ↔
20: Corrugator supercilii
21: Nasal bone →
22: Middle nasal meatus ←
23: Nasal septum ←
24: Nasal mucosa
25: Ethmoidal air cells ↔

26: Retrobulbar vein
27: Superior orbital fissure →
28: Sphenoidal sinus ↔
29: Cavernous sinus
30: Trigeminal cave ←
31: Internal carotid artery ↔
32: Basilar artery →
33: Ethmoidal bulla
34: Retrobulbar fat ↔
35: Sphenoidal sinus ↔
36: Internal carotid artery (siphon) ←
37: Adenohypophysis
38: Neurohypophysis

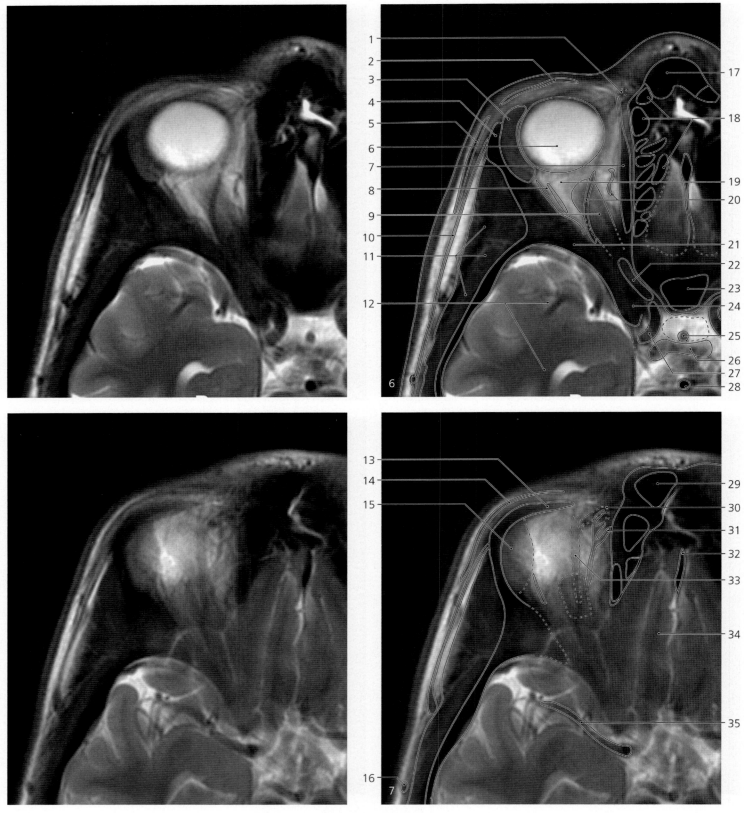

Orbita, axial MR

Scout view on page 225

1: Trochlea (of orbit)
2: Superior tarsus
3: Lacrimal gland ↔
4: Zygomatic process of frontal bone
5: Orbicularis oculi ↔
6: Vitreous body ←
7: Obliquus superior →
8: Lacrimal vessels
9: Rectus superior and levator palpebrae →
10: Superficial temporal fascia fused with temporo-parietal fascia →
11: Temporalis ↔

12: Temporal lobe ↔
13: Supraorbital margin of frontal bone
14: Orbicularis oculi ←
15: Lacrimal gland ←
16: Superficial temporal artery ←
17: Nasal bone ←
18: Ethmoidal air cells ↔
19: Retrobulbar fat ←
20: Retrobulbar veins ←
21: Lesser wing of sphenoidal bone ←
22: Optic nerve in optic canal ←
23: Sphenoidal sinus ←

24: Anterior clinoid process
25: Infundibulum of hypophysis
26: Dorsum sellae
27: Internal carotid artery ←
28: Basilar artery ←
29: Frontal sinus
30: Obliquus superior (tendon) ←
31: Anterior ethmoidal vessel
32: Crista galli
33: Superior ophthalmic vein
34: Gyrus rectus
35: Middle cerebral artery

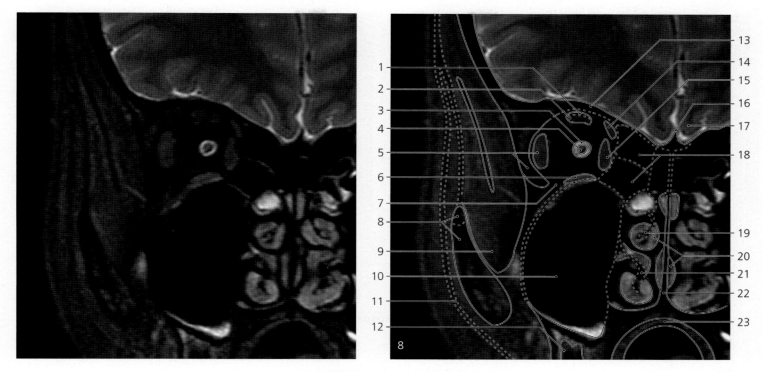

Orbita, coronal MR

Scout view on page 225

1: Levator palpebrae
2: Rectus superior
3: Subaracnoid space
4: Optic nerve
5: Rectus lateralis and greater wing of sphenoid bone
6: Rectus inferior
7: Inferior orbital fissure

8: Masseter and zygomatic arch
9: Temporalis
10: Maxillary sinus
11: Temporo-parietal fascia
12: Molar tooth
13: Orbital part of frontal bone
14: Obliquus superior
15: Rectus medialis
16: Crista galli

17: Gyrus rectus
18: Ethmoidal air cells
19: Middle nasal concha
20: Mucosa
21: Inferior nasal concha
22: Nasal septum
23: Mucosa of hard palate

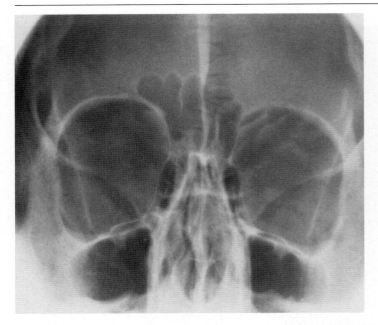

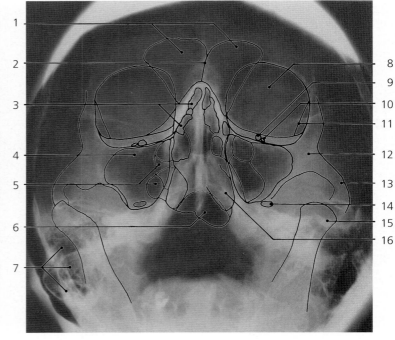

Paranasal sinuses, a-p X-ray

1: Falx cerebri (calcified)
2: Frontal sinus
3: Orbita
4: Ethmoidal air cells
5: Superior orbital fissure

6: Maxillary sinus
7: Sagittal suture
8: Innominate line (radiology term, tangential view of greater wing of sphenoid bone)

9: Hypophyseal fossa (bottom)
10: Nasal septum

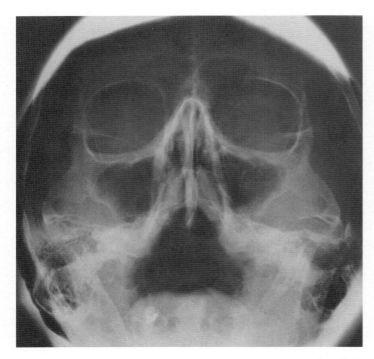

Paranasal sinuses, a-p, tilted X-ray

1: Frontal sinus
2: Septum of frontal sinus
3: Anterior ethmoidal air cells
4: Maxillary sinus
5: Posterior ethmoidal air cells
6: Sphenoid sinus

7: Mastoid air cells
8: Orbita
9: Foramen rotundum
10: Infra-orbital foramen
11: Innominate line (radiology term)
12: Body of zygomatic bone

13: Zygomatic arch
14: Oval foramen
15: Head of mandible
16: Inferior nasal concha

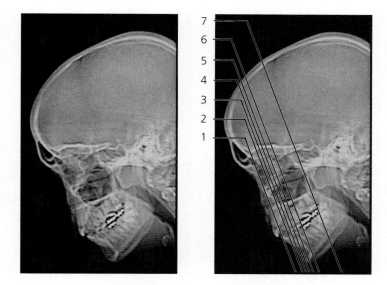

Paranasal sinuses, scout view

Lines #1–7 indicate positions of sections in the following CT series. Sections are 1 mm thick. Prone position with hyperextended neck. Sections #2–6 display the "ostiomeatal complex/unit" comprising the maxillary sinus ostium, infundibulum, uncinate process, hiatus semilunaris, ethmoidal bulla, middle concha and middle meatus. Arrows ←, → and ↔ indicate that a structure can be seen on a previous or following section or both.

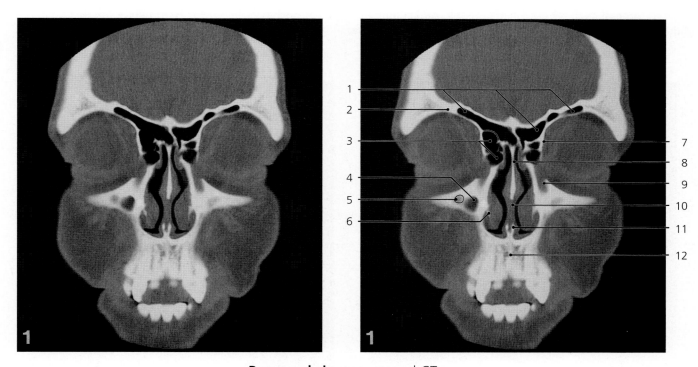

Paranasal sinuses, coronal CT

1: Frontal sinus →
2: Orbital part of frontal bone →
3: Anterior ethmoidal air cells →
4: Maxillary sinus →
5: Infraorbital foramen

6: Inferior nasal concha →
7: Lacrimal bone →
8: Perpendicular plate of ethmoidal bone →
9: Nasolacrimal duct

10: Cartilaginous part of nasal septum →
11: Vomer →
12: Incisive bone

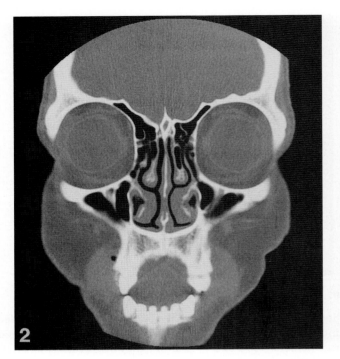

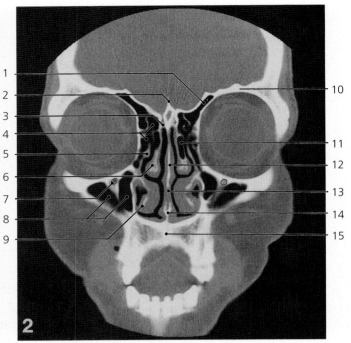

Paranasal sinuses, coronal CT

1: Frontal sinus ↔
2: Crista galli →
3: Cribriform plate →
4: Anterior ethmoidal air cells ↔
5: Uncinate process →
6: Middle nasal concha →

7: Infraorbital canal →
8: Maxillary sinus ↔
9: Inferior nasal concha ↔
10: Orbital part of frontal bone ↔
11: Air cell in middle nasal concha (concha bullosa) →

12: Perpendicular plate of ethmoidal bone ↔
13: Cartilaginous part of nasal septum ↔
14: Vomer ↔
15: Hard palate →

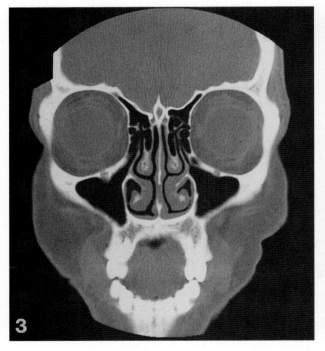

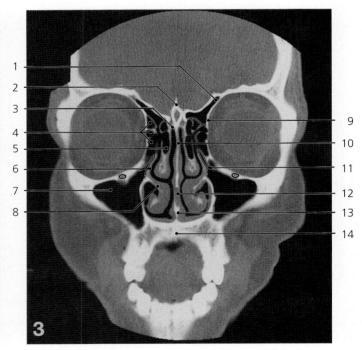

Paranasal sinuses, coronal CT

1: Frontal sinus ↔
2: Crista galli ↔
3: Cribriform plate ↔
4: Anterior ethmoidal air cells ↔
5: Air cell in middle concha (concha bullosa) ↔

6: Uncinate process ↔
7: Maxillary sinus ↔
8: Inferior nasal concha ↔
9: Lamina papyracea of ethmoidal bone →
10: Perpendicular plate of ethmoidal bone ↔

11: Duct between maxillary sinus and nasal cavity →
12: Cartilaginous part of nasal septum ↔
13: Vomer ↔
14: Hard palate ↔

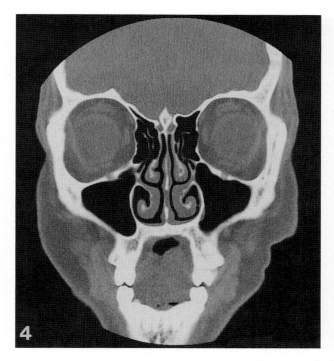

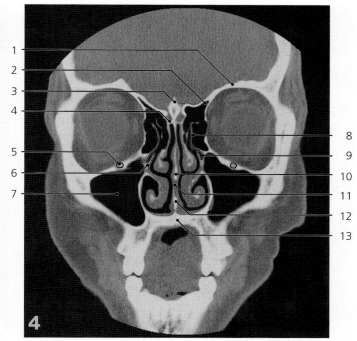

Paranasal sinuses, coronal CT

Position of sections is indicated on scout view on page 231

1: Orbital part of frontal bone ↔
2: Frontal sinus ↔
3: Crista galli ↔
4: Cribriform plate ↔
5: Infraorbital canal ↔

6: Uncinate process ↔
7: Maxillary sinus ↔
8: Ethmoidal bulla →
9: Duct between maxillary sinus and nasal cavity ↔

10: Perpendicular plate of ethmoidal bone ↔
11: Cartilaginous part of nasal septum ↔
12: Vomer ↔
13: Hard palate ↔

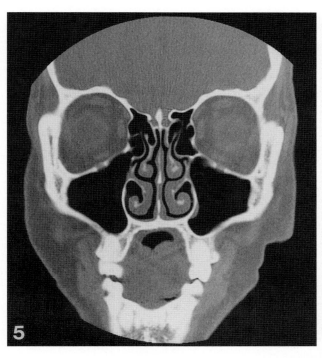

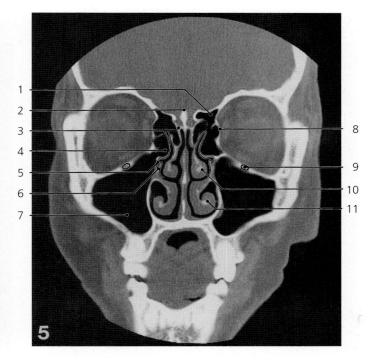

Paranasal sinuses, coronal CT

1: Frontal sinus ←
2: Crista galli ↔
3: Cribriform plate ↔
4: Ethmoidal bulla ←
5: Opening of duct from maxillary sinus in hiatus semilunaris ←

6: Uncinate process ←
7: Maxillary sinus ↔
8: Lamina papyracea of ethmoidal bone ↔

9: Infraorbital canal ↔
10: Middle nasal concha ↔
11: Inferior nasal concha ↔

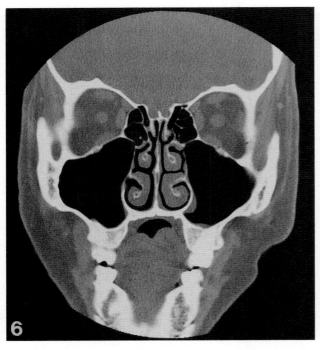

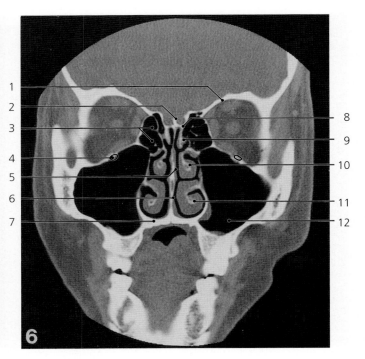

Paranasal sinuses, coronal CT

Position of sections is indicated on scout view on page 231

1: Orbital part of frontal bone ←
2: Crista galli ←
3: Anterior ethmoidal air cells ←
4: Infraorbital canal ←
5: Perpendicular plate of ethmoidal
   bone ←

6: Vomer ↔
7: Hard palate ←
8: Cribriform plate ←
9: Superior nasal concha

10: Middle nasal concha ←
11: Inferior nasal concha ←
12: Maxillary sinus ←

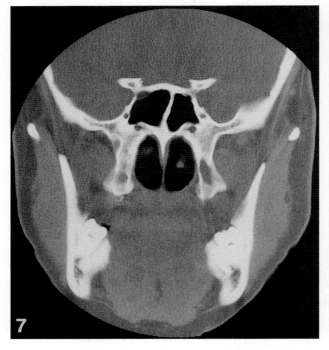

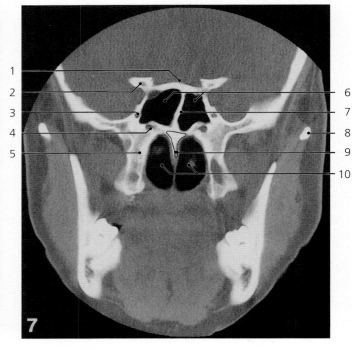

Paranasal sinuses, coronal CT

1: Prechiasmic sulcus
2: Anterior clinoid process
3: Foramen rotundum
4: Pterygoid canal

5: Pterygoid process
6: Sphenoidal sinus
7: Septum of sphenoidal sinus
8: Zygomatic arch

9: Vomer ←
10: Choanae

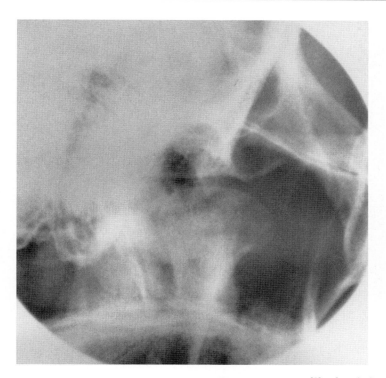
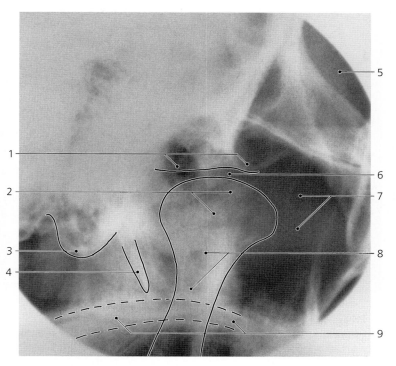

Temporomandibular joint, oblique X-ray, transmaxillary

1: Articular tubercle	4: Styloid process	7: Maxillary sinus
2: Head of mandible	5: Orbita	8: Neck of mandible
3: Mastoid process	6: Temporomandibular joint (with disc)	9: Hard palate

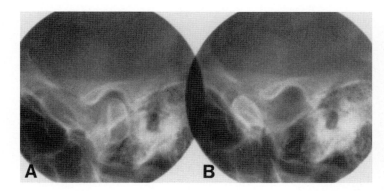
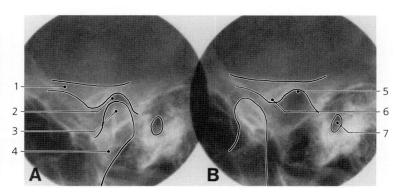

Temporomandibular joint, oblique X-ray

A: mouth closed. B: mouth open

1: Zygomatic arch	4: Neck of mandible	7: External acoustic meatus
2: Temporomandibular joint (with disc)	5: Mandibular fossa	
3: Head of mandible	6: Articular tubercle	

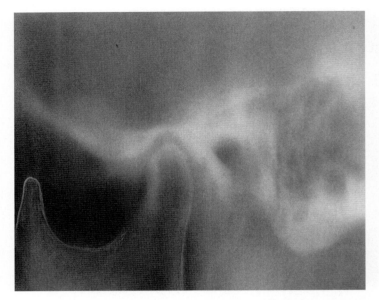
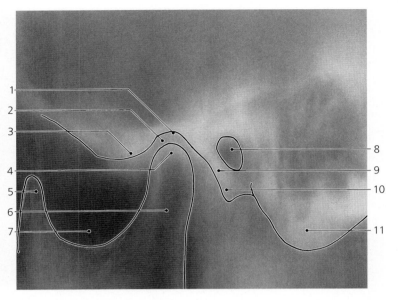

Temporomandibular joint, lateral X-ray, tomography

1: Mandibular fossa
2: Articular disc
3: Articular tubercle
4: Head of mandible
5: Coronoid process

6: Neck of mandible
7: Mandibular incisure
8: External acoustic meatus
9: Tympanic part (plate) of temporal bone

10: Styloid process (root)
11: Mastoid process

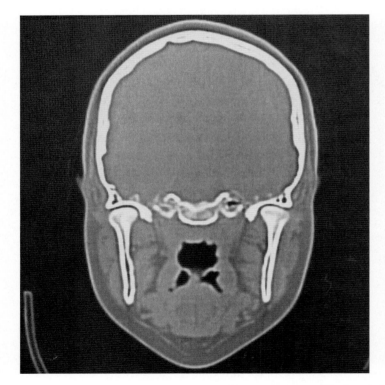
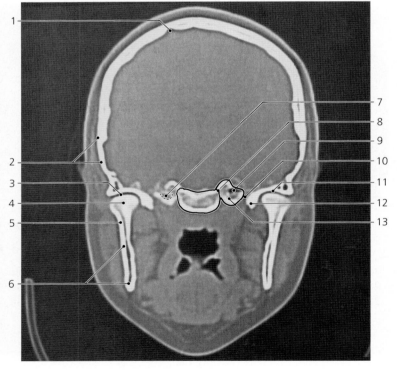

Temporomandibular joint, coronal CT (bone settings)

1: Granular foveola
2: Squamous part of temporal bone
3: Temporomandibular joint
4: Head of mandible
5: Neck of mandible

6: Ramus of mandible
7: Carotid canal, anterior bend
8: Petro-occipital fissure
9: Air cell in petrous bone
10: Sphenopetrous fissure

11: Mandibular fossa
12: Spine of sphenoid bone
13: Apex of petrous bone

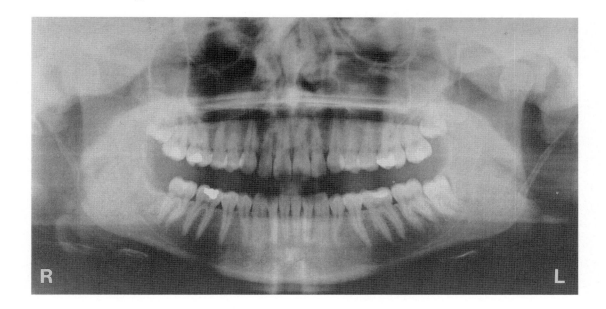

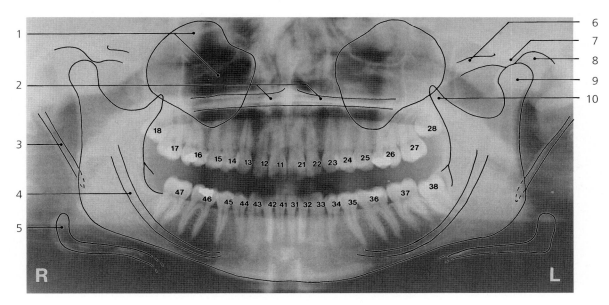

Teeth, adult, rotational panoramic X-ray

Teeth are numbered according to the Two Digit System of the Federation Dentaire Internationale (FDI)

1: Maxillary sinus
2: Hard palate
3: Styloid process
4: Mandibular canal

5: Great horn of hyoid bone
6: Zygomatic arch
7: Articular tubercle
8: Mandibular fossa

9: Head of mandible
10: Coronoid process of mandible

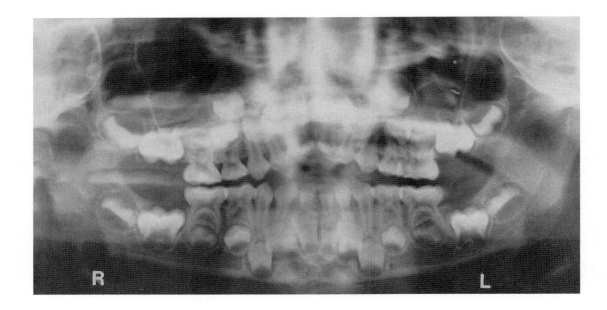

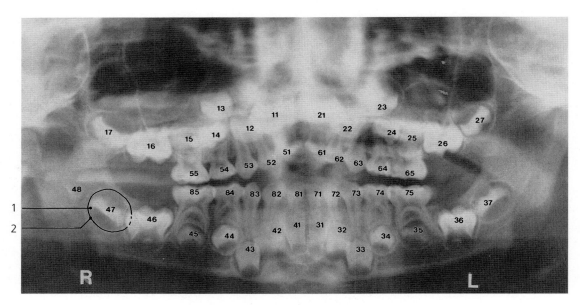

Teeth, child 5 years, rotational panoramic X-ray

Teeth are numbered according to the Two Digit System of the Federation Dentaire Internationale (FDI)

1: Periodontoblastic lamina
2: Dental sac

11: First permanent incisor tooth
12: Second permanent incisor tooth
13: Permanent canine tooth
14: First permanent premolar tooth
15: Second permanent premolar tooth
16: First permanent molar tooth
17: Second permanent molar tooth

48: Third permanent molar tooth
     (wisdom tooth)
51: First deciduous incisor tooth
52: Second deciduous incisor tooth
53: Deciduous canine tooth
54: First deciduous molar tooth
55: Second deciduous molar tooth

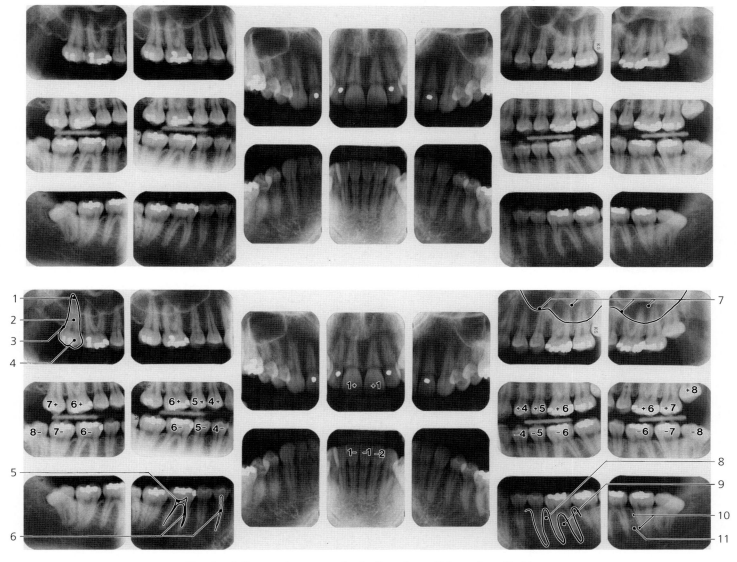

Teeth, full mouth survey (including four "bite-wings"), X-ray

Teeth are numbered according to the Haderup formula

1: Apex of root
2: Radix dentis (root)
3: Cervical margin
4: Crown

5: Pulp chamber
6: Pulp canal
7: Maxillary sinus
8: Interalveolar septum

9: Interradicular septum
10: Lamina dura of dental alveolus
11: Cancellous bone

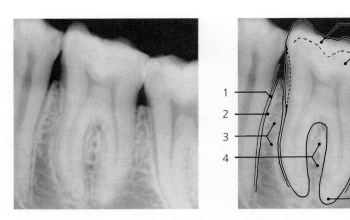

Tooth, first premolar, X-ray

1: Periodontal ligament space
2: Lamina dura
3: Interalveolar septum
4: Interradicular septum

5: Enamel
6: Dentine
7: Crown
8: Neck

9: Pulp cavity of crown
10: Root canal
11: Root
12: Root apex

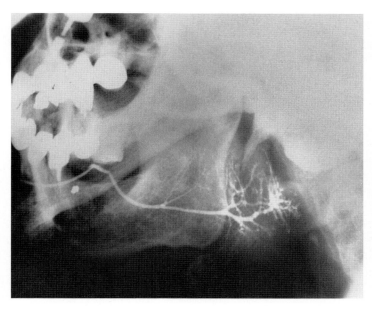

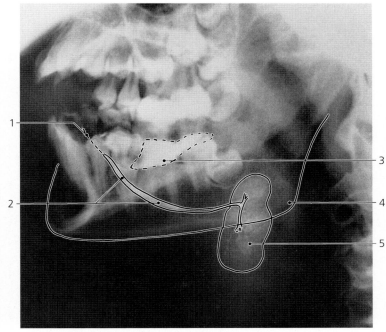

Parotid gland, oblique X-ray, sialography

1: Orifice of parotid duct
2: Cannula
3: Angle of mandible (contralateral)

4: Styloid process
5: Mastoid process
6: Parotid duct

7: Intraglandular ducts
8: Angle of mandible (ipsilateral)
9: Base of mandible

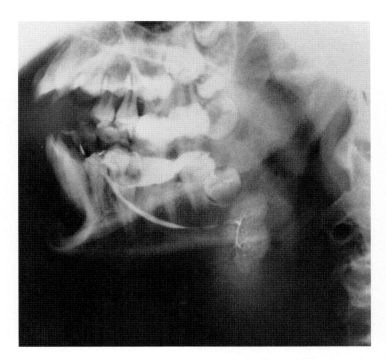

Submandibular gland, lateral X-ray, sialography

1: Cannula
2: Submandibular duct

3: Contrast medium in mouth
4: Angle of mandible

5: Submandibular gland

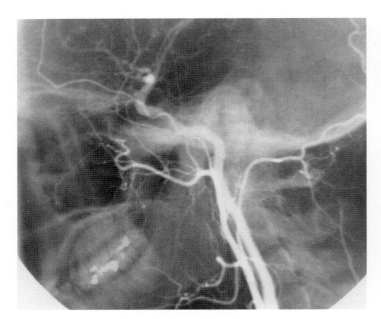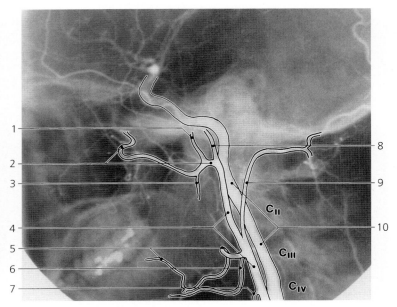

Carotid arteries, lateral X-ray, arteriography

1: Middle meningeal artery
2: Maxillary artery
3: Inferior alveolar artery
4: External carotid artery

5: Facial artery
6: Lingual artery
7: Superior thyroid artery
8: Superficial temporal artery

9: Occipital artery
10: Internal carotid artery

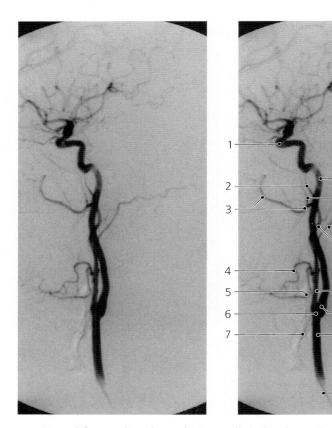

Carotid arteries, lateral X-ray, digital subtraction arteriography

1: Carotid "syphon"
2: Superficial temporal artery
3: Maxillary artery
4: Facial artery
5: Lingual artery

6: Carotid bifurcation
7: Superior thyroid artery
8: Internal carotid artery
9: Middle meningeal artery
10: Occipital artery

11: External carotid artery
12: Carotid sinus
13: Common carotid artery
14: Catheter

Brain

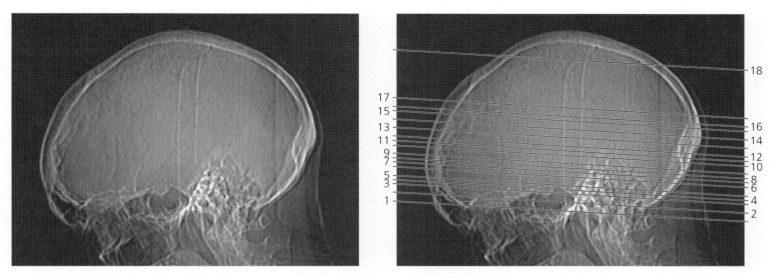

Scout view of brain

Lines #1–18 indicate position of sections in the following axial CT series.

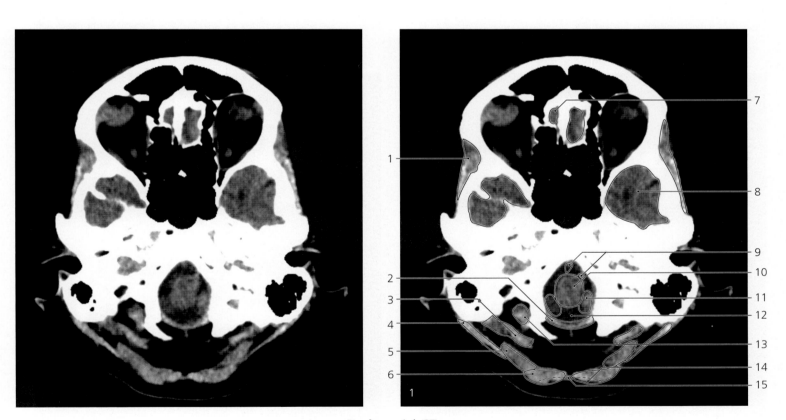

Brain, axial CT

The corresponding image of the skull base is shown on page 207, image #1.

1: Temporalis →
2: Posterior atlantooccipital membrane
3: Rectus capitis posterior major and minor
4: Sternocleidomastoideus →

5: Splenius capitis and obliuus capitis superior →
6: Semispinalis capitis →
7: Olfactory bulb
8: Temporal lobe →
9: Vertebral arteries in cisterna medullaris →

10: Medulla oblongata →
11: Tonsil of cerebellum →
12: Cisterna magna
13: Rectus capitis lateralis
14: Trapezius →
15: Nuchal ligament →

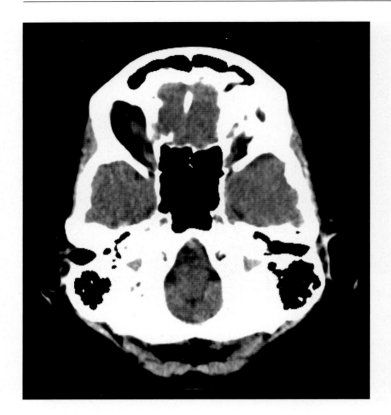
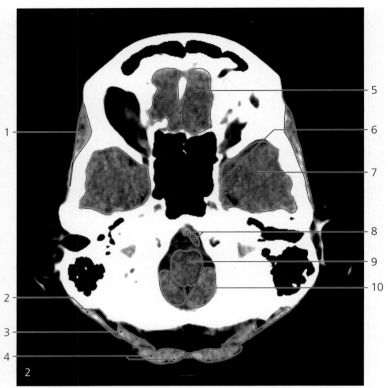
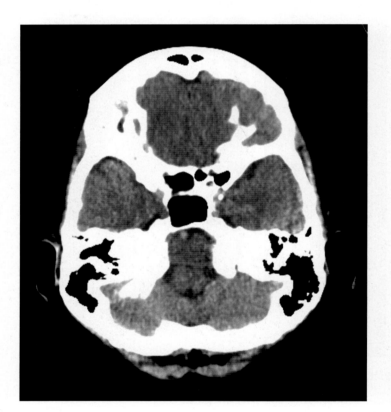
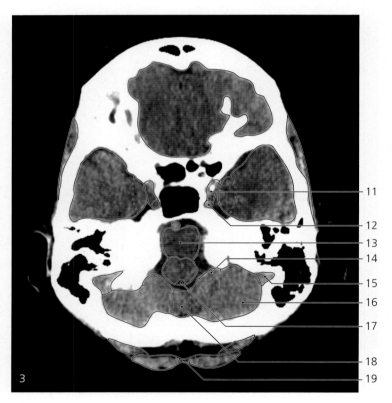

Brain, axial CT

Scout view on page 245. Image #2 of this series is shown in bone settings on page 208.
Image #3 is similarly shown on page 209.

1: Temporalis ↔
2: Sternocleidomastoideus ←
3: Splenius capitis and obliquus capitis superior ↔
4: Semispinalis capitis and trapezius ↔
5: Gyrus rectus
6: Uncus of temporal lobe →

7: Temporal lobe ↔
8: Vertebral arteries in cistern medullaris ←
9: Medulla oblongata ←
10: Cerebellum (tonsil) ←
11: Cavernous sinus →
12: Internal carotid artery →

13: Pons →
14: Flocculus →
15: Sigmoid sinus →
16: Cerebellar hemisphere →
17: Fourth ventricle (obex) →
18: Vermis (nodule) →
19: Nuchal ligament ←

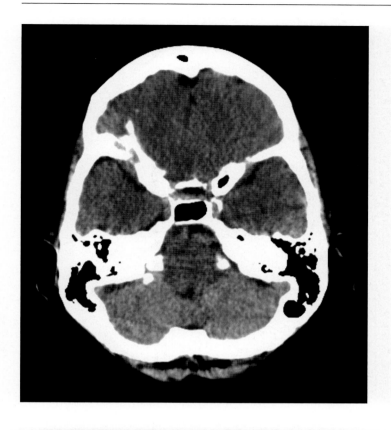
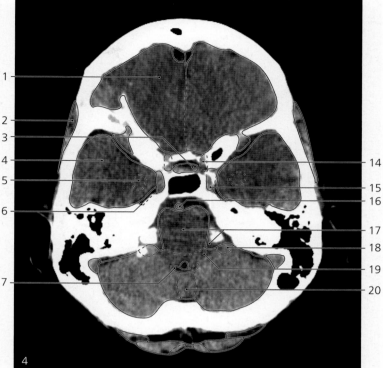
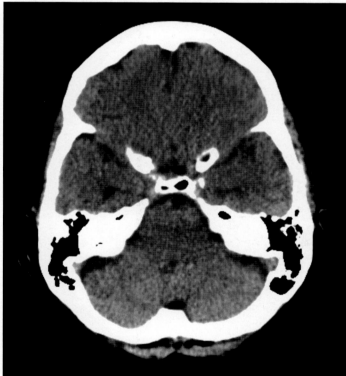
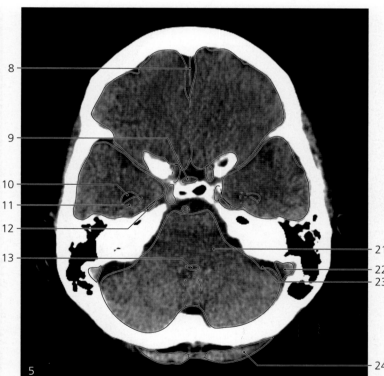

Brain, axial CT

Scout view on page 245. Images #4 and #5 of this series are shown in bone settings on page 210, images #6 and #7.

1: Frontal lobe →
2: Temporalis ←
3: Pituitary gland
4: Temporal lobe ↔
5: Amygdaloid nucleus
6: Trigeminal cave
7: Choroid plexus of fourth ventricle
8: Falx cerebri ↔
9: Infundibulum and pars tuberalis of pituitary gland

10: Lateral ventricle (temporal horn) →
11: Hippocampus →
12: Trigeminal ganglion
13: Fourth ventricle ↔
14: Internal carotid artery (siphon) ←
15: Cavernous sinus ←
16: Basilar artery in cicterna pontina ↔
17: Pons ↔ and cerebellopontine angle/cistern
18: Flocculus ←

19: Inferior cerebellar peduncle
20: Vermis (uvula) ↔
21: Middle cerebellar peduncle →
22: Sigmoid sinus ↔
23: Horizontal fissure →
24: Semispinalis capitis and trapezius ↔

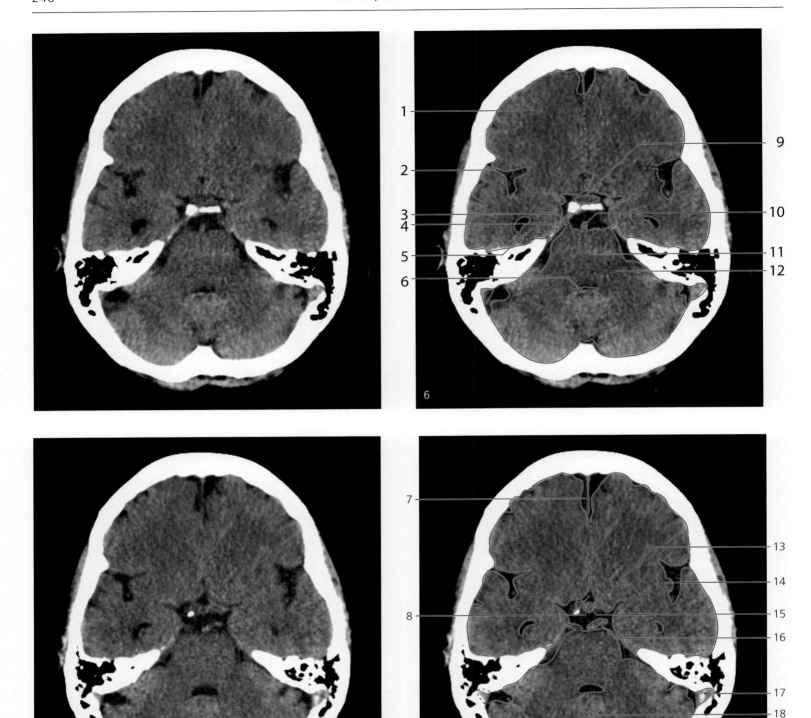

Brain, axial CT

Scout view on page 245

1: Frontal lobe ↔
2: Lateral sulcus (of Sylvius) →
3: Trigeminal nerve
4: Superior petrosal sinus in dura strap (petrosphenoidal ligament)
5: Hippocampus ↔
6: Fourth ventricle (rhomboid fossa) ↔
7: Falx cerebri ↔
8: Suprasellar ('pentagonal') cistern →

9: Optic chiasm
10: Basilar artery in cistern pontina ←
11: Pons ←
12: Middle cerebral peduncle ←
13: Middle cerebral artery
14: Insula →
15: Infundibulum (with infundibular recess) ←
16: Posterior cerebral artery

17: Sigmoid sinus ↔
18: Vermis (tuber) ↔
19: Cerebellar hemisphere ↔
20: Horizontal fissure ↔
21: Posterior belly of epicranius muscle

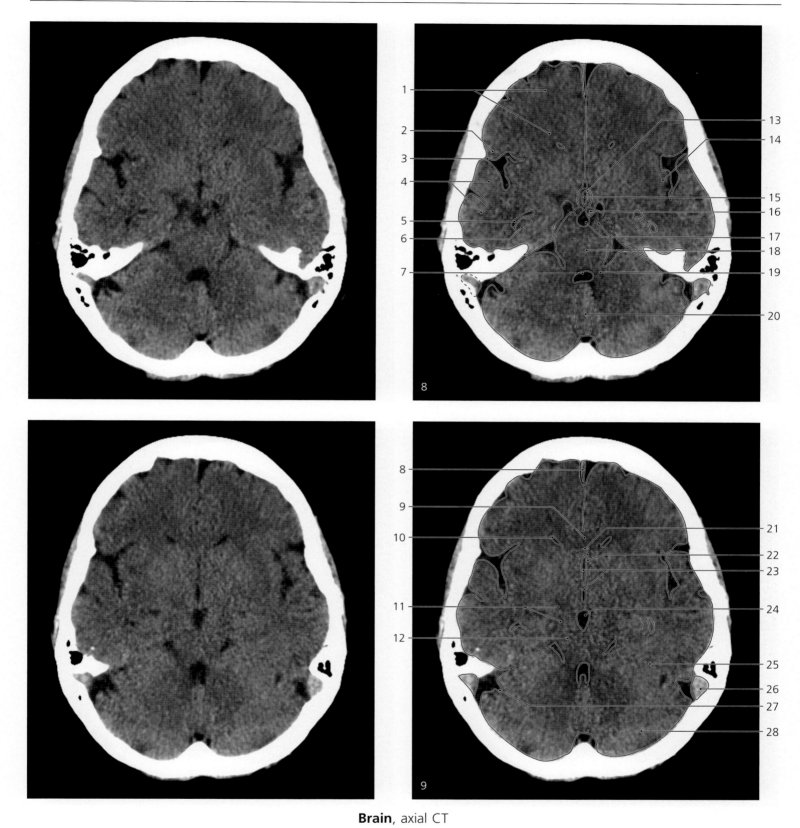

Brain, axial CT

Scout view on page 245

1: Frontal lobe ↔
2: Operculum ↔
3: Lateral sulcus (of Sylvius) ↔
4: Temporal lobe ↔
5: Lateral ventricle (temporal horn) ↔
6: Hippocampus ↔
7: Fourth ventricle (rhomboid fossa) ↔
8: Falx cerebri ↔
9: Corpus callosum (rostrum) →
10: Lateral ventricle (frontal horn) →

11: Cerebral peduncle
12: Red nucleus
13: Hypothalamus →
14: Insula ↔
15: Third ventricle →
16: Mammilary body
17: Cerebral peduncle and
    interpeduncular fossa ←
18: Mesencephalon (midbraim)
19: Superior cerebellar peduncle

20: Vermis (tuber) ↔
21: Anterior commissure
22: Hypothalamus ↔
23: Third ventricle ↔
24: Interpeduncular fossa ←
25: Tentorium cerebella →
26: Sigmoid sinus ←
27: Horizontal fissure ←
28: Cerebellar hemisphere ↔

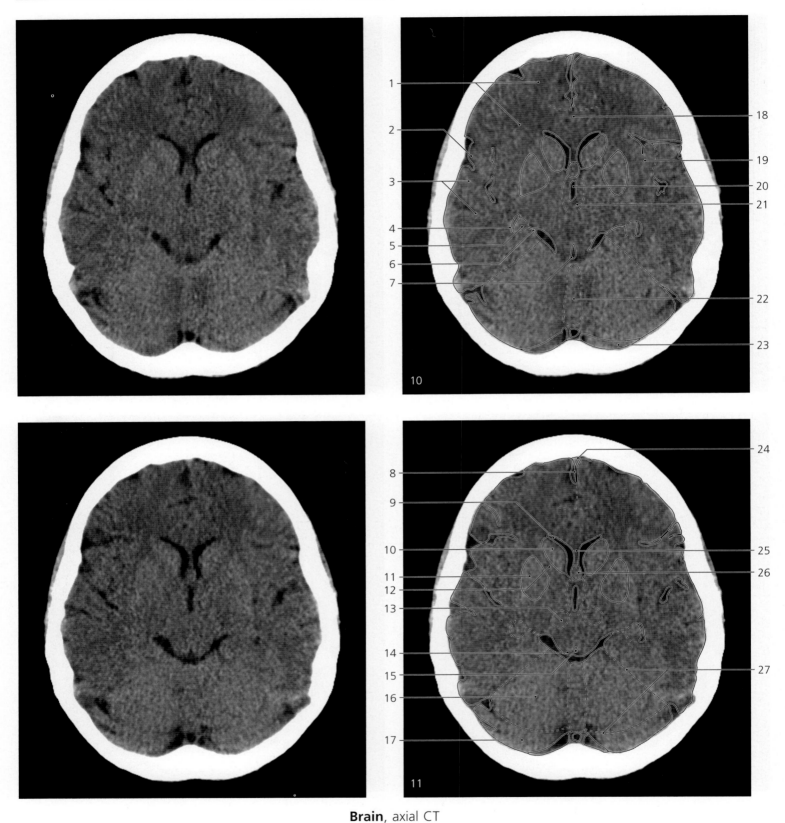

Brain, axial CT

Scout view on page 245

1: Frontal lobe ↔
2: Operculum ←
3: Temporal lobe ↔
4: Lateral ventricle (temporal horn) ↔
5: Hippocampus and choroid plexus ↔
6: Hippocampal sulcus
7: Fourth ventricle ←
8: Falx cerebri ↔
9: Lateral ventricle (frontal horn) ↔

10: Caudate nucleus (head)
11: Lentiform nucleus →
12: Internal capsule (anterior limb) ↔
13: Subthalamic area →
14: Inferior colliculus
15: Cerebral aqueduct
16: Cerebellar hemisphere ↔
17: Occipital lobe →
18: Corpus callosum (genu) →

19: Insula ↔
20: Third ventricle ↔
21: Hypothalamus ↔
22: Vermis ↔
23: Transverse sinus →
24: Superior sagittal sinus →
25: Septum pellucidum →
26: Column of fornix
27: Tentorium cerebelli ↔

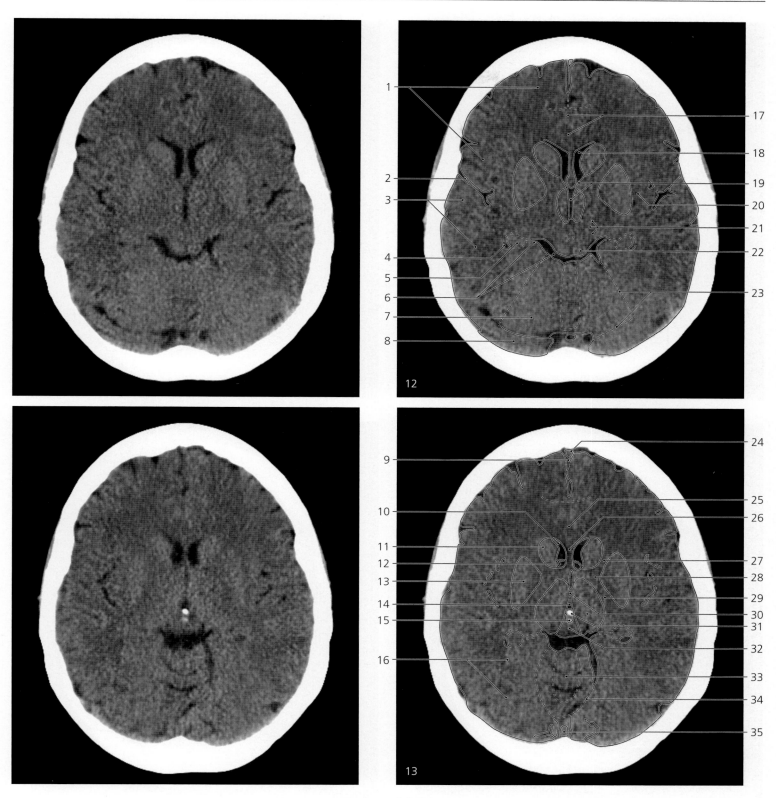

Brain, axial CT

Scout view on page 245

1: Frontal lobe ↔
2: Lateral sulcus (Sylvius)
3: Temporal lobe ↔
4: Lateral ventricle (temporal horn) ↔
5: Choroid plexus ↔
6: Hippocampal sulcus and quadrigeminal cistern →
7: Cerebellar hemisphere ↔
8: Occipital lobe ↔
9: Falx cerebri ↔
10: Lateral ventricle (central part) ↔
11: Caudate nucleus (body) ↔
12: Choroid plexus ↔

13: Lentiform nucleus ↔
14: Third ventricle ↔
15: Pineal body (with calcification)
16: Occipital lobe ↔
17: Corpus callosum (genu) ↔
18: Lateral ventricle (central part) ↔
19: Interventricular foramen (Monroi) and third ventricle →
20: Insula ↔
21: Subthalamic area ←
22: Superior colliculus
23: Tentorium cerebelli ↔
24: Superior sagittal sinus →

25: Corpus callosum (body) ↔
26: Septum pellucidum ←
27: Internal capsule (anterior limb) ←
28: Internal capsule (genu) ←
29: Internal capsule (posterior limb) ←
30: Thalamus → and interthalamic adhesion
31: Habenula (with calcification)
32: Tectal plate of midbrain
33: Vermis (culmen) ↔
34: Tentorium cerebelli ↔
35: Confluence of sinuses

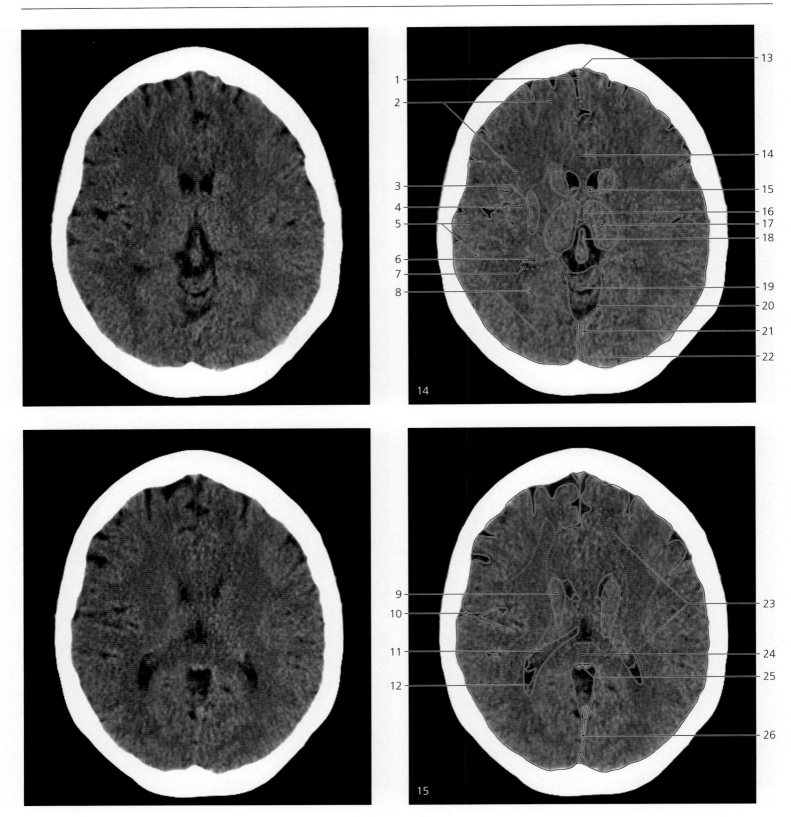

Brain, axial CT

Scout view on page 245

1: Falx cerebri ↔
2: Frontal lobe ↔
3: Lentiform nucleus ←
4: Insula ←
5: Temporal lobe ←
6: Choroid plexus ↔
7: Lateral ventricle (temporal horn) ←
8: Occipital lobe ↔
9: Caudate nucleus (body) ↔
10: Lateral sulcus (of Sylvius)

11: Choroid plexus (in atrium of lateral ventricle) ↔
12: Lateral ventricle (occipital horn) →
13: Superior sagittal sinus ↔
14: Corpus callosum (body) ↔
15: Choroid plexus (in central part of lateral ventricle) ↔
16: Third ventricle ←
17: Thalamus ←
18: Great cerebral vein (of Galen) in transverse cerebral fissure

19: Vermis (culmen) ←
20: Tentorium cerebelli ↔
21: Straight sinus →
22: Superior sagittal sinus ↔
23: Corona radiate (centrum semiovale) →
24: Corpus callosum (splenium) ↔
25: Superior cerebellar veins →
26: Falx cerebri ↔

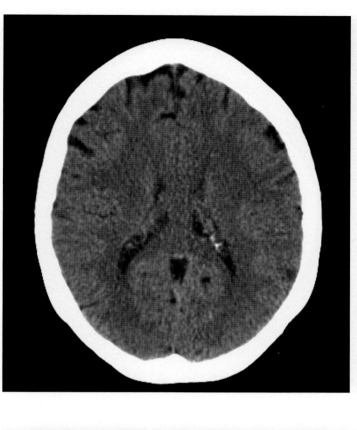

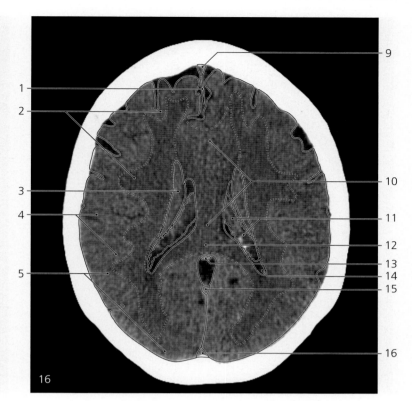

16

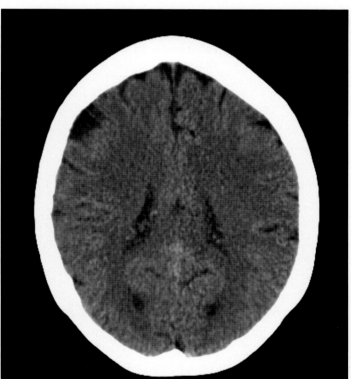

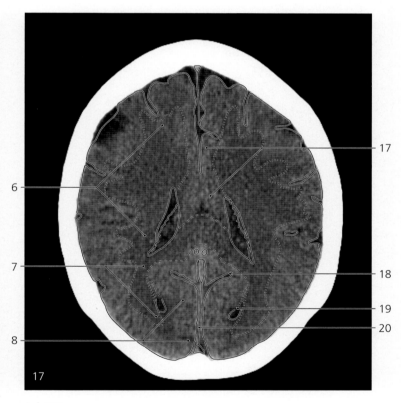

17

Brain, axial CT

Scout view on page 245

1: Falx cerebri ↔
2: Frontal lobe ↔
3: Caudate nucleus (body) ←
4: Parietal lobe →
5: Occcipital lobe ↔
6: Corona radiata ←
7: Optic radiation

8: Visual cortex
9: Superior sagittal sinus ↔
10: Corpus callosum (body) ←
11: Choroid plexus (with calcifications) ↔
12: Corpus callosum (splenium) ←
13: Superior cerebellar veins ←
14: Lateral ventricle (occipital horn) ↔

15: Straight sinus ←
16: Superior sagittal sinus ↔
17: Cingulate gyrus
18: Calcarine fissure
19: Lateral ventricle (occipital horn) ←
20: Falx cerebri (in longitudinal cerebral fissure) ↔

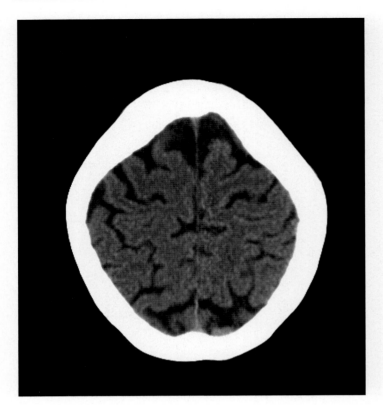
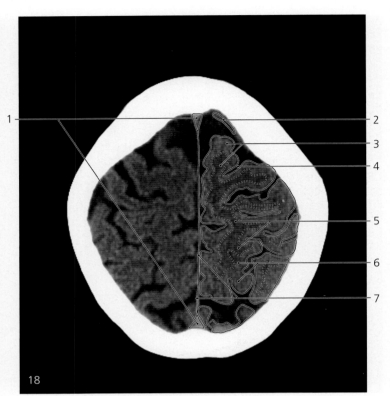

Brain, axial CT

Scout view on page 245

1: Superior sagittal sinus ←
2: Superior cerebral vein (in subarachnoid space)

3: Cerebral gyrus
4: Cerebral sulcus
5: White matter

6: Grey matter
7: Falx cerebri (in longitudinal cerebral fissure) ←

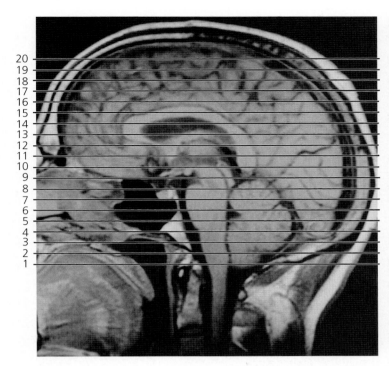
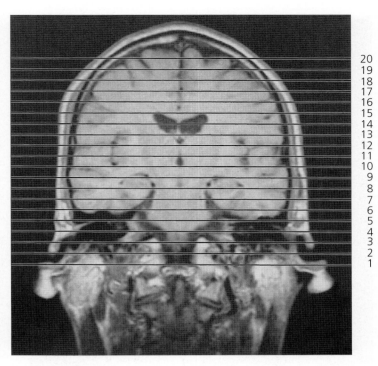

Scout views of axial MR series

Lines #1–20 indicate positions of axial sections in the following MR series.

Interpretations of the scout images are found on page 306 and page 290 in the corresponding sagittal and coronal series.

All sections are 5 mm thick and are spaced by 0.5 mm.

Each section is displayed in both T2 (above) and T1 (below) weighted imaging.

Bone structures are delineated by yellow lines on the T2 weighted images.

Arrows ←, → and ↔ indicate that a structure can be seen on a previous or following section, or both.

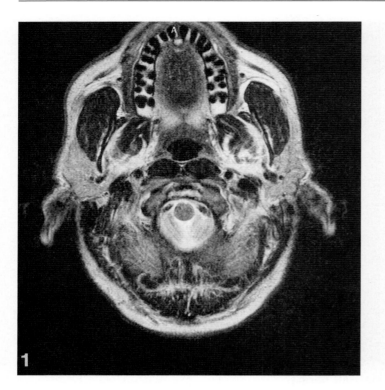

1
2
3
4
5
6
7
8
9
10
11
12
13
14
15
16
17

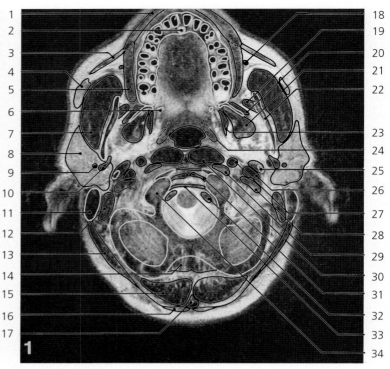

18
19
20
21
22
23
24
25
26
27
28
29
30
31
32
33
34

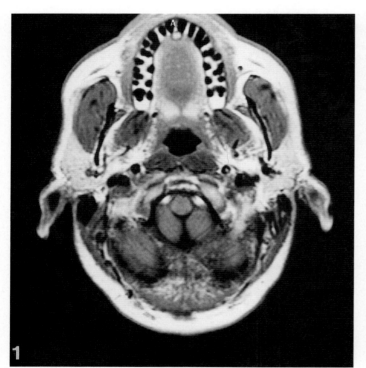

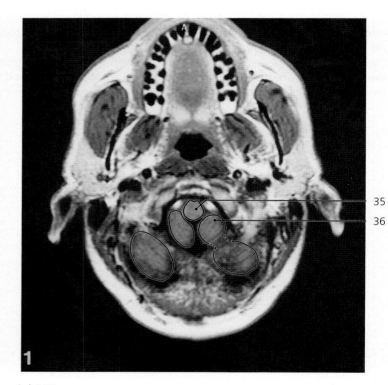

35
36

Brain, axial MR

Scout view on previous page

1: Orbicularis oris →
2: Incisive foramen →
3: Risorius
4: Accessory parotid gland →
5: Buccinator →
6: Pterygoid hamulus
7: Masseter →
8: Parotid gland →
9: Retromandibular vein →
10: Maxillary artery branching from external carotid artery
11: Mastoid process →
12: Digastricus, posterior belly →

13: Splenius capitis →
14: Rectus capitis posterior minor
15: Semispinalis capitis →
16: Trapezius →
17: Nuchal ligament →
18: Facial artery/vein →
19: Temporalis muscle (insertion) →
20: Lateral pterygoid muscle →
21: Medial pterygoid muscle →
22: Ramus of mandible →
23: Tensor veli palatini →
24: Levator veli palatini →
25: Styloid process →

26: Internal jugular vein →
27: Internal carotid artery →
28: Rectus capitis lateralis
29: Rectus capitis anterior →
30: Longus capitis →
31: Alar ligament
32: Vertebral artery →
33: Tectorial membrane
34: Occipital condyle
35: Medulla oblongata →
36: Cerebellar tonsil

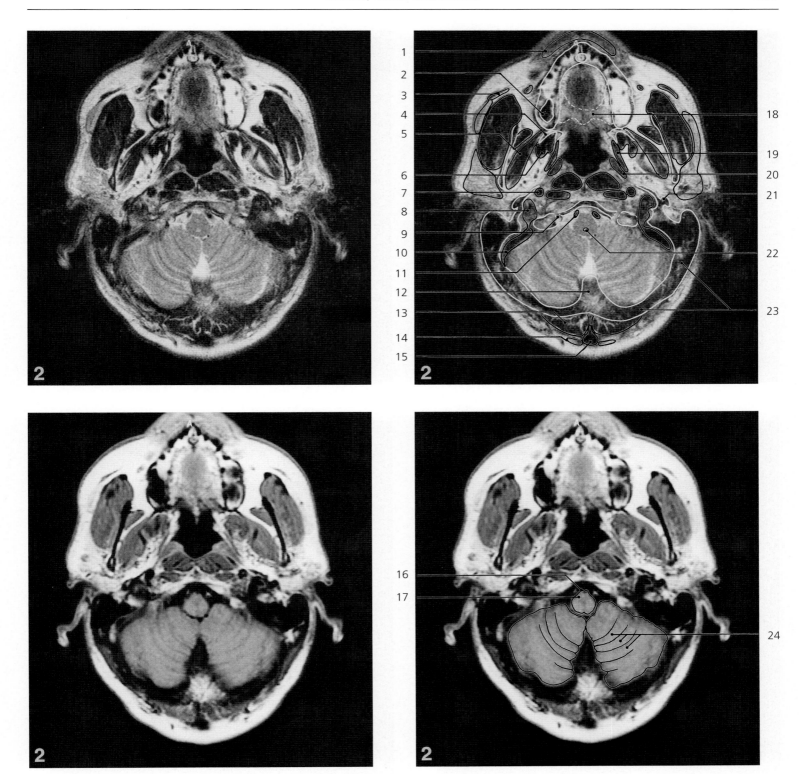

Brain, axial MR

Scout view on page 255

1: Orbicularis oris ←
2: Maxillary sinus →
3: Zygomaticus major muscle →
4: Pterygoid process ↔
5: Lateral pterygoid muscle ↔
6: Medial pterygoid muscle ←
7: Internal carotid artery ↔
8: Internal jugular vein (bulb) ↔

9: Hypoglossal canal
10: Sigmoid sinus →
11: Vertebral artery ↔
12: Internal occipital crest →
13: Semispinalis capitis ←
14: Trapezius ←
15: Nuchal ligament ←
16: Pyramis →

17: Medulla oblongata ↔
18: Hard palate
19: Tensor veli palatini ↔
20: Levator veli palatini ↔
21: Styloid process (root) ←
22: Central canal of medulla oblongata
23: Squamous part of occipital bone
24: Folia of cerebellum

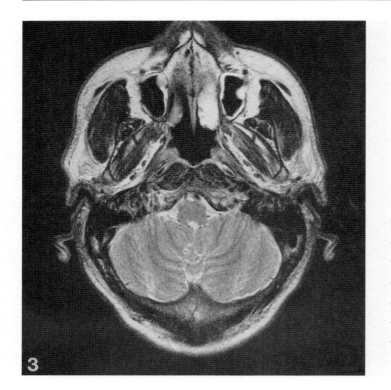

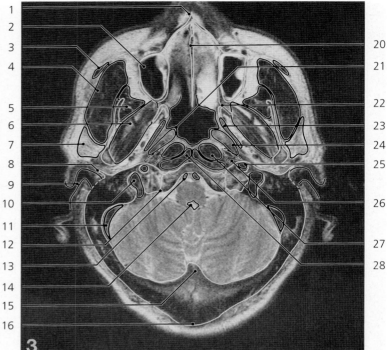

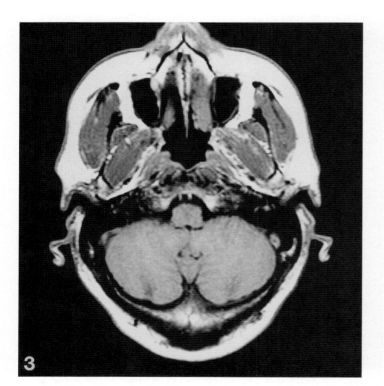

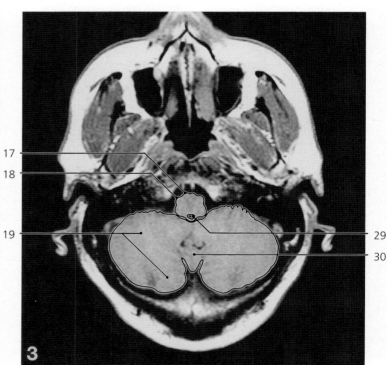

Brain, axial MR

Scout view on page 255

1: Anterior nasal spine
2: Maxillary sinus ↔
3: Zygomaticus major muscle ↔
4: Masseter ↔
5: Temporalis muscle ↔
6: Lateral pterygoid muscle ↔
7: Parotid gland ↔
8: Tympanic part of temporal bone
9: External acoustic meatus
10: Internal jugular vein (bulb) ←

11: Sigmoid sinus ↔
12: Petro-occipital fissure →
13: Vertebral artery ↔
14: Fourth ventricle →
15: Internal occipital protuberance
16: External occipital protuberance
17: Pyramis ↔
18: Oliva
19: Cerebellar hemisphere
20: Vomer →

21: Torus levatorius
22: Pterygoid process ←
23: Tensor veli palatini ←
24: Levator veli palatini ←
25: Internal carotid artery in carotid canal ↔
26: Auditory tube
27: Longus capitis ←
28: Rectus capitis anterior ←
29: Fourth ventricle →
30: Vermis of cerebellum →

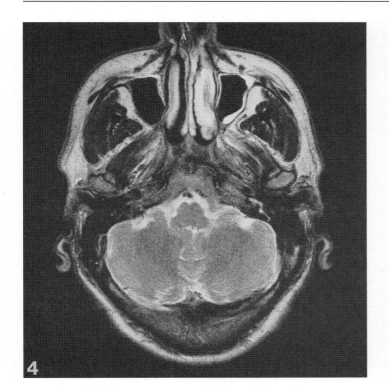

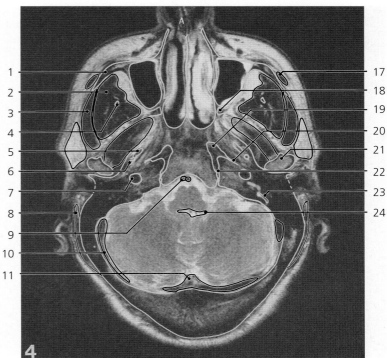

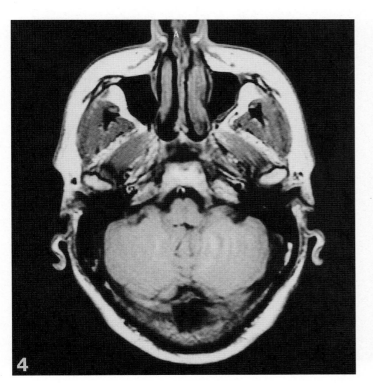

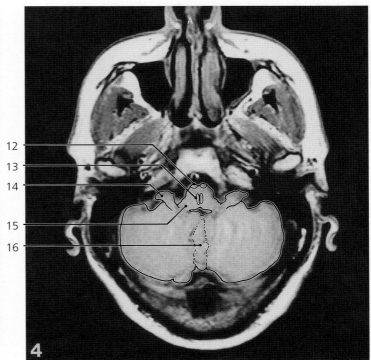

Brain, axial MR

Scout view on page 255

1: **Body of zygomatic bone** →
2: **Temporalis muscle** ↔
3: **Masseter** ←
4: **Coronoid process (tip) within temporalis muscle** ←
5: **Foramen ovale**
6: **Foramen spinosum**
7: **Carotid canal** ↔
8: **Posterior auricular muscle**

9: **Vertebral artery** ←
10: **Transverse sinus** ↔
11: **Confluence of sinuses** →
12: **Pyramis** ←
13: **Medial lemniscus** →
14: **Flocculus**
15: **Inferior cerebellar peduncle**
16: **Vermis of cerebellum** ←
17: **Zygomaticus major muscle** ←

18: **Pterygopalatine fossa** →
19: **Foramen lacerum**
20: **Sphenopetrous fissure**
21: **Head of mandible** →
22: **Petro-occipital fissure**
23: **Posterior semicircular canal**
24: **Fourth ventricle** ↔

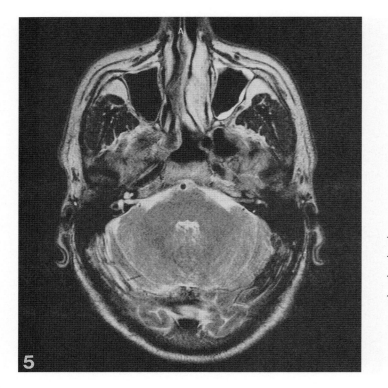

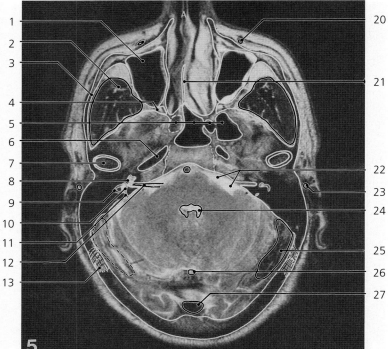

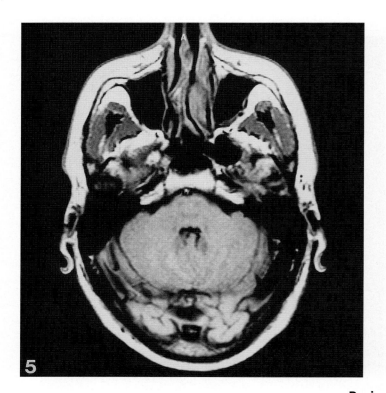

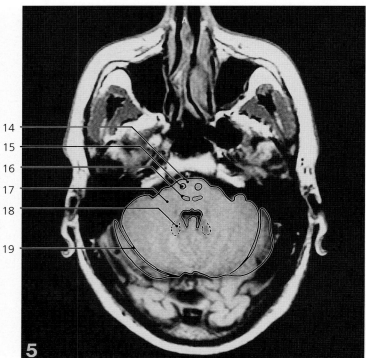

Brain, axial MR

Scout view on page 255

1: Maxillary sinus ↔
2: Temporalis muscle ↔
3: Zygomatic arch
4: Pterygopalatine fossa ↔
5: Sphenoidal sinus →
6: Carotid canal ↔
7: Head of mandible in mandibular fossa ←
8: Cochlea
9: Lateral semicircular canal
10: Vestibule

11: Perilymphatic duct
12: Internal acoustic porus with facial and vestibulocochlear nerve
13: Asterion
14: Pons →
15: Corticospinal tract →
16: Medial lemniscus ↔
17: Middle cerebellar peduncle
18: Olivary nucleus
19: Horizontal fissure

20: Facial artery/vein
21: Vomer ↔
22: Cerebellopontine cistern
23: Superficial temporal artery →
24: Fourth ventricle ↔
25: Transverse sinus ←
26: Straight sinus →
27: Confluence of sinuses ←

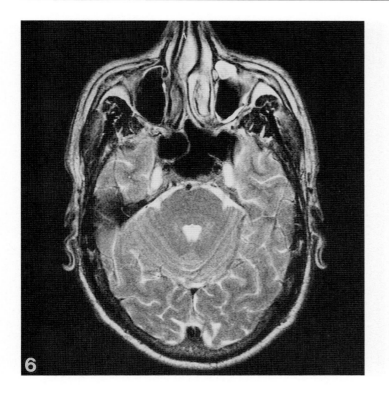

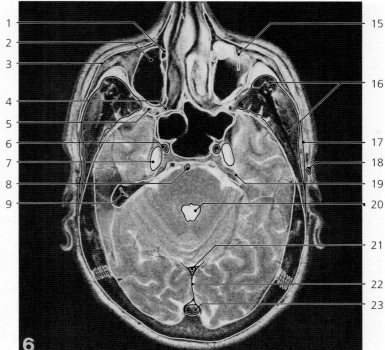

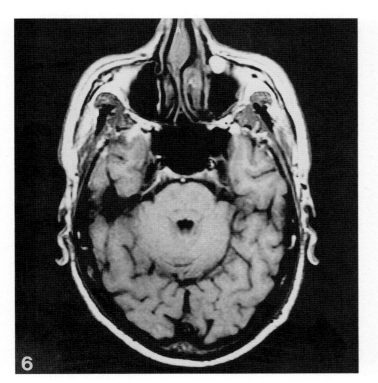

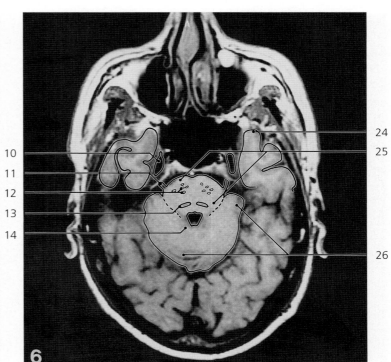

Brain, axial MR

Scout view of page 255

1: Nasolacrimal duct →
2: Maxillary sinus ↔
3: Body of zygomatic bone ↔
4: Foramen sphenopalatinum
5: Pterygopalatine fossa ↔
6: Internal carotid artery in carotid canal ↔
7: Trigeminal cave
8: Basilar artery ↔
9: Anterior semicircular canal

10: Trigeminal ganglion
11: Trigeminal nerve
12: Corticospinal tract ↔
13: Medial lemniscus ↔
14: Superior cerebellar peduncle →
15: Infraorbital canal
16: Temporalis muscle ↔
17: Temporal fascia
18: Superficial temporal artery ←

19: Superior margin of petrous bone
20: Fourth ventricle ↔
21: Straight sinus ↔
22: Falx cerebri
23: Superior sagittal sinus →
24: Anterior pole of temporal lobe
25: Pons ↔
26: Cerebellum ↔

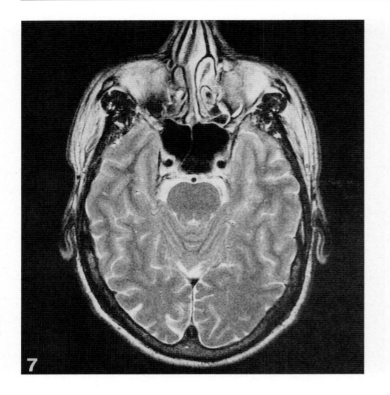

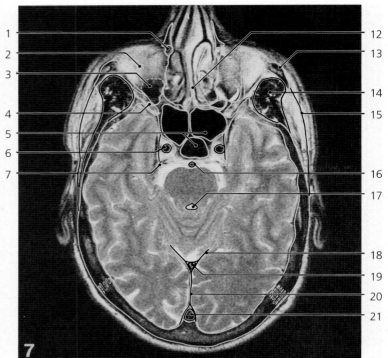

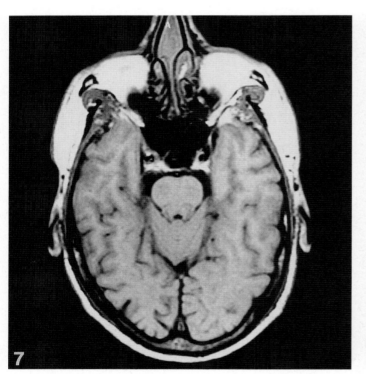

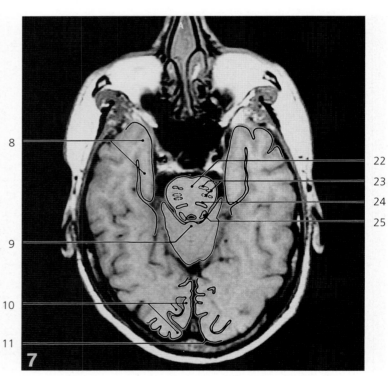

Brain, axial MR

Scout view on page 255

1: Nasolacrimal duct ←
2: Orbita
3: Maxillary sinus ←
4: Pterygopalatine fossa ←
5: Sphenoidal sinus ↔
6: Internal carotid artery
   in cavernous sinus ↔
7: Posterior clinoid process
8: Lateral occipitotemporal gyrus

9: Culmen of cerebellum ↔
10: Visual cortex around calcarine sulcus
11: Occipital pole of brain
12: Vomer ↔
13: Body of zygomatic bone ↔
14: Temporalis muscle ↔
15: Temporal fascia ↔
16: Basilar artery ↔
17: Fourth ventricle ↔

18: Tentorium cerebelli →
19: Straight sinus ↔
20: Falx cerebri ↔
21: Superior sagittal sinus ↔
22: Pons ←
23: Corticospinal tract ↔
24: Medial lemniscus ↔
25: Superior cerebellar peduncle ←

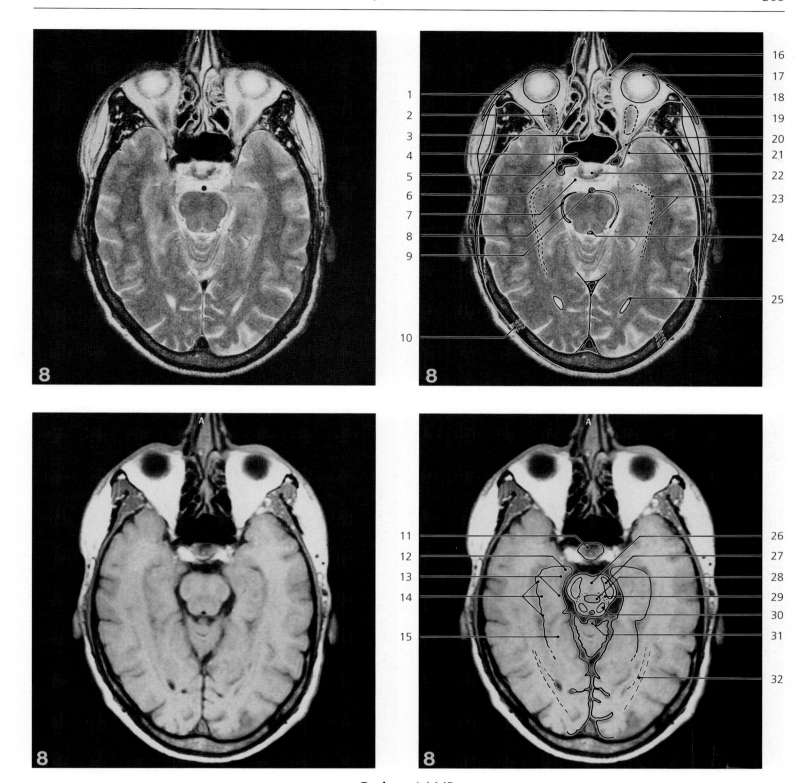

Brain, axial MR

Scout view on page 255

1: Frontal process of zygomatic bone →
2: Rectus inferior muscle
3: Ethmoidal air cells →
4: Sphenoidal sinus ←
5: Anterior clinoid process
6: Internal carotid artery ↔
7: Dorsum sellae
8: Superior cerebellar artery in cisterna ambiens
9: Basilar artery in cisterna pontina ←
10: Lambdoid suture ↔
11: Hypophysis

12: Uncus
13: Parahippocampal gyrus
14: Hippocampus →
15: Medial occipitotemporal gyrus
16: Lacrimal groove
17: Eyeball
18: Orbicularis oculi
19: Temporalis muscle ↔
20: Superior orbital fissure →
21: Lesser wing of sphenoid bone
22: Hypophysial fossa
23: Lateral ventricle, temporal horn →

24: Cerebral aqueduct →
25: Lateral ventricle occipital horn →
26: Mesencephalon →
27: Corticospinal tract →
28: Decussation of superior cerebellar peduncles
29: Medial lemniscus →
30: Nucleus of inferior colliculus
31: Culmen ←
32: Optic radiation

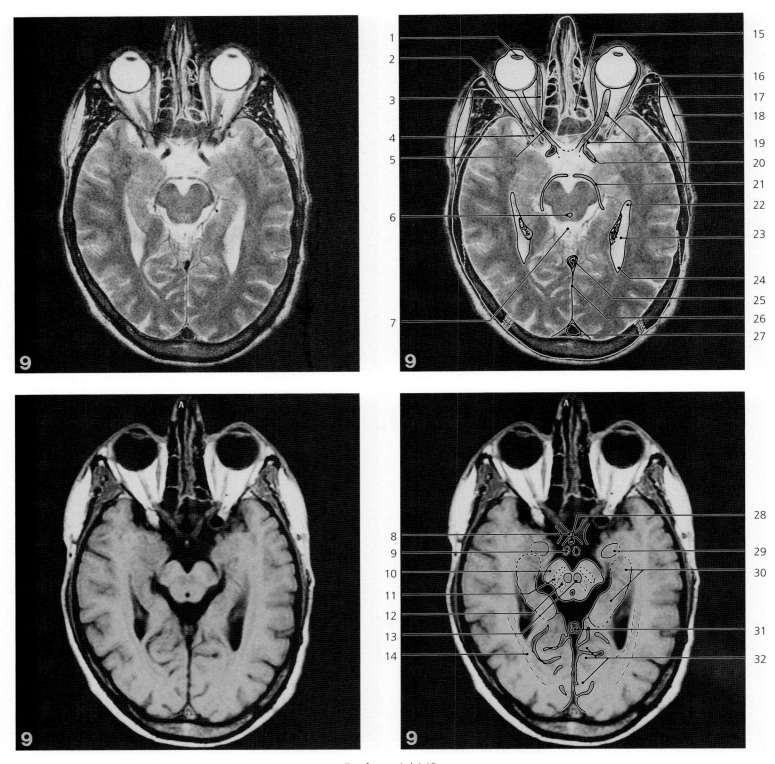

Brain, axial MR

Scout view on page 255

1: Lens
2: Rectus lateralis →
3: Rectus medialis →
4: Superior orbital fissure ←
5: Optic nerve in optic canal
6: Cerebral aqueduct ←
7: Quadrigeminal cistern
8: Optic chiasm
9: Mammillary bodies in interpeduncular cistern
10: Corticospinal tract in cerebral peduncle ↔

11: Substantia nigra
12: Medial lemniscus ←
13: Red nucleus
14: Optic radiation ↔
15: Ethmoidal air cells ↔
16: Frontal process of zygomatic bone ↔
17: Temporalis muscle ↔
18: Temporal fascia ↔
19: Ophthalmic artery →
20: Internal carotid artery ←
21: Posterior cerebral artery
22: Lateral ventricle, temporal horn ←

23: Lateral ventricle, atrium →
24: Lateral ventricle, occipital horn →
25: Straight sinus ↔
26: Falx cerebri ↔
27: Superior sagittal sinus ↔
28: Infundibulum of hypophysis in cisterna suprasellaris
29: Amygdaloid body
30: Hippocampus ←
31: Pia mater around great cerebral vein
32: Visual cortex around calcarine sulcus ←

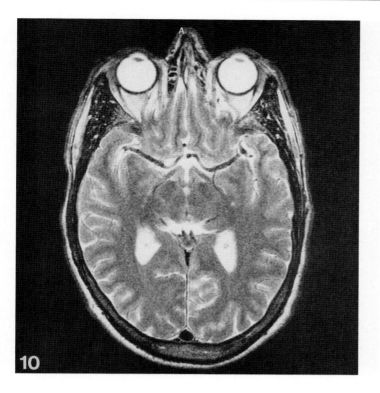

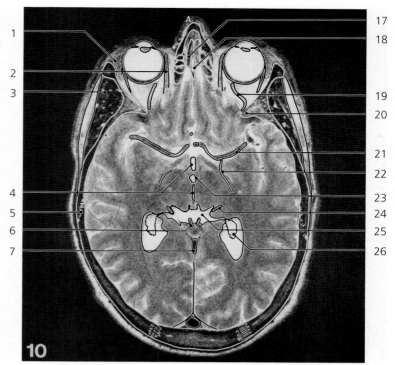

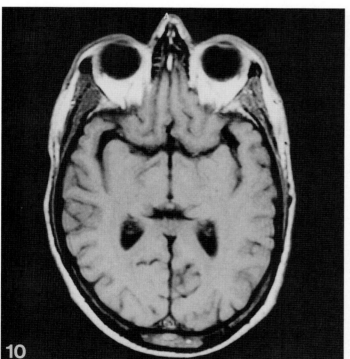

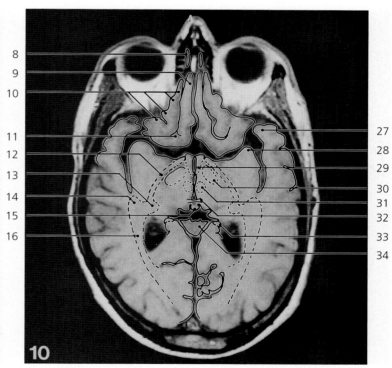

Brain, axial MR

Scout view on page 255

1: Lacrimal gland →
2: Obliquus superior muscle
3: Temporalis muscle ↔
4: Third ventricle →
5: Squamous suture ←
6: Internal cerebral vein →
7: Great cerebral vein ←
8: Olfactory bulb
9: Straight gyrus →
10: Orbital gyri →
11: Olfactory trigone
12: Optic tract

13: Lateral geniculate body
14: Optic radiation, sublentiform part
15: Pineal body
16: Optic radiation ↔
17: Cribriform plate
18: Crista galli
19: Ophthalmic artery ←
20: Lesser wing of sphenoid bone ←
21: Middle cerebral artery →
22: Anterior choroid artery
23: Interpeduncular cistern
24: Posterior cerebral artery ←

25: Transverse cerebral fissure
26: Choroid plexus of lateral ventricle ↔
27: Anterior pole of temporal lobe
28: Limen of insula
29: Hypothalamus
30: Cerebral peduncle ←
31: Red nucleus ←
32: Posterior commissure
33: Crus of fornix →/Fimbria of hippocampus
34: Corpus callosum, splenium →

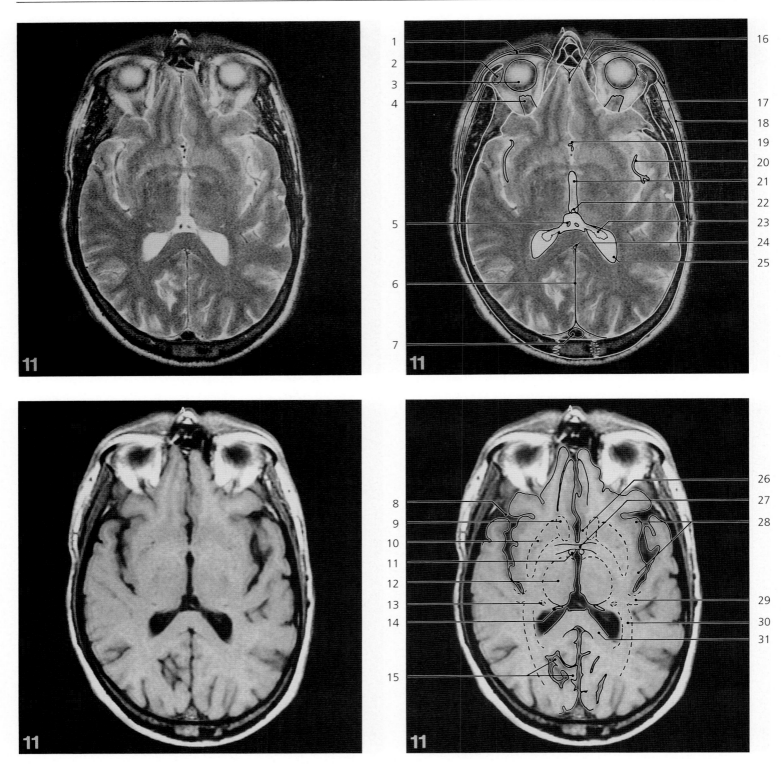

Brain, axial MR

Scout view on page 255

1: Orbicularis oculi
2: Lacrimal gland ←
3: Eyeball ←
4: Rectus superior/Levator palpebrae superioris
5: Internal cerebral vein ↔
6: Falx cerebri ↔
7: Superior sagittal sinus ↔
8: Lateral sulcus (Sylvian) →
9: Caudate nucleus, head →
10: Putamen →

11: Fornix, column →
12: Thalamus ↔
13: Caudate nucleus tail →
14: Crus of fornix →
15: Visual cortex in calcarine sulcus
16: Falx cerebri ↔
17: Temporalis muscle ↔
18: Temporal fascia ↔
19: Anterior cerebral artery in longitudinal fissure of brain →
20: Middle cerebral artery, branch ←

21: Third ventricle ↔
22: Choroid plexus of third ventricle →
23: Choroid plexus of lateral ventricle ↔
24: Inferior sagittal sinus →
25: Lateral ventricle, occipital horn →
26: Area subcallosa/Paraterminal gyrus →
27: Anterior commissure
28: Insula ↔
29: Acoustic radiation
30: Optic radiation ←
31: Occipital forceps →

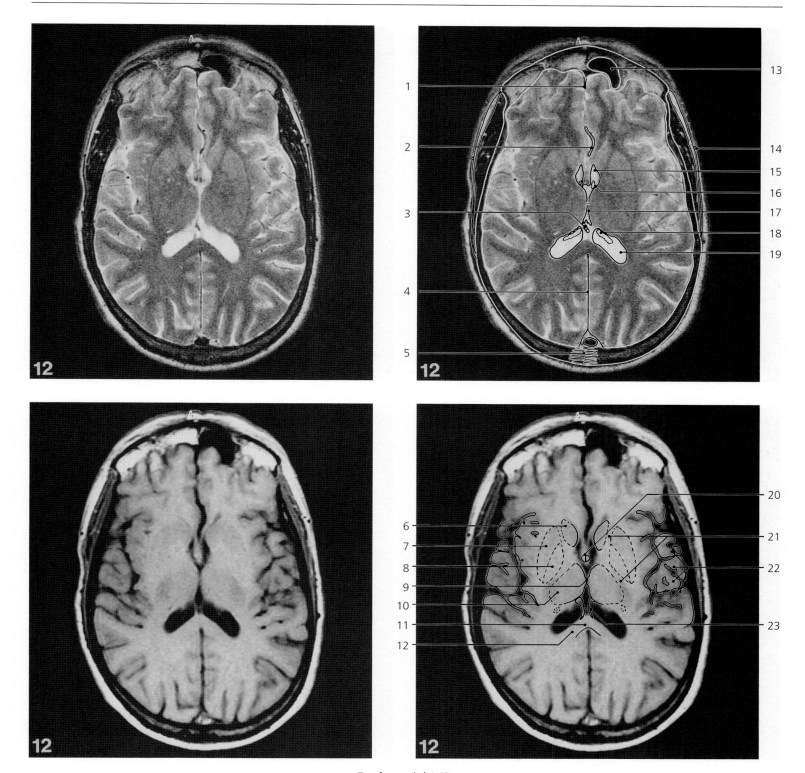

Brain, axial MR

Scout view on page 255

1: Falx cerebri ↔
2: Anterior cerebral artery ←
3: Internal cerebral vein ←
4: Falx cerebri ↔
5: Lambda
6: Caudate nucleus, head ↔
7: Putamen ↔
8: Globus pallidus

9: Interthalamic adhesion
10: Thalamus ↔
11: Corpus callosum, splenium ↔
12: Occipital forceps ↔
13: Frontal sinus
14: Superficial temporal artery
15: Lateral ventricle ↔
16: Interventricular foramen (Monroi)

17: Third ventricle ←
18: Choroid plexus of lateral ventricle ↔
19: Lateral ventricle, atrium ↔
20: Fornix, column ↔
21: Internal capsule →
22: Auditory cortex of temporal lobe
23: Fornix, crus ↔

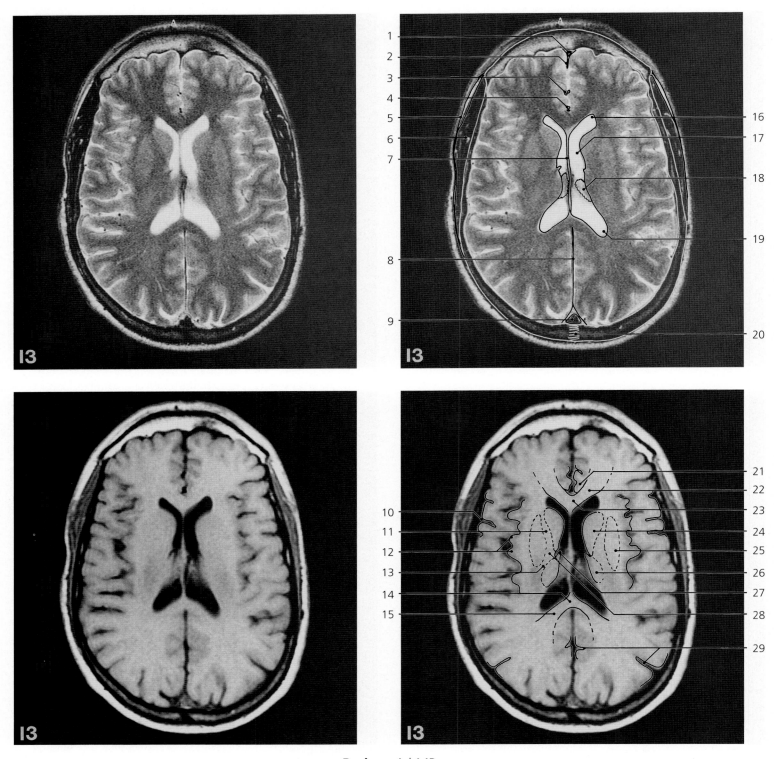

Brain, axial MR

Scout view on page 255

1: Superior sagittal sinus ↔
2: Falx cerebri ↔
3: Callosomarginal artery →
4: Pericallosal artery →
5: Temporal fascia ↔
6: Temporalis muscle ↔
7: Septum pellucidum →
8: Falx cerebri ↔
9: Superior sagittal sinus ↔
10: Central sulcus (Roland) →

11: Internal capsule, anterior limb ↔
12: Insula ↔
13: Internal capsule, posterior limb ↔
14: Corpus callosum, splenium ↔
15: Occipital forceps ↔
16: Lateral ventricle, frontal horn →
17: Lateral ventricle, central part →
18: Choroid plexus of lateral ventricle ←
19: Lateral ventricle, atrium ←
20: Sagittal suture →

21: Paraterminal gyrus ←/Area
    subcallosa ←
22: Frontal forceps →
23: Corpus callosum, genu →
24: Caudate nucleus, head ←
25: Putamen →
26: Thalamus ←
27: Fornix ←
28: Internal capsule, genu
29: Parieto-occipital sulcus →

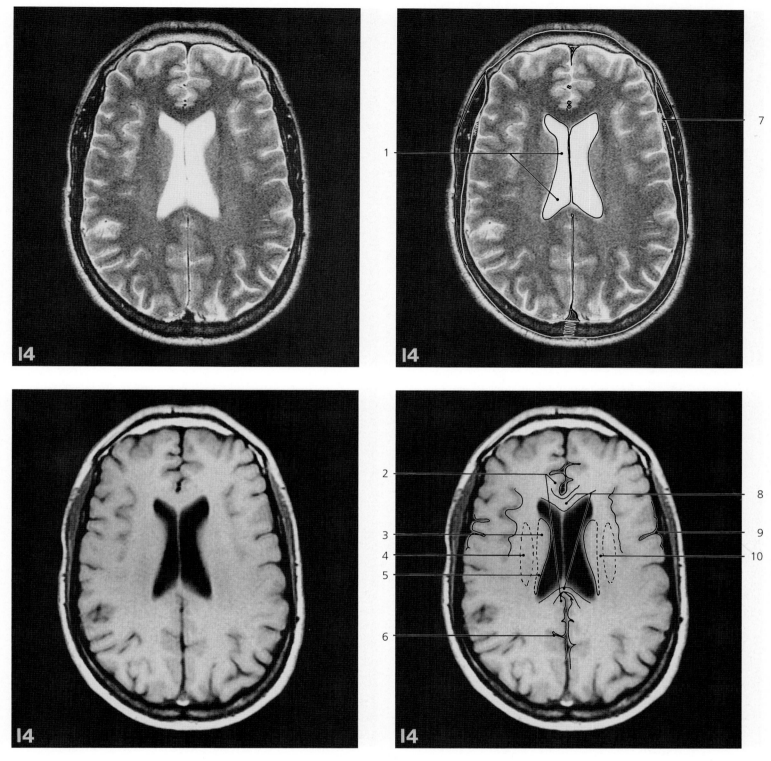

Brain, axial MR

Scout view on page 255

1: Lateral ventricle, central part ↔
2: Cingulate gyrus →
3: Caudate nucleus, body ←
4: Putamen ←
5: Caudate nucleus, tail ←
6: Parieto-occipital sulcus ↔
7: Coronal suture →
8: Corpus callosum, body →
9: Central sulcus (Roland) ↔
10: Internal capsule ←

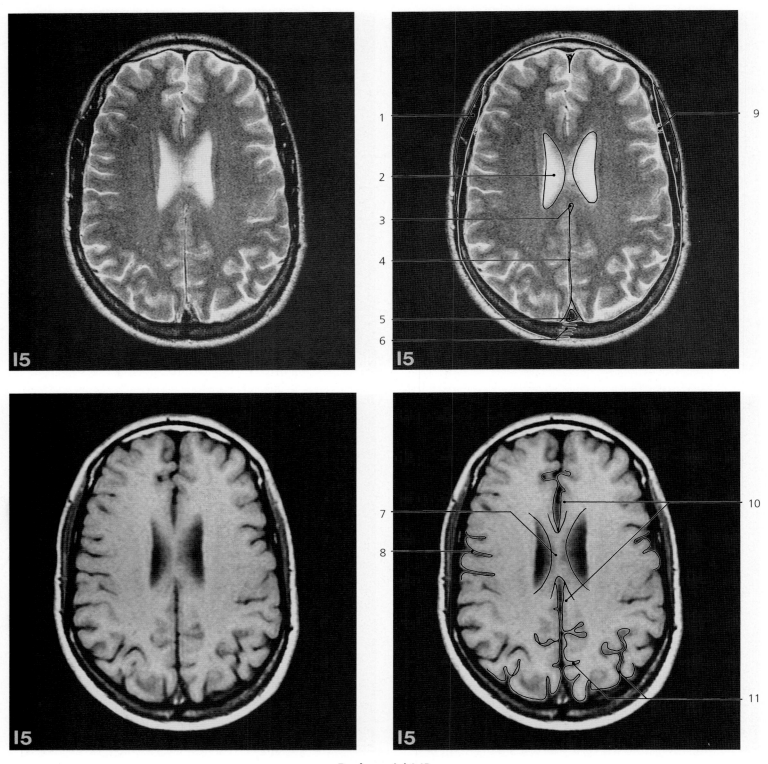

Brain, axial MR

Scout view on page 255

1: Temporalis muscle ↔
2: Lateral ventricle, central part ←
3: Inferior sagittal sinus
4: Falx cerebri ↔

5: Superior sagittal sinus ↔
6: Sagittal suture ↔
7: Corpus callosum, body ←
8: Central sulcus (Roland) ↔

9: Coronal suture ↔
10: Cingulate gyrus ↔
11: Parieto-occipital sulcus ←

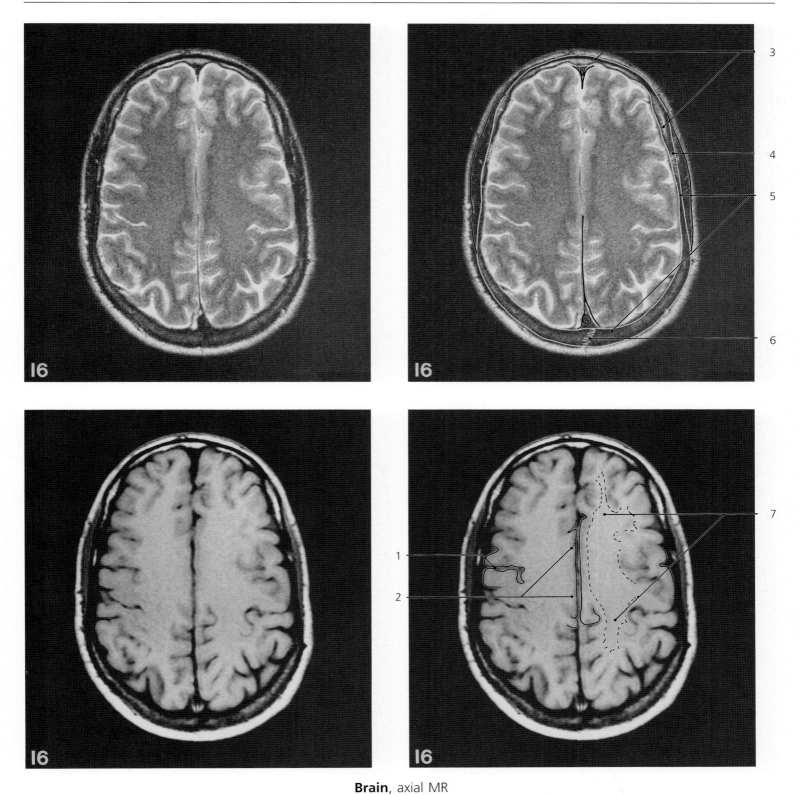

Brain, axial MR

Scout view on page 255

1: Central sulcus ↔
2: Cingulate gyrus ←
3: Frontal bone, squamous part ↔

4: Coronal suture ↔
5: Parietal bone ↔
6: Sagittal suture ↔

7: Corona radiata/centrum semiovale
   (radiology term) →

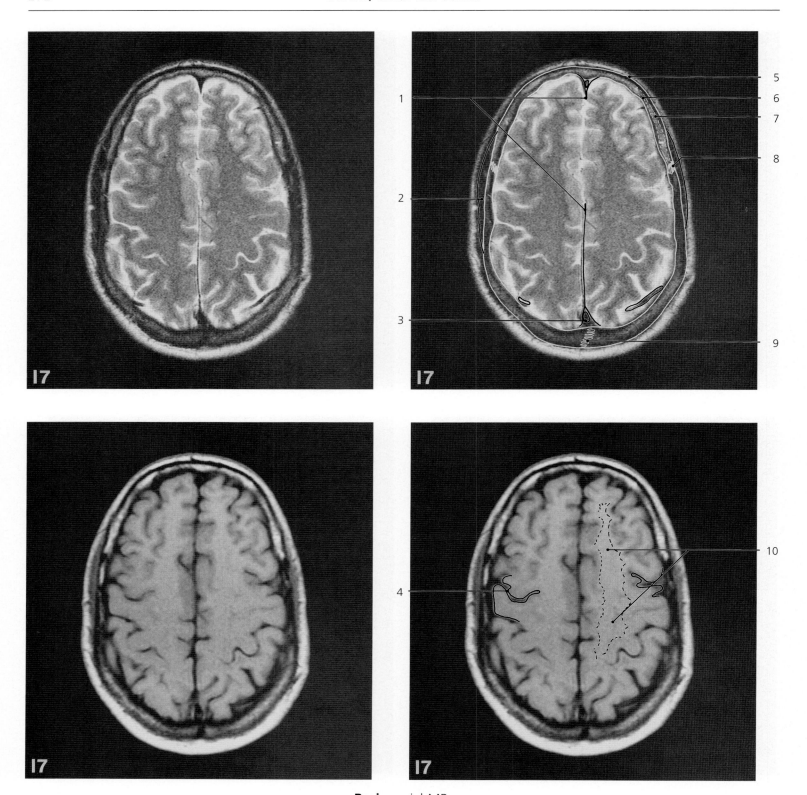

Brain, axial MR

Scout view on page 255

1: Falx cerebri ↔
2: Temporalis muscle ←
3: Superior sagittal sinus ↔
4: Central sulcus (Roland) ↔

5: Frontal bone, external lamina
6: Frontal bone, internal lamina
7: Frontal bone, diploë
8: Sutura coronalis ↔

9: Sutura sagittalis ↔
10: Corona radiata ←

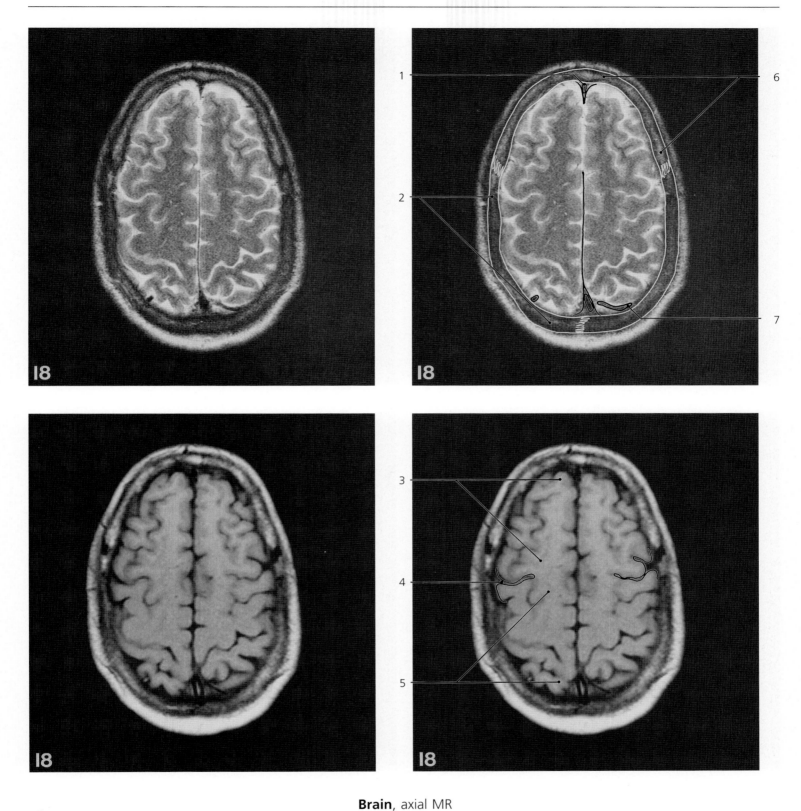

Brain, axial MR

Scout view on page 255

1: Superior sagittal sinus ↔   4: Central sulcus ↔   7: Superior cerebral vein →
2: Parietal bone ↔   5: Parietal lobe ↔
3: Frontal lobe ↔   6: Frontal bone, squamous part ↔

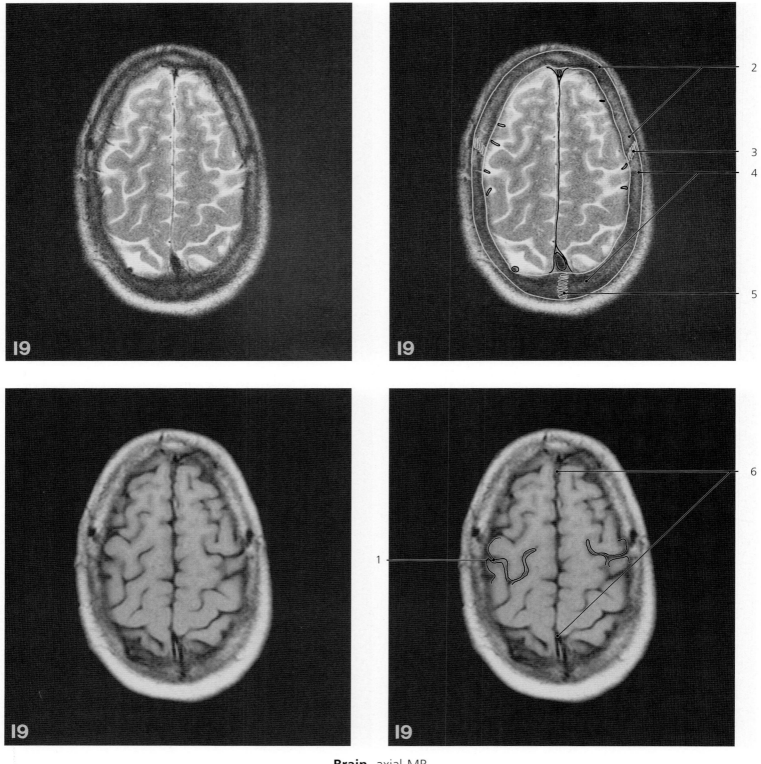

Brain, axial MR

Scout view on page 255

1: Central sulcus (Roland) ↔
2: Frontal bone, squamous part ↔

3: Coronal suture ↔
4: Parietal bone ↔

5: Sagittal suture ↔
6: Longitudinal fissure of brain ↔

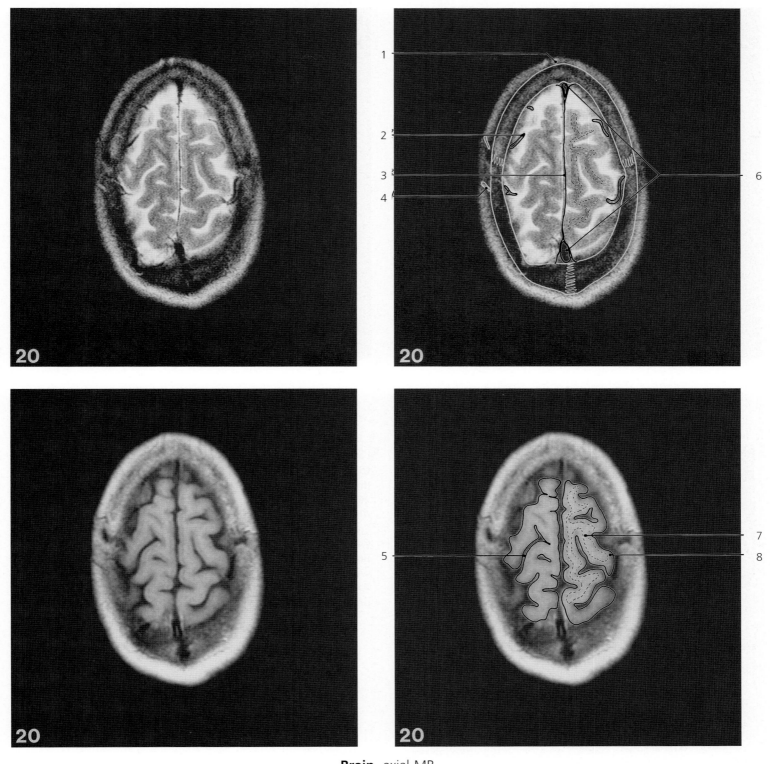

Brain, axial MR

Scout view on page 255

Scout view on page 255

1: Vena irae ←
2: Superior cerebral vein ←
3: Falx cerebri ←
4: Scalp veins ←
5: Sulcus of cerebral cortex
6: Superior sagittal sinus ←
7: White matter of cerebral gyrus
8: Grey matter of cerebral gyrus

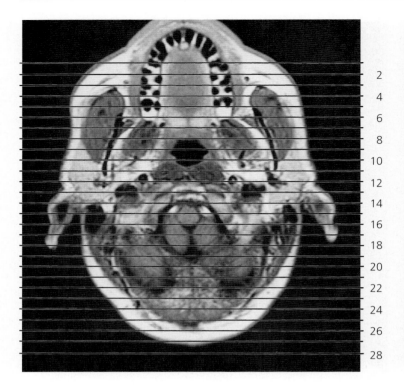

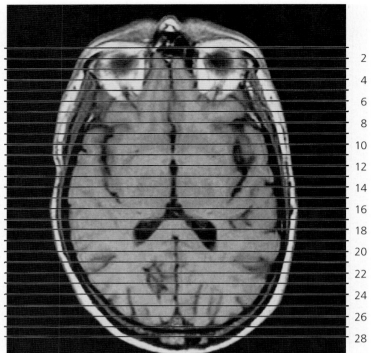

2	2
4	4
6	6
8	8
10	10
12	12
14	14
16	16
18	18
20	20
22	22
24	24
26	26
28	28

2 4 6 8 10 12 14 16 18 20 22 24 26 28

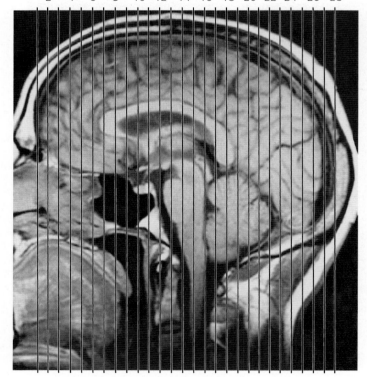

Scout views of coronal MR series

Lines #1–28 indicate positions of coronal sections in the following MR series.

Interpretation of the scout images are found on pages 256, 266 and 306 in the corresponding axial and sagittal series.

All sections are 5 mm thick and are spaced by 0.5 mm.

Each section is displayed in both T2 (above) and T1 (below) weighted imaging.

Bone structures are delineated by yellow lines on the T2 weighted images.

Arrows ←, → and ↔ indicate that a structure can be seen on a previous or following section, or both.

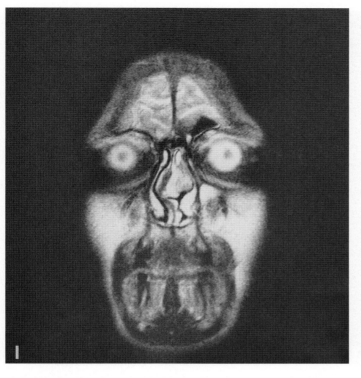

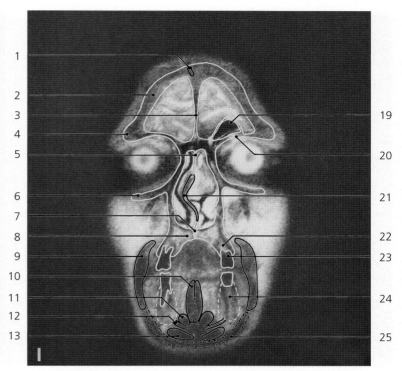

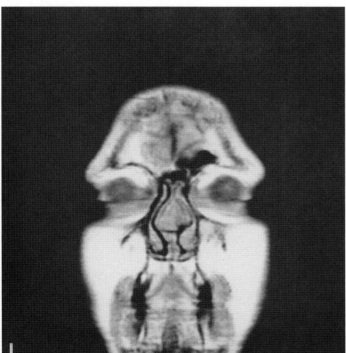

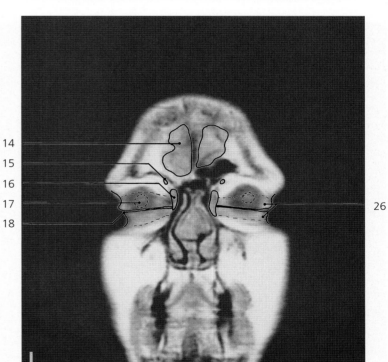

Brain, coronal MR

Scout view on previous page

1: Diploic vein →
2: Frontal bone, squamous part →
3: Frontal crest
4: Supraorbital margin of frontal bone →
5: Perpendicular plate of ethmoidal bone →
6: Infraorbital margin of maxilla →
7: Median palatine suture →
8: Hard palate →
9: Buccinator →

10: Genioglossus →
11: Geniohyoideus →
12: Mylohyoideus →
13: Digastricus, anterior belly →
14: Frontal pole of brain
15: Obliquus superior muscle in trochlea →
16: Lacrimal sac
17: Lens
18: Palpebral fissure

19: Frontal sinus
20: Orbital part of frontal bone →
21: Cartilaginous part of nasal septum →
22: Alveolar part of maxilla →
23: Second upper premolar tooth
24: Alveolar part of mandible →
25: Platysma →
26: Eyelids

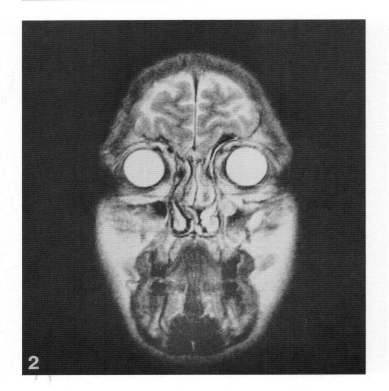

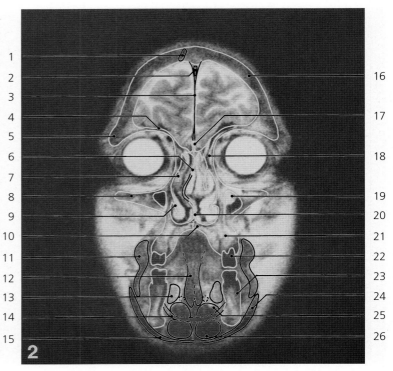

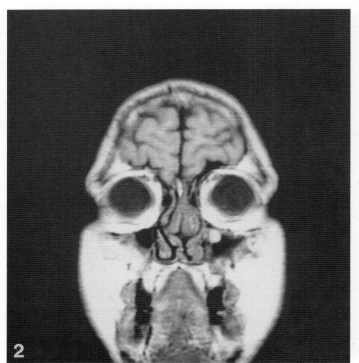

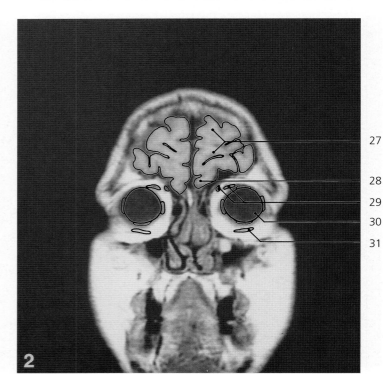

Brain, coronal MR

Scout view on page 276

1: Diploic vein ↔
2: Superior sagittal sinus →
3: Falx cerebri →
4: Orbital part of frontal bone ↔
5: Supra-orbital margin of frontal bone ←
6: Perpendicular plate of ethmoidal bone ↔
7: Middle concha →
8: Infra-orbital margin of maxilla ←
9: Inferior choncha ↔
10: Hard palate ↔

11: Buccinator ↔
12: Genioglossus ↔
13: Sublingual gland →
14: Mylohyoideus ↔
15: Platysma ↔
16: Squamous part of frontal bone ↔
17: Crista galli →
18: Ethmoidal air cells →
19: Maxillary sinus →
20: Vomer →
21: Alveolar part of maxilla ↔

22: First upper molar tooth
23: Alveolar part of mandibula ↔
24: Platysma ↔
25: Geniohyoideus ↔
26: Digastricus, anterior belly ↔
27: Frontal lobe ↔
28: Straight gyrus →
29: Obliquus superior muscle ↔
30: Eyeball ↔
31: Obliquus inferior muscle →

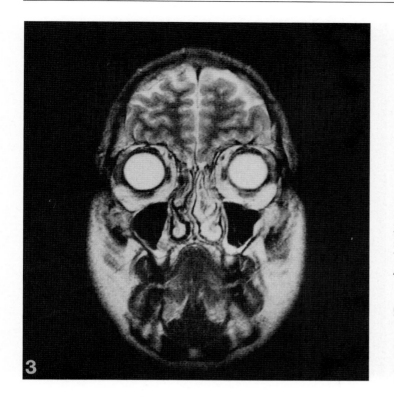

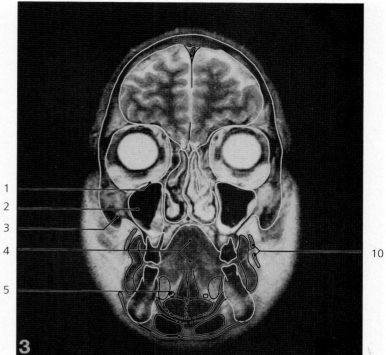

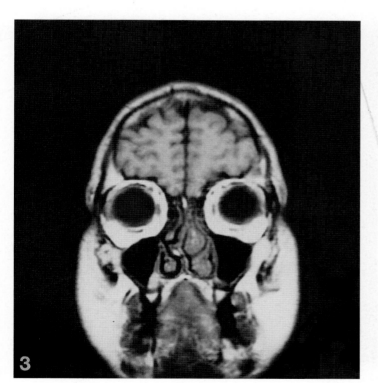

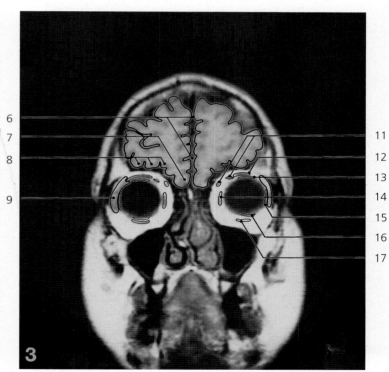

Brain, coronal MR

Scout view on page 276

1: Orbital plate of maxilla ↔
2: Maxillary sinus ↔(with oedematous mucous membrane)
3: Body of zygomatic bone →
4: Tongue ↔
5: Submandibular duct →

6: Longitudinal fissure of brain ↔
7: Straight gyrus ↔
8: Orbital gyri →
9: Lacrimal gland →
10: Facial artery/vein
11: Obliquus superior ↔

12: Levator palpebrae superioris ↔
13: Rectus superior ↔
14: Rectus medialis ↔
15: Rectus lateralis ↔
16: Rectus inferior ↔
17: Obliquus inferior ←

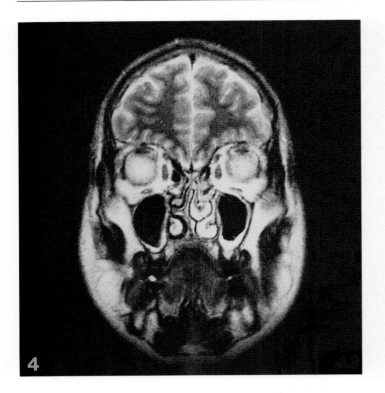

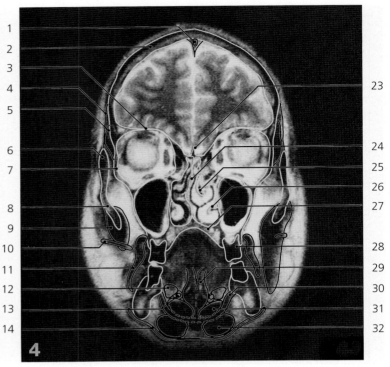

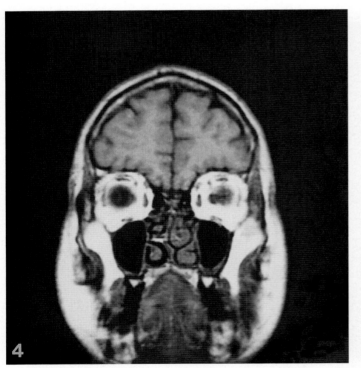

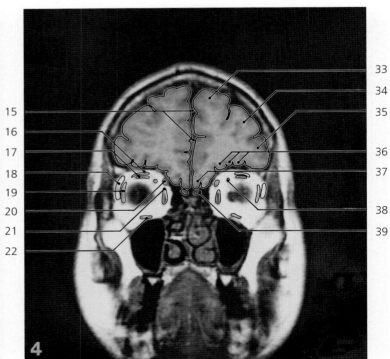

Brain, coronal MR

Scout view on page 276

1: Superior sagittal sinus ↔
2: Squamous part of frontal bone ↔
3: Orbital part of frontal bone ↔
4: Temporal fascia →
5: Temporalis muscle →
6: Frontal process of zygomatic bone
7: Greater wing of sphenoid bone in lateral wall of orbita →
8: Body of zygomatic bone ←
9: Masseter
10: Parotid duct →
11: Buccinator ↔
12: Sublingual gland ←

13: Submandibular duct surrounded by deep part of gland ↔
14: Platysma ↔
15: Longitudinal fissure of brain ↔
16: Levator palpebrae superioris ↔
17: Rectus superior ↔
18: Lacrimal gland ←
19: Rectus lateralis ↔
20: Obliquus superior ↔
21: Rectus medialis ↔
22: Rectus inferior ↔
23: Crista galli ↔
24: Nasal septum ↔
25: Middle concha ↔

26: Inferior concha ↔
27: Hard palate ↔
28: Second upper molar tooth
29: Genioglossus ↔
30: Mylohyoideus ↔
31: Geniohyoideus ↔
32: Digastricus, anterior belly ↔
33: Superior frontal gyrus →
34: Middle frontal gyrus →
35: Inferior frontal gyrus →
36: Orbital gyri ↔
37: Straight gyrus ↔
38: Ophthalmic artery →
39: Olfactory bulb

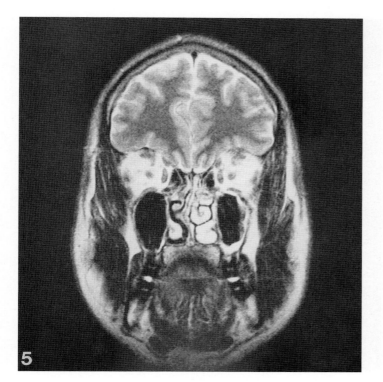

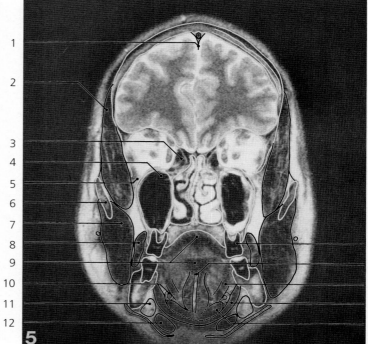

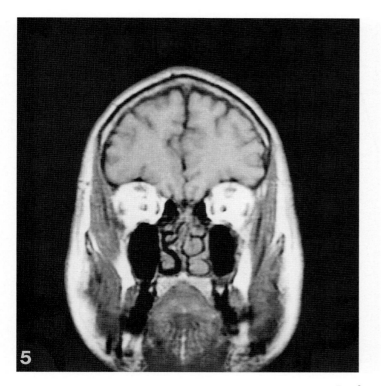

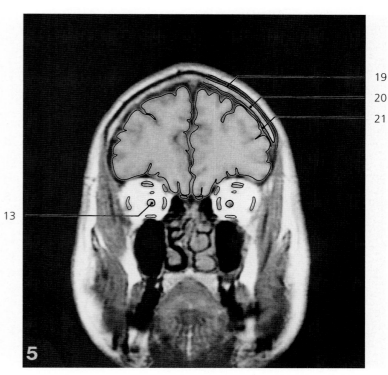

Brain, coronal MR

Scout view on page 276

1: Falx cerebri ↔
2: Temporalis muscle ↔
3: Ethmoid sinus ↔
4: Maxillary sinus ↔
5: Infra-orbital fissure →
6: Zygomatic arch →
7: Masseter ↔

8: Buccinator ↔
9: Tongue ↔
10: Submandibular duct ←
11: Submandibular gland ←
12: Digastricus, anterior belly ↔
13: Optic nerve →
14: Third upper molar tooth

15: Lingual septum
16: Hyoglossus →
17: Mylohyoideus ↔
18: Geniohyoideus ↔
19: Outer lamina of frontal bone
20: Diploë of frontal bone
21: Inner lamina of frontal bone

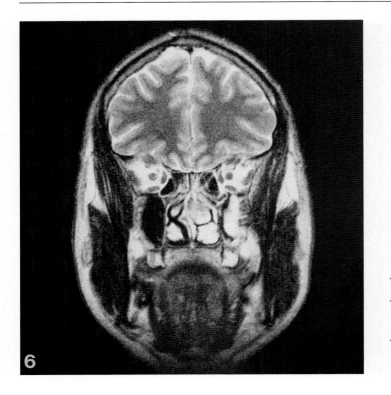

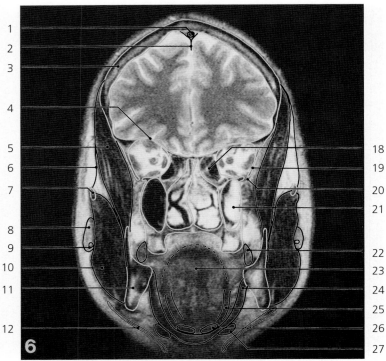

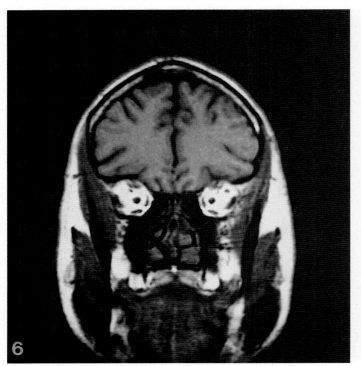

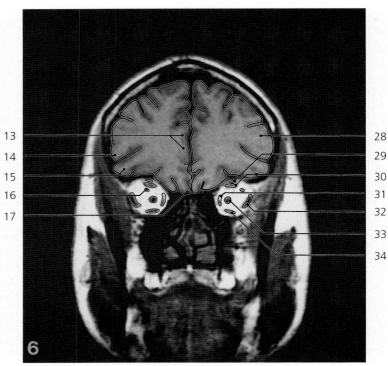

Brain, coronal MR

Scout view on page 276

1: Superior sagittal sinus ↔
2: Falx cerebri ↔
3: Squamous part of frontal bone ↔
4: Orbital part of frontal bone ↔
5: Temporalis muscle ↔
6: Temporal fascia ↔
7: Zygomatic arch ↔
8: Accessory parotid gland
9: Parotid duct ↔
10: Masseter ↔
11: Ramus of mandible →
12: Platysma ←

13: Cingulate gyrus →
14: Middle frontal gyrus ↔
15: Inferior frontal gyrus ↔
16: Ophthalmic artery ←
17: Straight gyrus ↔
18: Ethmoid sinus ↔
19: Greater wing of sphenoid bone ↔
20: Infra-orbital fissure ↔
21: Maxillary sinus ←(with oedematous mucous membrane)
22: Buccinator ←
23: Tongue ↔

24: Mylohyoideus ↔
25: Hyoglossus ↔
26: Geniohyoideus ←
27: Digastricus, anterior belly ←
28: Middle frontal gyrus ↔
29: Levator palpebrae superioris ↔
30: Rectus superior ↔
31: Rectus medialis ↔
32: Rectus lateralis ↔
33: Optic nerve ↔
34: Rectus inferior ↔

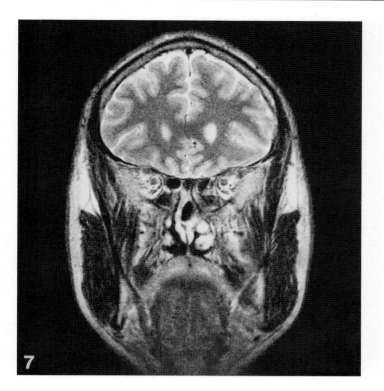

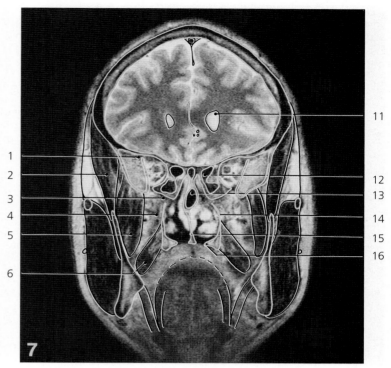

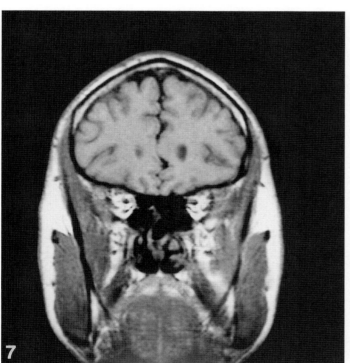

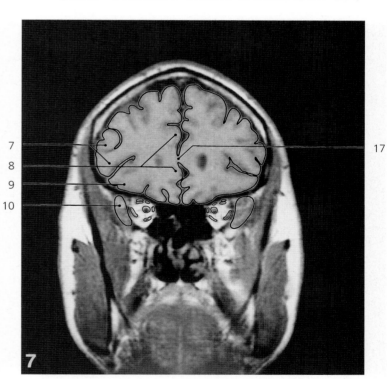

Brain, coronal MR

Scout view on page 276

1: Superior orbital fissure ↔
2: Temporalis muscle ↔
3: Foramen sphenopalatinum
4: Pterygopalatine fossa
5: Pterygoideus lateralis muscle →
6: Pterygoideus medialis muscle →

7: Middle frontal gyrus ↔
8: Cingulate gyrus ↔
9: Inferior frontal gyrus ↔
10: Anterior pole of temporal lobe →
11: Lateral ventricle, frontal horn →
12: Ethmoidal sinus ←

13: Sphenoidal sinus →
14: Perpendicular plate of palatine bone
15: Vomer
16: Pterygoid process
17: Corpus callosum, genu →

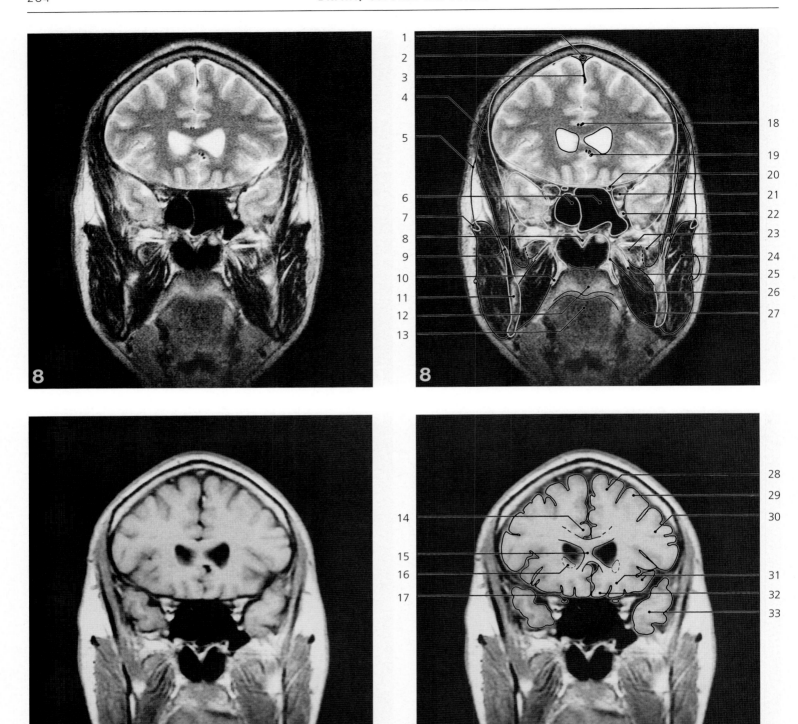

Brain, coronal MR

Scout view on page 276

1: Superior sagittal sinus ↔
2: Squamous part of frontal bone ↔
3: Falx cerebri ↔
4: Temporalis muscle ↔
5: Temporal fascia ↔
6: Sphenoidal sinus ↔
7: Zygomatic arch ↔
8: Vomer, attachment on sphenoidal bone ←
9: Coronoid process of mandible →
10: Pterygoid hamulus
11: Ramus of mandible →

12: Soft palate →
13: Tongue ←
14: Cingulate gyrus ↔
15: Corpus callosum, genu ↔
16: Caudate nucleus, head →
17: Optic nerve ↔
18: Pericallosal artery ↔
19: Anterior cerebral artery →
20: Optic canal
21: Apex of orbita
22: Foramen rotundum with maxillary nerve

23: Lateral pterygoid muscle ↔
24: Masseter ↔
25: Lateral lamina of pterygoid process
26: Medial lamina of pterygoid process ←
27: Pterygoideus medialis muscle ↔
28: Superior frontal gyrus ↔
29: Middle frontal gyrus ↔
30: Inferior frontal gyrus ↔
31: Gyri orbitales ←
32: Straight gyrus ↔
33: Temporal lobe ↔

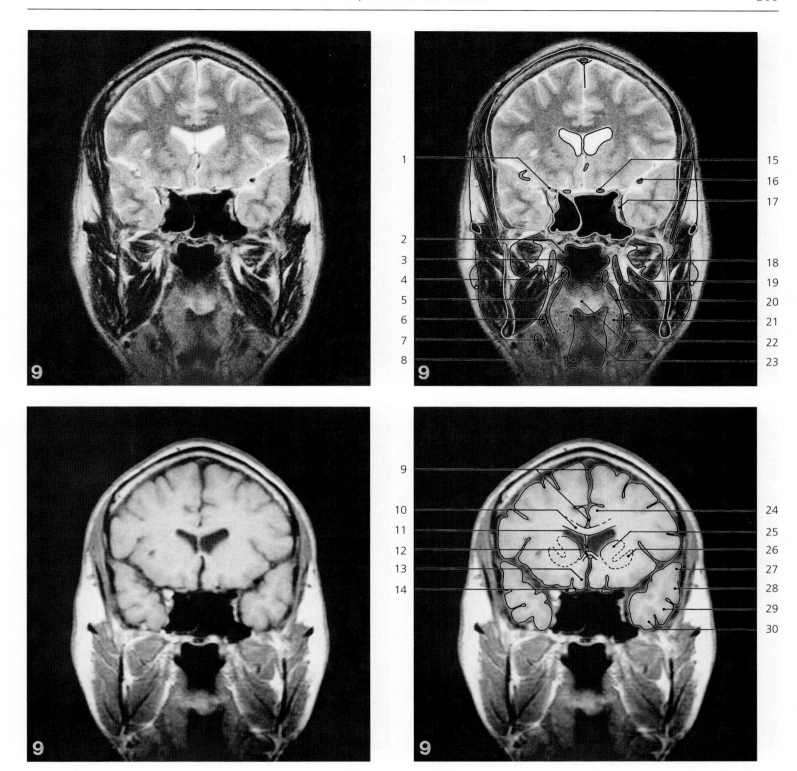

Brain, coronal MR

Scout view on page 276

1: Anterior clinoid process →
2: Torus tubarius
3: Pharyngeal opening of auditory tube
4: Tensor veli palatini
5: Levator veli palatini →
6: Stylohyoideus and styloglossus →
7: Digastricus, posterior belly →
8: Vallecula epiglottica
9: Longitudinal fissure of brain ↔
10: Corpus callosum ↔

11: Septum pellucidum →
12: Corpus callosum, rostrum →
13: Straight gyrus ←
14: Optic nerve ←
15: Optic nerve ←
16: Middle cerebral artery →
17: Cavernous sinus →
18: Lateral pterygoid muscle ↔
19: Medial pterygoid muscle ↔
20: Superior constrictor →

21: Palatine tonsil
22: Soft palate ←
23: Palatopharyngeal arch
24: Cingulate gyrus ↔
25: Caudate nucleus, head ↔
26: Putamen →
27: Superior temporal gyrus →
28: Middle temporal gyrus →
29: Inferior temporal gyrus →
30: Lateral occipitotemporal gyrus →

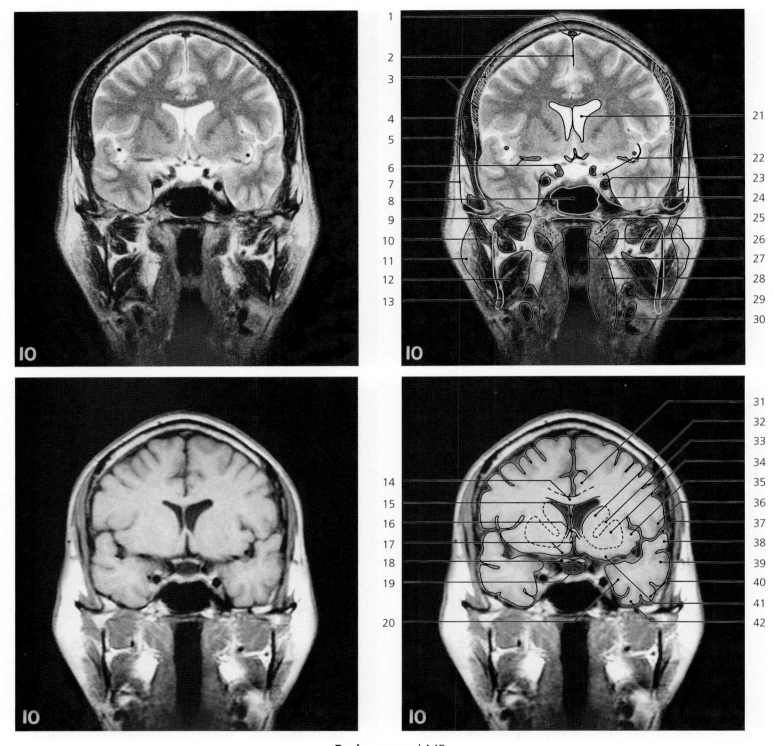

Brain, coronal MR

Scout view on page 276

1: Superior sagittal sinus ↔
2: Falx cerebri ↔
3: Coronal suture →
4: Temporalis muscle ↔
5: Pterion
6: Middle cerebral artery ↔
7: Temporal fascia ↔
8: Sphenoidal sinus ↔
9: Lateral pterygoid muscle
10: Masseter ←
11: Parotid gland →
12: Medial pterygoid muscle ←
13: Angle of mandible
14: Corpus callosum ↔
15: Septum pellucidum↔
16: Corpus callosum, rostrum ←

17: Paraterminal gyrus/Area subcallosa
18: Optic chiasm
19: Hypophysis
20: Parahippocampal gyrus →
21: Lateral ventricle, frontal horn ↔
22: Anterior clinoid process ←
23: Internal carotid artery in cavernous sinus →
24: Cavernous sinus ←
25: Auditory tube →
26: Levator veli palatini ↔
27: Nasopharynx
28: Superior constrictor ↔
29: "Stylomuscles", departure of stylopharyngeus ↔
30: Digastricus, posterior belly ↔

31: Cingulate gyrus ↔
32: Caudate nucleus, head ↔
33: Internal capsule, anterior limb ↔
34: Putamen ↔
35: Limen insulae
36: Operculum frontale
37: Lateral sulcus of brain (Sylvius) →
38: Superior temporal gyrus ↔
39: Middle temporal gyrus ↔
40: Inferior temporal gyrus ↔
41: Anterior perforated substance →
42: Lateral occipitotemporal gyrus ↔

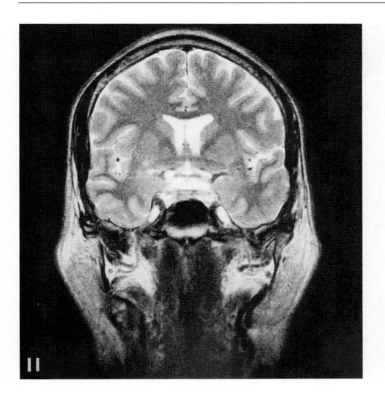

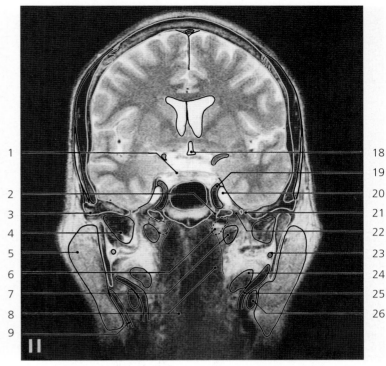

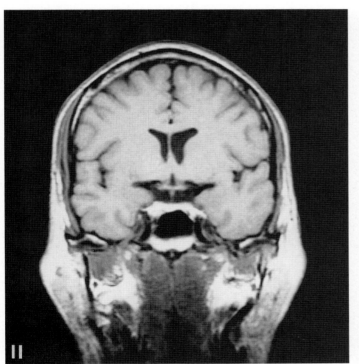

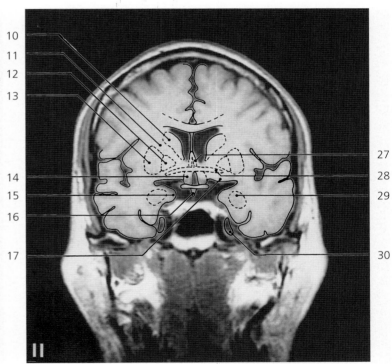

Brain, coronal MR

Scout view on page 276

1: Hypophysial fossa, floor
2: Foramen lacerum
3: Articular tubercle
4: Lateral pterygoid muscle ↔
5: Parotid gland ↔
6: Auditory tube ↔
7: Levator veli palatini ↔
8: Superior constrictor and longus colli/ capitis →
9: Retromandibular vein →
10: Caudate nucleus, body →

11: Internal capsule, anterior limb ↔
12: Globus pallidus →
13: Putamen →
14: Area subcallosa ←/hypothalamus →
15: Uncus →
16: Infundibulum of hypophysis
17: Anterior perforated substance ←
18: Third ventricle →
19: Internal carotid artery ↔
20: Trigeminal cave →

21: Foramen spinosum with middle meningeal artery
22: Foramen ovale
23: Maxillary artery →
24: "Stylo-muscles" ↔
25: External carotid artery
26: Digastricus, posterior belly ↔
27: Column of fornix →
28: Anterior commissure
29: Amygdaloid body →
30: Trigeminal ganglion →

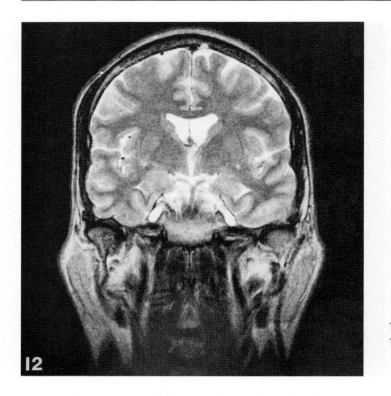

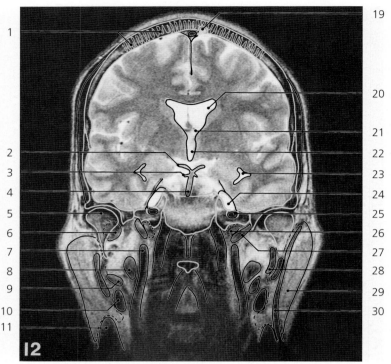

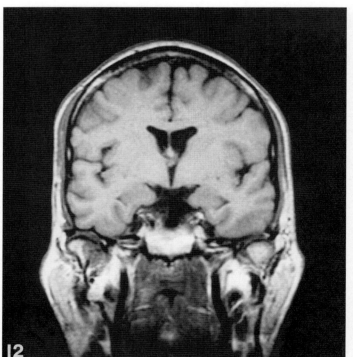

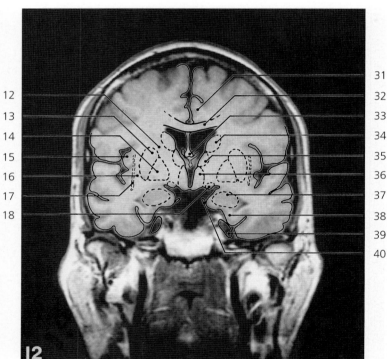

Brain, coronal MR

Scout view on page 276

1: Coronal suture ←
2: Posterior cerebral artery →
3: Superior cerebellar artery →
4: Basilar artery in pontine cistern →
5: Head of mandible
6: Lateral pterygoid muscle ← (insertion)
7: Internal carotid artery ↔
8: "Stylo-muscles" ↔
9: External carotid artery ←
10: Digastricus, posterior belly ↔
11: Sternocleidomastoideus →
12: Internal capsule ↔
13: Putamen ↔
14: Globus pallidus ↔

15: Insula ↔
16: External capsule →
17: Claustrum →
18: Optic tract →
19: Arachnoid granulation
20: Lateral ventricle →
21: Interventricular foramen (Monroi)
22: Third ventricle →
23: Lateral ventricle, temporal horn →
24: Trigeminal cave ←
25: Internal carotid artery in carotid canal ↔
26: Auditory tube ←
27: Levator veli palatini ←
28: Maxillary artery ←

29: Parotid gland ↔
30: Retromandibular vein ←
31: Cingulate gyrus ↔
32: Corpus callosum, body ↔
33: Column of fornix ↔
34: Caudate nucleus, body ↔
35: Thalamus →
36: Hypothalamus →
37: Amygdaloid body ←
38: Parahippocampal gyrus ↔
39: Trigeminal ganglion ←
40: Oculomotor nerve

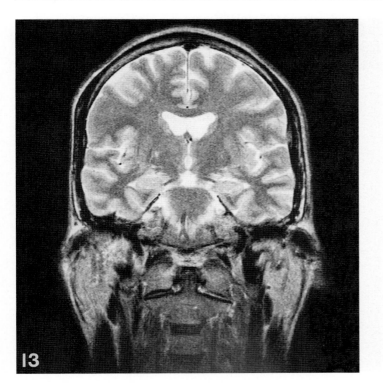

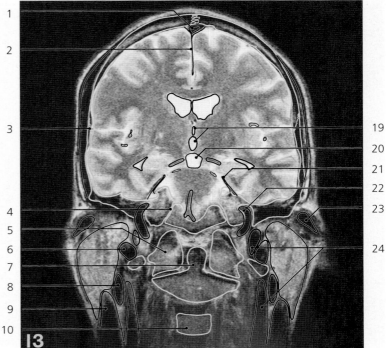

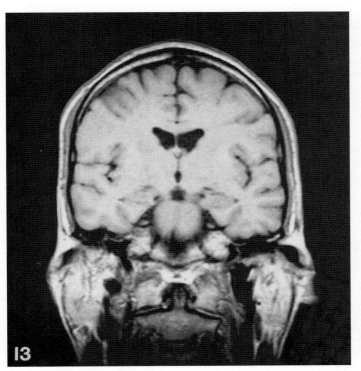

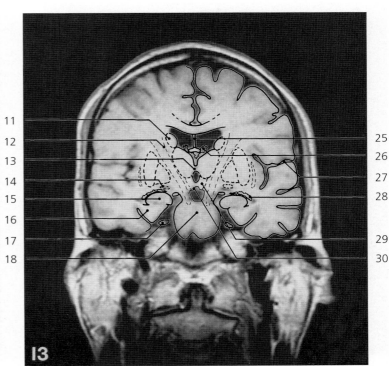

Brain, coronal MR

Scout view on page 276

1: Superior sagittal sinus ↔
2: Falx cerebri ↔
3: Squamous suture →
4: Petro-occipital fissure
5: Atlas, lateral mass →
6: "Stylo-muscles" ↔
7: Dens →
8: Digastricus, posterior belly ↔
9: Sternocleidomastoideus ↔
10: Body of third cervical vertebra →

11: Caudate nucleus, body ↔
12: Internal capsule, posterior limb ↔
13: Interthalamic adhesion
14: Caudate nucleus, tail
15: Hippocampus →
16: Parahippocampal gyrus ↔
17: Trigeminal nerve →
18: Pons →
19: Third ventricle ↔
20: Interpeduncular cistern →

21: Tentorium cerebelli →
22: Internal carotid artery in carotid canal ←
23: External acoustic meatus →
24: Internal jugular vein →
25: Septum pellucidum ↔
26: Choroid plexus of lateral ventricle ↔
27: Lateral sulcus (Sylvius) ↔
28: Choroid plexus in temporal horn ↔
29: Hypothalamus ←
30: Mammillary body (posterior edge)

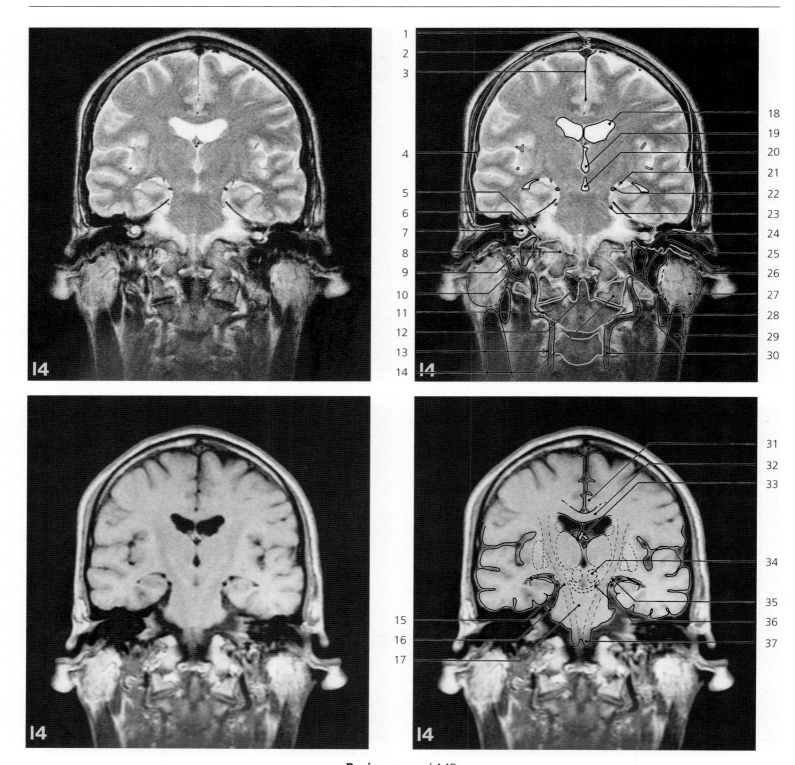

Brain, coronal MR

Scout view on page 276

1: Sagittal suture ↔
2: Superior sagittal sinus ↔
3: Falx cerebri ↔
4: Squamous suture ←
5: Internal acoustic opening (porus)
6: Jugular foramen
7: Cochlea
8: Hypoglossal canal
9: Styloid process
10: "Stylo-muscles" ←
11: Alar ligament
12: Dens ←
13: Foramen transversarium of C3

14: Lateral mass of atlas ↔
15: Corticospinal tract in cerebral peduncle
16: Trigeminal nerve in ambient cistern ←
17: Pons ↔
18: Lateral ventricle, central part ↔
19: Third ventricle ↔
20: Interpeduncular cistern ←
21: Anterior choroid artery
22: Posterior cerebral artery →
23: Superior cerebellar artery ←
24: Internal jugular vein, bulb ←
25: External auditory meatus ←
26: Tympanic part of temporal bone

27: Parotid gland ←
28: Digastricus, posterior belly ↔
29: Sternocleidomastoideus ↔
30: Vertebral artery →
31: Cingulate gyrus ↔
32: Corpus collosum, body ↔
33: Body of fornix ↔
34: Red nucleus →
35: Optic tract ←
36: Substantia nigra
37: Corticospinal tract in pyramis

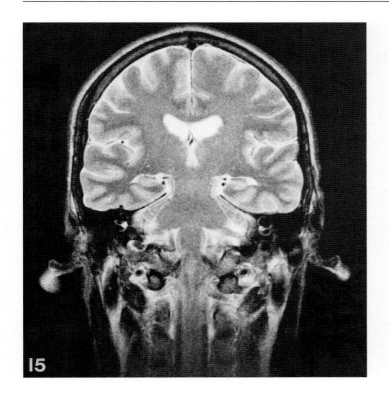

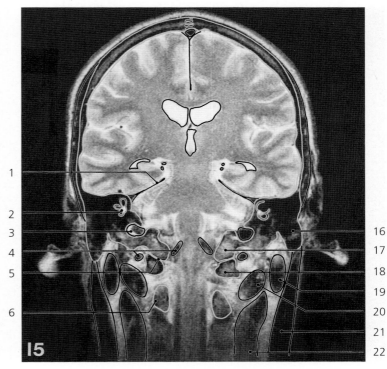

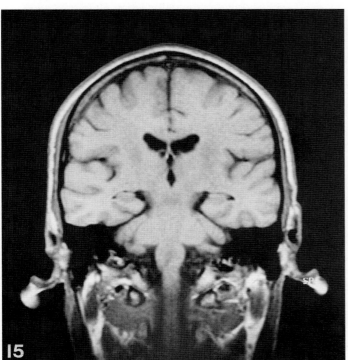

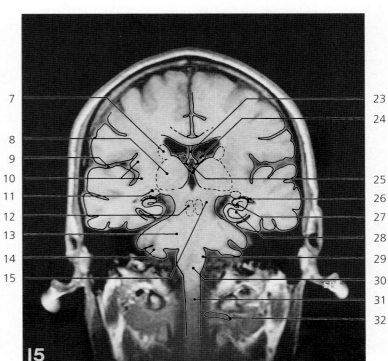

Brain, coronal MR

Scout view on page 276

1: Tentorium cerebelli ↔
2: Vestibule of bony labyrinth
3: Sigmoid sinus →
4: Vertebral artery ↔
5: Atlanto-occipital joint
6: Arch of axis
7: Caudate nucleus, body ↔
8: Thalamus ↔
9: Lateral sulcus (Sylvian) ↔
10: Insula ↔
11: Lateral geniculate body
12: Red nucleus ←

13: Middle cerebellar peduncle →
14: Flocculus
15: Pedunculus cerebri ←
16: Mastoid process →
17: Occipital condyle ←
18: Lateral mass of atlas ←
19: Digastricus, posterior belly ↔
20: Obliquus capitis inferior →
21: Sternocleidomastoideus ↔
22: Scalenus muscles →
23: Septum pellucidum ←

24: Choroid plexus of lateral ventricle, central part ↔
25: Choroid plexus of third ventricle
26: Choroid plexus of lateral ventricle, temporal horn →
27: Hippocampus ↔
28: Parahippocampal gyrus ↔
29: Olive
30: Medulla oblongata ↔
31: Spinal cord →
32: Second cervical spinal nerve

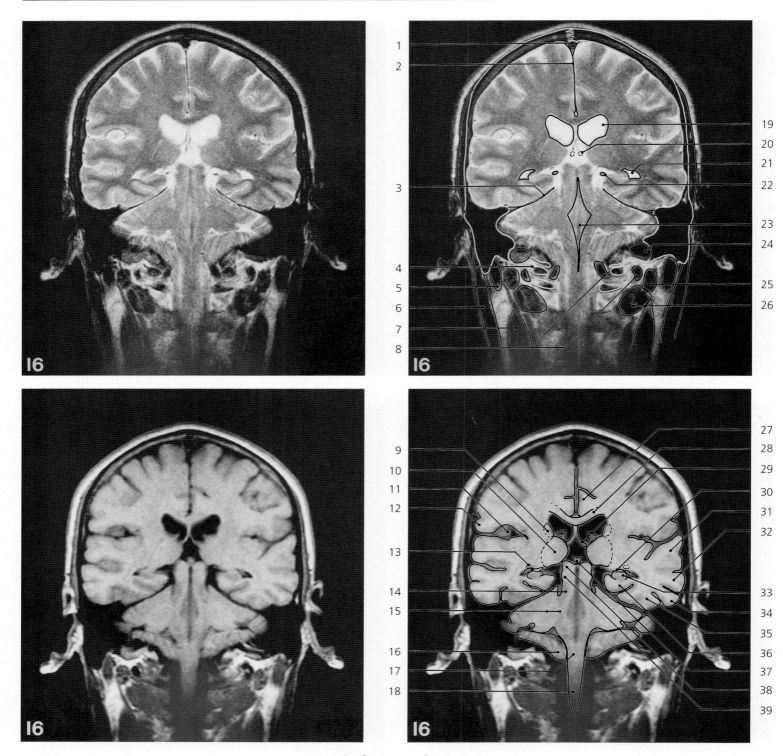

Brain, coronal MR

Scout view on page 276

1: Superior sagittal sinus ↔
2: Falx cerebri ↔
3: Tentorium cerebelli ↔
4: Lateral mass of atlas (posterior edge) ←
5: Digastricus, posterior belly (insertion) ←
6: Sternocleidomastoideus ↔
7: Scalenus muscles ←
8: Vertebral artery ↔
9: Caudate nucleus, body ↔
10: Thalamus (pulvinar) ↔
11: Lateral sulcus (Sylvian) ↔
12: Operculum frontoparietale
13: Caudate nucleus, tail ↔
14: Superior cerebellar peduncle

15: Middle cerebellar peduncle ←
16: Cerebellar tonsil →
17: Medulla oblongata ←
18: Spinal cord ←
19: Lateral ventricle, central part ←
20: Internal cerebral vein →
21: Lateral ventricle, temporal horn ↔
22: Posterior cerebral artery in ambient cistern →
23: Fourth ventricle /Fossa rhomboidea →
24: Sigmoid sinus →
25: Obliquus capitis superior →
26: Obliquus capitis inferior ↔
27: Cingulate gyrus ↔

28: Corpus callosum, body ↔
29: Crus of fornix →
30: Fimbria hippocampi
31: Superior temporal gyrus ↔
32: Middle temporal gyrus ↔
33: Hippocampus ↔
34: Inferior temporal gyrus ↔
35: Lateral occipitotemporal gyrus ↔
36: Parahippocampal gyrus ↔
37: Pineal body →
38: Superior colliculus
39: Inferior colliculus

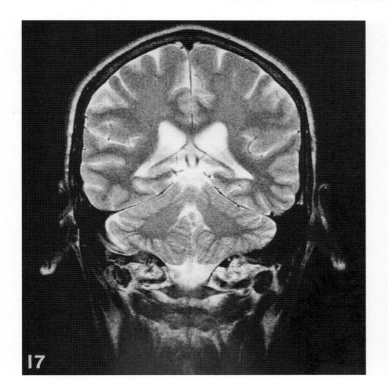

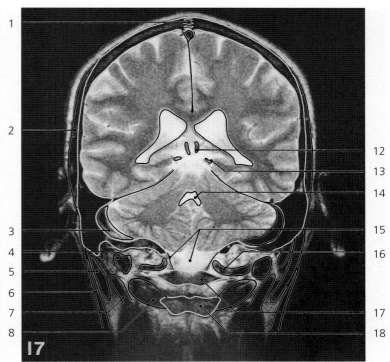

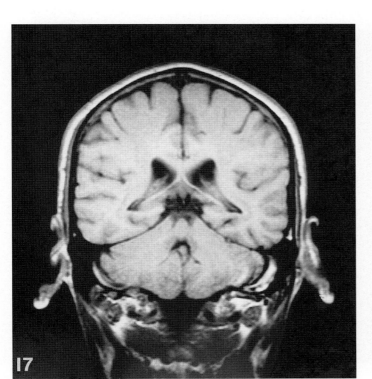

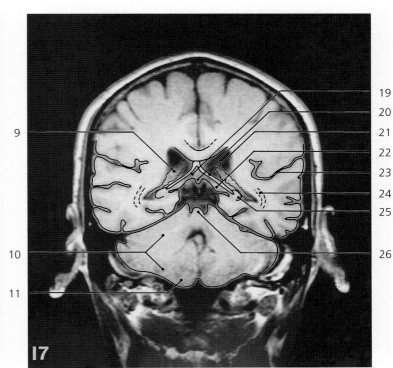

Brain, coronal MR

Scout view on page 276

1: Sagittal suture ↔
2: Temporalis muscle ←
3: Sigmoid sinus ↔
4: Obliquus capitis superior ↔
5: Splenius capitis →
6: Sternocleidomastoideus ↔
7: Longissimus capitis →
8: Obliquus capitis inferior ↔
9: Choroid plexus in atrium of lateral ventricle ↔

10: Cerebellar hemisphere ↔
11: Cerebellar tonsil ↔
12: Internal cerebral vein ↔
13: Posterior cerebral artery in quadrigeminal cistern ↔
14: Fourth ventricle ←
15: Tectorial membrane and cerebellomedullary cistern
16: Vertebral artery ←
17: Posterior arch of atlas →

18: Arch of axis
19: Habenula
20: Pineal body ←
21: Crus of fornix ←
22: Thalamus, posterior pole ←
23: Lateral sulcus (Sylvian)↔
24: Optic radiation →
25: Hippocampus ←
26: Culmen

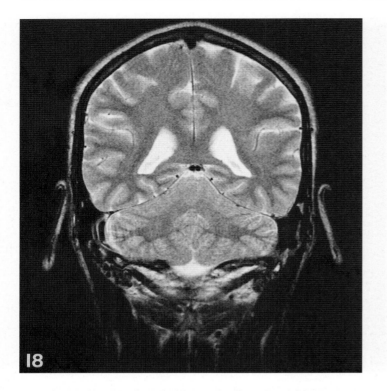

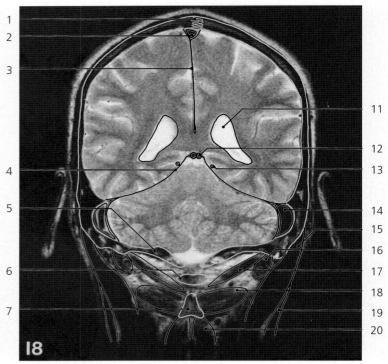

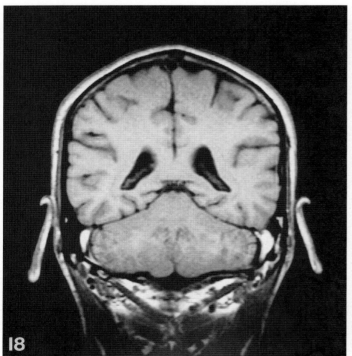

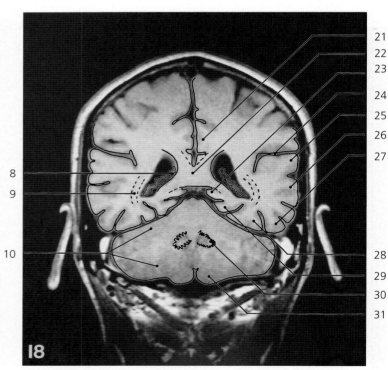

Brain, coronal MR

Scout view on page 276

1: Sagittal suture ↔
2: Superior sagittal sinus ↔
3: Falx cerebri ↔
4: Tentorium cerebelli ↔
5: Squamous part of occipital bone →
6: Posterior arch of atlas ↔
7: Spinous process of axis →
8: Choroid plexus in atrium of lateral ventricle ←
9: Optic radiation ↔
10: Cerebellar hemisphere ↔

11: Lateral ventricle, atrium ↔
12: Internal cerebral vein ←
13: Posterior cerebral artery ←
14: Sigmoid sinus ←
15: Splenius capitis ↔
16: Longissimus capitis (insertion) ←
17: Rectus capitis posterior major →
18: Obliquus capitis inferior →
19: Sternocleidomastoideus ←
20: Semispinalis cervicis
21: Cingulate gyrus ↔

22: Corpus callosum, splenium ←
23: Cingulate gyrus, isthmus →
24: Lateral sulcus (Sylvian) ↔
25: Superior temporal gyrus ↔
26: Middle temporal gyrus ↔
27: Inferior temporal gyrus ↔
28: Lateral occipitotemporal gyrus ↔
29: Medial occipitotemporal gyrus ↔
30: Dentate nucleus
31: Cerebellar tonsil ←

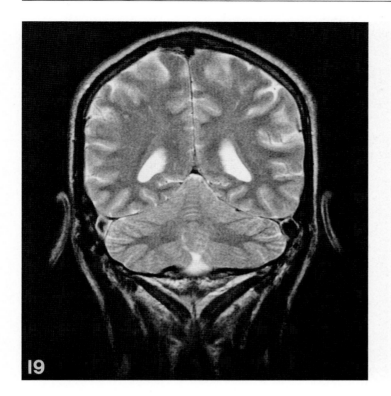

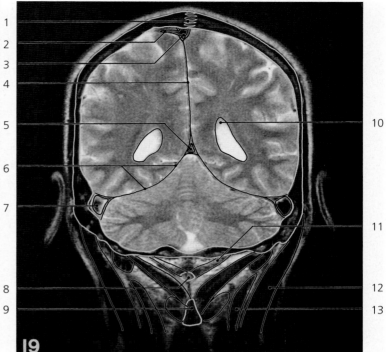

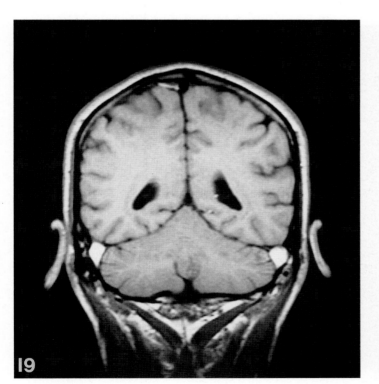

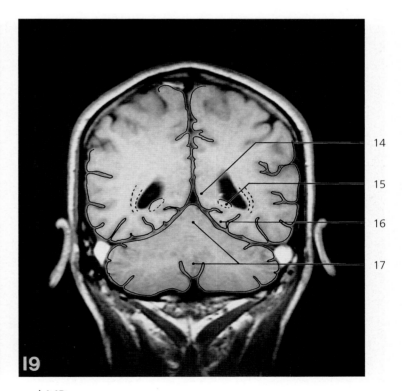

Brain, coronal MR

Scout view on page 276

1: Sagittal suture ↔
2: Superior cerebral vein →
3: Superior sagittal sinus ↔
4: Falx cerebri ↔
5: Straight sinus →
6: Tentorium cerebelli ↔

7: Transverse sinus →
8: Posterior tubercle of atlas ←
9: Spinous process of axis ←
10: Lateral ventricle, atrium ←
11: Rectus capitis posterior minor →
12: Splenius capitis →

13: Splenius cervicis
14: Cingulate gyrus, isthmus ←
15: Occipital forceps bulging into occipital
     horn of ventricle as calcar avis
16: Medial occipitotemporal gyrus ↔
17: Vermis of cerebellum →

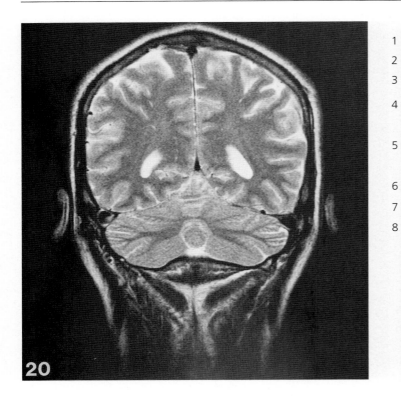

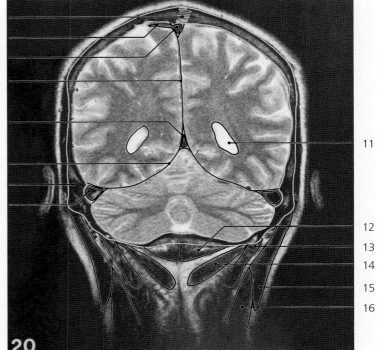

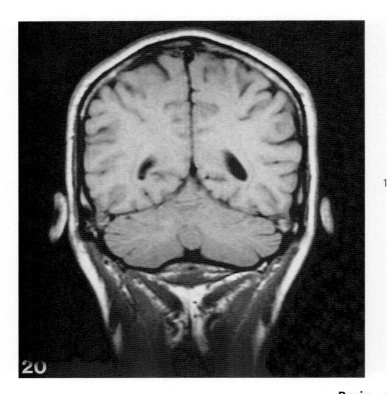

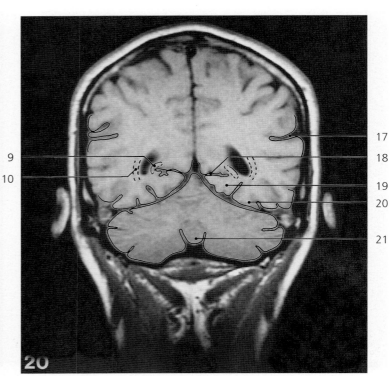

Brain, coronal MR

Scout view on page 276

1: Sagittal suture ↔
2: Superior cerebral vein ←
3: Superior sagittal sinus ↔
4: Falx cerebri ↔
5: Straight sinus ↔
6: Tentorium cerebelli ↔
7: Asterion

8: Transverse sinus ↔
9: Occipital forceps ←
10: Optic radiation ↔
11: Lateral ventricle, occipital horn →
12: Rectus capitis posterior minor ↔
13: Obliquus capitis superior (insertion) ←
14: Rectus capitis posterior major ↔

15: Splenius capitis ↔
16: Semispinalis capitis →
17: Lateral sulcus (Sylvian) ←
18: Calcarine sulcus ↔
19: Medial occipitotemporal gyrus ↔
20: Lateral occipitotemporal gyrus
21: Vermis of cerebellum ↔

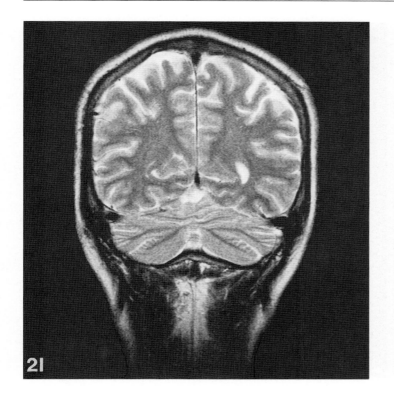

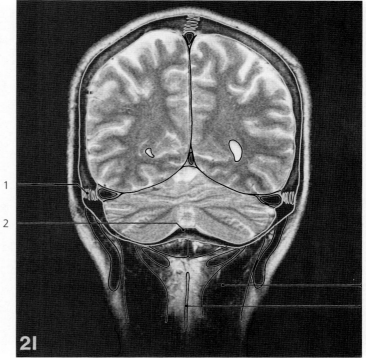

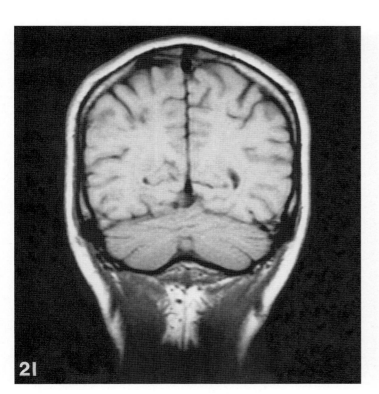

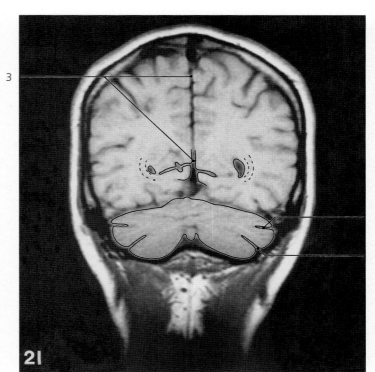

Brain, coronal MR

Scout view on page 276

1: Lambdoid suture →
2: Internal occipital crest →
3: Longitudinal fissure of brain ↔

4: Semispinalis capitis ↔
5: Nuchal ligament →
6: Horizontal fissure of cerebellum →

7: Posterolateral fissure of cerebellum

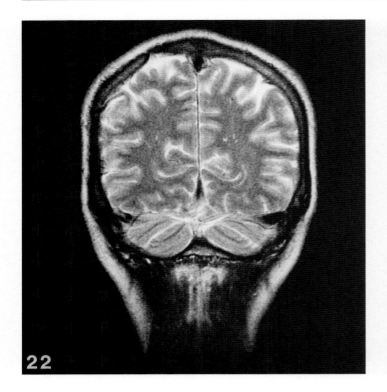

22

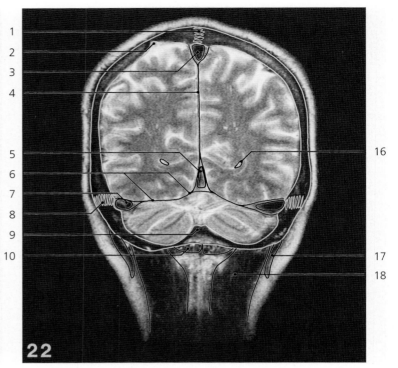

22

1
2
3
4
5
6
7
8
9
10

16

17
18

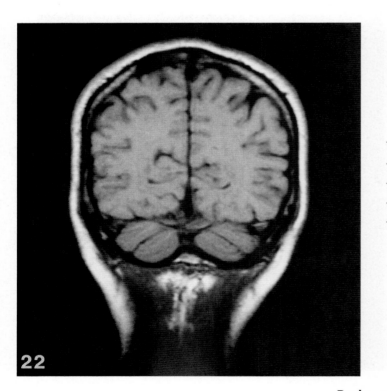

22

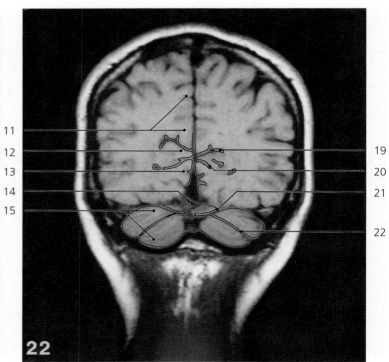

22

11
12
13
14
15

19
20
21

22

Brain, coronal MR

Scout view on page 276

1: Sagittal suture ↔
2: Arachnoid granulation
3: Superior sagittal sinus ↔
4: Falx cerebri ↔
5: Straight sinus ↔
6: Tentorium cerebelli ↔
7: Transverse sinus ↔
8: Lambdoid suture ↔

9: Internal occipital crest ←
10: Rectus capitis posterior minor ←
11: Precuneus ↔
12: Cuneus →
13: Medial occipitotemporal gyrus ↔
14: Vermis of cerebellum ←
15: Cerebellar hemisphere ↔
16: Lateral ventricle, occipital horn ↔

17: Splenius capitis ←
18: Semispinalis capitis ↔
19: Parieto-occipital sulcus ↔
20: Calcarine sulcus ↔
21: Primary fissure of cerebellum
22: Horizontal fissure ↔

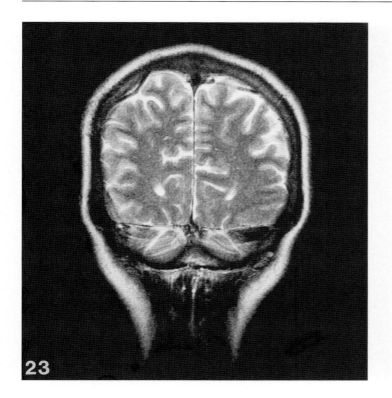

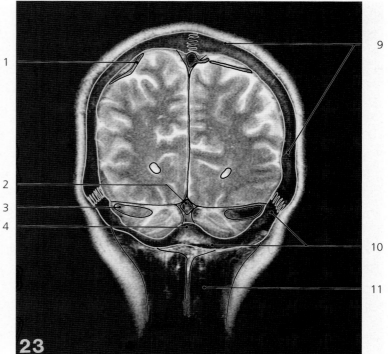

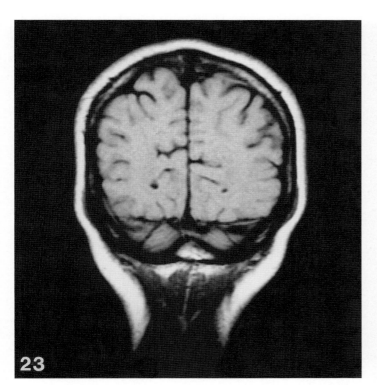

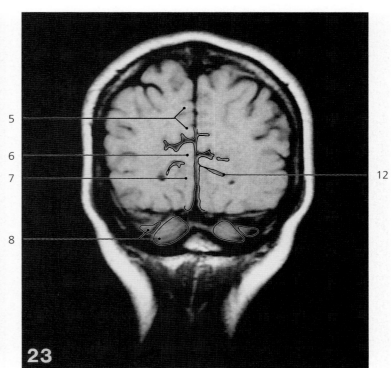

Brain, coronal MR

Scout view on page 276

1: Superior cerebral vein
2: Straight sinus ←
3: Transverse sinus ↔
4: Internal occipital protuberance

5: Precuneus ↔
6: Cuneus ↔
7: Medial occipitotemporal gyrus ←
8: Cerebellar hemisphere ←

9: Parietal bone ↔
10: Squamous part of occipital bone ↔
11: Semispinalis capitis ↔
12: Calcarine sulcus ↔

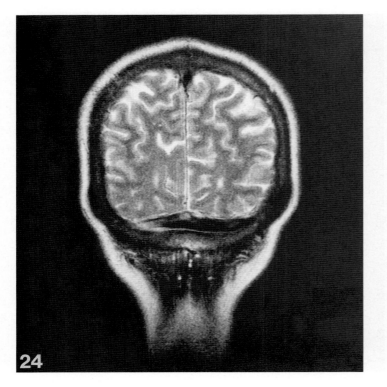

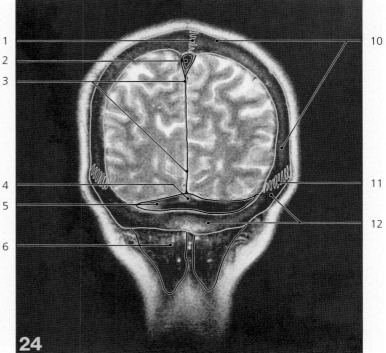

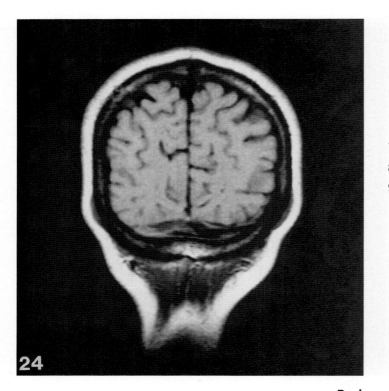

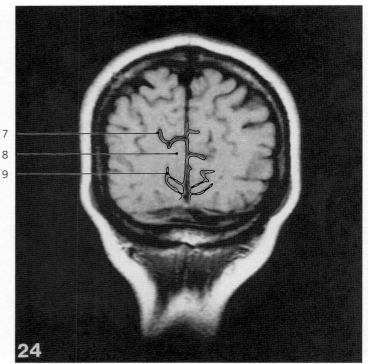

Brain, coronal MR

Scout view on page 276

1: Sagittal suture ↔
2: Superior sagittal sinus ↔
3: Falx cerebri ↔
4: Confluence of sinuses →

5: Transverse sinus ←
6: Semispinalis capitis ↔
7: Parieto-occipital sulcus ←
8: Cuneus ↔

9: Calcarine sulcus ↔
10: Parietal bone ↔
11: Lambdoid suture ↔
12: Squamous part of occipital bone ↔

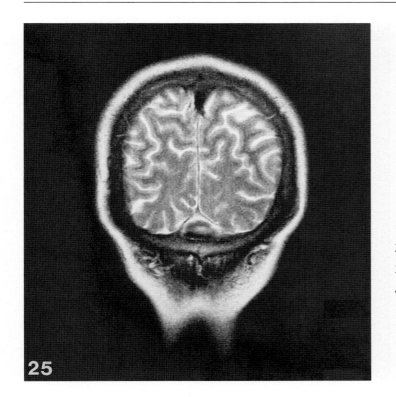

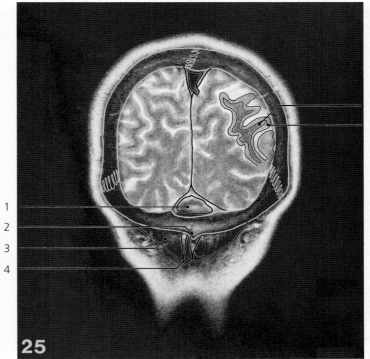

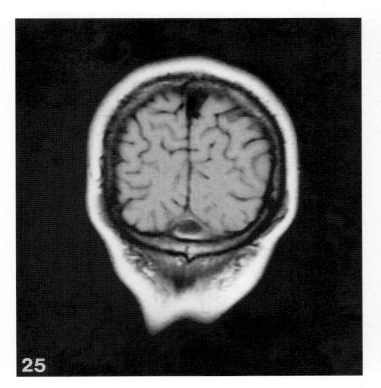

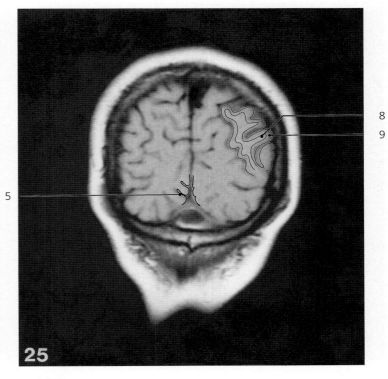

Brain, coronal MR

Scout view on page 276

1: Confluence of sinuses ←
2: External occipital crest →
3: Semispinalis capitis ←
4: Nuchal ligament →
5: Calcarine sulcus ↔
6: White matter
7: Grey matter
8: White matter
9: Grey matter

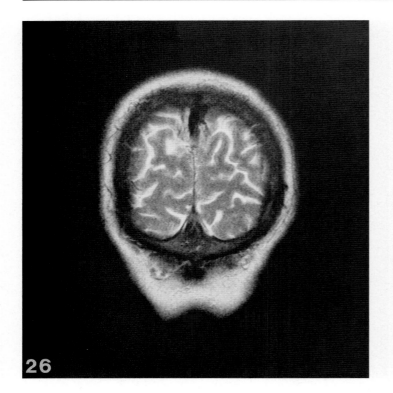

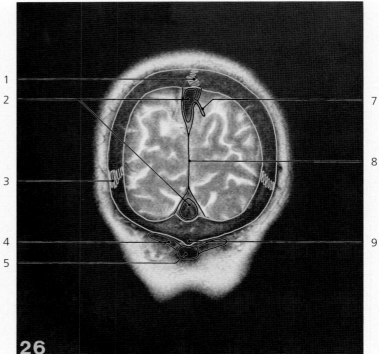

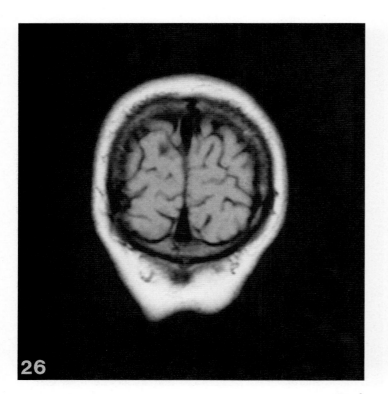

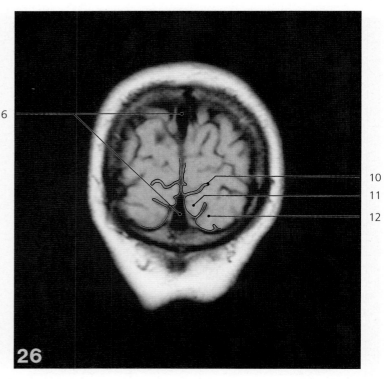

Brain, coronal MR

Scout view on page 276

1: Sagittal suture ↔
2: Superior sagittal sinus ↔
3: Lambdoid suture ↔
4: Trapezius

5: Nuchal ligament ←
6: Longitudinal fissure of brain ←
7: Superior cerebral vein
8: Falx cerebri ←

9: External occipital crest
10: Calcarine sulcus ↔
11: Medial occipitotemporal gyrus ←
12: Lateral occipitotemporal gyrus ←

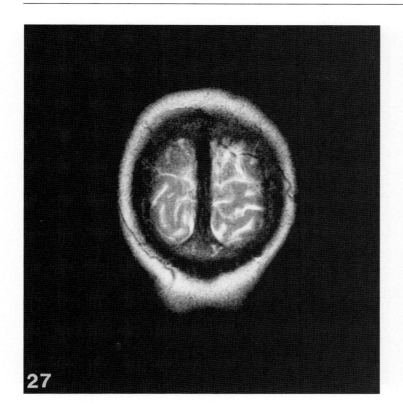

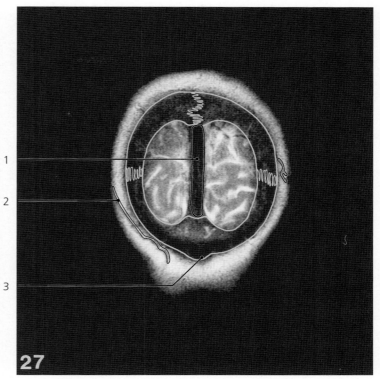

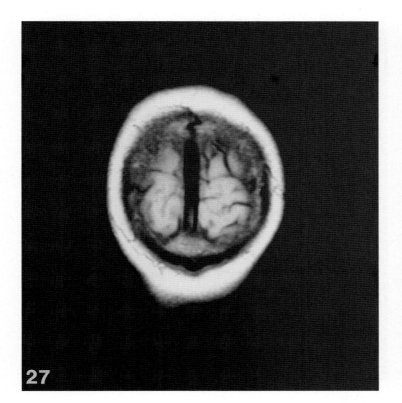

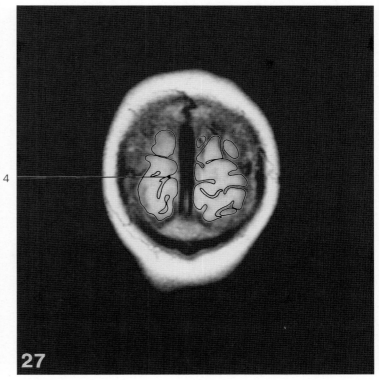

Brain, coronal MR

Scout view on page 276

1: Superior sagittal sinus ←   3: External occipital protuberance
2: Scalp vein   4: Calcarine sulcus ←

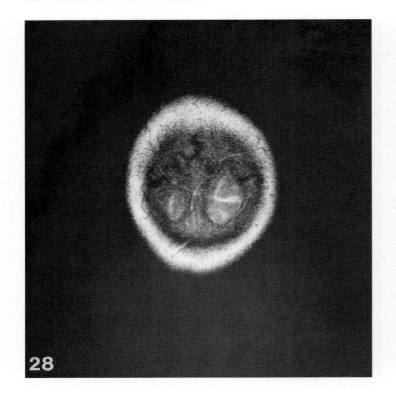

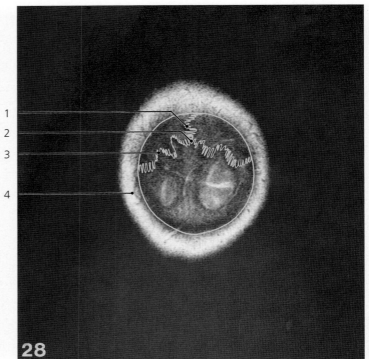

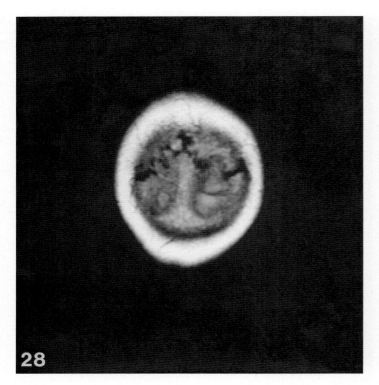

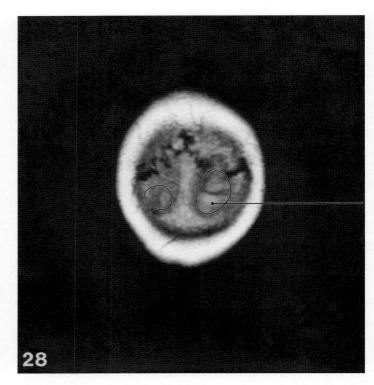

Brain, coronal MR

Scout view on page 276

1: Sagittal suture ←   3: Lambdoid suture ←   5: Occipital pole of brain
2: Lambda   4: Scalp

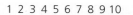

1 2 3 4 5 6 7 8 9 10

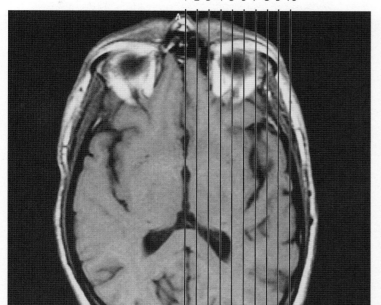

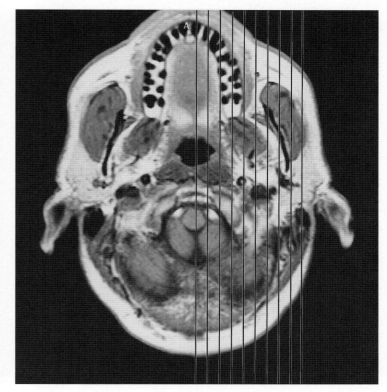

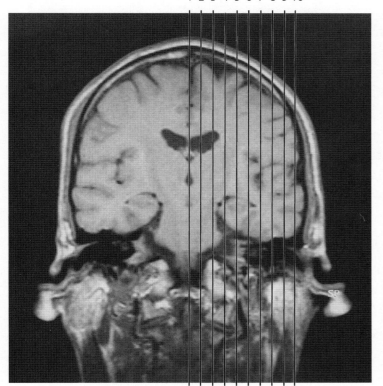

Scout views of sagittal MR series

Lines #1–10 indicate positions of sagittal sections in the following MR series.

Interpretation of the scout images are found on pages 266, 256 and 290 in the corresponding axial and coronal series.

All sections are 5 mm thick and are spaced by 1.5 mm.

Each section is displayed in both T2 (above) and T1 (below) weighted imaging.

Bone structures are delineated by yellow lines on the T2 weighted images.

Arrows ←, → and ↔ in the legends indicate that a structure can be seen on a previous or following section, or both.

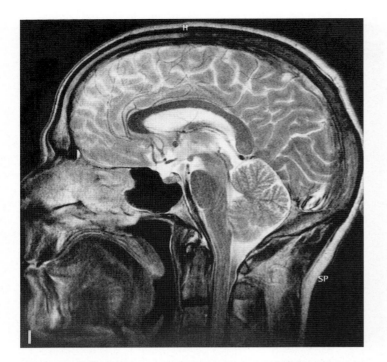

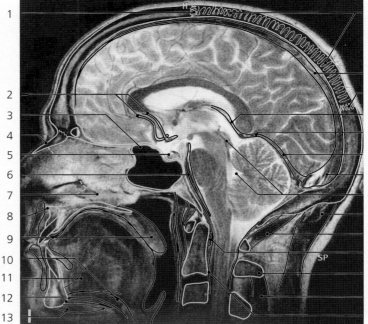

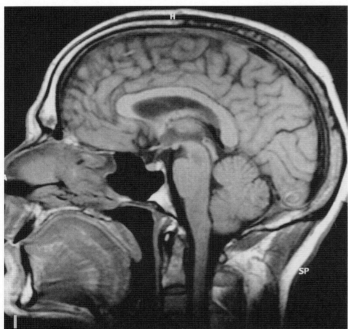

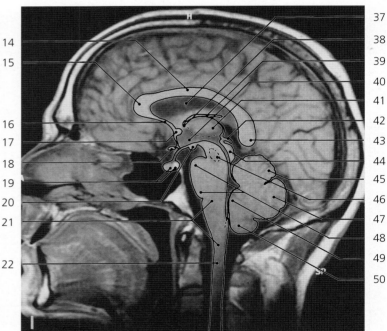

Brain, sagittal MR

Scout view on previous page

1: Coronal suture →
2: Anterior cerebral arteries
3: Sphenoidal sinus →
4: Nasal bone →
5: Hypophysial fossa
6: Basilar artery
7: Vomer
8: Anterior nasal spine
9: Uvula →
10: Geniohyoideus →
11: Genioglossus
12: Mylohyoideus →
13: Digastricus, anterior belly →
14: Corpus callosum, body →
15: Corpus callosum, genu →
16: Corpus callosum, rostrum
17: Anterior commissure →
18: Optic chiasm

19: Hypophysis (anterior and posterior lobe)
20: Mammillary body
21: Medulla oblongata →
22: Spinal cord →
23: Sagittal suture
24: Superior sagittal sinus →
25: Lambda
26: Internal cerebral vein →
27: Great cerebral vein →
28: Straight sinus
29: Confluence of sinuses →
30: Cerebral aqueduct and fourth ventricle →
31: Semispinalis capitis →
32: Rectus capitis posterior minor →
33: Transverse ligament of atlas →
34: Spinous process of axis →

35: Semispinalis cervicis
36: Tectorial membrane →
37: Septum pellucidum
38: Interventricular foramen
39: Body of fornix →
40: Hypothalamus →
41: Thalamus →
42: Pineal body
43: Corpus callosum splenium
44: Mesencephalon, tectum →
45: Cerebellum, lobulus quadrangularis →
46: Red nucleus
47: Cerebellum, lobulus simplex →
48: Pons
49: Cerebellum, uvula vermis
50: Cerebellum, tonsil →

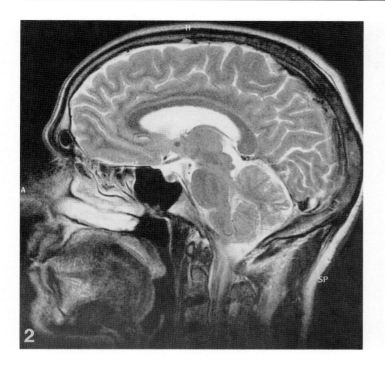

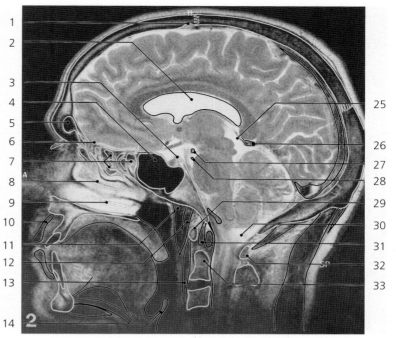

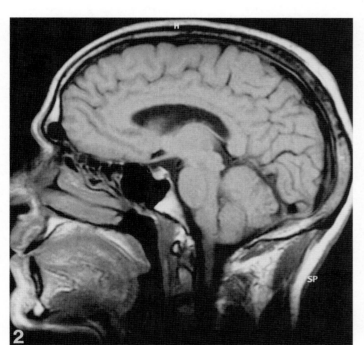

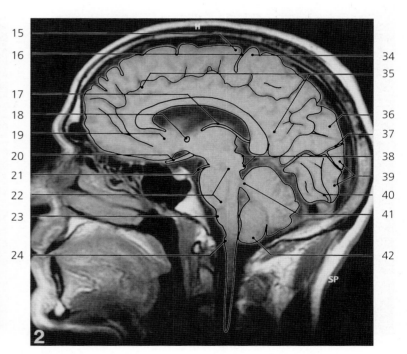

Brain, sagittal MR

Scout view on page 305

1: Arachnoid granulation
2: Lateral ventricle, central part →
3: Dorsum sellae ←
4: Sphenoidal sinus ↔
5: Frontal sinus →
6: Cribriform plate
7: Ethmoidal air cells →
8: Middle concha
9: Inferior concha
10: Orbicularis oris →
11: Longus capitis →
12: Rectus capitis anterior
13: Longus colli
14: Epiglottis

15: Precentral gyrus →
16: Central sulcus (Roland) →
17: Body of fornix ↔
18: Anterior commissure ↔
19: Area subcallosa
20: Optic tract →
21: Oculomotor nerve
22: Pons →
23: Olive
24: Pyramis
25: Quadrigeminal cistern ←
26: Great cerebral vein ←
27: Posterior cerebral artery →
28: Superior cerebellar artery →

29: Anterior arch of atlas ←
30: Cisterna magna ↔
31: Alar ligament
32: Posterior arch of atlas ↔
33: Dens ←
34: Postcentral gyrus →
35: Cingulate gyrus →
36: Precuneus →
37: Parieto-occipital sulcus →
38: Colliculus superior and inferior
39: Cuneus →
40: Calcarine sulcus ↔
41: Superior cerebellar peduncle →
42: Cerebellar tonsil ←

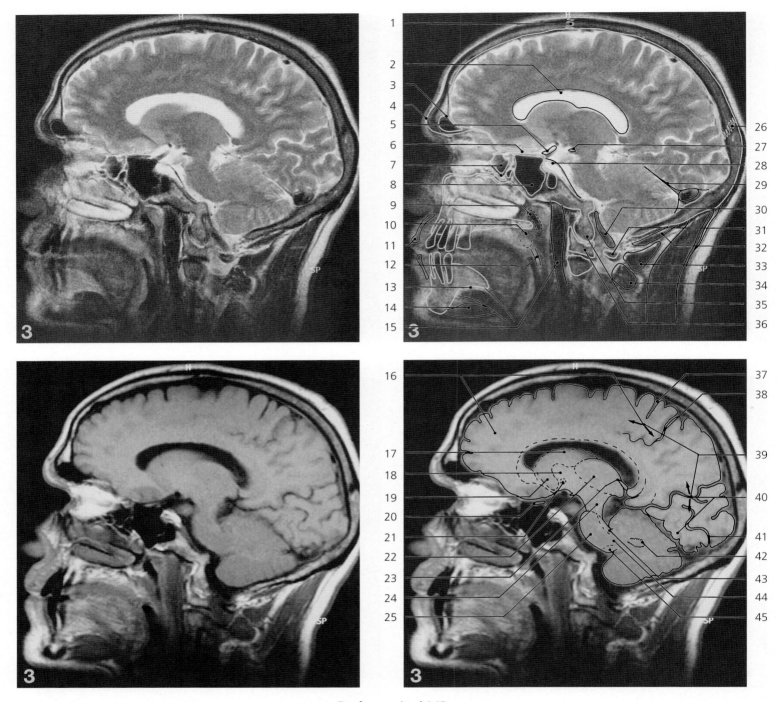

Brain, sagittal MR

Scout view on page 305

1: Coronal suture ↔
2: Lateral ventricle, central part ↔
3: Frontal sinus ←
4: Superciliary arch →
5: Middle cerebral artery →
6: Optic canal with optic nerve
7: Ethmoidal air cells ←
8: Sphenoidal sinus ↔
9: Pharyngeal recess
10: Palatine tonsil
11: Orbicularis oris ←
12: Palatopharyngeal arch
13: Mylohyoideus ↔
14: Digastricus, anterior belly ↔
15: Longus capitis ↔

16: Frontal lobe ↔
17: Caudate nucleus, body ←
18: Internal capsule →
19: Putamen →
20: Optic nerve →
21: Anterior commissure ↔
22: Thalamus ↔
23: Crus of fornix ↔
24: Cerebral peduncle ←
25: Pons ←
26: Lambdoid suture ↔
27: Posterior cerebral artery ←
28: Cavernous sinus/Trigeminal cave
29: Tentorium cerebelli →
30: Vertebral artery →

31: Posterior arch of atlas ←
32: Rectus capitis posterior minor ←
33: Rectus capitis posterior major →
34: Obliquus capitis inferior →
35: Occipital condyle →
36: Lateral mass of atlas →
37: Central sulcus ↔
38: Cingulate sulcus
39: Parietal lobe ↔
40: Occipital lobe ↔
41: Calcarine sulcus ↔
42: Dentate nucleus
43: Superior cerebellar peduncle ←
44: Middle cerebellar peduncle
45: Inferior cerebellar peduncle

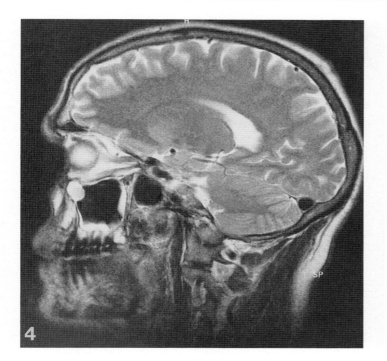

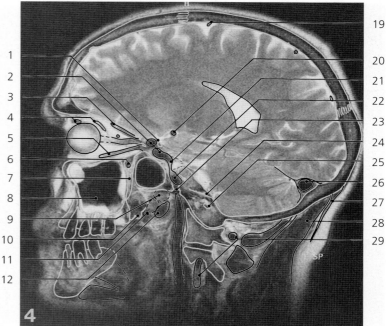

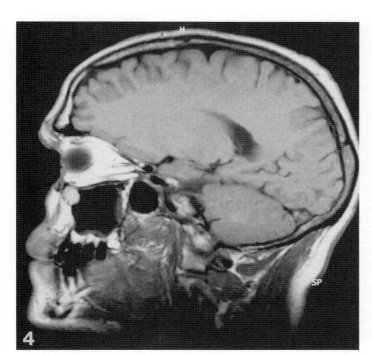

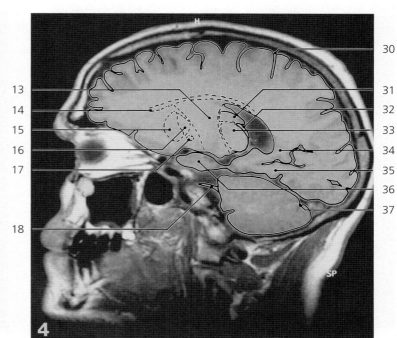

Brain, sagittal MR

Scout view on page 305

1: Anterior clinoid process
2: Internal carotid artery, "siphon" →
3: Rectus superior/levator palpebrae superioris →
4: Obliquus superior
5: Rectus inferior →
6: Maxillary artery
7: Pterygopalatine fossa →
8: Maxillary sinus →(with oedematous mucosa)
9: Auditory tube
10: Pterygoid hamulus
11: Tensor veli palatini
12: Levator veli palatini

13: Internal capsule ↔
14: Corpus callosum ←
15: Putamen ←
16: Global pallidus →
17: Anterior commissure ↔
18: Trigeminal nerve
19: Superior cerebral vein →
20: Middle cerebral artery ↔
21: Internal carotid artery in cavernous sinus
22: Internal carotid artery in carotid canal ↔
23: Foramen lacerum
24: Petro-occipital fissure →
25: Hypoglossal canal →

26: Transverse sinus ↔
27: Trapezius ↔
28: Semispinalis capitis ↔
29: Vertebral artery ↔
30: Central sulcus ↔
31: Caudate nucleus ←
32: Fornix, crus ←
33: Thalamus ←
34: Isthmus of cingulate gyrus
35: Medial occipitotemporal gyrus
36: Uncus
37: Horizontal fissure of cerebellum

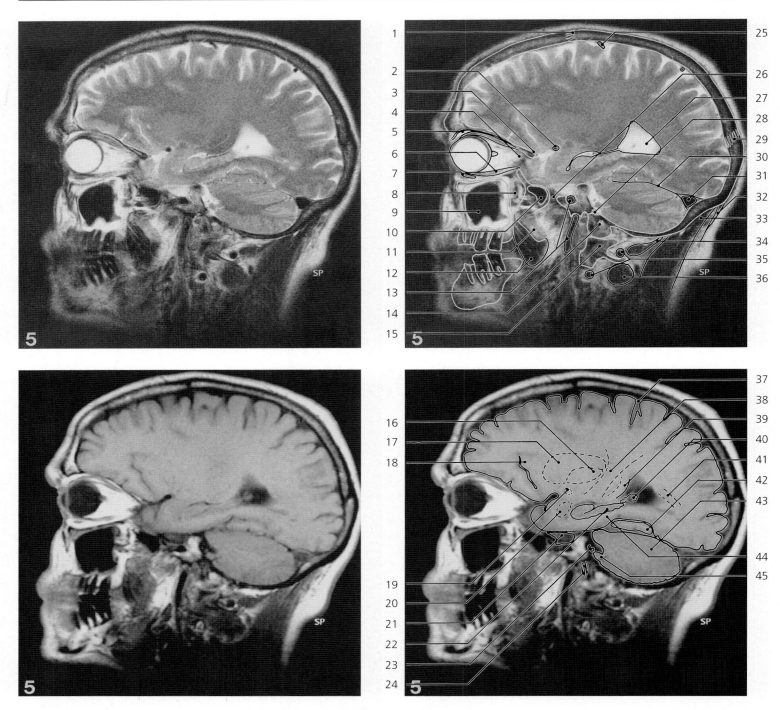

Brain, sagittal MR

Scout view on page 305

1: Coronal suture ↔
2: Middle cerebral artery ↔
3: Lesser wing of sphenoidal bone →
4: Superior orbital fissure
5: Levator palpabrae superioris ↔
6: Rectus inferior ←
7: Obliquus inferior →
8: Pterygopalatine fossa ←
9: Maxillary sinus ↔
10: Sphenoidal sinus ←
11: Pterygoid process ←
12: Medial pterygoid muscle →
13: Internal carotid artery ↔
14: Hypoglossal canal ←
15: Lateral mass of atlas ←
16: Globus pallidus ←

17: Putamen ←
18: Insula, limen →
19: Anterior commissure ←
20: Amygdaloid body
21: Trigeminal ganglion
22: Hippocampus →
23: Acoustic and facial nerve
24: Vagus, glossopharyngeal and
    accessory nerves
25: Superior cerebral vein ↔
26: Foramen ovale with mandibular nerve
27: Lateral ventricle, atrium ↔
28: Petro-occipital fissure ←
29: Lambdoid suture ↔
30: Tentorium cerebelli ↔
31: Transverse sinus ↔

32: Trapezius ←
33: Semispinalis capitis ↔
34: Rectus capitis posterior major ↔
35: Vertebral artery ↔
36: Obliquus capitis inferior ↔
37: Central sulcus ↔
38: Internal capsule, posterior limb ←
39: Occipital forceps
40: Choroid plexus ↔
41: Optic radiation
42: Lateral occipitotemporal gyrus →
43: Cerebellum ↔
44: Medial occipitotemporal
    (parahippocampal) gyrus ←
45: Flocculus

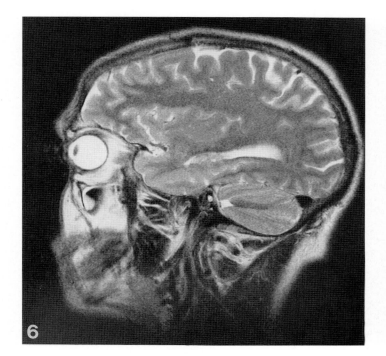

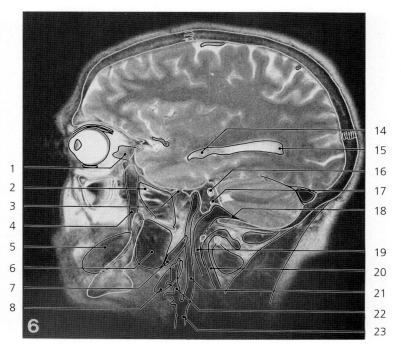

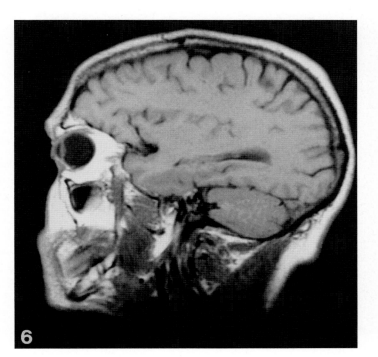

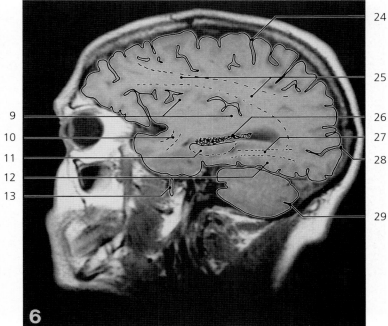

Brain, sagittal MR

Scout view on page 305

1: Rectus lateralis →
2: Lateral pterygoid muscle →
3: Foramen spinosum
4: Temporalis muscle →
5: Masseter →
6: Medial pterygoid muscle ↔
7: "Stylo-muscles" →
8: Digastricus, posterior belly →
9: Insula ↔
10: Uncinate fasciculus

11: Hippocampus ←
12: Lateral occipitotemporal gyrus →
13: Mandibular nerve
14: Lateral ventricle, temporal horn →
15: Lateral ventricle, occipital horn
16: Internal acoustic opening
17: Perilymphatic duct
18: Sigmoid sinus →
19: Internal jugular vein →
20: Vertebral artery ←

21: Internal carotid artery ←
22: External carotid artery
23: Common carotid artery
24: Central sulcus ↔
25: Superior longitudinal fasciculus (arcuatus)
26: Choroid plexus of lateral ventricle
27: Inferior longitudinal fasciculus
28: Calcarine sulcus ↔
29: Horizontal fissure of cerebellum ↔

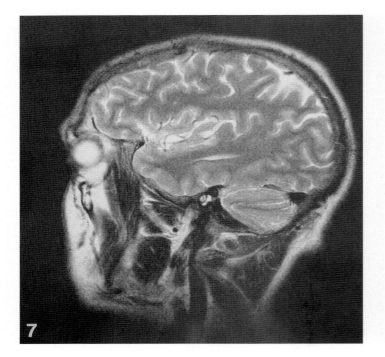

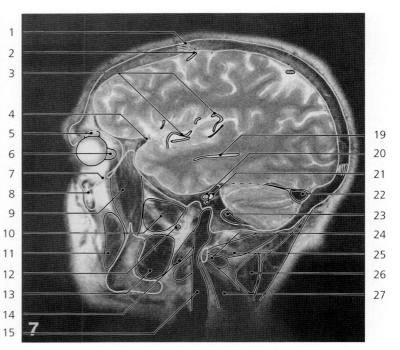

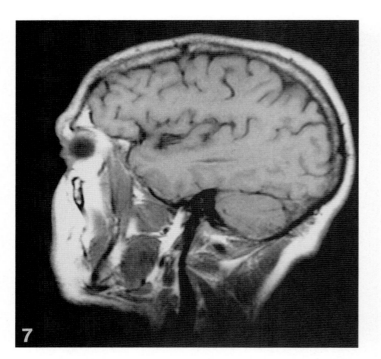

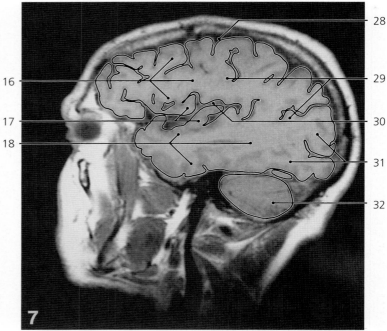

Brain, sagittal MR

Scout view on page 305

1: Coronal suture ↔
2: Superior cerebral vein ↔
3: Insular branches of middle cerebral artery ←
4: Lesser wing of sphenoidal bone ←
5: Lacrimal gland
6: Rectus lateralis ←
7: Inferior orbital fissure
8: Maxilla, body
9: Temporalis muscle ↔
10: Lateral pterygoid muscle ↔

11: Masseter ↔
12: Maxillary artery ↔
13: Medial pterygoid muscle ↔
14: "Stylo-muscles" ↔
15: Internal jugular vein
16: Frontal lobe ↔
17: Insular gyri ←
18: Temporal lobe ↔
19: Lateral ventricle, temporal horn ←
20: Cochlea
21: Vestibule

22: Transverse sinus ↔
23: Sigmoid sinus ↔
24: Obliquus capitis inferior ←
25: Obliquus capitis superior →
26: Splenius capitis →
27: Levator scapulae
28: Central sulcus ↔
29: Parietal lobe ↔
30: Lateral sulcus (Sylvian)
31: Occipital lobe ↔
32: Cerebellum ↔

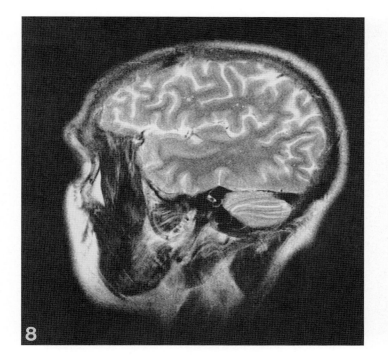

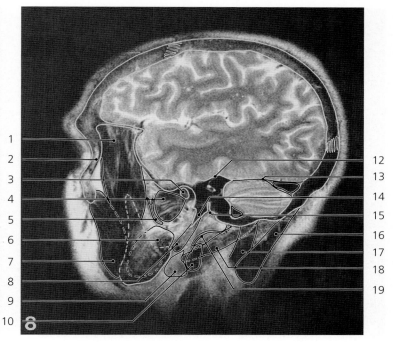

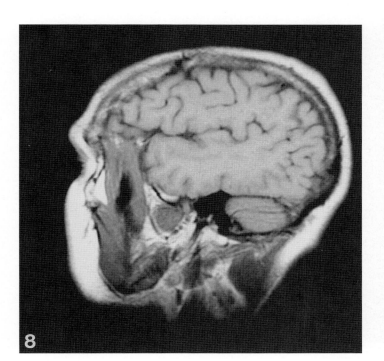

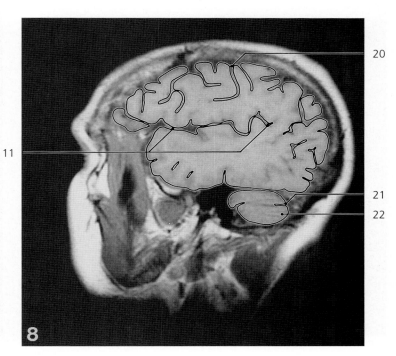

Brain, sagittal MR

Scout view on page 305

1: Temporalis muscle ↔
2: Frontal process of zygomatic bone →
3: Head of mandible →
4: Lateral pterygoid muscle →
5: Maxillary artery ←
6: Medial pterygoid muscle ←
7: Masseter ↔
8: "Stylo-muscles" ←

9: Parotid gland →
10: Internal jugular vein ←
11: Lateral sulcus (Sylvian) ↔
12: Tegmen tympani
13: Tentorium cerebelli ↔
14: Styloid process
15: Foramen stylomastoideum with facial nerve

16: Splenius capitis ↔
17: Obliquus capitis superior ←
18: Digastricus, posterior belly ←
19: Occipital artery
20: Central sulcus ↔
21: Horizontal fissure of cerebellum ←
22: Cerebellar hemisphere ↔

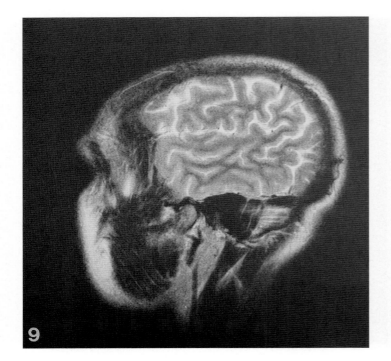

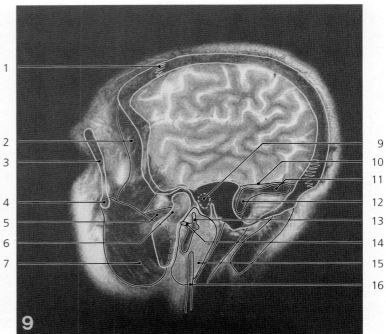

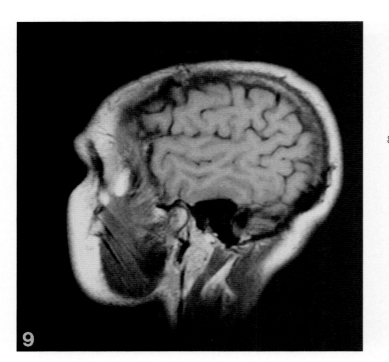

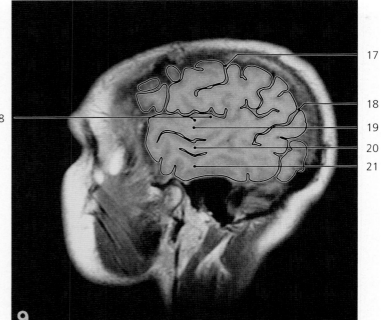

Brain, sagittal MR

Scout view on page 305

1: Coronal suture ←
2: Temporalis muscle ↔
3: Frontal process of zygomatic bone ←
4: Zygomatic arch →
5: Lateral pterygoid muscle (insertion) ←
6: Neck of mandible
7: Masseter ↔

8: Auditory cortex
9: Middle ear
10: Tentorium cerebelli ←
11: Transverse sinus ←
12: Sigmoid sinus ←
13: Superficial temporal artery
14: Maxillary artery ←

15: Parotid gland ↔
16: Retromandibular vein →
17: Central sulcus ↔
18: Parieto-occipital sulcus ←
19: Superior temporal gyrus
20: Middle temporal gyrus
21: Inferior temporal gyrus

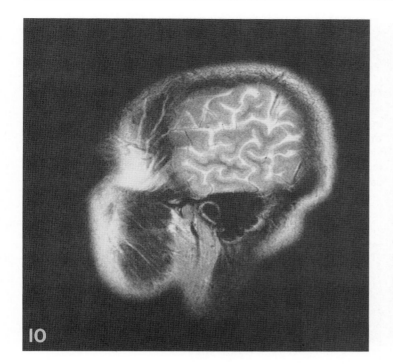

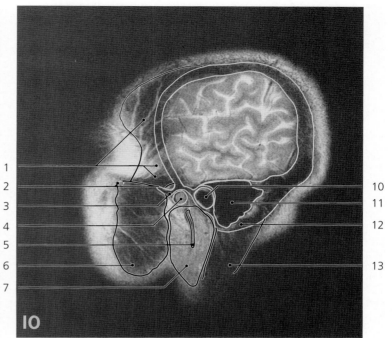

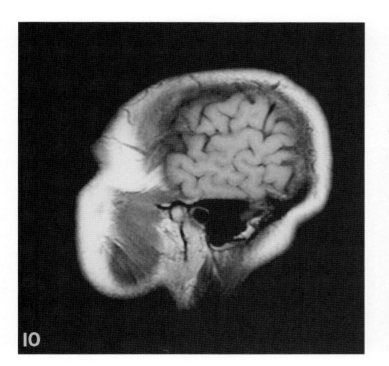

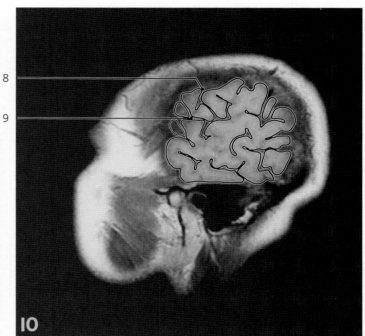

Brain, sagittal MR

Scout view on page 305

1: Temporalis muscle ←
2: Zygomatic arch ←
3: Articular tubercle
4: Head of mandible ←
5: Retromandibular vein ←
6: Masseter ←
7: Parotid gland ←
8: Central sulcus (Roland) ←
9: Lateral sulcus (Sylvian) ←
10: External acoustic meatus
11: Mastoid air cells
12: Mastoid process
13: Sternocleidomastoideus

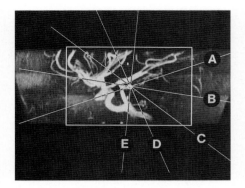

Scout view for MR angiography series

The following MR angiography series shows the bilateral set of cerebral arteries in a volume of brain, limited anteriorly and posteriorly, cranially and caudally as indicated by the frame on the scout view. The individual images A-E are the projected views perpendicular to the planes indicated by A-E on the scout view.

See corresponding series on pages 318–319.

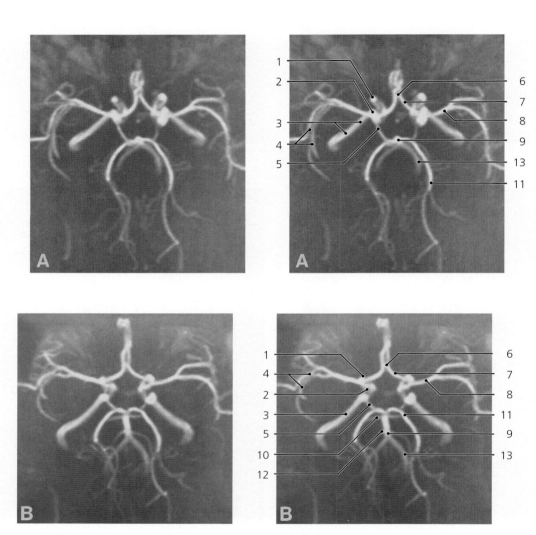

Brain arteries, MR angiography, circle of Willis

1: Internal carotid artery, "siphon"
2: Internal carotid artery in cavernous sinus
3: Internal carotid artery in carotid canal
4: Insular branches of middle cerebral artery

5: Posterior communicating artery
6: Anterior communicating artery
7: Anterior cerebral artery
8: Middle cerebral artery
9: Basilar artery
10: Superior cerebellar artery

11: Posterior cerebral artery
12: Anterior inferior cerebellar artery (AICA)
13: Vertebral artery

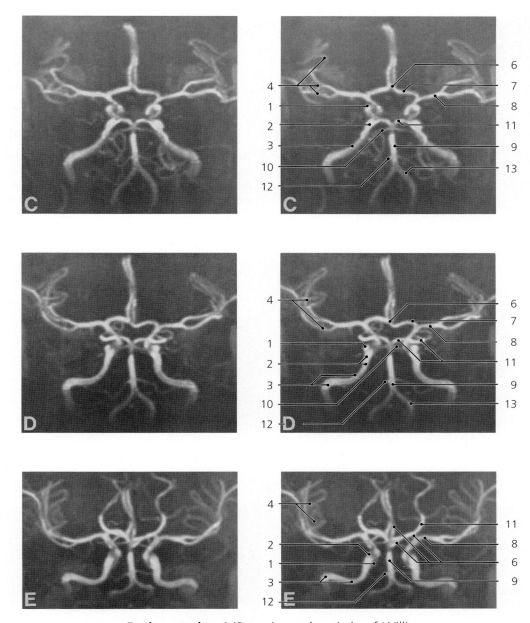

Brain arteries, MR angiography, circle of Willis

1: Internal carotid artery, "siphon"
2: Internal carotid artery in cavernous sinus
3: Internal carotid artery in carotid canal
4: Insular branches of middle cerebral artery

5: Posterior communicating artery
6: Anterior communicating artery
7: Anterior cerebral artery
8: Middle cerebral artery
9: Basilar artery
10: Superior cerebellar artery

11: Posterior cerebral artery
12: Anterior inferior cerebellar artery (AICA)
13: Vertebral artery

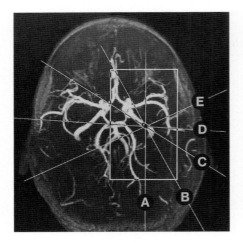

Scout view for MR angiography series

The following MR angiography series shows the cerebral arteries in a volume of the left hemisphere, reaching just across the midline and limited anteriorly and posteriorly, medially and laterally as indicated by the frame on the scout view.

See corresponding series on the previous pages.

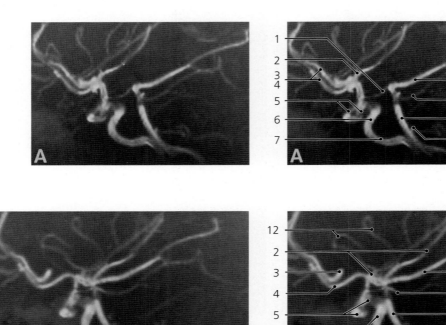

Brain arteries, MR angiography, circle of Willis

1: Posterior communicating artery
2: Middle cerebral artery
3: Right anterior cerebral artery
4: Left anterior cerebral artery
5: Internal carotid artery ("siphon")

6: Internal carotid artery in cavernous sinus
7: Internal carotid artery in carotid canal
8: Posterior cerebral artery
9: Superior cerebellar artery

10: Basilar artery
11: Anterior inferior cerebellar artery (AICA)
12: Insular branches of middle cerebral artery

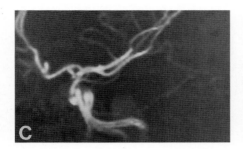
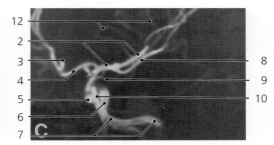

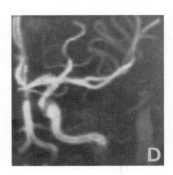
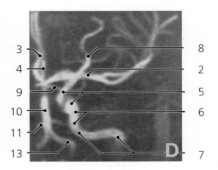

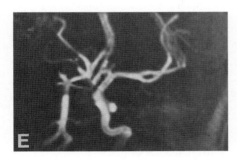
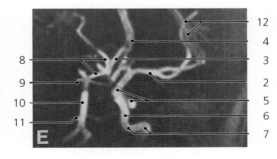

Brain arteries, MR angiography, circle of Willis

1: Posterior communicating artery
2: Middle cerebral artery
3: Right anterior cerebral artery
4: Left anterior cerebral artery
5: Internal carotid artery ("siphon")
6: Internal carotid artery in cavernous sinus

7: Internal carotid artery in carotid canal
8: Posterior cerebral artery
9: Superior cerebellar artery
10: Basilar artery
11: Anterior inferior cerebellar artery (AICA)

12: Insular branches of middle cerebral artery
13: Vertebral artery

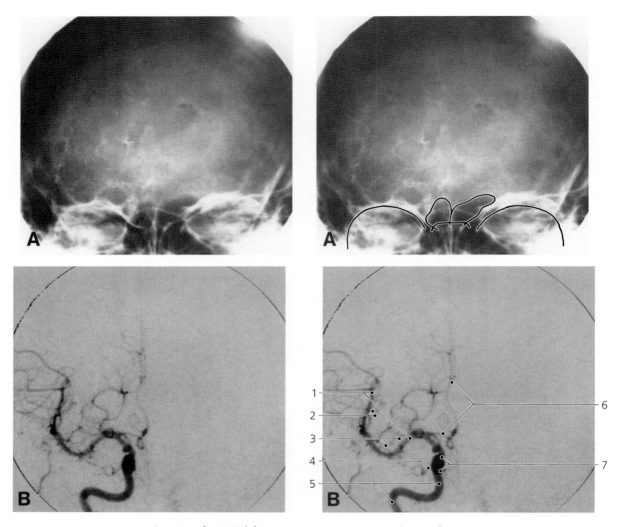

Internal carotid artery, a-p X-ray, arteriography

A: Unprocessed X-ray. B: After digital subtraction

1: Middle cerebral artery
2: Insular arteries
3: Lateral thalamostriate arteries

4: Ophthalmic artery
5: Internal carotid artery in carotid canal
6: Anterior cerebral artery

7: Carotid "syphon"

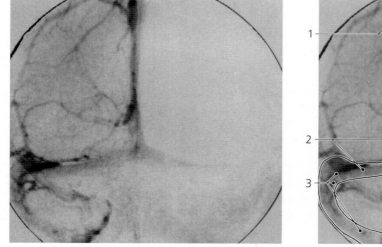

Cerebral veins, a-p X-ray, venous phase of arteriography (digital subtraction)

1: Superior cerebral veins
2: Transverse sinus

3: Sigmoid sinus
4: Superior sagittal sinus

5: Confluens of sinuses
6: Inferior petrous sinus

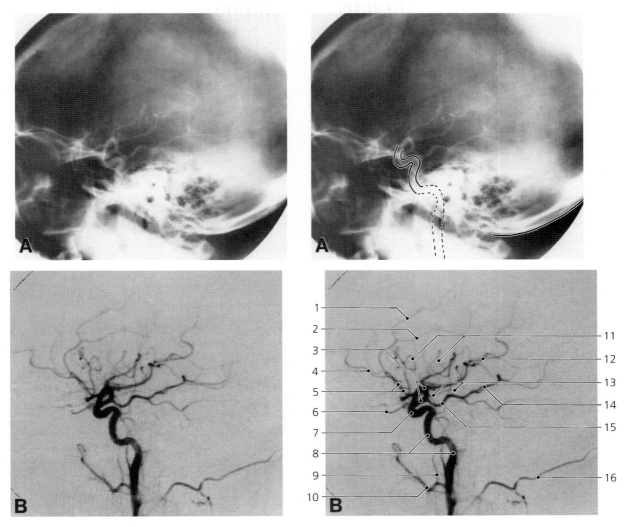

Internal carotid artery, lateral X-ray, arteriography A: Unprocessed X-ray. B: After digital subtraction

1: Callosomarginal artery
2: Pericallosal artery
3: Middle cerebral artery
4: Frontopolar artery
5: Anterior cerebral artery
6: Ophthalmic artery

7: Carotid "syphon"
8: Internal carotid artery in carotid canal
9: Middle meningeal artery
10: Maxillary artery
11: Insular arteries

12: Middle cerebral artery, parietal branches
13: Anterior choroid artery
14: Posterior cerebral artery
15: Posterior communicating artery
16: Occipital artery

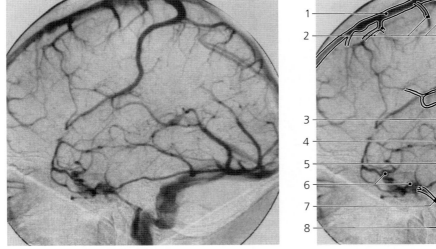

Cerebral veins, lateral X-ray, venous phase of arteriography (digital subtraction)

1: Superior sagittal sinus
2: Superior cerebral veins
3: Great cerebral vein (Galen)
4: Basal vein (Rosenthal)
5: Superior petrous sinus

6: Cavernous sinus
7: Inferior petrous sinus
8: Bulb of internal jugular vein
9: Thalamostriate vein
10: Internal cerebral vein

11: Straight sinus
12: Transverse sinus
13: Sigmoid sinus

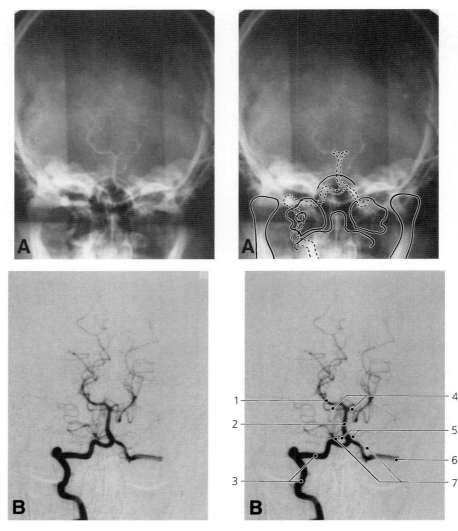

Vertebral artery, a-p X-ray, arteriography

A: Unprocessed X-ray. B: After digital subtraction

1: Posterior cerebral artery
2: Basilar artery
3: Vertebral artery
4: Superior cerebellar arteries

5: Anterior inferior cerebellar arteries ("AICA")
6: Overflow in contralateral vertebral artery

7: Posterior inferior cerebellar arteries ("PICA")

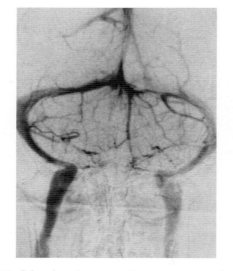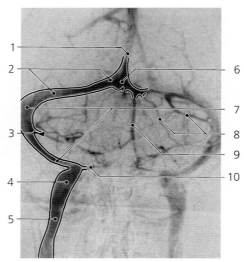

Cerebral veins, a-p X-ray, venous phase of arteriography (digital subtraction)

1: Superior sagittal sinus
2: Transverse sinus
3: Superior petrous sinus
4: Bulb of internal jugular vein

5: Internal jugular vein
6: Confluence of sinuses
7: Sigmoid sinus
8: Inferior veins of cerebellar hemisphere

9: Inferior vermis vein
10: Inferior petrous sinus

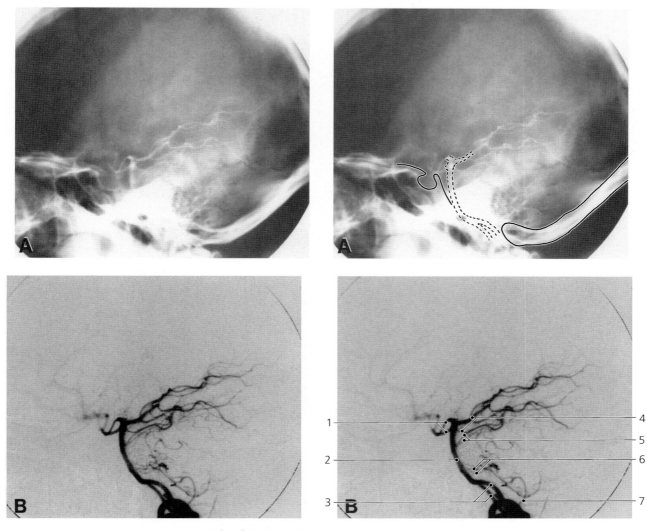

Vertebral artery, lateral X-ray, arteriography

A: Unprocessed X-ray. B: After digital subtraction

1: Posterior communicating arteries
2: Basilar artery
3: Vertebral arteries
4: Posterior cerebral arteries

5: Superior cerebellar arteries
6: Anterior inferior cerebellar arteries ("AICA")

7: Posterior inferior cerebellar artery ("PICA")

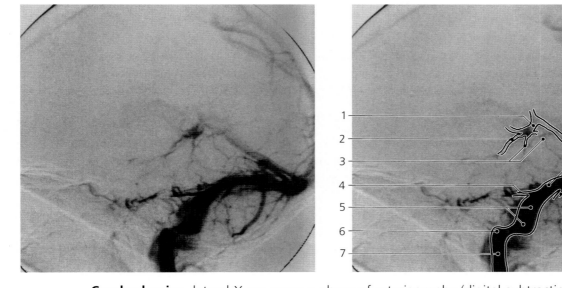

Cerebral veins, lateral X-ray, venous phase of arteriography (digital subtraction)

1: Great cerebral vein
2: Basal vein (Rosenthal)
3: Superior cerebellar veins
4: Superior petrous sinus

5: Sigmoid sinus
6: Bulb of the internal jugular vein
7: Internal jugular vein
8: Superior sagittal sinus

9: Straight sinus
10: Transverse sinus
11: Confluence of sinuses
12: Inferior cerebellar veins

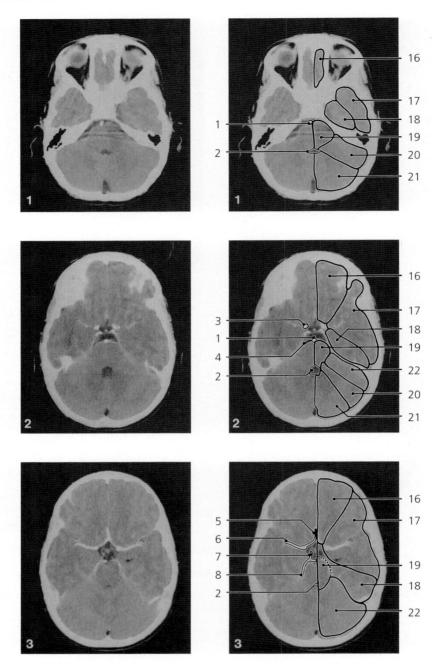

Brain, child, CT angiography

The typical distribution pattern of the cerebral arteries is marked on the left hemisphere

1: Basilar artery
2: Fourth ventricle
3: Internal carotid artery
4: Anterior inferior cerebellar artery
5: Anterior cerebral artery
6: Middle cerebral artery
7: Posterior communicating artery
8: Posterior cerebral artery

9: Lateral ventricle, anterior horn
10: Caudate nucleus
11: Lentiform nucleus
12: Third ventricle
13: Lateral ventricle, temporal horn
14: Superior collicle
15: Cerebellum
16: Anterior cerebral artery

17: Middle cerebral artery
18: Posterior cerebral artery
19: Basilar artery
20: Anterior inferior cerebellar artery ("AICA")
21: Posterior inferior cerebellar artery ("PICA")
22: Superior cerebellar artery

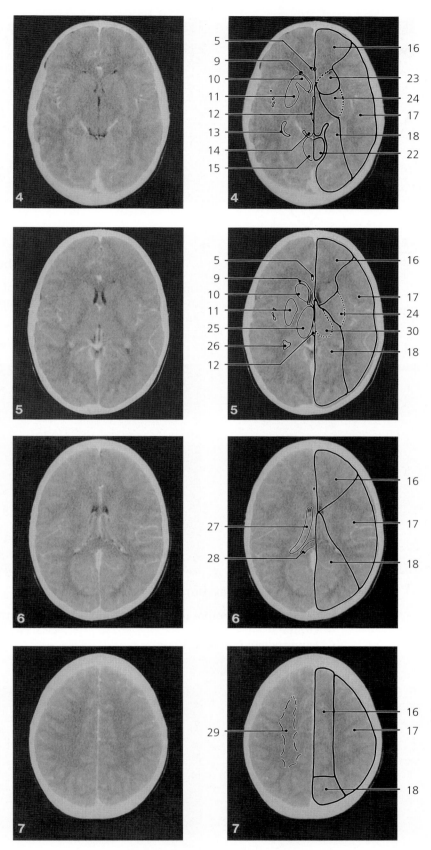

Brain, child, CT angiography

The typical distribution pattern of the cerebral arteries is marked on the left hemisphere
Numbering is transferred from the previous page

23: Striate branches of anterior cerebral
    artery
24: Striato-lenticular branches of middle
    cerebral artery

25: Thalamus
26: Lateral ventricle, atrium
27: Lateral ventricle, central part
28: Occipital forceps

29: Corona radiata
30: Thalamic branches of posterior
    cerebral artery

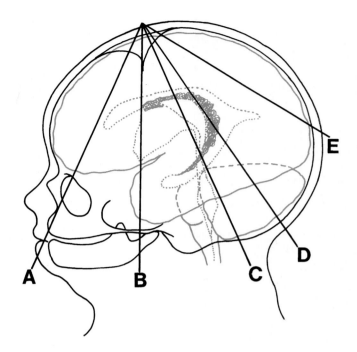

Brain, newborn, US

Lines A–E indicate the positions of tilted coronal sections in the following ultrasonographic series, recorded through the anterior fontanelle

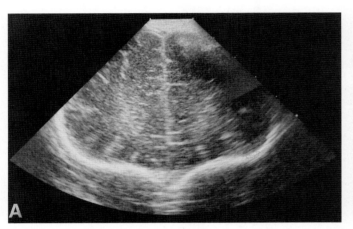

Brain, newborn, US

1: Anterior fontanelle
2: Superior sagittal sinus
3: Frontal lobe
4: Orbital part of frontal bone
5: Orbita
6: Longitudinal fissure of brain
7: Straight gyrus/olfactory bulb
8: Nasal cavity

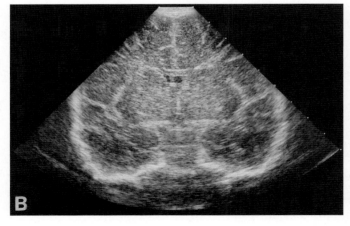

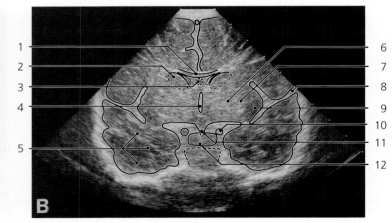

Brain, newborn, US

1: Corpus callosum
2: Caudate nucleus
3: Cave of septum pellucidum
4: Third ventricle
5: Temporal lobe
6: Internal capsule
7: Lentiform nucleus
8: Lateral sulcus (Sylvian)
9: Insula
10: Internal carotid artery
11: Hypophysis
12: Body of sphenoidal bone

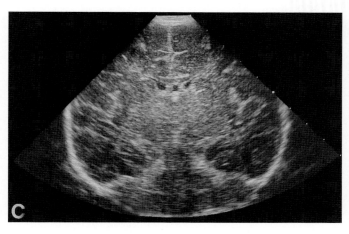
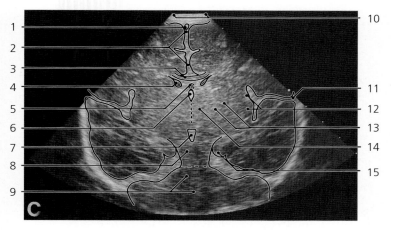

Brain, newborn, US

1: Superior sagittal sinus
2: Longitudinal fissure of brain
3: Corpus callosum
4: Lateral ventricle, central part
5: Cave of septum pellucidum

6: Third ventricle
7: Interpeduncular fossa
8: Mesencephalon
9: Cerebellum
10: Anterior fontanelle

11: Lateral sulcus (Sylvian)
12: Insula
13: Lentiform nucleus and internal capsule
14: Thalamus
15: Hippocampus

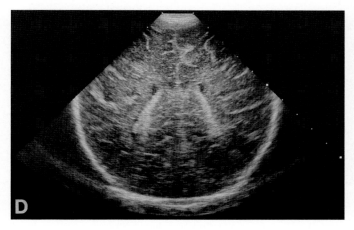
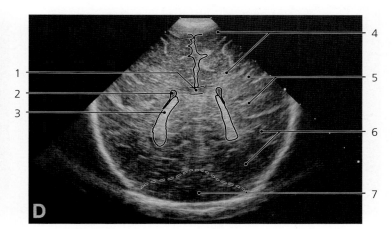

Brain, newborn, US

1: Corpus callosum
2: Lateral ventricle

3: Choroid plexus in atrium of lateral
   ventricle
4: Frontal lobe

5: Parietal lobe
6: Temporal lobe
7: Cerebellum

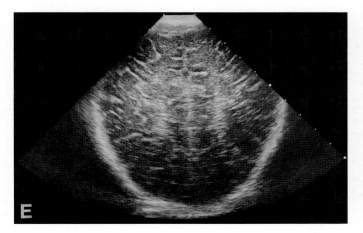
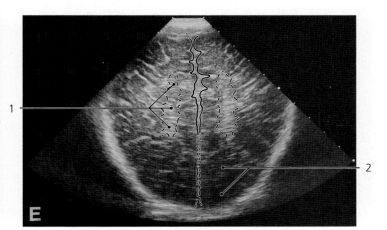

Brain, newborn, US

1: Corona radiata

2: Occipital lobe

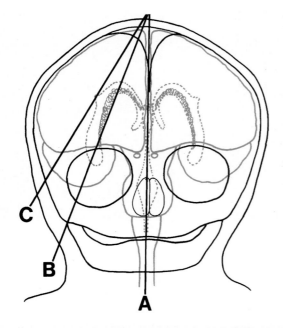

Brain, newborn, US

Lines A–C indicate the positions of sections in the following ultrasonographic series, recorded through the anterior fontanelle.

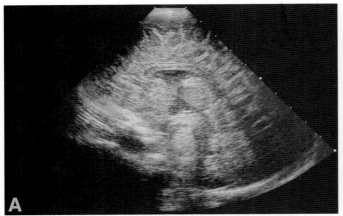

Brain, newborn, median, US

1: Corpus callosum	6: Pons	11: Cerebral aqueduct
2: Septum pellucidum (with cave)	7: Medulla oblongata	12: Fourth ventricle
3: Third ventricle	8: Anterior fontanelle	13: Cerebellum
4: Hypophysis	9: Thalamus	
5: Mesencephalon	10: Tectum of mesencephalon	

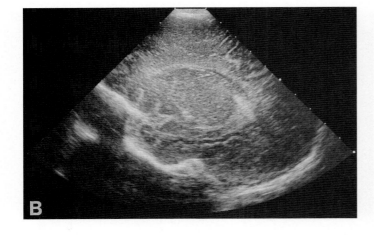
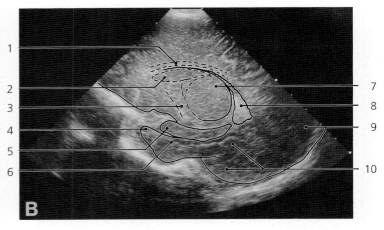

Brain, newborn, US

1: Corpus callosum	5: Hippocampus	8: Choroid plexus in atrium of lateral ventricle
2: Lateral ventricle	6: Parahippocampal gyrus	9: Occipital lobe
3: Internal capsule	7: Thalamus	10: Temporal lobe
4: Uncus of temporal lobe		

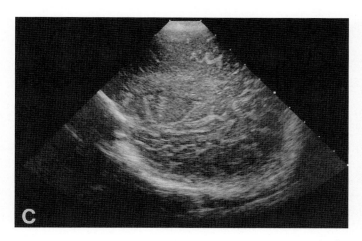

Brain, newborn, US

1: Frontal lobe
2: Corona radiata
3: Insula

4: Operculum frontale
5: Operculum temporale below lateral sulcus

6: Parietal lobe
7: Occipital lobe
8: Temporal lobe

Neck

Larynx
Pharynx
Axial CT series
Thyroid gland

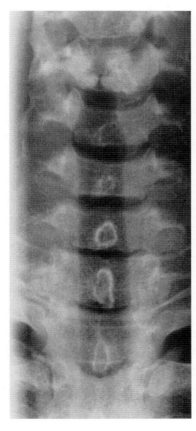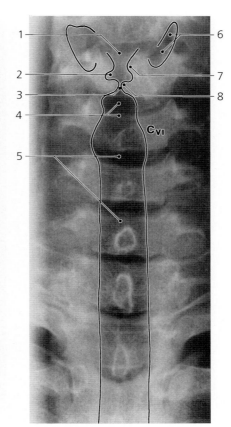

Larynx, a-p X-ray

1: Vestibule of larynx
2: Sinus (ventricle) of the larynx
3: Rima glottidis
4: Infraglottic cavity
5: Trachea
6: Piriform fossa
7: Vestibular fold
8: Vocal fold

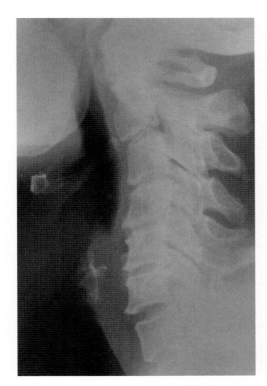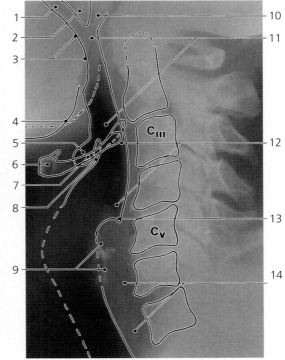

Larynx, lateral X-ray

1: Oral cavity
2: Uvula
3: Root of tongue
4: Angle of mandible
5: Vallecula
6: Body of hyoid bone
7: Greater cornu of hyoid bone
8: Epiglottis
9: Lamina of cricoid cartilage (calcified)
10: Nasal part of pharynx
11: Oral part of pharynx
12: Laryngeal part of pharynx
13: Entrance to esophagus
14: Esophagus

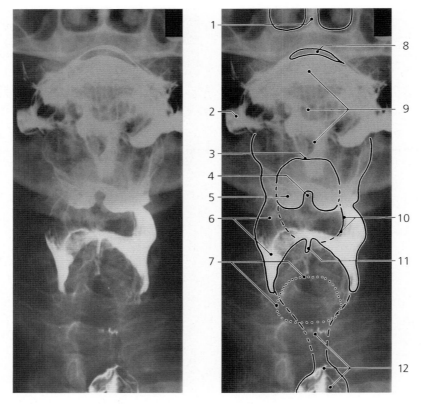

Pharynx, a-p X-ray, barium swallow

1: Nasal septum
2: Vestibule of the mouth
3: Epiglottis
4: Median glosso-epiglottic fold

5: Vallecula
6: Piriform fossa
7: Contour of lamina of cricoid cartilage
8: Air between tongue and palate

9: Barium in mouth and pharynx
10: Ary-epiglottic fold
11: Interarytenoid notch
12: Esophagus

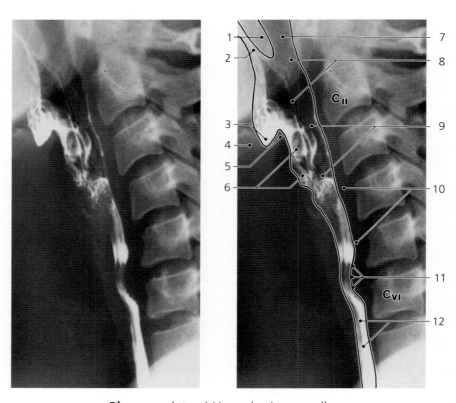

Pharynx, lateral X-ray, barium swallow

1: Uvula
2: Oral cavity
3: Vallecula
4: Hyoid bone
5: Epiglottis

6: Piriform fossa
7: Nasal part of pharynx (nasopharynx)
8: Oral part of pharynx (oropharynx)
9: Laryngeal part of pharynx (laryngopharynx)

10: Retropharyngeal space
11: Impression of cricopharyngeus muscle
12: Esophagus

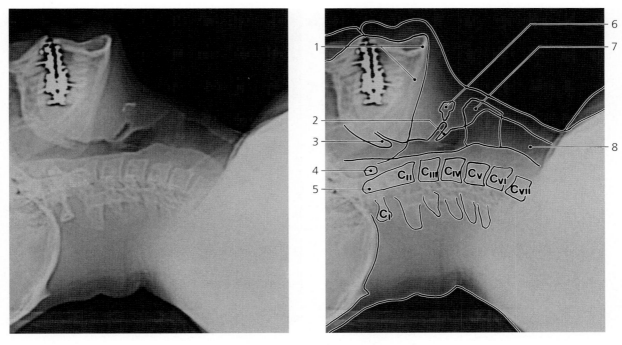

Scout view

1: Mandible   4: Anterior arch of atlas   7: Thyroid cartilage
2: Epiglottis   5: Dens axis   8: Trachea
3: Uvula   6: Hyoid bone

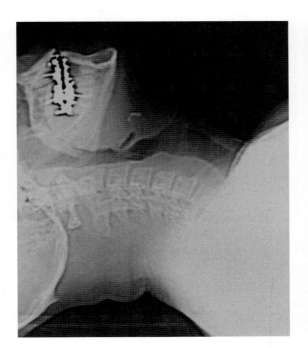
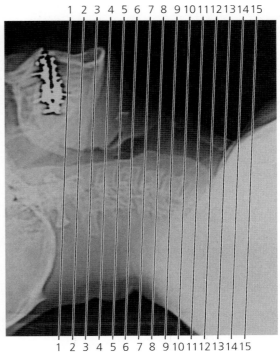

Scout view

Lines #1–15 indicate positions of sections in the following CT-series. Consecutive sections, 10 mm thick

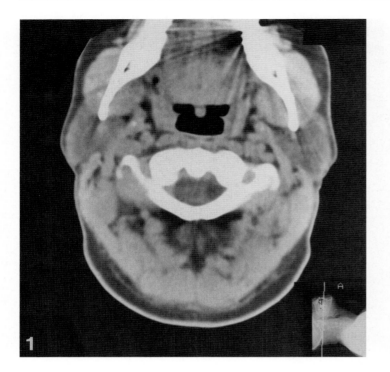

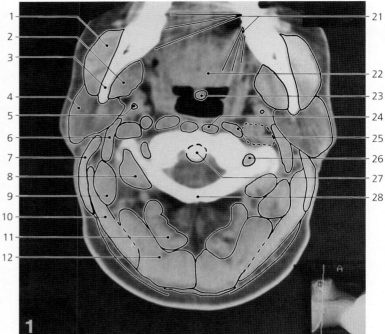

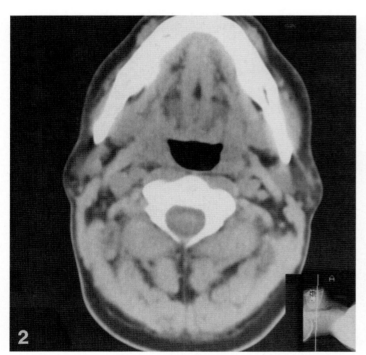

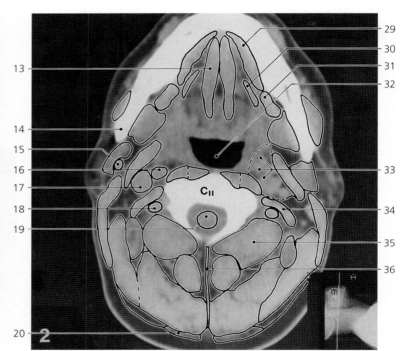

Neck, axial CT

Scout view on previous page

1: Masseter
2: Medial pterygoid muscle
3: Ramus of mandible
4: Parotid gland
5: Styloid process
6: Posterior belly of digastricus
7: Sternocleidomastoid
8: Obliquus capitis inferior
9: Longissimus capitis
10: Splenius capitis
11: Rectus capitis posterior major
12: Semispinalis capitis
13: Genioglossus

14: Angle of mandible
15: Retromandibular vein
16: Internal carotid artery
17: Internal jugular vein
18: Vertebral artery
19: Spinal cord
20: Trapezius
21: Artefacts from dental filling
22: Tongue
23: Uvula
24: Longus colli
25: Longus capitis
26: Foramen transversarium of atlas

27: Dens axis
28: Posterior arch of atlas
29: Mylohyoideus
30: Hyoglossus
31: Submandibular gland
32: Oral part of pharynx
33: Lateropharyngeal space
34: Levator scapulae, and splenius cervicis
35: Obliquus capitis inferior
36: Lig. nuchae

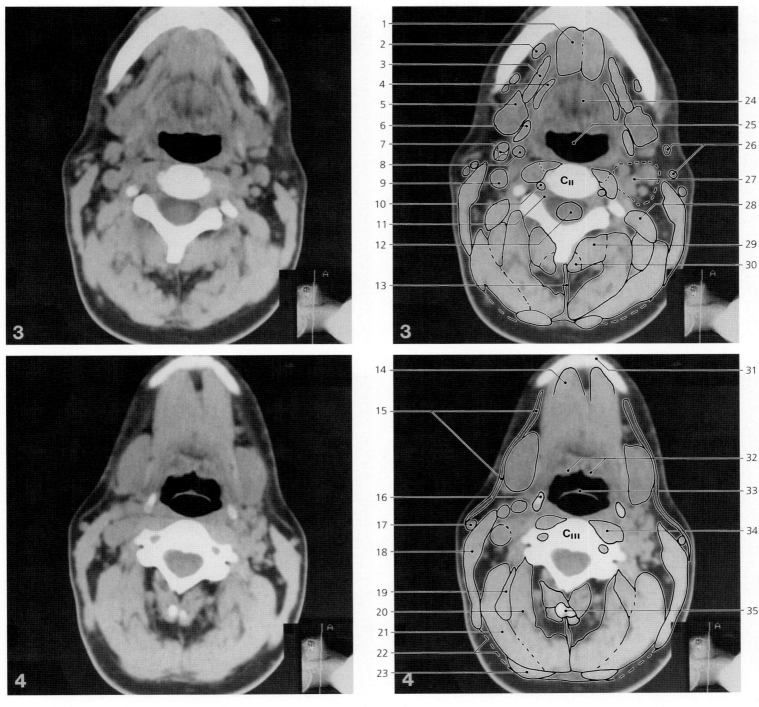

Neck, axial CT

Scout view on page 335

1: Geniohyoideus
2: Submandibular lymph node
3: Mylohyoideus
4: Hyoglossus
5: Submandibular gland
6: Digastricus and stylohyoideus
7: External carotid artery (branching)
8: Internal carotid artery
9: Internal jugular vein
10: Vertebral artery
11: Intervertebral foramen with spinal nerve
12: Spinal cord

13: Lig. nuchae
14: Digastricus, anterior belly
15: Platysma
16: Greater cornu of hyoid bone
17: External jugular vein
18: Sternocleidomastoid
19: Longissimus capitis
20: Semispinalis capitis
21: Splenius capitis
22: Superficial lamina of deep cervical fascia
23: Trapezius
24: Root of tongue

25: Oral part of pharynx
26: External jugular lymph nodes
27: Lateropharyngeal space with vessels, nerves and internal jugular lymph nodes
28: Splenius cervicis, and levator scapulae
29: Obliquus capitis inferior
30: Rectus capitis posterior major
31: Mental tuberosity
32: Lingual tonsil
33: Epiglottis
34: Longus colli, and longus capitis
35: Spinous process of C II

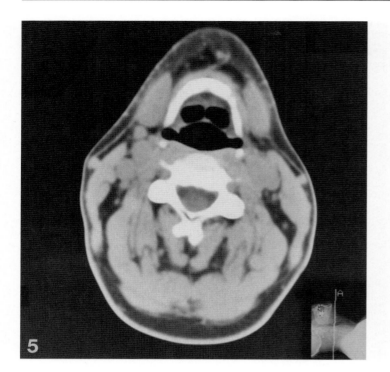

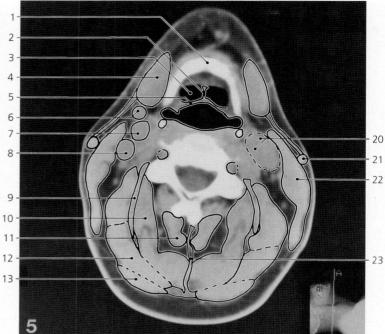

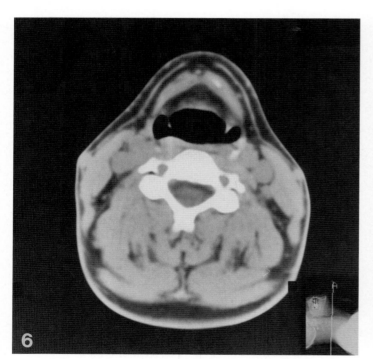

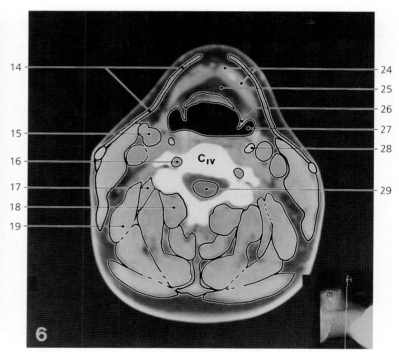

Neck, axial CT

Scout view on page 335

1: Body of hyoid bone
2: Median glosso-epiglottic fold
3: Vallecula
4: Submandibular gland
5: Epiglottis
6: External carotid artery
7: Carotid sinus
8: Internal jugular vein
9: Longissimus capitis
10: Semispinalis capitis

11: Semispinalis cervicis
12: Splenius capitis
13: Trapezius
14: Platysma
15: Carotid bifurcation
16: Vertebral artery
17: Longissimus cervicis
18: Rotator and multifidus muscles
19: Levator scapulae
20: Lateropharyngeal space

21: External jugular vein
22: Sternocleidomastoid
23: Lig. nuchae
24: Infrahyoid muscles
25: Laryngeal fat pad
26: Ary-epiglottic fold
27: Piriform fossa
28: Superior cornu of thyroid cartilage
29: Spinal cord

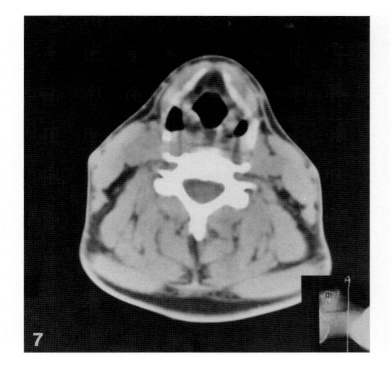

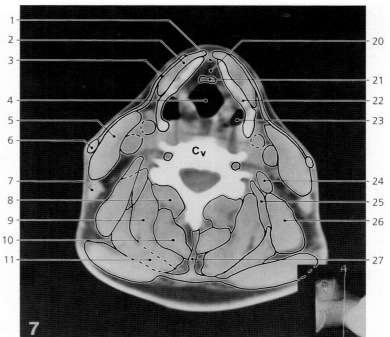

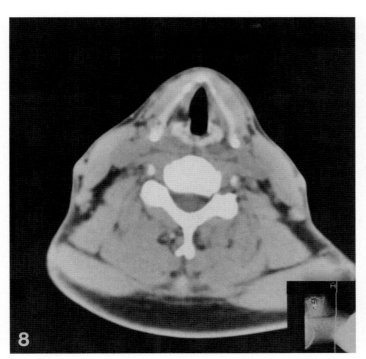

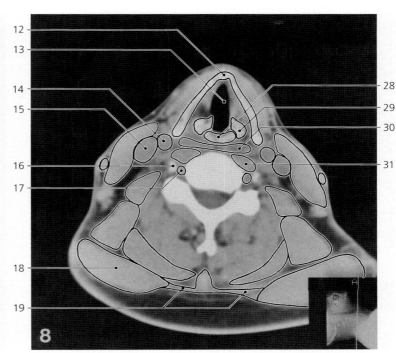

Neck, axial CT

Scout view on page 335

1: Thyroid notch
2: Infrahyoid muscles
3: Platysma
4: Vestibule of larynx
5: Sternocleidomastoid
6: External jugular vein
7: Lymph node
8: Rotatores and multifidi muscles
9: Semispinalis capitis
10: Semispinalis cervicis
11: Splenius capitis

12: Laryngeal prominence
13: Rima glottidis bordered by vocal muscle
14: Common carotid artery
15: Internal jugular vein
16: Anterior tubercle of transverse process
17: Vertebral artery
18: Trapezius
19: Speculum rhomboideum
20: Laryngeal fat pad

21: Epiglottis
22: Lamina of thyroid cartilage
23: Piriform fossa
24: Scalenus medius
25: Longissimus cervicis
26: Levator scapulae
27: Lig. nuchae
28: Lamina of cricoid cartilage
29: Arythenoid cartilage
30: Laryngeal part of pharynx
31: Longus colli and longus capitis

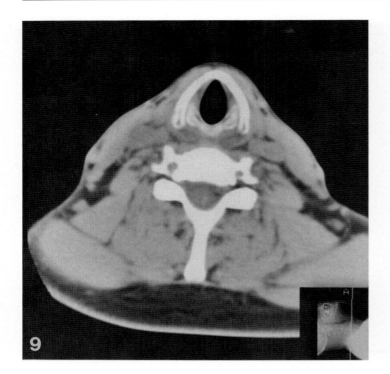

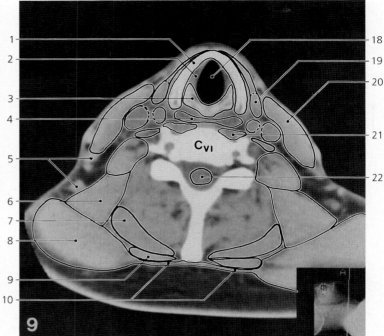

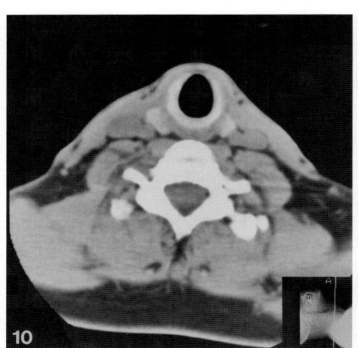

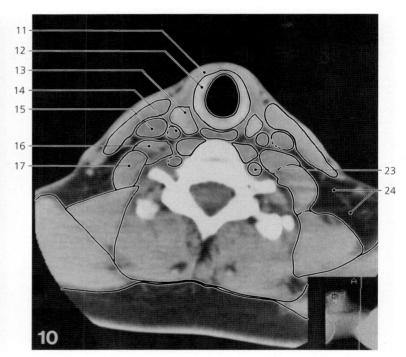

Neck, axial CT

Scout view on page 335

1: Lamina of thyroid cartilage
2: Conus elasticus
3: Lamina of cricoid cartilage
4: Laryngeal part of pharynx
5: Superficial cervical lymph nodes
6: Levator scapulae
7: Splenius
8: Trapezius

9: Rhomboideus
10: Speculum rhomboideum
11: Infrahyoid muscles
12: Arch of cricoid cartilage
13: Thyroid gland
14: Common carotid artery
15: Internal jugular vein
16: Scalenus anterior

17: Scalenus medius
18: Cavitas infraglottica
19: Omohyoideus, superior belly
20: Sternocleidomastoid
21: Longus colli and longus capitis
22: Spinal cord
23: Vertebral artery and vein
24: Lateral cervical region

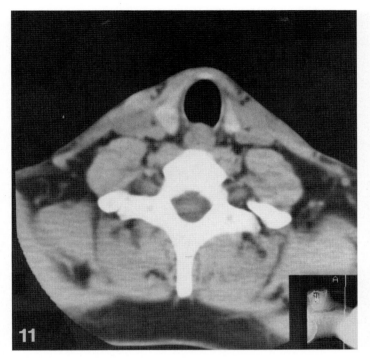

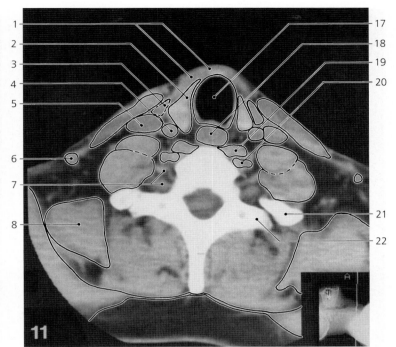

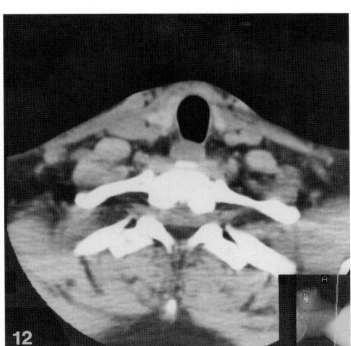

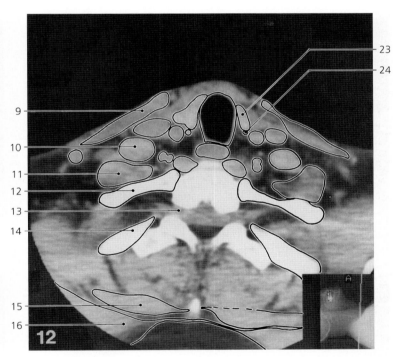

Neck, axial CT

Scout view on page 335

1: Sternohyoid, and sternothyroid muscles
2: Right lobe of thyroid gland
3: Omohyoideus, superior belly
4: Common carotid artery
5: Internal jugular vein
6: External jugular vein
7: Roots of brachial plexus
8: Levator scapulae

9: Sternocleidomastoid
10: Scalenus anterior
11: Scalenus medius
12: Neck of first rib
13: First thoracic spinal nerve
14: Second rib
15: Rhomboideus
16: Trapezius
17: Trachea

18: Esophagus
19: Longus colli
20: Vertebral artery and vein
21: Tubercle of first rib
22: Transverse process of Th I
23: Left lobe of thyroid gland
24: Inferior thyroid artery

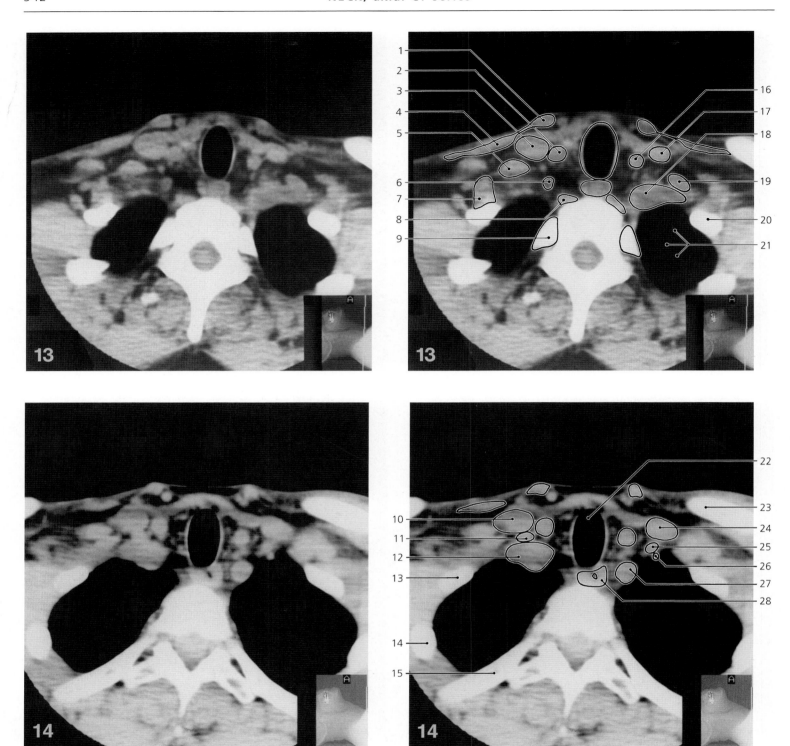

Neck, axial CT

Scout view on page 335

1: Sternal head of sternocleidomastoid
2: Right common carotid artery
3: Right internal jugular vein joining with right subclavian vein
4: Clavicular head of sternocleidomastoid
5: Right scalenus anterior
6: Right vertebral artery
7: Scalenus medius
8: Longus colli

9: Head of second rib
10: Right subclavian vein
11: Right vertebral vein
12: Right subclavian artery
13: First rib
14: Second rib
15: Third rib
16: Left common carotid artery
17: Left internal jugular vein
18: Left subclavian artery

19: Left scalenus anterior
20: First rib
21: Apex of lung
22: Trachea
23: Clavicle
24: Left subclavian vein
25: Left vertebral vein
26: Internal thoracic artery
27: Left subclavian artery
28: Esophagus

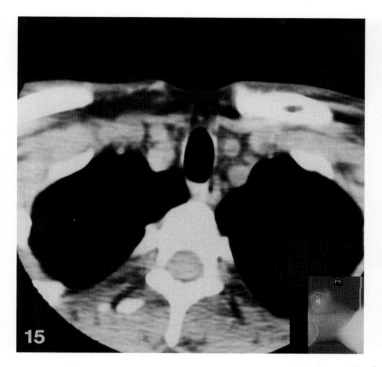

Neck, axial CT

Scout view on page 335

1: Clavicle
2: Infrahyoid muscles
3: Right subclavian vein
4: Right common carotid artery

5: Brachiocephalic trunk
6: Trachea
7: Left subclavian vein
8: Internal thoracic artery

9: First rib
10: Left common carotid artery
11: Left subclavian artery
12: Esophagus

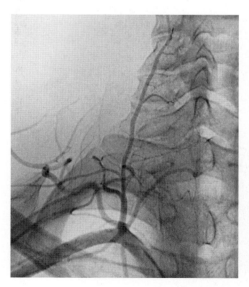

Thyrocervical trunk, X-ray, arteriography

1: First rib
2: Transverse cervical artery
3: Suprascapular artery

4: Thyrocervical trunk
5: Axillary artery
6: Ascending cervical artery

7: Inferior thyroid artery
8: Subclavian artery
9: Internal thoracic artery

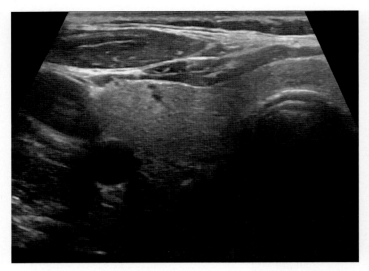
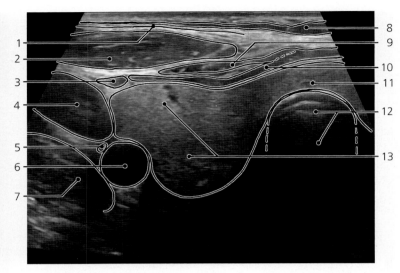

Thyroid gland, transverse section, US

1: Cervical fascia (superficial layer)
2: Sternocleidomastoideus
3: Omohyoideus
4: Internal jugular vein
5: Vagal nerve

6: Common carotid artery
7: Scalenus anterior
8: Platysma
9: Sternohyoideus
10: Sternothyroideus

11: Isthmus of thyroid gland
12: Trachea (with acoustic shadow)
13: Thyroid gland (right lobe)

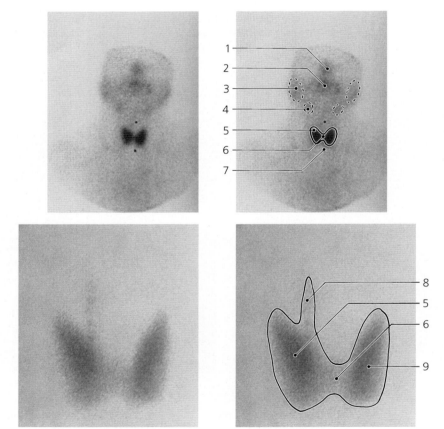

Thyroid gland, anterior view, ^{131}J-scintigraphy

(Note: salivary glands and mucous glands of the nose excrete iodine)

1: Nose
2: Mouth
3: Parotid gland
4: Submandibular gland

5: Right lobe of thyroid gland
6: Isthmus of thyroid gland
7: Marker at jugular incisure and on
   laryngeal prominence (above)

8: Pyramidal lobe of thyroid gland
9: Left lobe of thyroid gland

Thorax

Thoracic cage
Axial CT series
Heart and great vessels
Esophagus
Breast
Thoracic duct

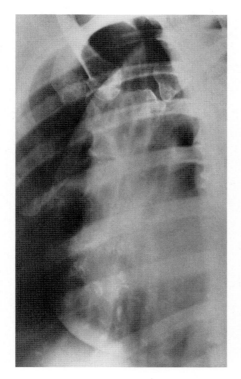
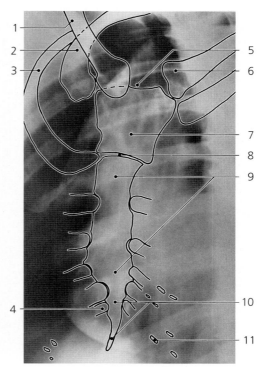

Sternum, oblique X-ray

1: Body of clavicle
2: First rib
3: Second rib
4: Seventh rib

5: Jugular incisure
6: Sternal end of clavicle
7: Manubrium of sternum
8: Sternal angle

9: Body of sternum
10: Xiphoid process
11: Calcified costal cartilage

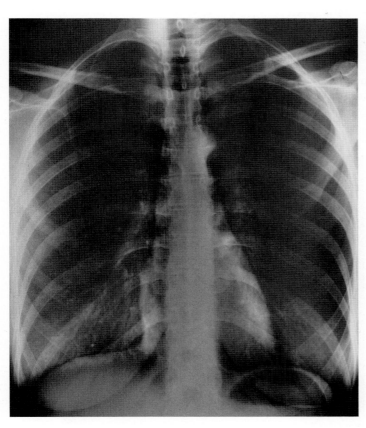
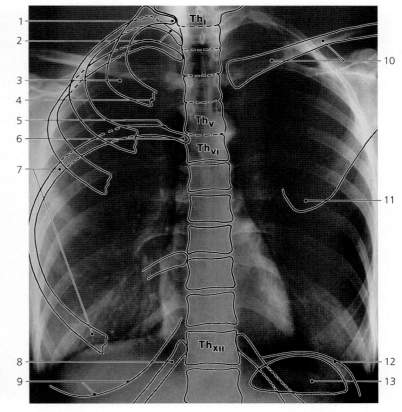

Thoracic cage, a-p X-ray

1: Head of first rib
2: Neck of second rib
3: Shaft of first rib
4: Osteochondral junction
5: Tuberculum of costa VI

6: Head of sixth rib
7: Shaft of sixth rib
8: 12th rib
9: Mamma
10: Clavicle

11: Inferior angle of scapula
12: Diaphragm
13: Gastric air

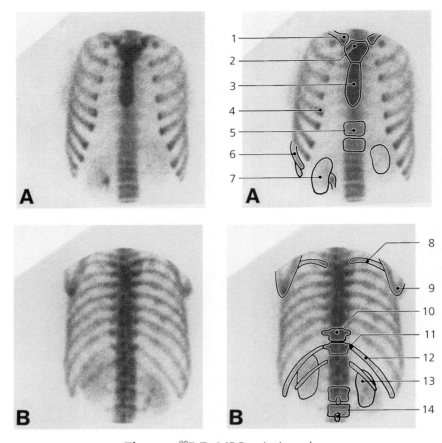

Thorax, ^{99m}Tc-MDP, scintigraphy

A: Anterior view. B: Posterior view

1: Sternal end of clavicle
2: Manubrium of sternum
3: Body of sternum
4: Osteochondral junction (5th rib)
5: Body of thoracic vertebra (Th X)

6: Ninth rib
7: Right kidney
8: Fourth rib
9: Inferior angle of scapula
10: Body of thoracic vertebra (Th X)

11: Transverse process of vertebra, and neck of rib
12: 11th rib
13: Right kidney
14: Spinous process of lumbar vertebra

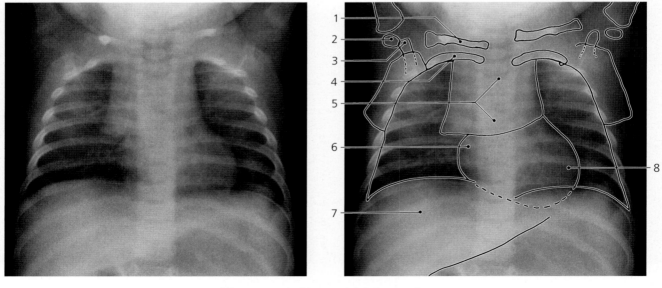

Thorax, a-p X-ray, child 1 month

1: Clavicle
2: Humeral head (ossification center)
3: Acromion

4: First rib
5: Thymus
6: Right atrium

7: Liver
8: Left ventricle

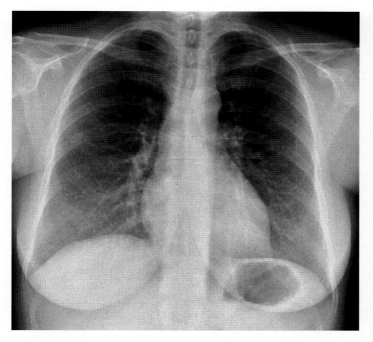
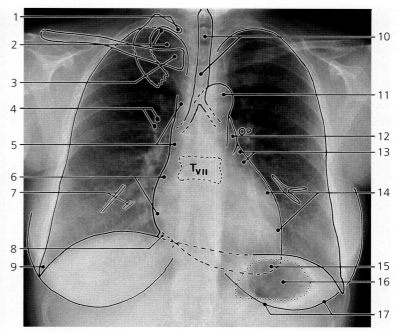

Thorax, p-a X-ray, deep inspiration

1: Head of first rib
2: Apex of lung
3: Sternal end of clavicle
4: Bronchus and lung vessel ("end-on")
5: Superior caval vein
6: Right atrium

7: Lung vessels
8: Inferior caval vein
9: Costodiaphragmatic sulcus
10: Trachea
11: Aortic arch
12: Pulmonary trunk

13: Left auricle
14: Left ventricle
15: Apex of heart
16: Air in fundus of stomach
17: Mamma

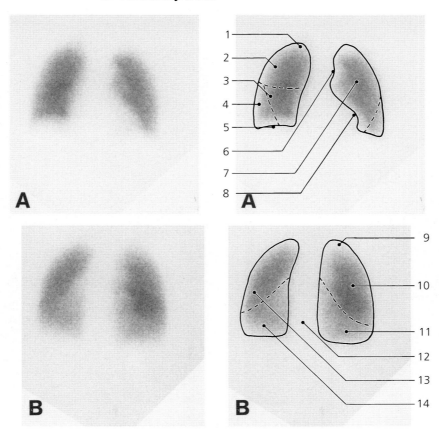

Lungs, ^{133} Xe inhalation, scintigraphy

A: Anterior view. B: Posterior view

1: Apex of right lung
2: Superior lobe of right lung
3: Middle lobe of right lung
4: Inferior lobe of right lung
5: Base of right lung

6: Impression from aorta
7: Superior lobe of left lung
8: Cardiac incisure
9: Apex of right lung
10: Superior lobe of right lung

11: Inferior lobe of right lung
12: Mediastinum
13: Superior lobe of left lung
14: Inferior lobe of left lung

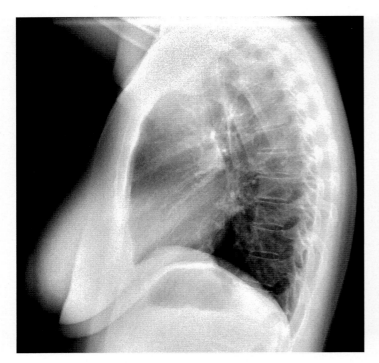
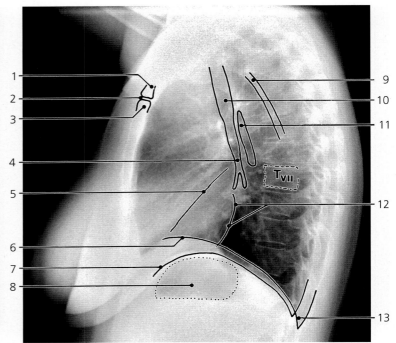

Thorax, lateral X-ray

1: Sternum (manubrium)
2: Sternum (angle)
3: Sternum (body)
4: Bronchus
5: Oblique fissure of lung

6: Diaphragma (right dome)
7: Diaphragma (left dome)
8: Air in fundus of stomach
9: Scapula
10: Trachea

11: Esophagus (with air)
12: Left atrium
13: Costodiaphragmatic sulcus

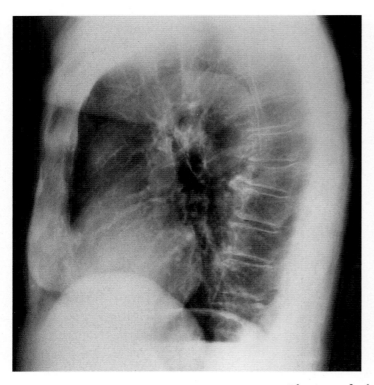
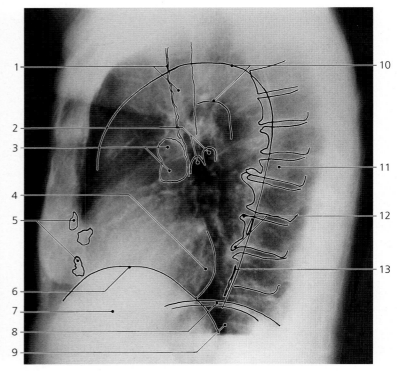

Thorax of old age, lateral X-ray

1: Trachea with calcified cartilage
2: Principal bronchi
3: Pulmonary arteries
4: Left ventricle (enlarged)
5: Calcified costal cartilage

6: Right dome of diaphragm (relaxed)
7: Liver
8: Left dome of diaphragm
9: Gastric air
10: Aortic arch (dilated)

11: Body of vertebra (collapsed)
12: Osteophytes
13: Calcification of aortic wall

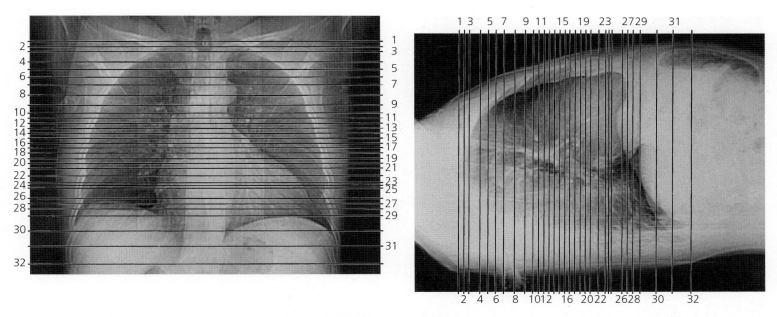

Scout views of axial CT series

Lines #1–32 indicate positions of axial sections in the following CT series.

All sections are 5mm thick and are spaced by 5–20mm.
Each section is displayed with bone settings (above), soft tissue settings (middle), and lung settings (below). Arms are raised above head. Intravenous contrast was given in the right cubital vein.
Vertebrae are numbered with romans and costae with arabics on the bone image.
Lung segments are numbered with arabics on the lung image.

Right lung segments

Superior lobe:
1: Apical segment
2: Posterior segment
3: Anterior segment

Middle lobe:
4: Lateral segment
5: Medial segment

Inferior lobe:
6: Superior segment
7: Medial basal segment
8: Anterior basal segment
9: Lateral basal segment
#10: Posterior basal segment

Left lung segments

Superior lobe:
1: Apical segment
2: Posterior segment
3: Anterior segment
4: Superior lingular segment
5: Inferior lingular segment

Inferior Lobe:
6: Superior segment
7: Medial basal segment
8: Anterior basal segment
9: Lateral basal segment
#10: Posterior basal segment

#1 and #2 of left lung usually arise from a common apicoposterior segmental bronchus.
Note that the diameter of bronchi appear very narrow in the lung image due to the partial volume effect in CT imaging.
Arrows ←, → and ↔ in the legends indicate that a structure can be seen on a previous or following section, or both.

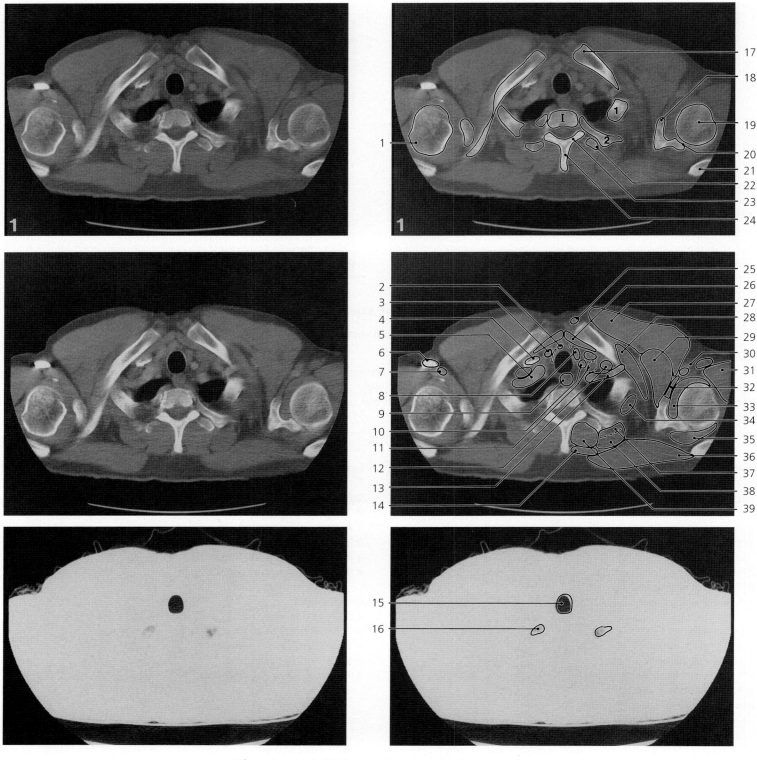

Thorax, axial CT (scout view on previous page)

1: Greater tubercle of humerus →
2: Anterior jugular vein
3: Right common carotid artery →
4: Internal jugular vein (with contrast)
5: Right subclavian artery →
6: Axillary vein (with contrast) →
7: Axillary artery →
8: Lower pole of thyroid lobe
9: Esophagus →
10: Left internal carotid artery →
11: Lymph node
12: Scalenus anterior muscle →
13: Left subclavian artery →
14: Rhomboideus →

15: Trachea →
16: Apex of lung →
17: Sternal end of clavicle →
18: Coracoid process →
19: Head of humerus →
20: Glenoid cavity →
21: Acromion →
22: Transverse process of Th II
23: Lamina of vertebral arch
24: Spinous process of Th I
25: Sternocleidomastoideus,
    sternal head →
26: Sternothyroideus and
    sternohyoideus →

27: Pectoralis major →
28: Subclavius muscle →
29: Pectoralis minor →
30: Axillary fossa →
31: Teres major →
32: Biceps brachii, short head
33: Subscapularis muscle →
34: Iliocostalis cervicis →
35: Supraspinatus →
36: Trapezius →
37: Longissimus →
38: Levator scapulae →
39: Transversospinal muscles →

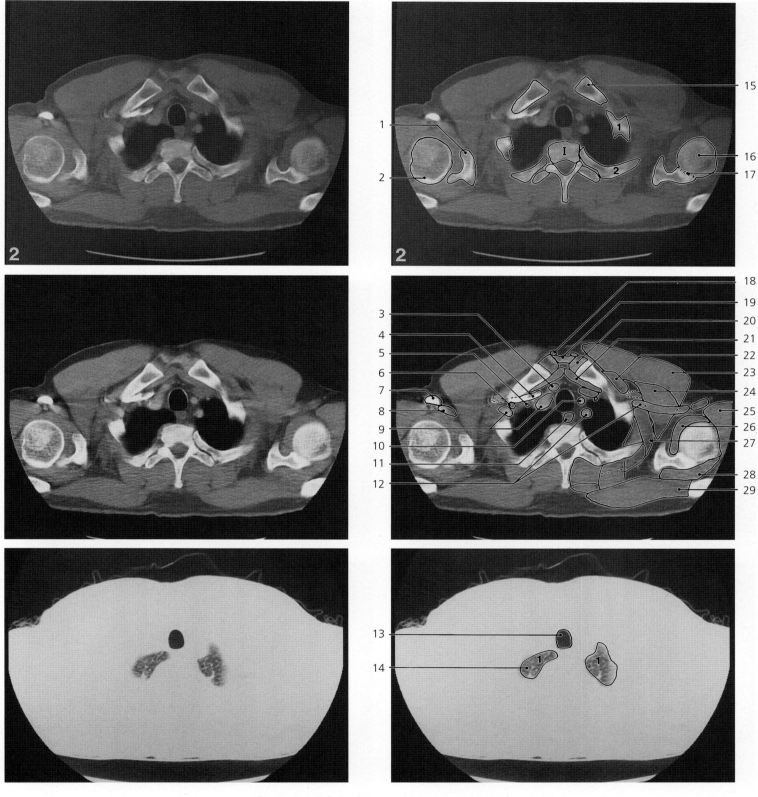

Thorax, axial CT (scout view on page 351)

1: **Processus coracoideus** ←
2: **Greater tubercle of humerus** ←
3: **Right common carotid artery** ←
4: **Subclavian and internal jugular vein, confluence** ↔
5: **Internal thoracic artery** →
6: **Scalenus anterior (insertion)** ←
7: **Axillary vein (with contrast)** ↔
8: **Axillary artery** ↔
9: **Right subclavian artery** ←
10: **Left common carotid artery** ↔
11: **Esophagus** ↔

12: **Left subclavian artery** ↔
13: **Trachea** ↔
14: **Apex of lung** ←
15: **Sternal end of clavicle** ↔
16: **Head of humerus** ↔
17: **Glenohumeral joint** ↔
18: **Sternocleidomastoideus, sternal head** ↔
19: **Interclavicular ligament**
20: **Articular disc of sternoclavicular joint** →

21: **Sternohyoid and sternothyroid muscles** ↔
22: **Subclavius muscle** ←
23: **Pectoralis major** ↔
24: **Pectoralis minor** ↔
25: **Teres major** ↔
26: **Subscapularis** ↔
27: **Serratus anterior** →
28: **Supraspinatus** ↔
29: **Trapezius** ↔

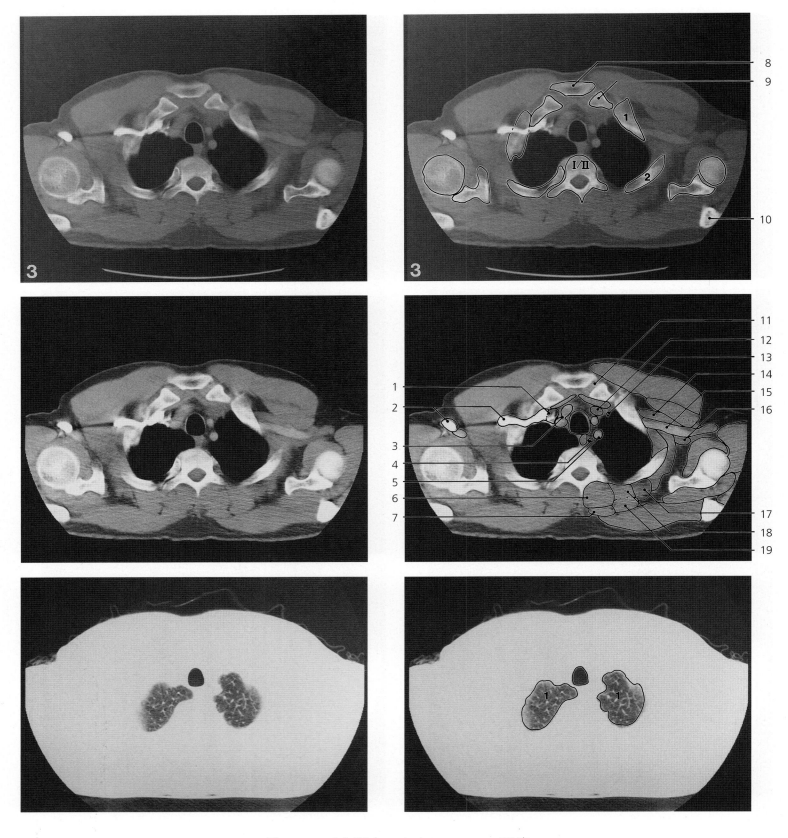

Thorax, axial CT (scout view on page 351)

1: Confluence of subclavian and internal jugular veins ←
2: Axillary vein (with contrast) ↔
3: Division of brachiocephalic trunk →
4: Thoracic duct →
5: Left subclavian artery ↔
6: Transversospinal muscles ↔
7: Rhomboideus ↔
8: Manubrium of sternum →
9: Sternal end of clavicle ←
10: Acromion ←
11: Articular disc of sternoclavicular joint ←
12: Left brachiocephalic vein ←
13: Internal thoracic artery ↔
14: Right axillary vein ↔
15: Right axillary artery ↔
16: Omohyoideus, inferior belly ←
17: Iliocostalis ↔
18: Longissimus ↔
19: Levator scapulae ↔

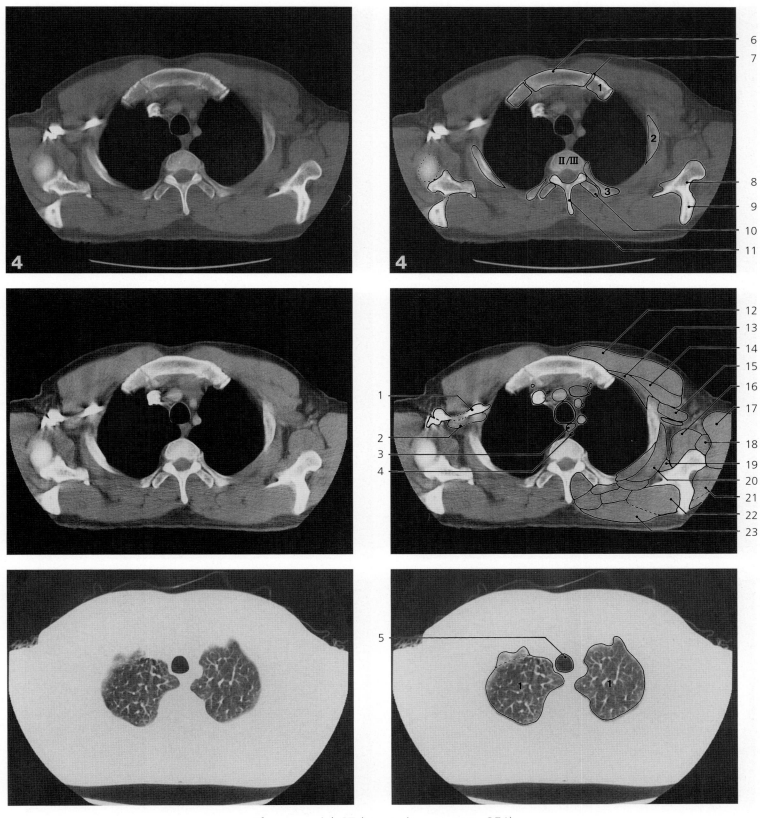

Thorax, axial CT (scout view on page 351)

1: Right axillary vein with contrast ↔
2: Axillary artery ←
3: Esophagus ↔
4: Thoracic duct ↔
5: Trachea ↔
6: Manubrium of sternum ↔
7: Synchondrosis of first rib
8: Neck of scapula

9: Spine of scapula →
10: Transverse process of Th III
11: Spinous process of Th II
12: Pectoralis major ↔
13: Intercostal muscles ↔
14: Pectoralis minor ↔
15: Left axillary vein ←
16: Subscapularis ↔

17: Teres major ↔
18: Teres minor →
19: Omohyoideus, inferior belly ←
20: Serratus anterior ↔
21: Infraspinatus →
22: Supraspinatus ↔
23: Trapezius ↔

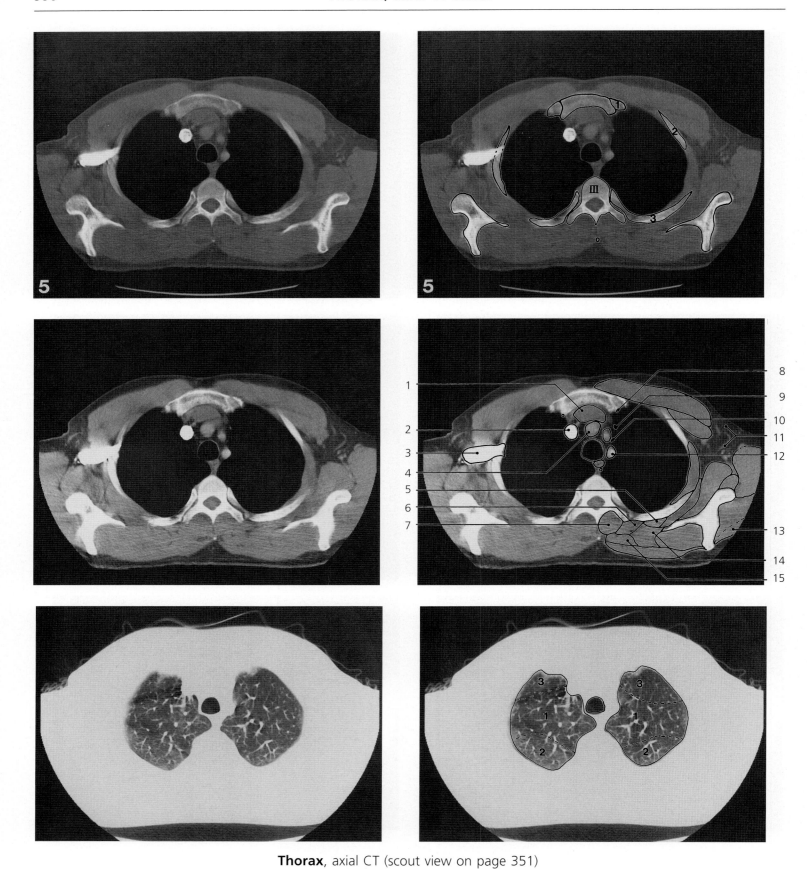

Thorax, axial CT (scout view on page 351)

1: Left brachiocephalic vein ↔
2: Right brachiocephalic vein ↔
3: Right axillary vein →
4: Brachiocephalic trunk ↔
5: Iliocostalis ↔
6: Longissimus ↔

7: Transversospinal muscles ↔
8: Internal thoracic artery ↔
9: Left phrenic nerve →
10: Left vagus nerve →
11: Axillary fossa with nerves, vessels and lymph nodes ↔

12: Left subclavian artery ←
13: Deltoideus ↔
14: Levator scapulae ↔
15: Rhomboideus ↔

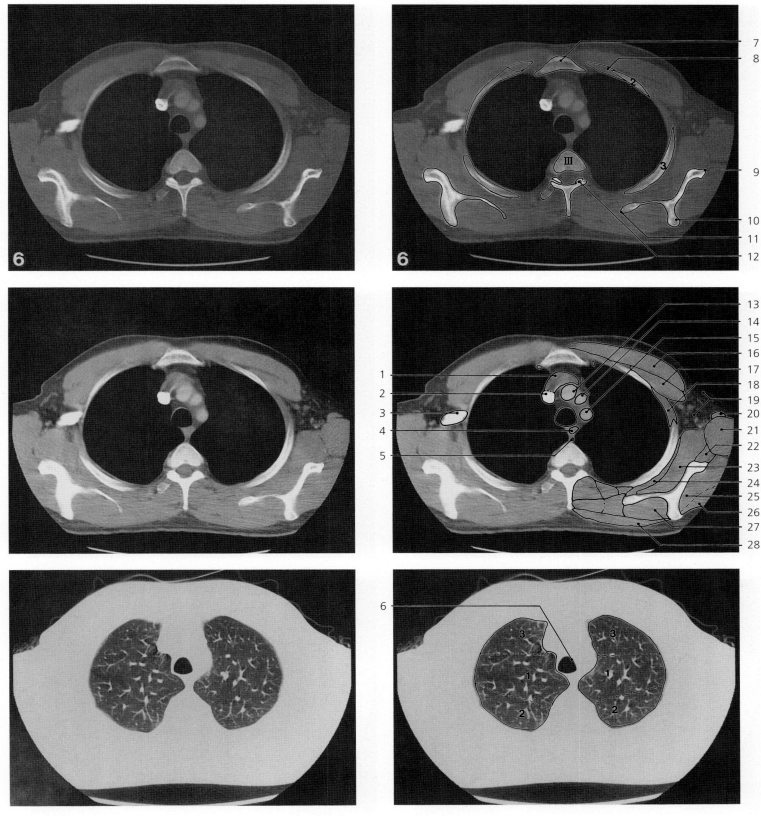

Thorax, axial CT (scout view on page 351)

1: Left brachiocephalic vein ↔	11: Medial margin of scapula	20: Latissimus dorsi →
2: Right brachiocephalic vein ↔	12: Zygapophyseal joint Th III-IV	21: Teres major ↔
3: Right axillary vein ←	13: Brachiocephalic trunk ←	22: Teres minor ↔
4: Esophagus ↔	14: Left common carotid artery ←	23: Subscapularis ↔
5: Thoracic duct ↔	15: Left subclavian artery ←	24: Serratus anterior ↔
6: Trachea ↔	16: Pectoralis major ↔	25: Infraspinatus ↔
7: Manubrium of sternum ↔	17: Pectoralis minor ↔	26: Deltoideus ←
8: Costal cartilage ↔	18: Intercostal muscles ↔	27: Supraspinatus ↔
9: Lateral margin of scapula	19: Axillary fossa with nerves, vessels	28: Trapezius ↔
10: Spine of scapula ↔	and lymph nodes ↔	

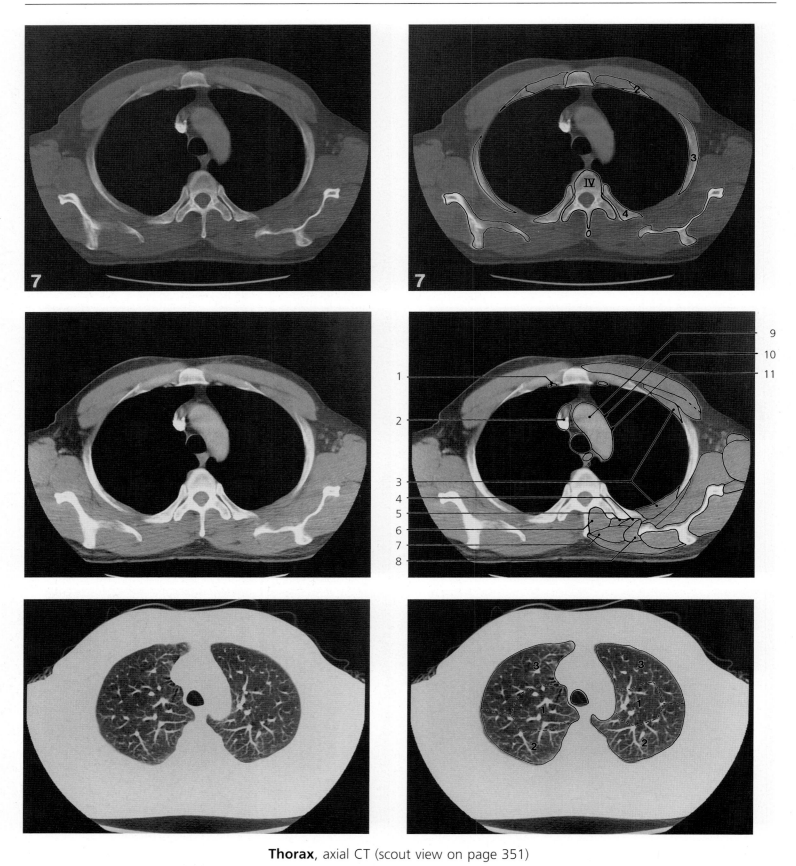

Thorax, axial CT (scout view on page 351)

1: Internal thoracic artery and vein ↔
2: Confluence of right and left
   brachiocephalic veins ←
3: Intercostal muscles ↔

4: Iliocostalis ↔
5: Longissimus ↔
6: Transversospinal muscles ↔
7: Rhomboideus ↔

8: Levator scapulae ↔
9: Aortic arch →
10: Left phrenic nerve ↔
11: Left vagus nerve ↔

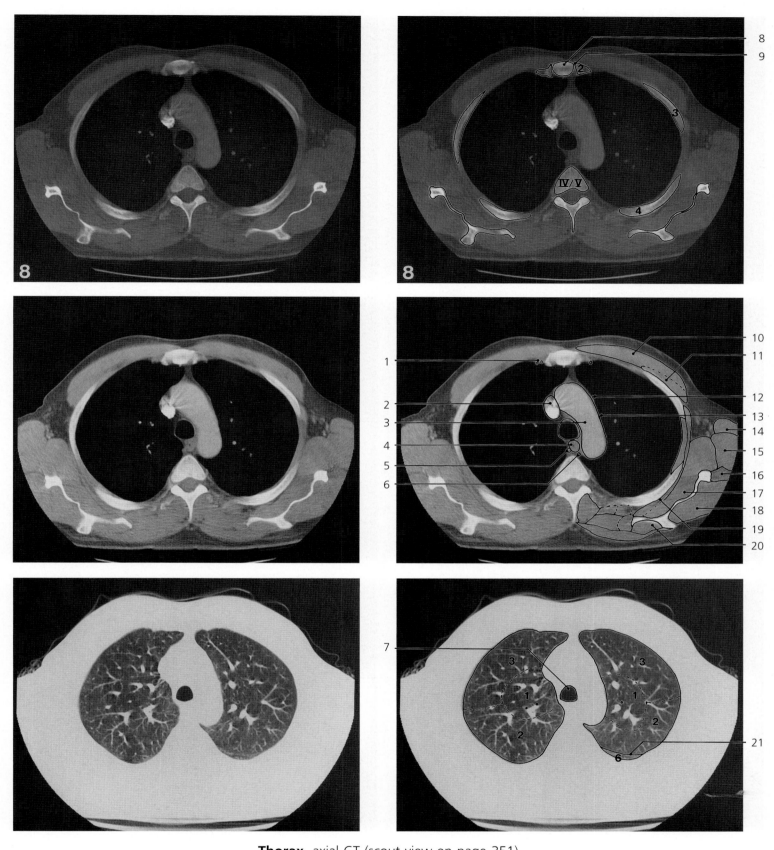

Thorax, axial CT (scout view on page 351)

1: Internal thoracic artery and vein ↔
2: Superior caval vein →
3: Aortic arch ←
4: Esophagus ↔
5: Azygos vein (right superior intercostal vein) →
6: Thoracic duct ↔
7: Trachea ↔

8: Body of sternum →
9: Sternocostal joint of second rib
10: Pectoralis major ↔
11: Pectoralis minor ↔
12: Left phrenic nerve ↔
13: Left vagus nerve ↔
14: Latissimus dorsi ↔
15: Teres major ↔

16: Teres minor ↔
17: Subscapularis ↔
18: Infraspinatus ↔
19: Serratus anterior ↔
20: Supraspinatus ↔
21: Oblique fissure of left lung →

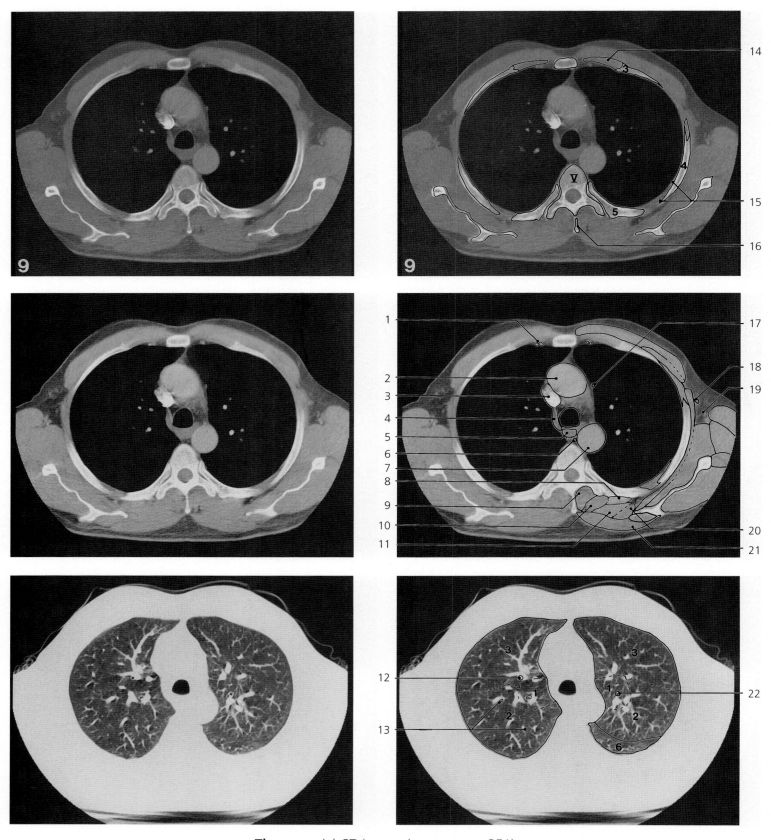

Thorax, axial CT (scout view on page 351)

1: Internal thoracic artery and vein ↔
2: Ascending aorta →
3: Superior caval vein ↔
4: Azygos vein (arch) →
5: Esophagus ↔
6: Thoracic duct ↔
7: Descending aorta →
8: Iliocostalis

9: Transversospinal muscles ↔
10: Longissimus ↔
11: Rhomboideus ↔
12: Branch of anterior segmental
   bronchus B III →
13: Branches of posterior segmental
   bronchus B II
14: Costal cartilage ↔

15: Costal sulcus
16: Spinous process of Th IV
17: Left phrenic nerve ↔
18: Lateral thoracic artery →
19: Axillary fossa ↔
20: Levator scapulae ↔
21: Trapezius ↔
22: Apical segmental bronchus B I

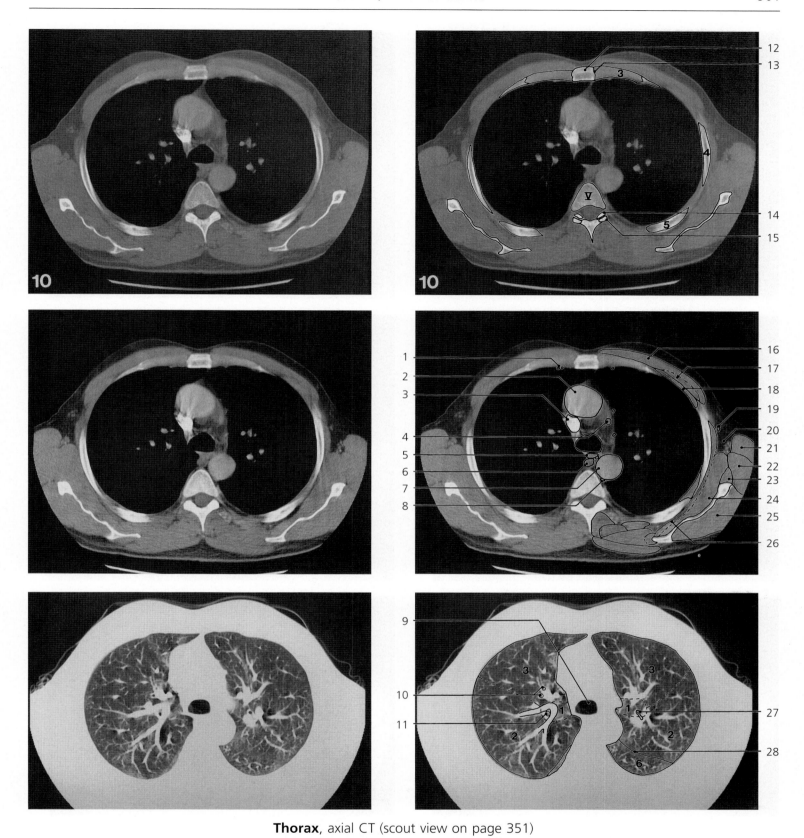

Thorax, axial CT (scout view on page 351)

1: Internal thoracic artery and vein ↔
2: Ascending aorta ↔
3: Superior caval vein ↔
4: Ligamentum arteriosum (ductus arteriosus) in "aortopulmonary window"
5: Esophagus ↔
6: Azygos vein ↔
7: Descending aorta ↔
8: Hemiazygos vein →
9: Trachea ↔

10: Branches of anterior segmental bronchus B III →
11: Apical segmental bronchus B I ↔
12: Body of sternum ↔
13: Sternocostal joint of third rib
14: Superior articular process of Th VI
15: Inferior articular process of Th V
16: Pectoralis major ↔
17: Pectoralis minor ↔
18: Intercostal muscles ↔
19: Lateral thoracic artery ↔

20: Axillary fossa ↔
21: Latissimus dorsi ↔
22: Teres major ↔
23: Teres minor ↔
24: Subscapularis ↔
25: Infraspinatus ↔
26: Serratus anterior ↔
27: Common segmental bronchus of B I and B II of left lung →
28: Oblique fissure ↔

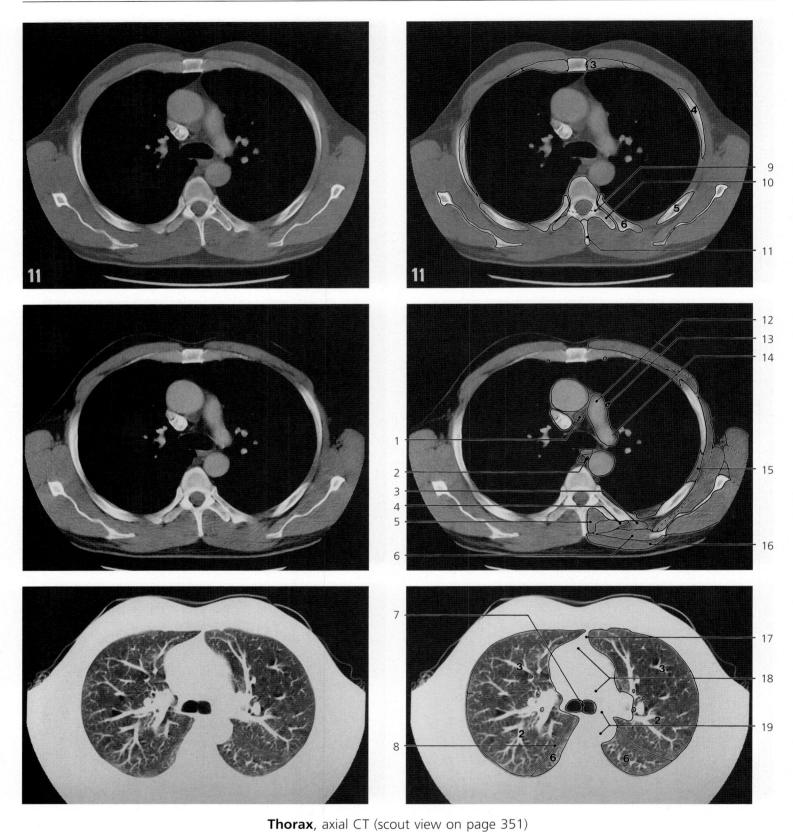

Thorax, axial CT (scout view on page 351)

1: Precarinal lymph node
2: Thoracic duct ↔
3: Iliocostalis ↔
4: Longissimus ↔
5: Transversospinal muscles ↔
6: Rhomboideus ↔
7: Carina (Bifurcatio tracheae) →

8: Oblique fissure of right lung ↔
9: Zygapophyseal joint Th V/VI
10: Transverse process of Th VI
11: Spinous process of Th V
12: Pulmonary trunk →
13: Left phrenic nerve →
14: Left pulmonary artery →

15: Intercostal muscles ↔
16: Trapezius ↔
17: Anterior mediastinum →
18: Middle mediastinum →
19: Posterior mediastinum →

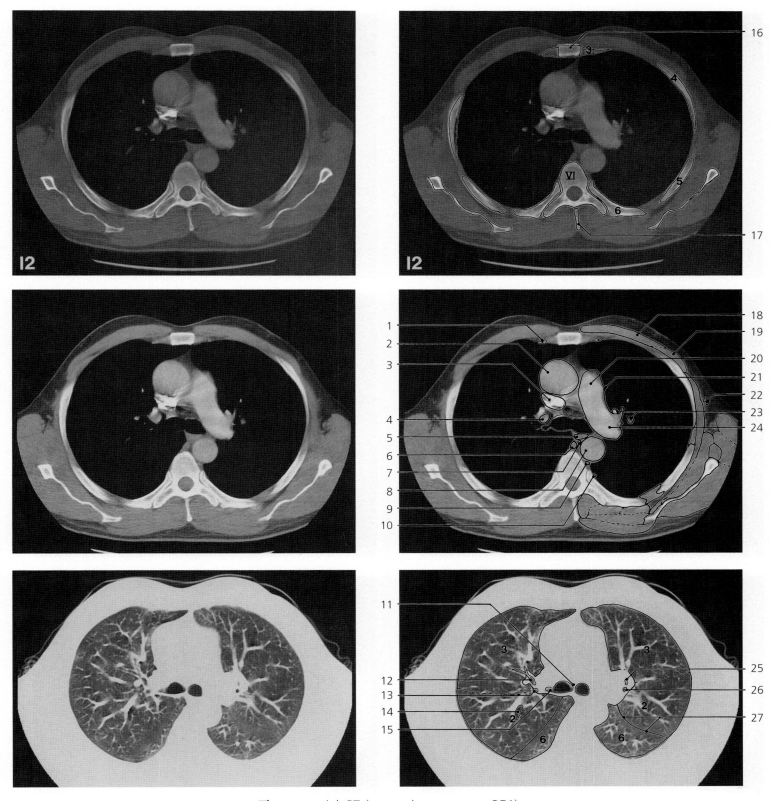

Thorax, axial CT (scout view on page 351)

1: Internal thoracic artery and vein ↔

2: Ascending aorta ↔

3: Superior caval vein ↔

4: Superior lobal branch of right pulmonary artery →

5: Esophagus ↔

6: Azygos vein ↔

7: Thoracic duct ↔

8: Descending aorta ↔

9: Hemiazygos vein ↔

10: Sympathetic trunk →

11: Carina ←

12: Anterior segmental bronchus B III of right upper lobe

13: Apical segmental bronchus B I of right upper lobe ←

14: Posterior segmental bronchus B II of right upper lobe

15: Right superior lobar bronchus →

16: Body of sternum ↔

17: Spinous process of Th V

18: Pectoralis major ↔

19: Pectoralis minor ↔

20: Pulmonary trunk ↔

21: Left phrenic nerve ↔

22: Lateral thoracic artery and vein ↔

23: Branches of upper left pulmonary vein →

24: Left pulmonary artery ↔

25: Anterior segmental bronchus B III of left upper lobe ←

26: Apicoposterior segmental bronchus B I + II of left upper lobe

27: Oblique fissure of left lung ↔

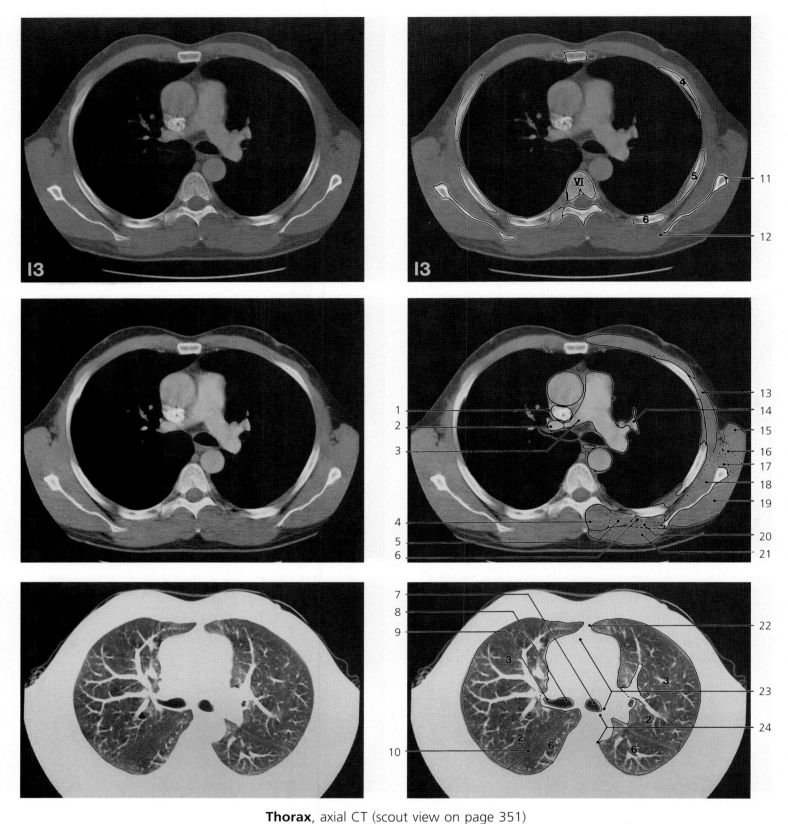

Thorax, axial CT (scout view on page 351)

1: Right phrenic nerve →
2: Superior lobar branch of right pulmonary artery
3: Right pulmonary artery →
4: Transversospinal muscles ↔
5: Longissimus ↔
6: Iliocostalis ↔
7: Left main bronchus →
8: Right main bronchus →

9: Right superior lobar bronchus ←
10: Oblique fissure of right lung ↔
11: Lateral margin of scapula ↔
12: Medial margin of scapula ↔
13: Serratus anterior ↔
14: Branches of left upper pulmonary vein
15: Latissimus dorsi ↔
16: Teres major ↔

17: Teres minor ↔
18: Subscapularis ↔
19: Infraspinatus ↔
20: Rhomboideus ↔
21: Trapezius ↔
22: Anterior mediastinum ↔
23: Middle mediastinum ↔
24: Posterior mediastinum ↔

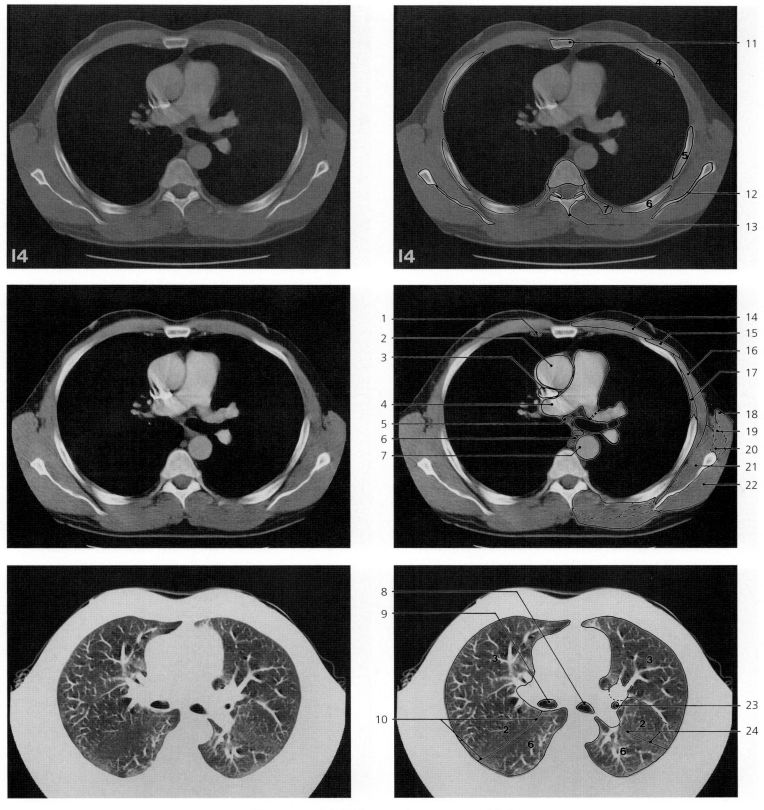

Thorax, axial CT (scout view on page 351)

1: Internal thoracic artery and vein ↔
2: Ascending aorta ↔
3: Superior caval vein ↔
4: Right pulmonary artery ↔
5: Subcarinal (bifurcal) lymph node
6: Thoracic duct ↔
7: Descending aorta ↔
8: Left main bronchus ↔
9: Right main bronchus ↔

10: Oblique fissure of right lung ↔
11: Body of sternum ↔
12: Scapula ↔
13: Spinous process of Th VI
14: Pectoralis major ↔
15: Pectoralis minor ↔
16: Serratus anterior ↔
17: Intercostal muscles
18: Latissimus dorsi ↔

19: Teres major ↔
20: Teres minor ↔
21: Subscapularis ↔
22: Infraspinatus ↔
23: Upper left lobar bronchus, superior division
24: Oblique fissure of left lung ↔

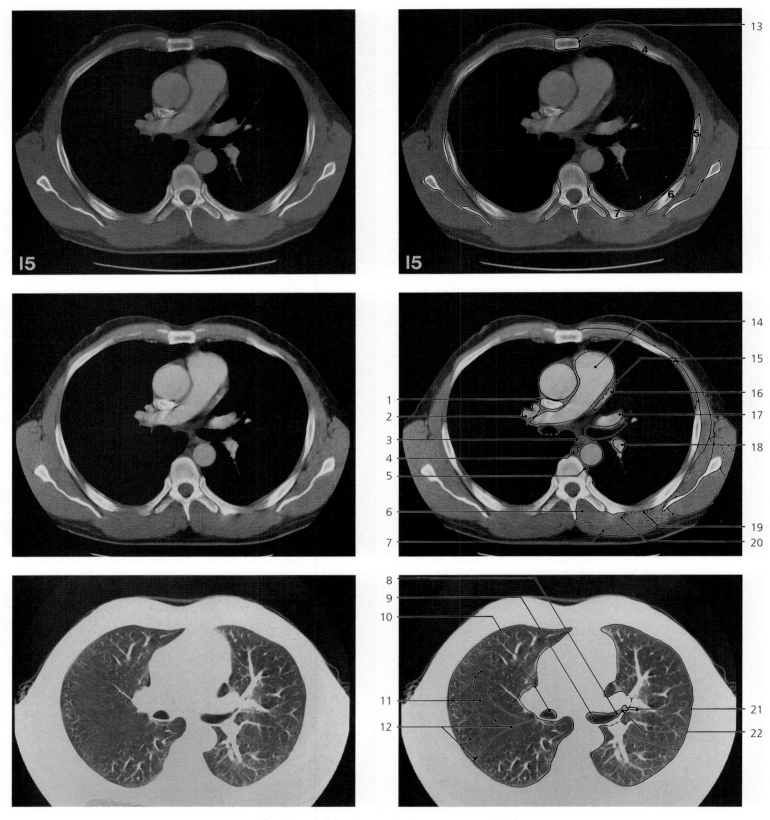

Thorax, axial CT (scout view on page 351)

1: Right phrenic nerve ↔
2: Right superior pulmonary vein →
3: Esophagus ↔
4: Azygos vein ↔
5: Hemiazygos vein ↔
6: Transversospinal muscles ↔
7: Trapezius ↔
8: Left upper lobar bronchus
9: Left main bronchus ←

10: Right main bronchus ←
11: Horizontal fissure (in plane of sectioning)
12: Oblique fissure of right lung ↔
13: Sternocostal joint of fourth rib
14: Pulmonary trunk ↔
15: Left phrenic nerve ↔
16: Left auricle →
17: Left upper pulmonary vein →

18: Inferior branch of left pulmonary artery →
19: Iliocostalis ↔
20: Longissimus ↔
21: Superior lingular segmental bronchus B IV
22: Lingular division of left superior lobar bronchus

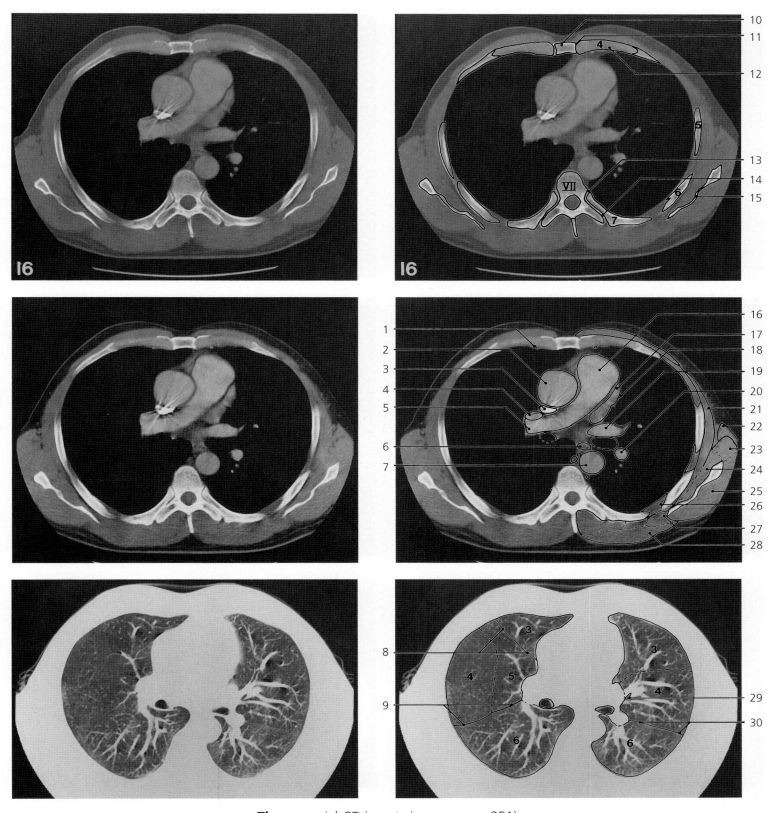

Thorax, axial CT (scout view on page 351)

1: Internal thoracic artery and vein ←
2: Ascending aortae ↔
3: Superior caval vein ↔
4: Right superior pulmonary vein ↔
5: Right pulmonary artery ←
6: Esophagus ↔
7: Descending aorta ↔
8: Horizontal fissure of right lung ↔
9: Oblique fissure of right lung ↔
10: Body of sternum ↔
11: Sternocostal joint of fourth rib

12: Costal cartilage
13: Costovertebral joint
14: Costotransverse joint
15: Scapula ↔
16: Pulmonary trunk ↔
17: Left auricle ↔
18: Left phrenic nerve ↔
19: Left superior pulmonary vein ↔
20: Inferior branch of left pulmonary artery ↔
21: Serratus anterior ↔

22: Latissimus dorsi ↔
23: Teres major ↔
24: Subscapularis ↔
25: Infraspinatus ↔
26: Intercostal muscles ↔
27: Rhomboideus ↔
28: Trapezius ↔
29: Inf. lingular segmental bronchus B V →
30: Oblique fissure of left lung ↔

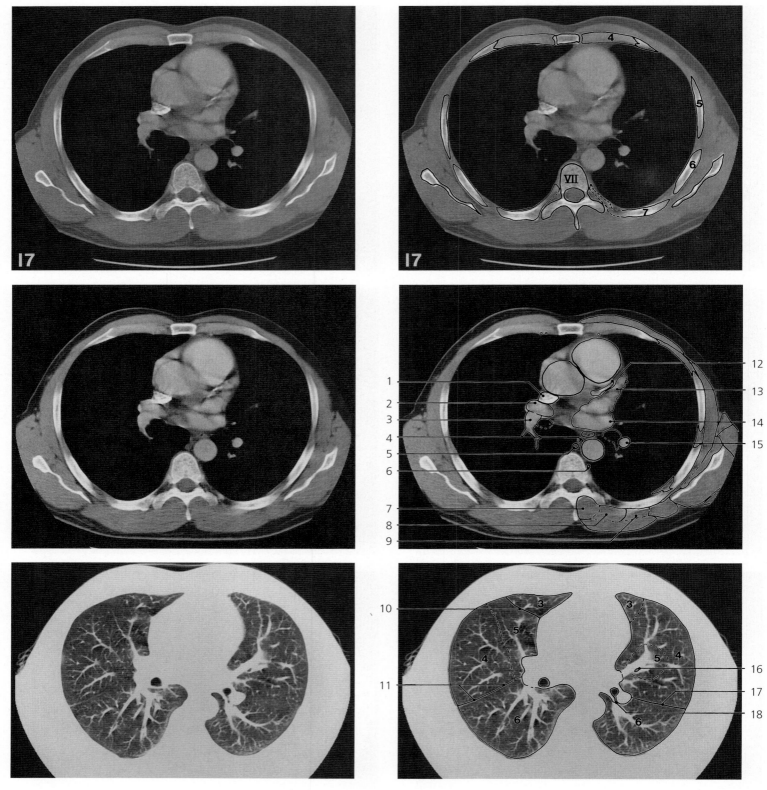

Thorax, axial CT (scout view on page 351)

1: Superior caval vein ←
2: Right superior pulmonary vein ←
3: Inferior branch of right
   pulmonary a. ↔
4: Thoracic duct ↔
5: Azygos vein ↔
6: Hemiazygos vein ↔
7: Transversospinal muscles ↔

8: Longissimus ↔
9: Iliocostalis ↔
10: Horizontal fissure ↔
11: Oblique fissure of right lung ↔
12: Left coronary artery (calcified) →
13: Left auricle ↔
14: Entrance of left superior pulmonary
    vein in left atrium ←

15: Inferior branch of left pulmonary
    artery ↔
16: Inf. lingular segmental
    bronchus B V ↔
17: Oblique fissure of left lung ↔
18: Superior segmental bronchus of left
    lower lobe B VI

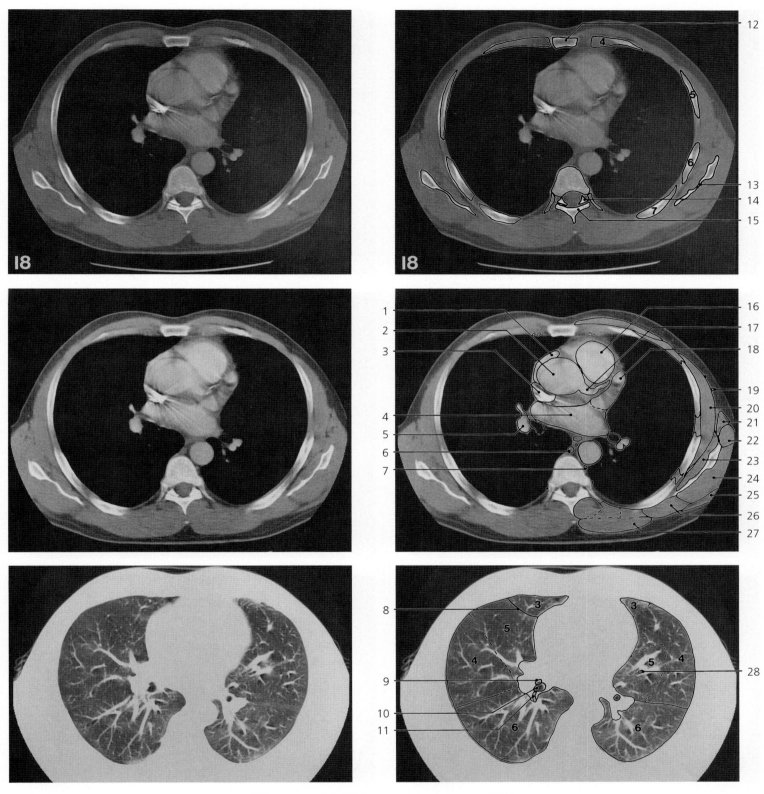

Thorax, axial CT (scout view on page 351)

1: Right auricle →
2: Ascending aorta (bulb) ←
3: Entrance of superior caval vein in right atrium ←
4: Left atrium →
5: Inf. branch of right pulmonary artery ↔
6: Azygos vein ↔
7: Hemiazygos vein ↔
8: Horizontal fissure ↔
9: Middle lobar bronchus

10: Inferior lobar bronchus
11: Superior segmental bronchus B VI of right lower lobe
12: Body of sternum ↔
13: Scapula ↔
14: Upper articular process of Th VIII
15: Lamina of vertebral arch Th VII
16: Pulmonary trunk ←
17: Left coronary artery ←
18: Left auricle ←
19: Lateral thoracic artery ↔

20: Serratus anterior ↔
21: Latissimus dorsi ↔
22: Teres major ↔
23: Subscapularis ↔
24: Infraspinatus ↔
25: Latissimus dorsi ↔
26: Rhomboideus ↔
27: Trapezius ↔
28: Inf. lingular segmental bronchus B V ←

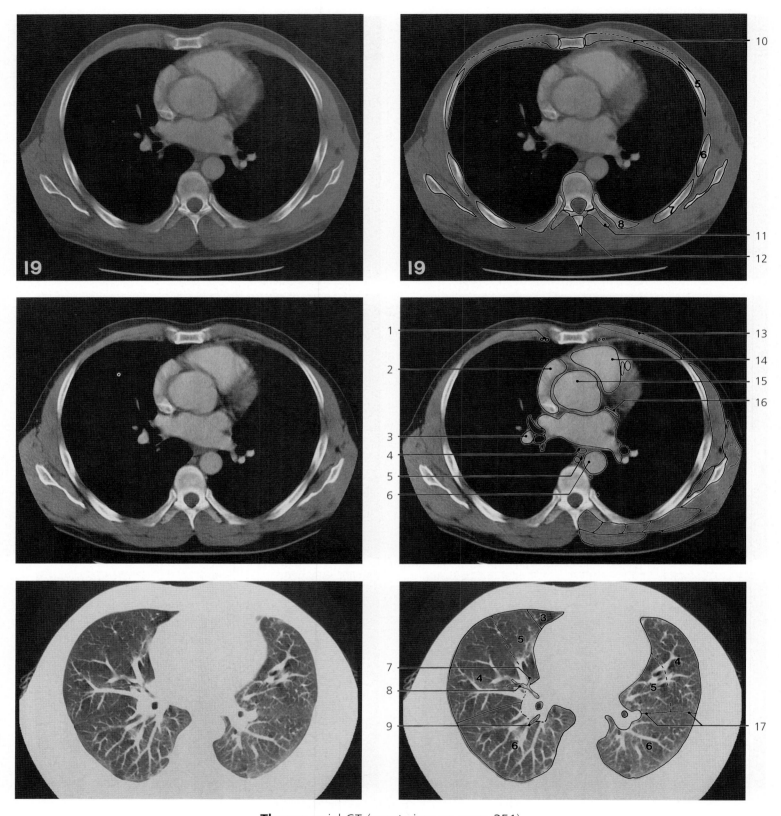

Thorax, axial CT (scout view on page 351)

1: Internal thoracic artery and vein ↔
2: Right auricle ↔
3: Inf. branch of right pulmonary artery ↔
4: Esophagus ↔
5: Thoracic duct ↔
6: Descending aorta ↔

7: Medial segmental bronchus B V of middle lobe
8: Lateral segmental bronchus B IV of middle lobe
9: Superior segmental bronchus B VI of lower lobe
10: Costal cartilage
11: Transverse process of Th VIII

12: Spinous process of Th VII
13: Pectoralis major ↔
14: Conus arteriosus →
15: Aortic bulb ↔
16: Circumflex branch of left coronary a. →
17: Oblique fissure of left lung ↔

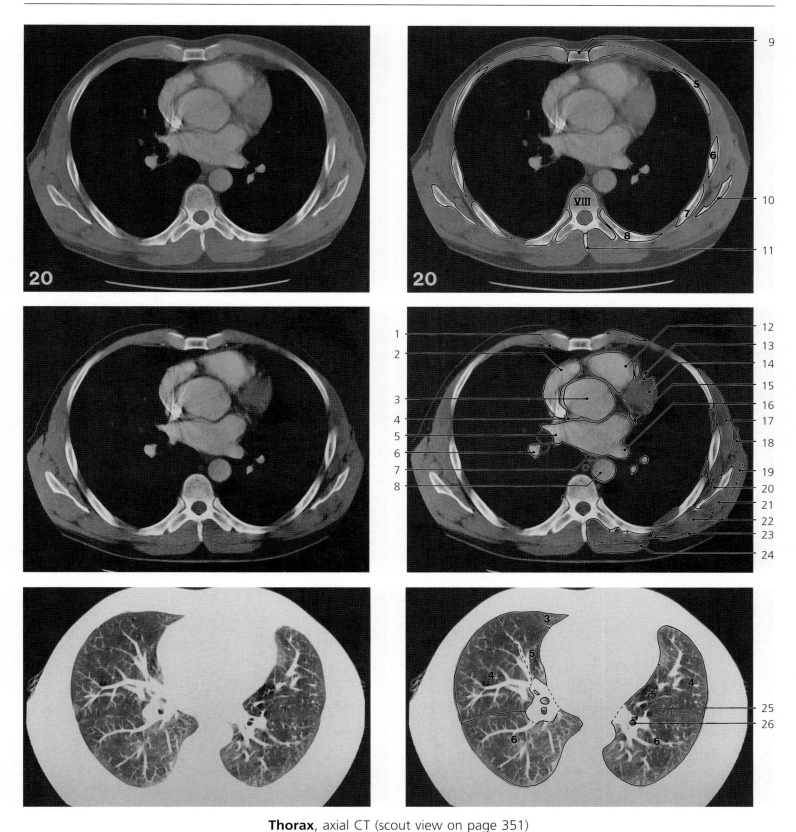

Thorax, axial CT (scout view on page 351)

1: Internal thoracic artery and vein ↔
2: Right auricle ↔
3: Aortic bulb ↔
4: Right coronary artery →
5: Right superior pulmonary vein ←
6: Inferior branch of right pulmonary artery →
7: Esophagus ↔
8: Descending aorta ↔
9: Body of sternum ↔
10: Scapulae ↔

11: Spinous process of Th VII
12: Conus arteriosus ↔
13: Anterior interventricular branch of left coronary artery →
14: Left ventricle (grazing section)
15: Circumflex branch of left coronary a. ↔
16: Left inferior pulmonary vein →
17: Serratus anterior ↔
18: Latissimus dorsi ↔
19: Teres major ↔

20: Subscapularis ←
21: Infraspinatus ↔
22: Rhomboideus ↔
23: Latissimus dorsi ↔
24: Trapezius ↔
25: Anteromedial segmental bronchus B VII + B VIII of left lower lobe →
26: Basolateral segmental bronchus B IX + B X of left lower lobe →

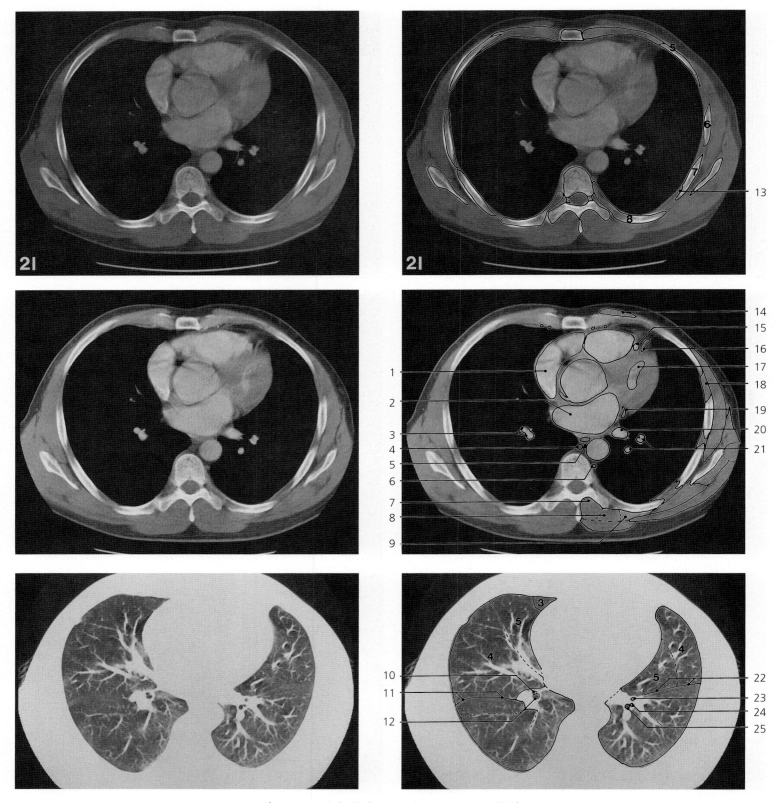

Thorax, axial CT (scout view on page 351)

1: Right atrium ↔
2: Left atrium ↔
3: Branches of pulmonary artery to right lower lobe ↔
4: Azygos vein ↔
5: Thoracic duct ↔
6: Hemiazygos vein ↔
7: Transversospinal muscles ↔
8: Longissimus ↔
9: Iliocostalis ↔
10: Medial and anterior segmental bronchus B VII + B VIII of right lower lobe

11: Oblique fissure of right lung ↔
12: Lateral and posterior segmental bronchus B IX + B X of right lower lobe
13: Sulcus costae
14: Pectoralis major ↔
15: Great cardiac vein
16: Anterior interventricular branch of left coronary artery ↔
17: Left ventricular lumen (grazing section) →
18: Intercostal muscles ↔

19: Circumflex branch of left coronary artery ←
20: Left inferior pulmonary vein ←
21: Branches of left pulmonary artery to lower lobe ↔
22: Oblique fissure of left lung ↔
23: Anteromedial segmental bronchus B VII + B VIII of left lower lobe ↔
24: Lateral segmental bronchus B IX of left lower lobe ↔
25: Posterior segmental bronchus B X of left lower lobe ↔

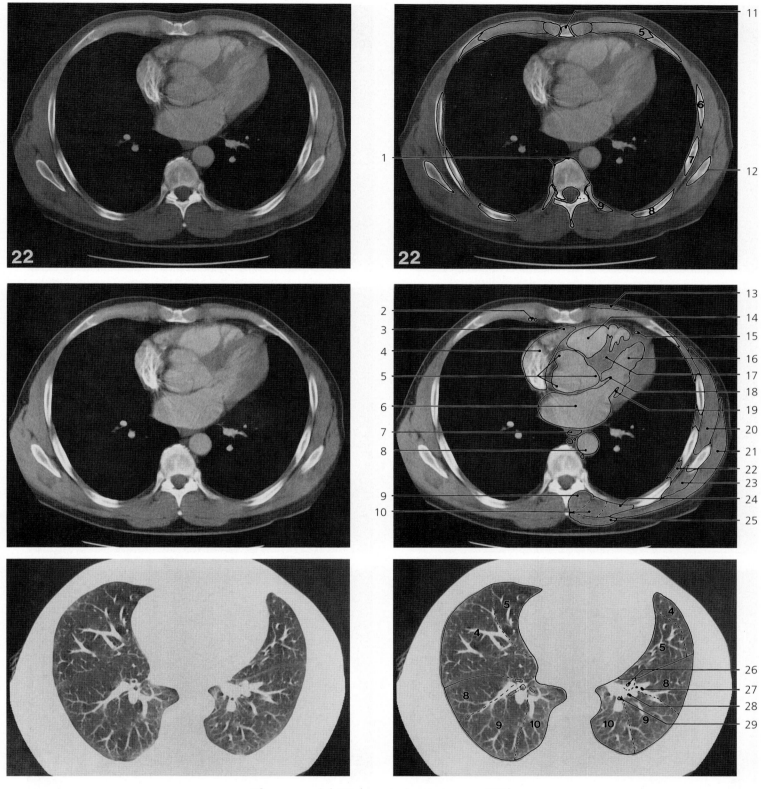

Thorax, axial CT (scout view on page 351)

1: Calcification (osteophyte)
2: Internal thoracic artery and vein ↔
3: Right auricle ←
4: Right atrium ↔
5: Aortic sinuses
6: Left atrium ↔
7: Esophagus ↔
8: Descending aorta ↔
9: Transversospinal muscles ↔
10: Longissimus ↔
11: Body of sternum ←
12: Inferior angle of scapula ←

13: Pectoralis major ←
14: Conus arteriosus ↔
15: Anterior interventricular branch of
    left coronary artery ↔
16: Left ventricle ↔
17: Interventricular septum ↔
18: Anterior cusp of mitral valve
19: Posterior cusp of mitral valve
20: Serratus anterior ↔
21: Latissimus dorsi ↔
22: Intercostal muscles ↔
23: Rhomboideus ↔

24: Iliocostalis ↔
25: Trapezius ↔
26: Medial segmental bronchus B VII of
    lower lobe ←
27: Anterior segmental bronchus B VIII of
    lower lobe (branch) ←
28: Lateral segmental bronchus B IX of
    lower lobe ←
29: Posterior segmental bronchus B X of
    lower lobe ←

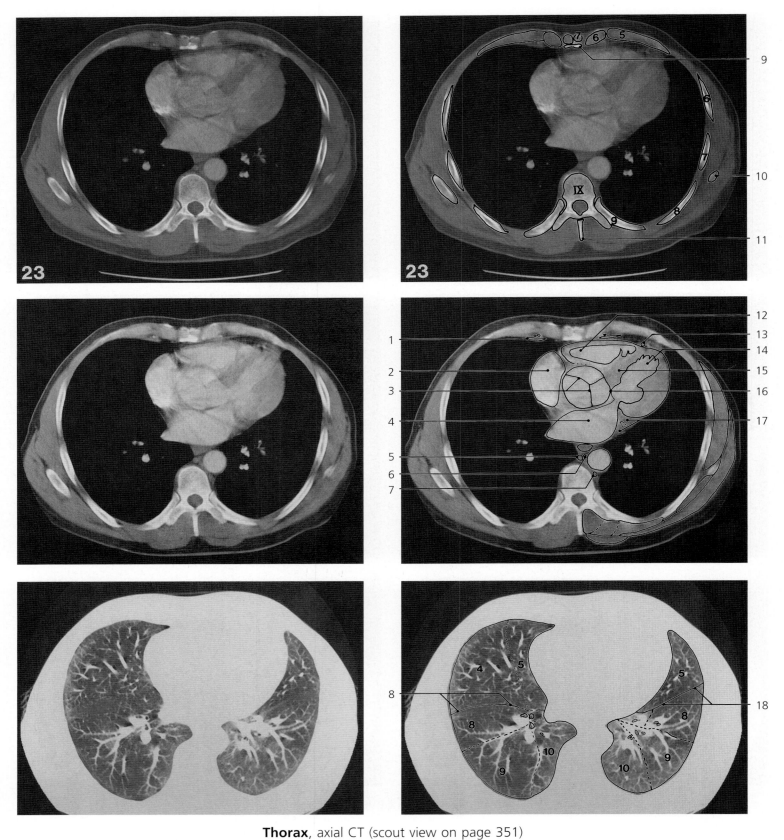

Thorax, axial CT (scout view on page 351)

1: Transversus thoracis muscle →
2: Right atrium ↔
3: Semilunar valves of aortic valve (closed)
4: Left atrium ↔
5: Azygos vein ↔
6: Thoracic duct ↔
7: Hemiazygos vein ↔

8: Oblique fissure of right lung ↔
9: Xiphoid process →
10: Inferior angle of scapula ←
11: Spinous process of Th VIII
12: Conus arteriosus ←
13: Anterior interventricular branch of left coronary artery →
14: Left ventricle ↔

15: Interventricular septum ↔
16: Left semilunar valve attaching to upper edge of membranous part of interventricular septum
17: Coronary sulcus with circumflex branch and fat ↔
18: Oblique fissure of left lung ↔

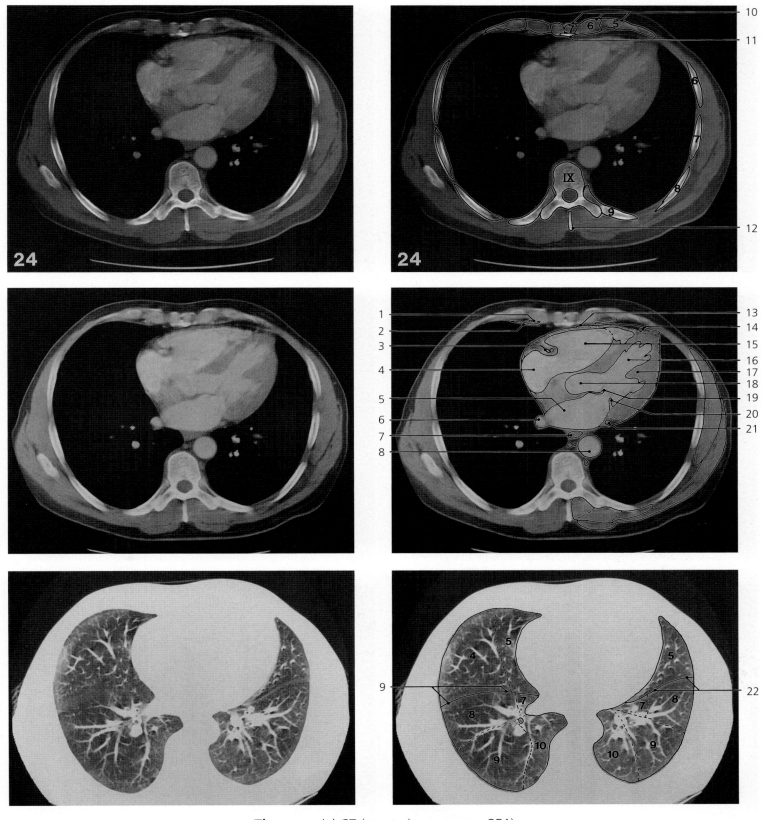

Thorax, axial CT (scout view on page 351)

1: Internal thoracic artery and vein ↔
2: Transversus thoracis muscle ↔
3: Right coronary artery and great cardiac vein ↔
4: Right atrium ↔
5: Left atrium ↔
6: Right inferior pulmonary vein →
7: Esophagus ↔
8: Descending aorta ↔

9: Oblique fissure of right lung ↔
10: Fused costal cartilages
11: Xiphoid process ↔
12: Spinous process of Th VIII
13: Fibrous pericardium
14: Anterior interventricular branch of left coronary artery ↔
15: Right ventricle →
16: Left ventricle ↔

17: Post. papillary muscle of left ventricle ↔
18: Left ventricular outflow tract →
19: Anterior cusp of mitral valve ↔
20: Posterior cusp of mitral valve ↔
21: Circumflex branch of left coronary a. ↔
22: Oblique fissure of left lung ↔

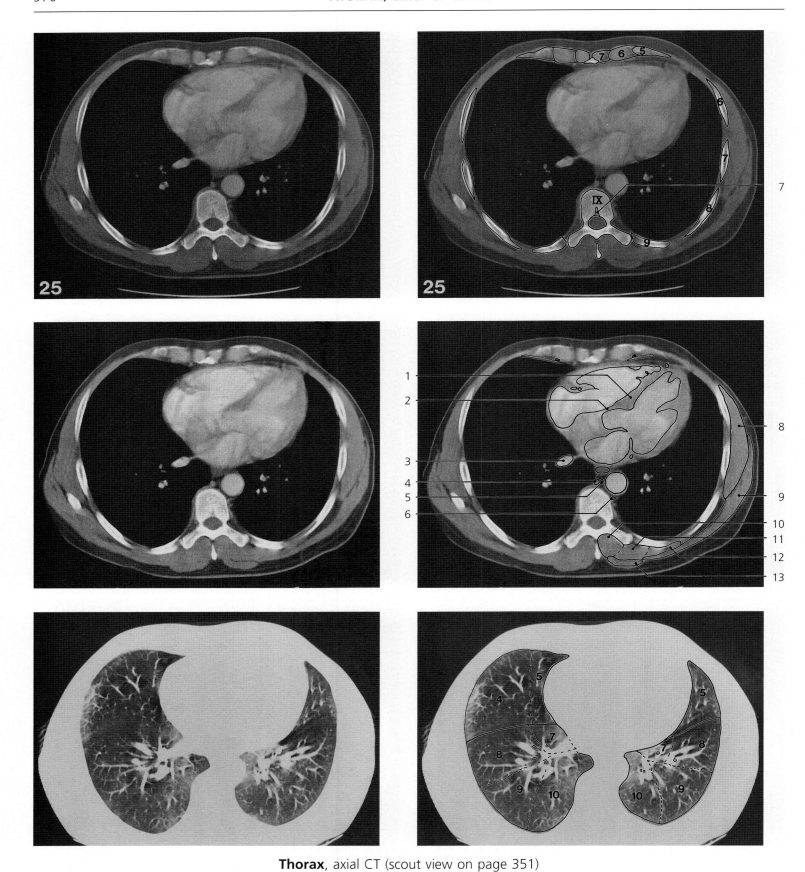

Thorax, axial CT (scout view on page 351)

1: Interventricular septum ↔
2: Membranous part of interventricular
   septum ←
3: Left inferior pulmonary vein ←
4: Azygos vein ↔

5: Thoracic duct ↔
6: Hemiazygos vein ↔
7: Basivertebral vein
8: Serratus anterior ↔
9: Latissimus dorsi ↔

10: Transversospinal muscles ↔
11: Longissimus ↔
12: Iliocostalis ↔
13: Trapezius ↔

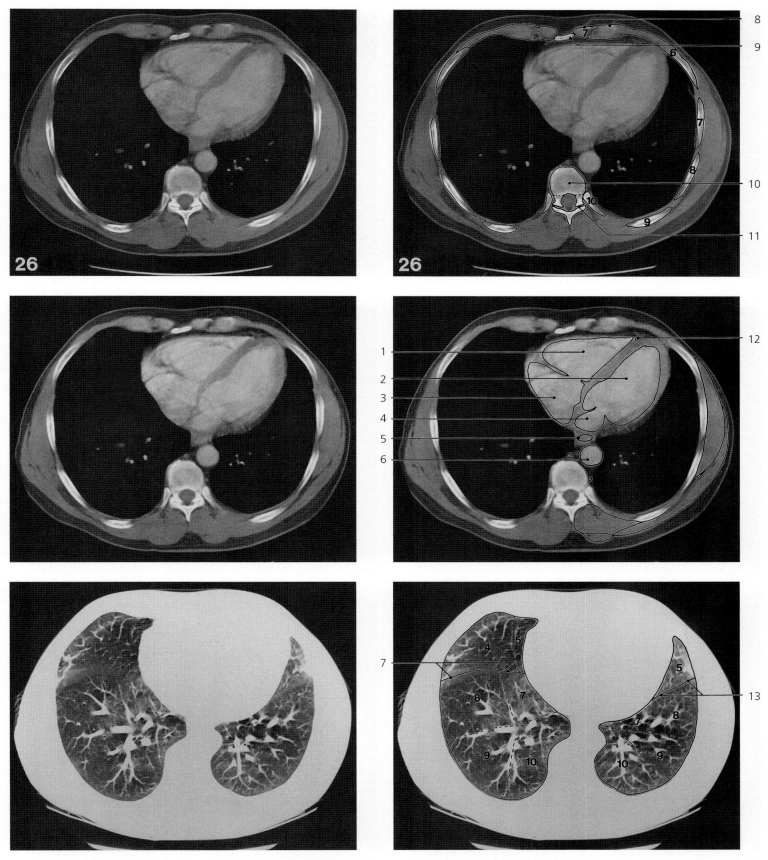

Thorax, axial CT (scout view on page 351)

1: Right ventricle ↔
2: Left ventricle ↔
3: Right atrium ↔
4: Left atrium ←
5: Esophagus ↔

6: Descending aorta ↔
7: Oblique fissure of right lung ↔
8: Fused costal cartilages ↔
9: Xiphoid process ↔
10: Intervertebral disc Th IX – Th X

11: Zygopophysial joint Th IX – Th X
12: Anterior interventricular branch of
    left coronary artery ↔
13: Oblique fissure of left lung ↔

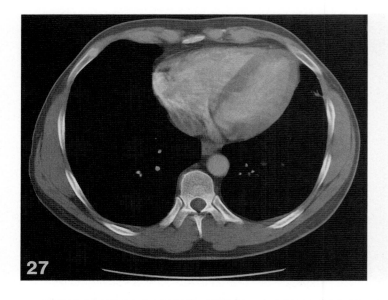

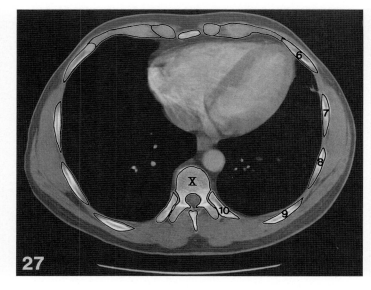

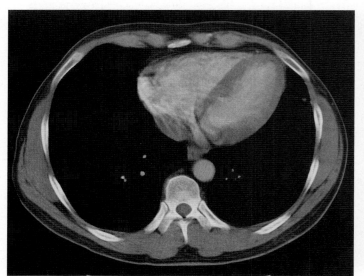

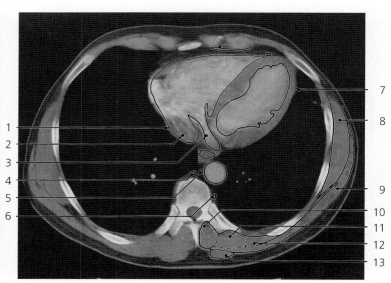

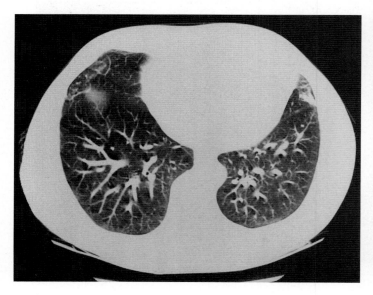

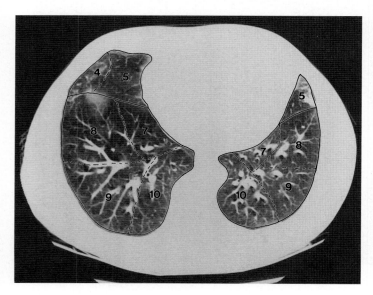

Thorax, axial CT (scout view on page 351)

1: Right phrenic nerve ↔

2: Inferior caval vein, inlet in right atrium →

3: Coronary sinus

4: Azygos vein ↔

5: Thoracic duct ↔

6: Hemiazygos vein ↔

7: Left phrenic nerve ↔

8: Serratus anterior ↔

9: Latissimus dorsi ↔

10: Transversospinal muscles ↔

11: Longissimus ↔

12: Iliocostalis ↔

13: Trapezius ↔

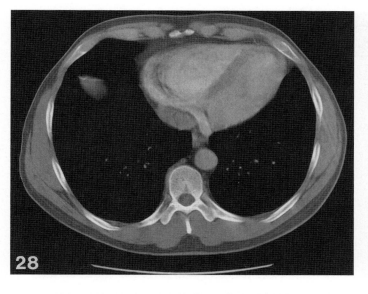

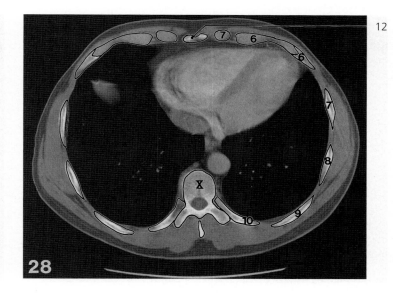

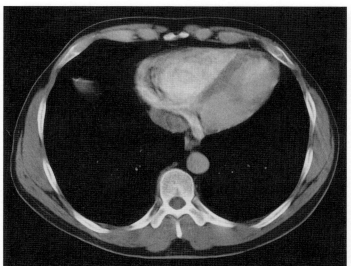

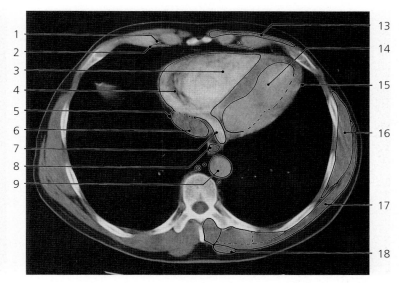

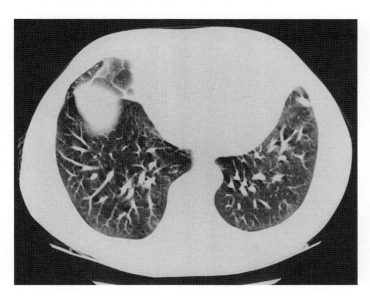

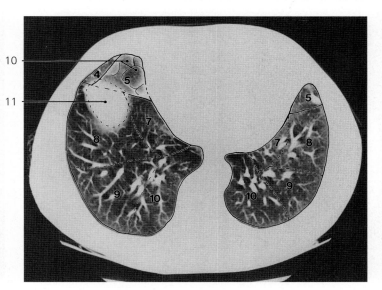

Thorax, axial CT (scout view on page 351)

1: Internal thoracic artery ↔
2: Transversus thoracis muscle ↔
3: Right ventricle ↔
4: Right atrium ←
5: Right phrenic nerve ←
6: Inferior caval vein ↔

7: Coronary sinus ←
8: Esophagus ↔
9: Descending aorta ↔
10: Bullae
11: Diaphragm
12: Xiphoid process →

13: Rectus abdominis →
14: Left ventricle ↔
15: Left phrenic nerve ←
16: Serratus anterior ↔
17: Latissimus dorsi ↔
18: Trapezius ↔

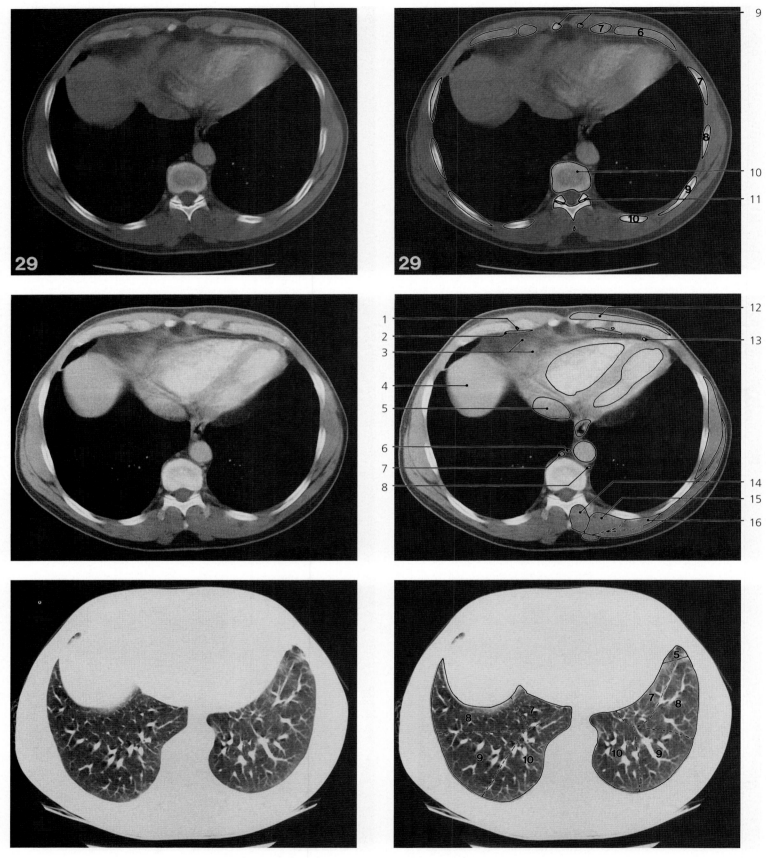

Thorax, axial CT (scout view on page 351)

1: Internal thoracic artery ←
2: Transversus thoracis muscle ←
3: Epicardial fat pad
4: Liver →
5: Inferior caval vein ↔
6: Thoracic duct ↔

7: Azygos vein ↔
8: Hemiazygos vein ↔
9: Xiphoid process (forked) ←
10: Intervertebral disc Th X – Th XI
11: Zygapophysial joint Th X – Th XI
12: Rectus abdominis ↔

13: Anterior interventricular branch of left coronary artery ←
14: Transversospinal muscles ↔
15: Longissimus ↔
16: Iliocostalis ↔

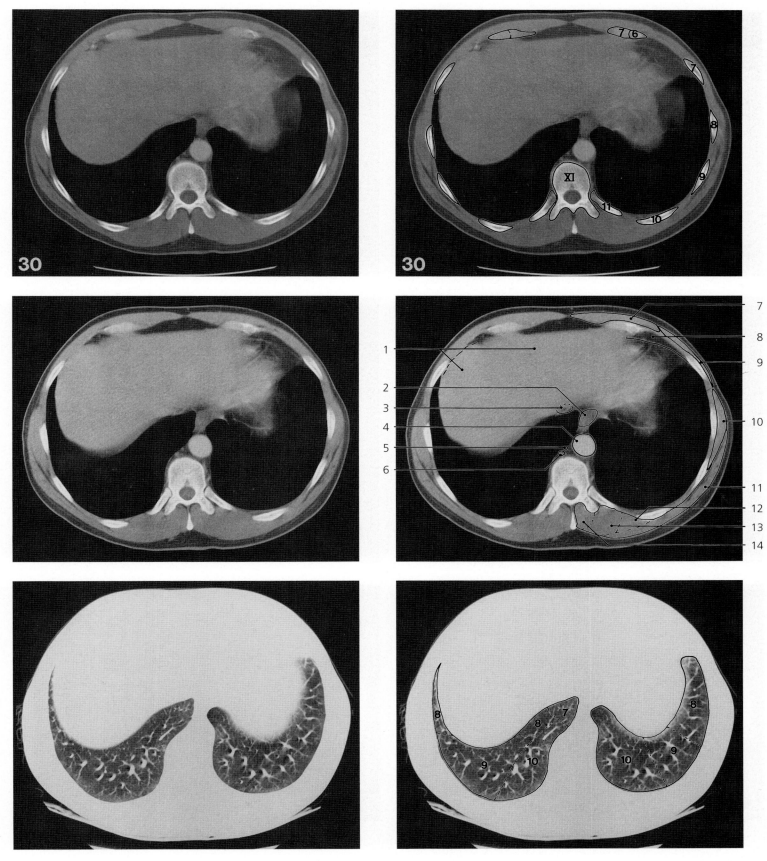

Thorax, axial CT (scout view on page 351)

1: Liver ↔
2: Esophagus ↔
3: Inferior caval vein ↔
4: Descending aorta ↔
5: Thoracic duct ↔

6: Azygos vein ↔
7: Rectus abdominis ↔
8: Costodiaphragmatic recess →
9: Obliquus externus abdominis →
10: Serratus anterior ↔

11: Latissimus dorsi ↔
12: Iliocostalis ↔
13: Longissimus ↔
14: Transversospinal muscles ↔

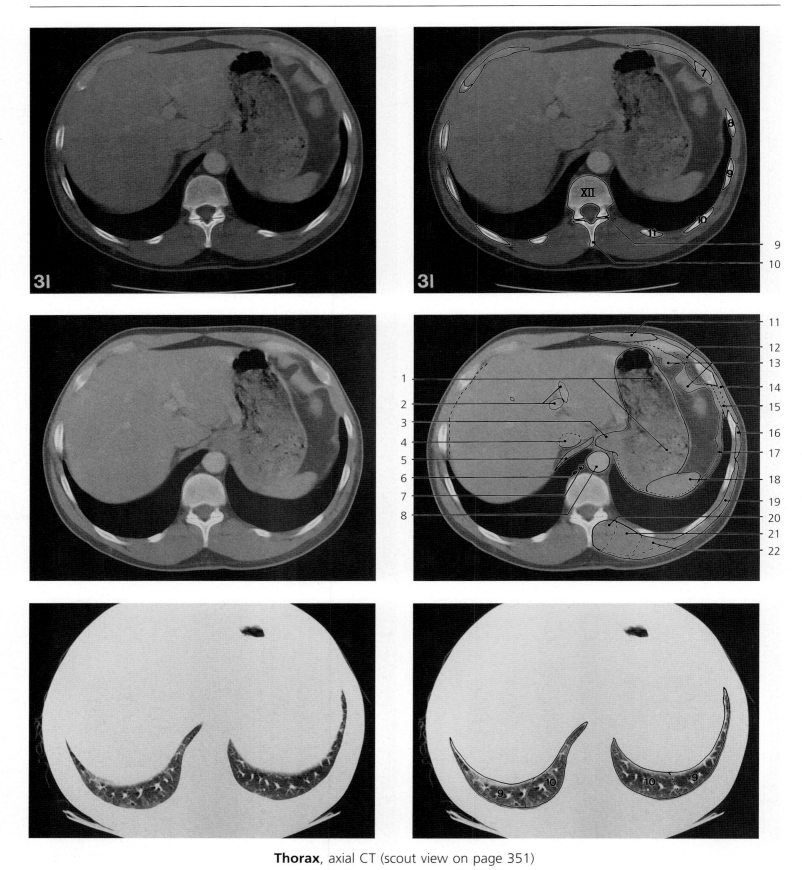

Thorax, axial CT (scout view on page 351)

1: Stomach →
2: Portal veins
3: Esophagus, abdominal part ←
4: Inferior caval vein ↔
5: Right crus of diaphragm →
6: Azygos vein ↔
7: Thoracic duct/Cisterna chyli ↔
8: Descending aorta ↔

9: Zygapophysial joint Th XI – Th XII
10: Spinous process of Th XI
11: Rectus abdominis ↔
12: Costodiaphramatic recess ←
13: Contraction furrows in diaphragm →
14: Obliquus externus abdominis ↔
15: Intercostal muscles ↔
16: Serratus anterior ←

17: Diaphragm ↔
18: Spleen →
19: Latissimus dorsi ↔
20: Transversospinal muscles ↔
21: Longissimus ↔
22: Iliocostalis ↔

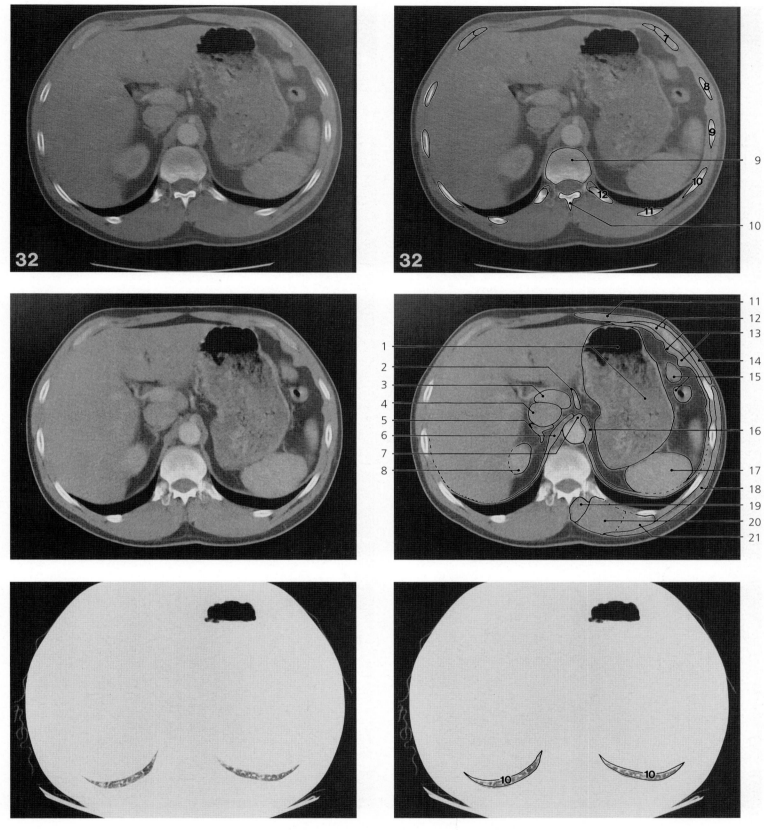

Thorax, axial CT (scout view on page 351)

1: Stomach ←	**8: Upper pole of right kidney**	**15: Left flexure of colon**
2: Left gastric artery	**9: Intervertebral disc Th XII – L I**	**16: Left crus of diaphragm** ←
3: Portal vein	**10: Spinous process Th XII**	**17: Spleen** ←
4: Inferior caval vein ←	**11: Rectus abdominis** ←	**18: Latissimus dorsi** ←
5: Right suprarenal gland	**12: Costodiaphragmatic recess** ←	**19: Transversospinal muscles** ←
6: Right crus of diaphragm ←	**13: Contraction furrows in diaphragm** ←	**20: Longissimus** ←
7: Celiac trunk	**14: Obliquus externus abdominis** ←	**21: Iliocostalis** ←

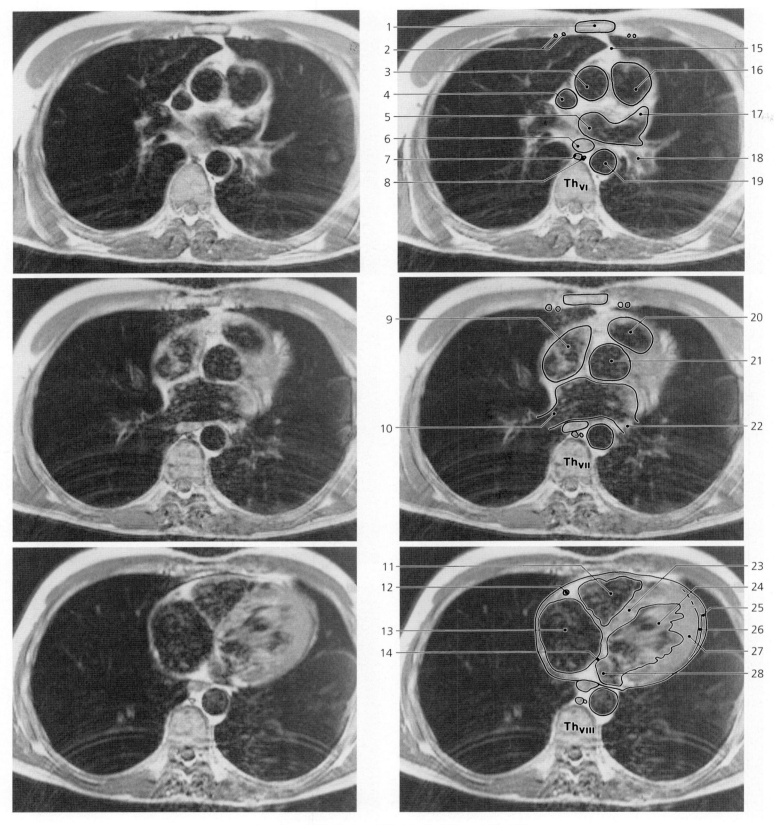

Heart, axial MR, level Th VI, Th VII and Th VIII

T1 weighted recording

1: Body of sternum
2: Internal thoracic artery and vein
3: Ascending aorta
4: Superior caval vein
5: Left atrium
6: Esophagus
7: Azygos vein
8: Thoracic duct
9: Right atrium
10: Right inferior pulmonary vein

11: Right ventricle
12: Right coronary artery
13: Right atrium
14: Interatrial septum
15: Anterior mediastinum
    (sternopericardial ligament)
16: Pulmonary trunk
17: Left auricle
18: Root of left lung
19: Thoracic aorta

20: Conus arteriosus
21: Bulb of aorta
22: Left inferior pulmonary vein
23: Interventricular septum
24: Left ventricle
25: Pericardial sac
26: Pericardial cavity
27: Myocardium of left ventricle
28: Left atrium

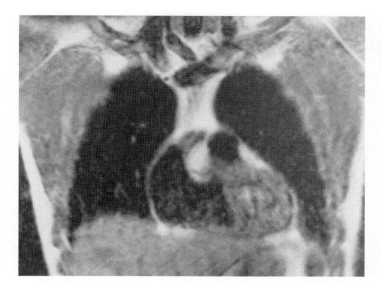
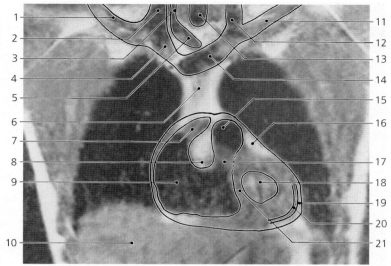

Heart, coronal MR

T1 weighted recording

1: Right subclavian vein
2: Right internal jugular vein
3: Right common carotid artery
4: Right brachiocephalic vein
5: Brachiocephalic trunk
6: Superior mediastinum with thymus
7: Right atrium
8: Supraventricular crest
9: Right ventricle
10: Liver
11: Left subclavian vein
12: Left internal jugular vein
13: Trachea
14: Left brachiocephalic vein
15: Pulmonary trunk
16: Epicardial fat
17: Conus arteriosus
18: Left ventricular cavity
19: Pericardial sac
20: Pericardial cavity
21: Interventricular septum

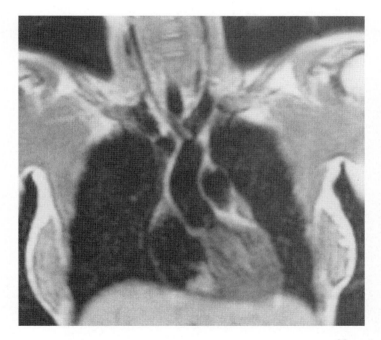
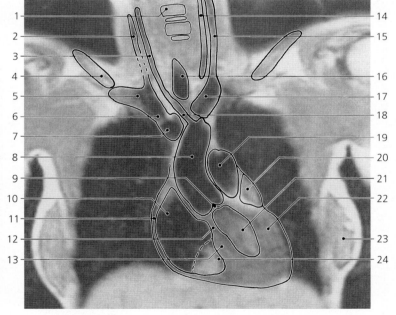

Heart, coronal MR

T1 weighted recording

1: Body of cervical vertebra
2: Right internal jugular vein
3: Right common carotid artery
4: Clavicle
5: Right subclavian vein
6: Right brachiocephalic vein
7: Superior caval vein
8: Ascending aorta
9: Aortic valve
10: Right atrium
11: Right atrial wall, pericardium and pleura
12: Interventricular septum, membranous part
13: Interventricular septum, muscular part
14: Left common carotid artery
15: Left internal jugular vein
16: Trachea
17: Left brachiocephalic vein
18: Brachiocephalic trunk
19: Pulmonary trunk
20: Left auricle
21: Left ventricle
22: Myocardium of left ventricle
23: Mamma
24: Right ventricle

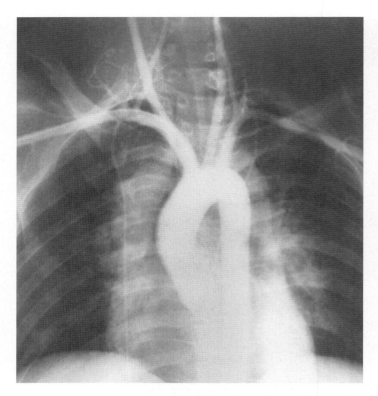
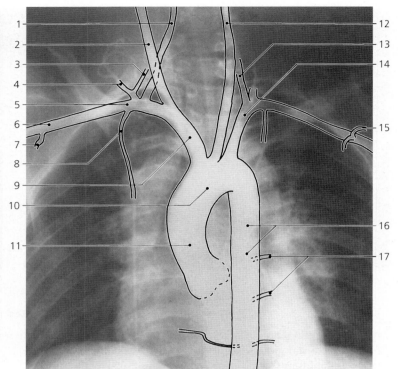

Aortic arch and great arteries, a-p X-ray (slightly oblique), aortography

1: Right vertebral artery
2: Right common carotid artery
3: Inferior thyroid artery
4: Transverse cervical artery
5: Right subclavian artery
6: Axillary artery

7: Subscapular artery
8: Internal thoracic artery
9: Brachiocephalic trunk
10: Aortic arch
11: Ascending aorta
12: Left common carotid artery

13: Left vertebral artery
14: Left subclavian artery
15: Thoraco-acromial artery
16: Thoracic aorta
17: Intercostal arteries

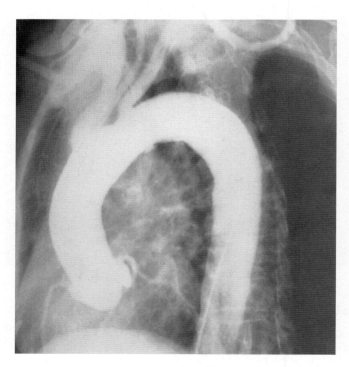
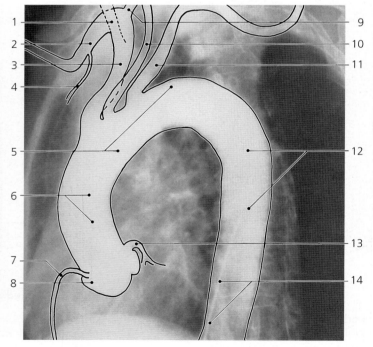

Aortic arch and great arteries, oblique X-ray, aortography

1: Right common carotid artery
2: Right subclavian artery
3: Brachiocephalic trunk
4: Internal thoracic artery
5: Aortic arch

6: Ascending aorta
7: Right coronary artery
8: Aortic sinus
9: Right vertebral artery
10: Left common carotid artery

11: Left subclavian artery
12: Thoracic aorta
13: Left coronary artery
14: Catheter

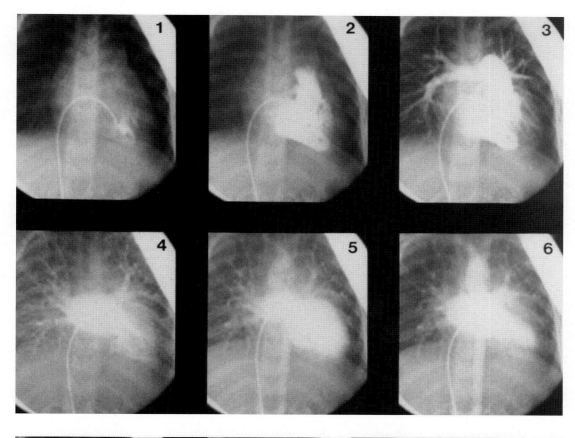

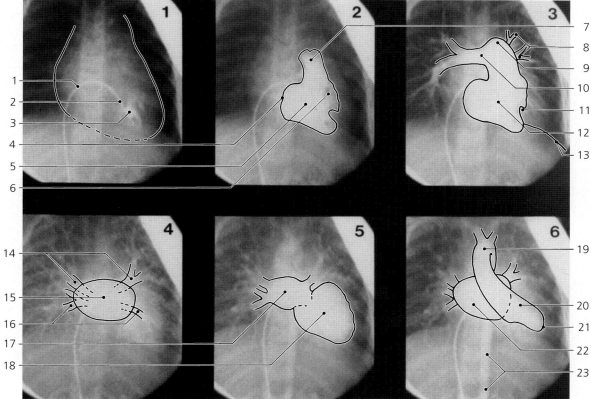

Heart, a-p, cardiac cineangiography, child

Six frames of a cardiac angiography sequence

1: Catheter in right atrium
2: Tip of catheter in right ventricle
3: Initial outflow of contrast medium
4: Tricuspid valve (closed)
5: Right ventricle (early systole)
6: Trabeculae carneae
7: Pulmonary trunk
8: Branches of left pulmonary artery

9: Left pulmonary artery
10: Right pulmonary artery
11: Anterior papillary muscle of right ventricle
12: Right ventricle (systole)
13: Diaphragm
14: Superior pulmonary veins
15: Left atrium (diastole)

16: Inferior pulmonary veins
17: Left atrium (systole)
18: Left ventricle (diastole)
19: Aortic arch
20: Left ventricle (systole)
21: Apex of left ventricle
22: Left atrium (diastole)
23: Abdominal aorta

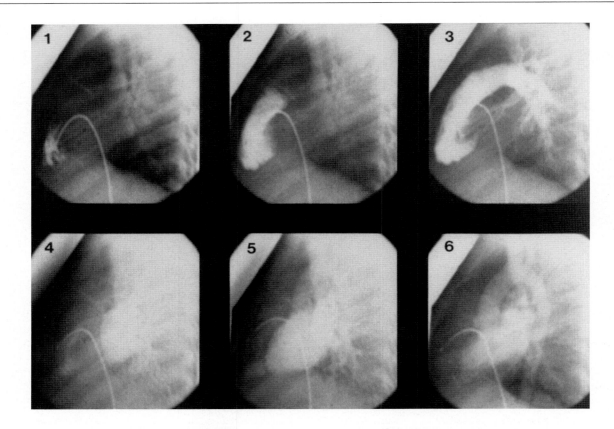

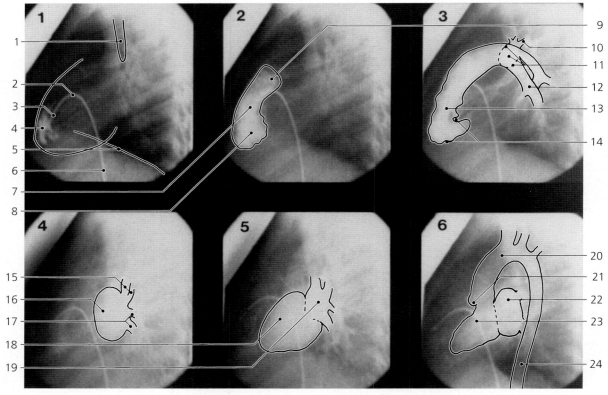

Heart, lateral, cardiac cineangiography, child

Six frames of a cardiac angiography sequence

1: Trachea
2: Catheter in right atrium
3: Tip of catheter in right ventricle
4: Initial outflow of contrast medium
5: Diaphragm
6: Catheter in inferior caval vein
7: Conus arteriosus (infundibulum)
8: Right ventricle (early systole)
9: Pulmonary trunk

10: Pulmonary artery branches to upper lobes
11: Right pulmonary artery (longitudinal view)
12: Branches of left pulmonary artery
13: Right ventricle (systole)
14: Trabeculae carneae
15: Superior pulmonary veins
16: Left atrium (diastole)

17: Inferior pulmonary veins
18: Left ventricle (diastole)
19: Left atrium (systole)
20: Aortic arch
21: Aortic sinus
22: Left atrium (diastole)
23: Left ventricle (systole)
24: Descending aorta

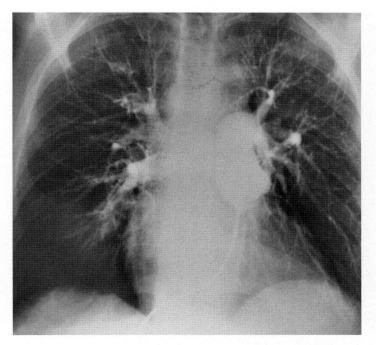

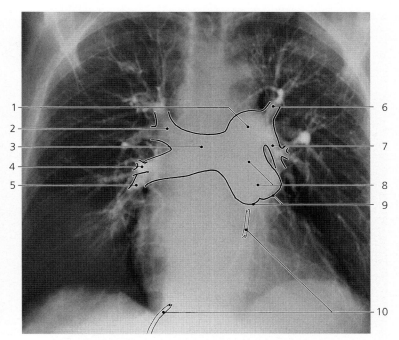

Pulmonary arteries, a-p X-ray, arteriography

1: Left pulmonary artery
2: Right upper lobe artery
3: Right pulmonary artery
4: Middle lobe artery

5: Right lower lobe artery
6: Left upper lobe artery
7: Left lower lobe artery
8: Pulmonary trunk

9: Pulmonary valve
10: Catheter

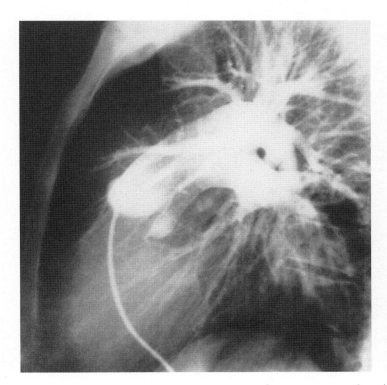

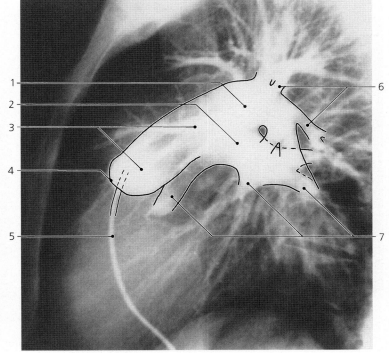

Pulmonary arteries, lateral X-ray, arteriography

1: Left pulmonary artery
2: Right pulmonary artery
3: Pulmonary trunk

4: Pulmonary valve
5: Catheter in right ventricle
6: Branches of left pulmonary artery

7: Branches of right pulmonary artery

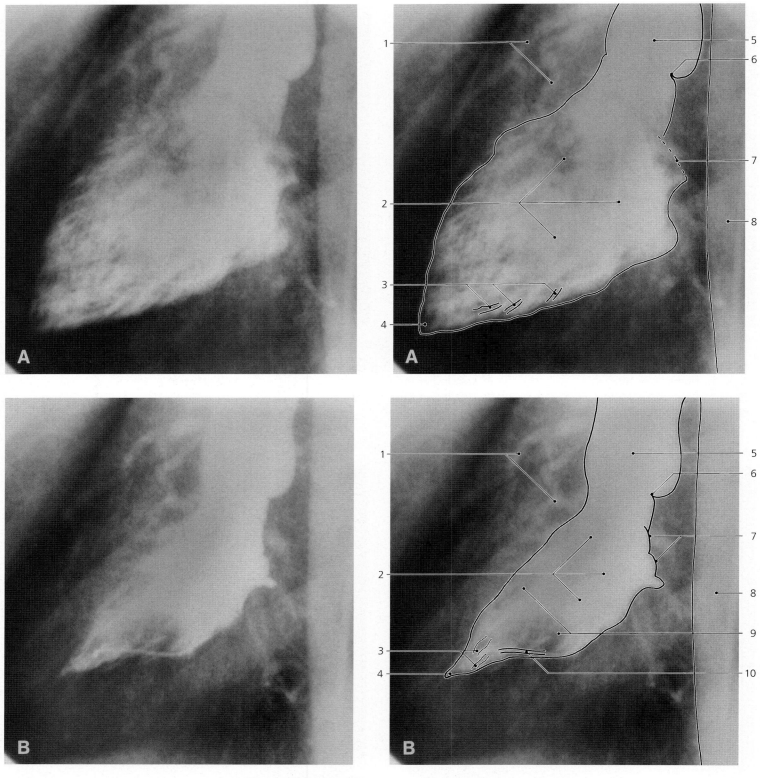

Left ventricle, lateral X-rays, cardiac angiography

A: Diastole. B: Systole

1: Coronary arteries
2: Left ventricle
3: Trabeculae carneae
4: Apex of left ventricle

5: Aortic bulb
6: Semilunar valve of aortic ostium
7: Mitral valve
8: Thoracic aorta

9: Anterior and posterior papillary
muscle
10: Catheter

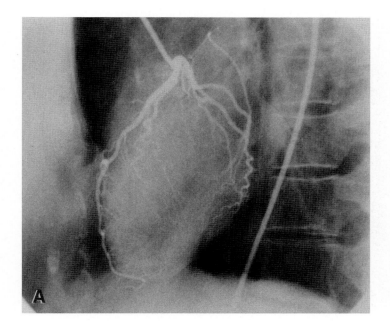
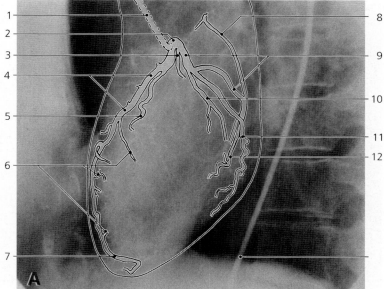
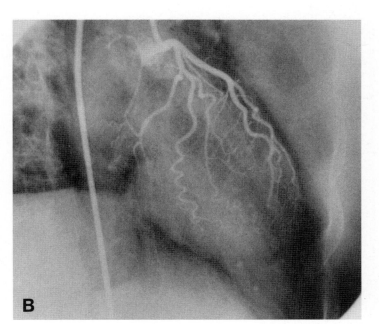
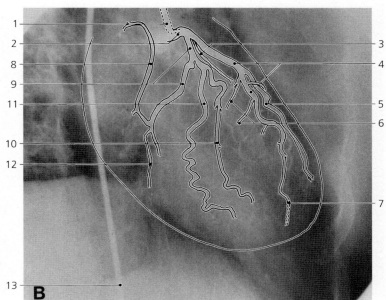

Left coronary artery, arteriography

A: left lateral X-ray. B: right anterior oblique (RAO) X-ray

1: Catheter with tip in orifice of left coronary artery
2: Left coronary artery, main stem
3: Intermediate ramus
4: Anterior interventricular artery (left anterior descendent, LAD)
5: Left diagonal artery
6: Anterior septal rami
7: LAD at apex of the heart
8: Atrial ramus
9: Circumflex artery
10: Anterior left ventricular branch (anterior marginal branch)
11: Obtuse marginal branch
12: Posterior left ventricular branch (posterior marginal branch)
13: Catheter in aorta

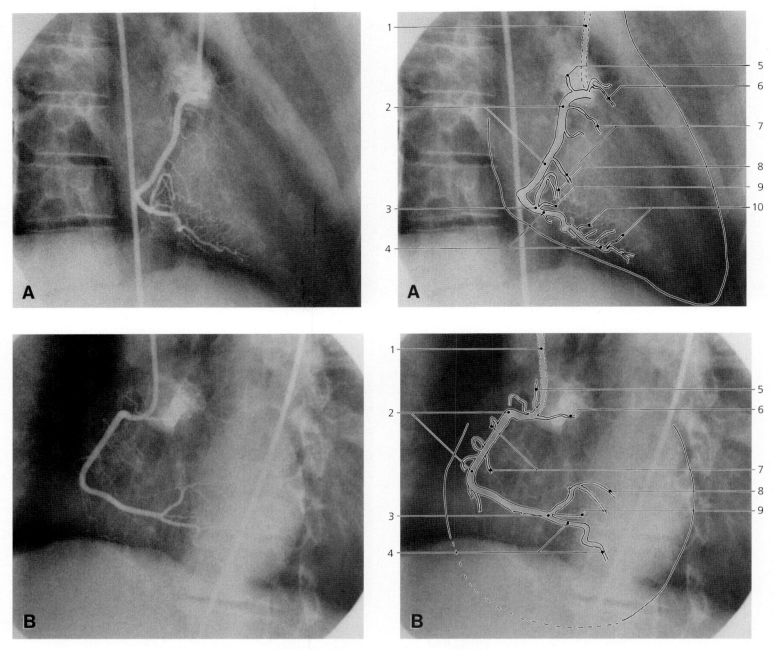

Right coronary artery, arteriography

A: right anterior oblique (RAO) X-ray. B: left anterior oblique (LAO) X-ray

1: Catheter with tip in orifice of right
   coronary artery
2: Right coronary artery
3: Crux of heart
4: Posterior interventricular artery

5: Sinus node artery
6: Conus artery
7: Anterior right ventricular rami
   (marginal branches)
8: Terminal left ventricular ramus

9: Atrio-ventricular node artery
10: Posterior septal rami

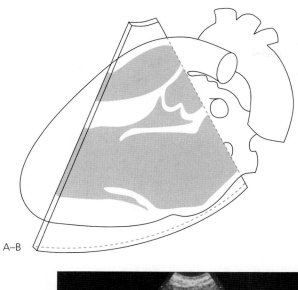

Orientation of parasternal, long axis sections A and B, parallel to axis of the heart.

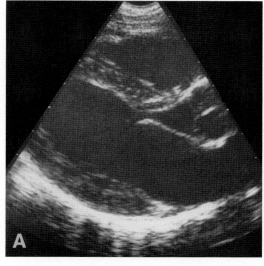

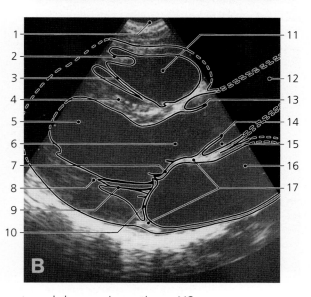

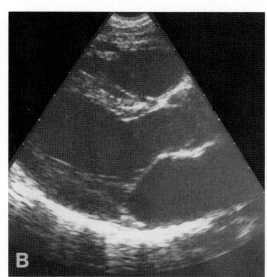

Mitral and aortic valve, parasternal, long axis sections, US

A: diastole. B: systole

1: Probe over fourth left intercostal space
2: Anterior papillary muscle of right ventricle
3: Septomarginal trabecula (inconstant)
4: Interventricular septum
5: Left ventricle
6: Left ventricular outflow tract
7: Anterior cusp of mitral valve
8: Papillary muscle
9: Chorda tendinea
10: Posterior cusp of mitral valve
11: Right ventricle
12: Ascending aorta
13: Right semilunar cusp of aortic valve
14: Posterior semilunar cusp of aortic valve
15: Aortic sinus
16: Left atrium
17: Fibrous annulus of mitral ostium

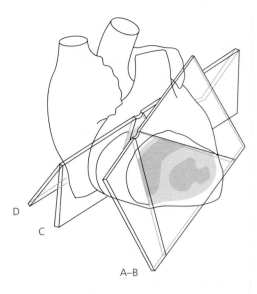

Orientation of parasternal, short axis sections A-D, perpendicular to axis of the heart

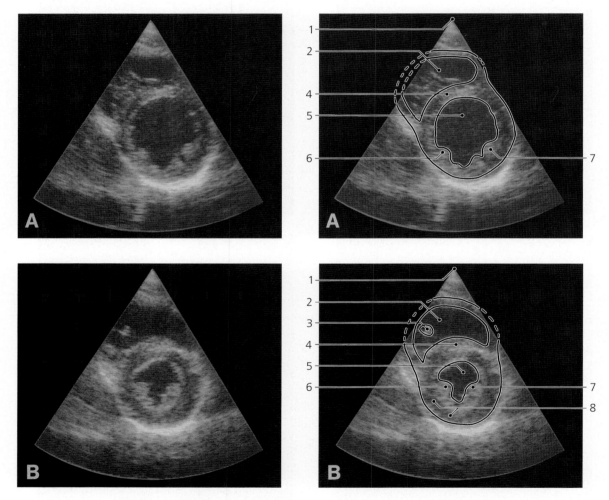

Right and left ventricle, parasternal, short axis sections, US

A: diastole. B: systole

1: Probe over third left intercostal space
2: Right ventricle
3: Septomarginal trabecula (moderator band)
4: Interventricular septum
5: Left ventricle
6: Posterior papillary muscle of left ventricle
7: Anterior papillary muscle of left ventricle
8: Posterior wall of left ventricle

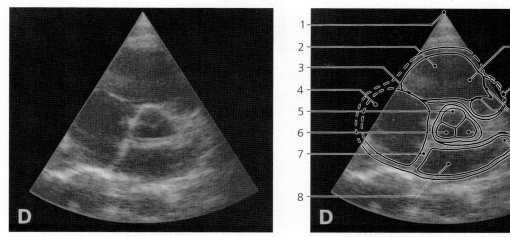

Mitral valve, parasternal, short axis section, US

Position of section C explained on previous page

1: Probe over third intercostal space
2: Right ventricle
3: Interventricular septum

4: Left ventricular outflow tract
5: Anterior cusp of mitral valve
6: Mitral ostium

7: Posterior cusp of mitral valve
8: Blood between ventricular wall, and posterior cusp

Aortic valve, parasternal, short axis section, US

Position of section D explained on previous page

1: Probe over third intercostal space
2: Right ventricle
3: Tricuspid valve
4: Right atrium
5: Right semilunar cusp of aortic valve

6: Posterior semilunar cusp of aortic valve
7: Interatrial septum
8: Left atrium
9: Conus arteriosus

10: Pulmonary trunk
11: Pulmonary valve
12: Left semilunar cusp of aortic valve
13: Left auricle

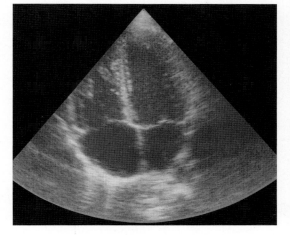

Cardiac four chambers, probe over apex, US

1: Apex of heart
2: Interventricular septum
3: Right ventricle with moderator band
4: Anterior papillary muscle

5: Tricuspid valve
6: Membraneous part of interventricular septum
7: Right atrium

8: Left ventricle
9: Mitral valve
10: Interatrial septum
11: Left atrium

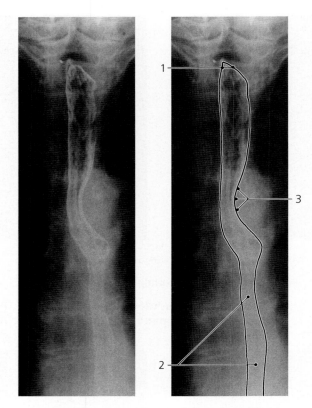

Esophagus, a-p X-ray, barium swallow

1: Cricoesophageal sphincter   2: Esophagus, thoracic part   3: Impression from aortic arch

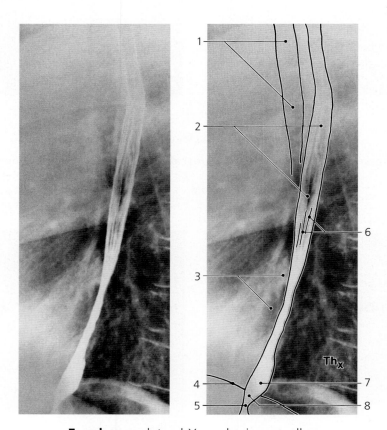

Esophagus, lateral X-ray, barium swallow

1: Trachea   4: Diaphragm   7: "Ampulla phrenica" (radiology term)
2: Esophagus   5: Cardia   8: Abdominal part of esophagus
3: Left atrium   6: Mucosal folds

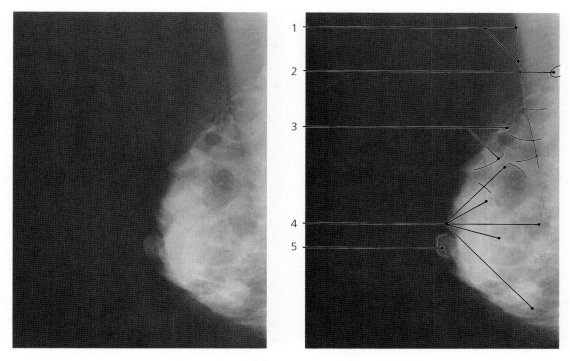

Breast, young, oblique X-ray, mammography

1: Pectoralis major
2: Axillary lymph node

3: Suspensory ligaments (Cooper)
4: Fibroglandular tissue

5: Nipple

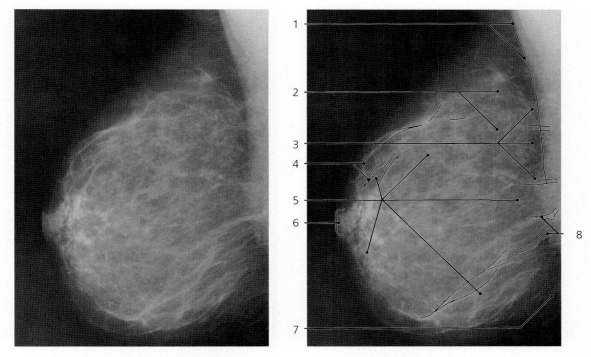

Breast, middle-age, oblique X-ray, mammography

1: Pectoralis major
2: Axillary process of mammary gland
3: Retroglandular fat

4: Suspensory ligaments (Cooper)
5: Fibroglandular tissue
6: Nipple

7: Inframammary sulcus
8: Vessels

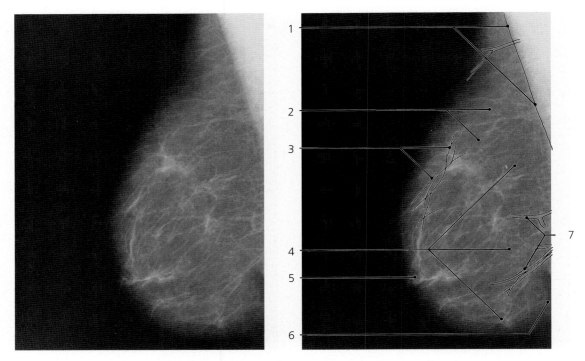

Breast, senescent, oblique X-ray, mammography

1: Pectoralis major
2: Axillary process of mamma
3: Suspensory ligaments (Cooper)

4: Fat involuted glandular tissue
5: Nipple
6: Inframammary sulcus

7: Vessels

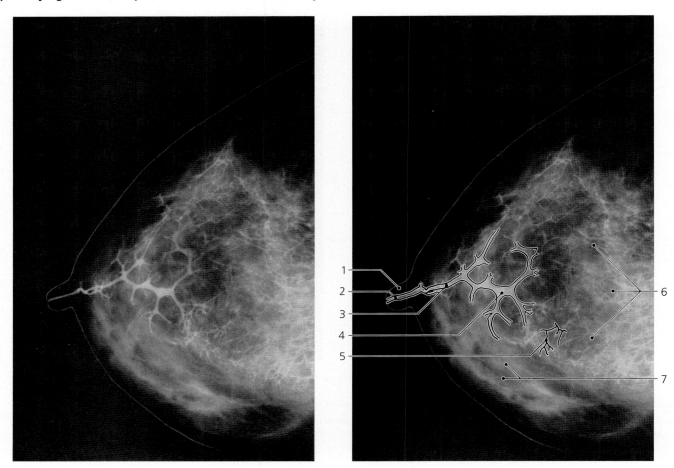

Breast, lateral X-ray, ductography

1: Nipple
2: Lactiferous duct
3: Lactiferous sinus

4: Major excretory duct
5: Minor excretory duct
6: Glandular tissue with contrast filling

7: Glandular tissue without contrast filling

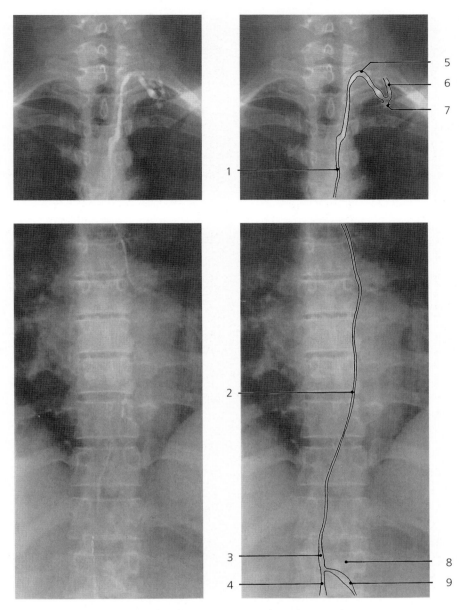

Thoracic duct, a-p X-ray lymphography

1: Thoracic duct at level of Th IV
2: Thoracic duct at level of Th IX – Th X
3: Cisterna chyli
4: Right lumbar trunk

5: Arch of thoracic duct
6: Jugular trunk (overflow)
7: Opening of thoracic duct into
   subclavian vein

8: First lumbar vertebra
9: Left lumbar trunk

Abdomen

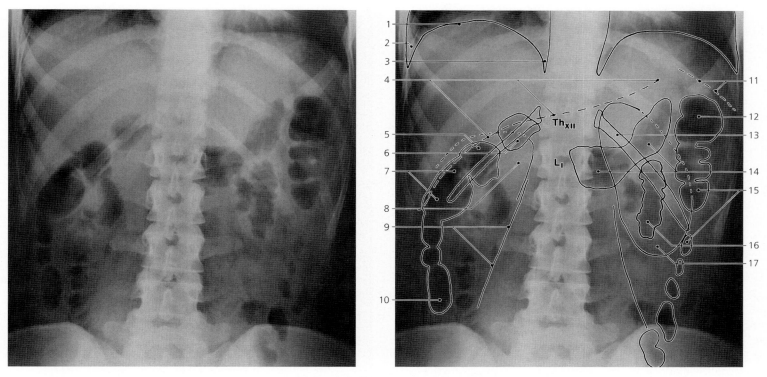

Abdomen, a-p X-ray, erect

The gastro-intestinal tract is outlined by its natural gas content

1: Diaphragm	7: Ascending colon	13: 12th rib
2: Costodiaphragmatic sulcus	8: Upper pole of right kidney	14: Stomach
3: Mediastinodiaphragmatic sulcus	9: Psoas major (lateral contour)	15: Descending colon
4: Lower border of liver	10: Cecum	16: Jejunum
5: Hepatic flexure of colon	11: Lower border of spleen	17: Lower pole of left kidney
6: Duodenal cap (radiology term)	12: Splenic flexure of colon	

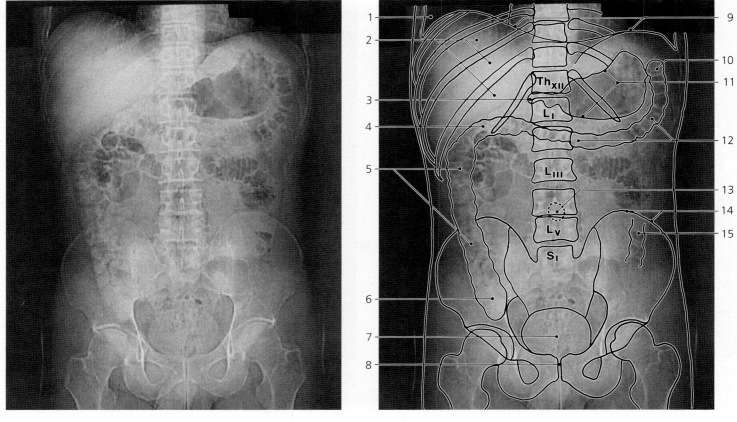

Scout view

1: Costodiaphragmatic sulcus
2: Liver
3: Duodenal cap
4: Hepatic flexure of colon
5: Ascending colon

6: Cecum
7: Urinary bladder
8: Symphysis pubis
9: Diaphragm
10: Splenic flexure of colon

11: Curvatures of stomach
12: Transverse colon
13: Position of umbilicus
14: Iliac crest
15: Descending colon

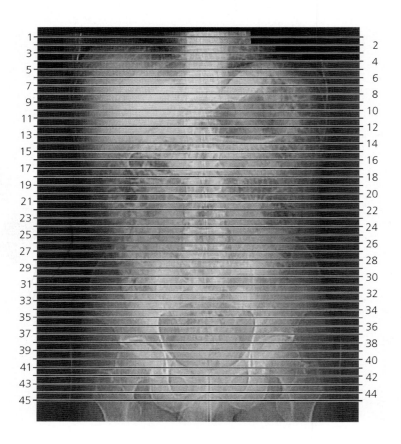

Scout view

Lines #1–45 indicate position of sections in the following CT series.

Consecutive sections, 10 mm thick.

The gastrointestinal tract is outlined by peroral contrast medium.

The urinary tract is outlined by excretion of intravenous watersoluble contrast medium.

Residues of contrast from an earlier lymphography are present in some iliac and lumbar lymph nodes.

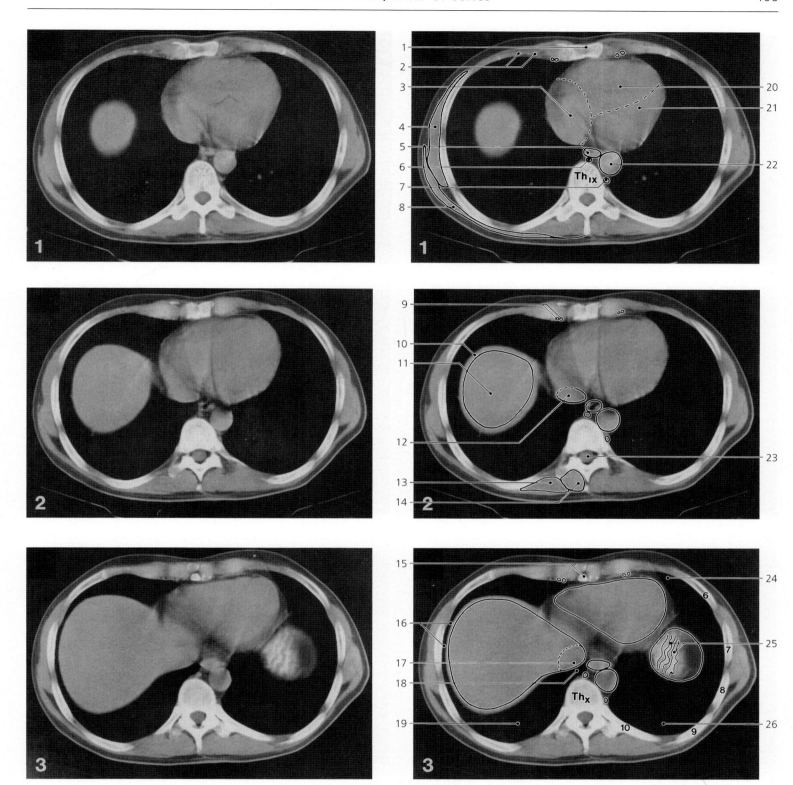

Abdomen, axial CT

Scout view on opposite page

1: Body of sternum
2: Calcified costal cartilage
3: Right atrium
4: Serratus anterior
5: Esophagus
6: Azygos vein
7: Hemiazygos vein
8: Latissimus dorsi
9: Internal thoracic artery and vein
10: Diaphragm

11: Right lobe of liver
12: Inferior caval vein
13: Iliocostalis thoracis, and longissimus thoracis
14: Transversospinal muscles
15: Xiphoid process
16: Costodiaphragmatic groove
17: Inferior caval vein
18: Phrenico-mediastinal groove
19: Lower lobe of right lung

20: Right ventricle
21: Left ventricle
22: Thoracic aorta
23: Spinal cord
24: Lingula of left lung
25: Rugae in fundus of stomach
26: Lower lobe of left lung
Ribs are numbered.

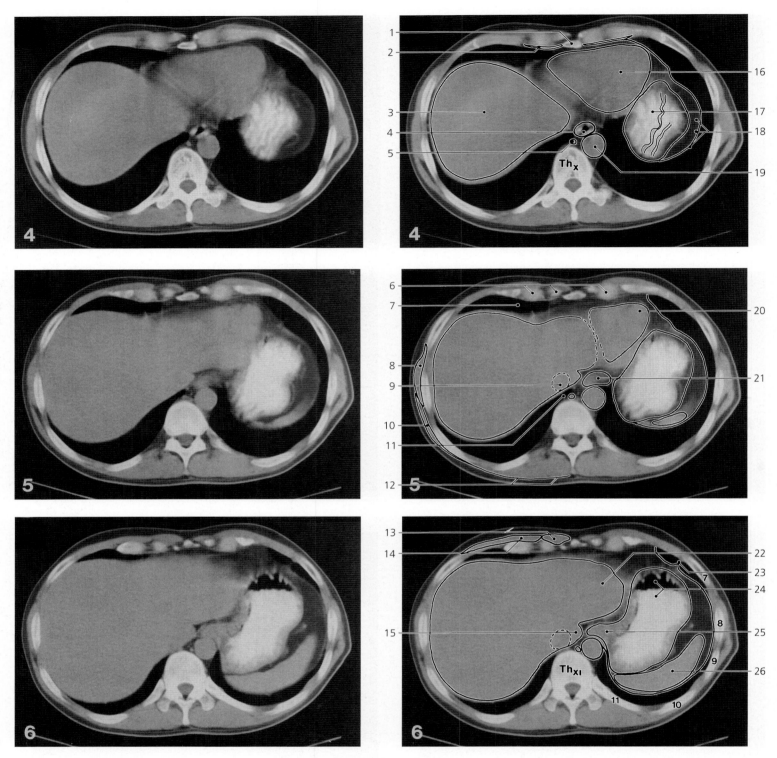

Abdomen, axial CT

Scout view on page 404

1: Xiphoid process
2: Transversus thoracis
3: Right lobe of liver
4: Esophagus
5: Azygos vein
6: Costal cartilage
7: Costo-diaphragmatic groove with inferior margin of right lung
8: Serratus anterior
9: Inferior caval vein

10: Latissimus dorsi
11: Phrenico-mediastinal groove
12: Thoracolumbar fascia
13: Rectus abdominis
14: Obliquus externus abdominis
15: Caudate lobe of liver
16: Heart
17: Fundus of stomach with rugae
18: Parietal pleura, diaphragm, and parietal peritoneum

19: Thoracic aorta
20: Apex of heart
21: Esophagus, abdominal part
22: Left lobe of liver
23: Oblique fissure of left lung
24: Fundus of stomach with air and barium
25: Cardia
26: Spleen
Ribs are numbered.

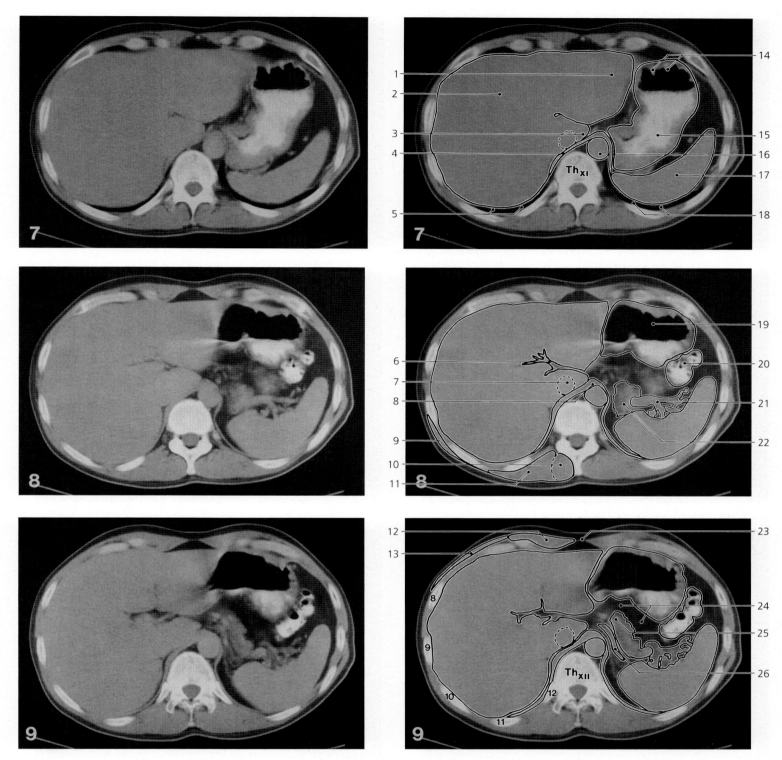

Abdomen, axial CT

Scout view on page 404

1: Left lobe of liver
2: Right lobe of liver
3: Caudate lobe of liver
4: Lumbar part of diaphragm
5: Inferior margin of left lung
6: Porta hepatis
7: Inferior caval vein
8: Right crus of diaphragm
9: Latissimus dorsi
10: Transversospinal muscles

11: Iliocostalis and longissimus
12: Rectus abdominis
13: Obliquus externus abdominis
14: Rugae in fundus of stomach
15: Body of stomach
16: Thoracic aorta
17: Spleen
18: Inferior margin of left lung
19: Air in body of stomach
20: Splenic flexure of colon

21: Splenic vessels
22: Tail of pancreas
23: Linea alba
24: Omental bursa with surrounding peritoneal fat
25: Body of pancreas
26: Splenic artery
Ribs are numbered.

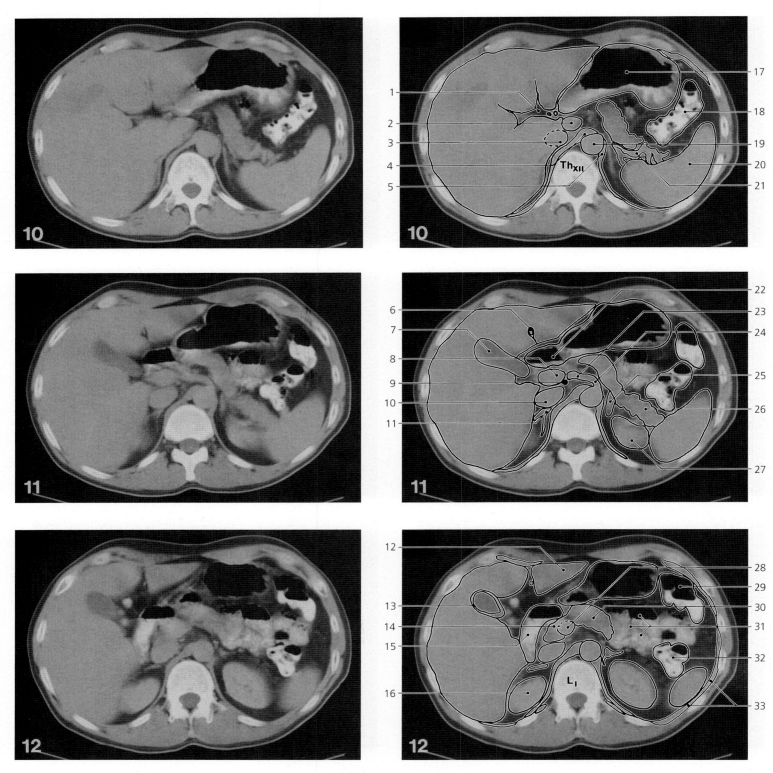

Abdomen, axial CT

Scout view on page 404

1: Porta hepatis
2: Portal vein
3: Inferior caval vein
4: Right crus of diaphragm
5: Left crus of diaphragm
6: Lig. teres hepatis
7: Gall bladder
8: Portal vein
9: Bile duct (choledochus)
10: Inferior caval vein
11: Right suprarenal gland

12: Left lobe of liver
13: Wall of gall bladder
14: Head of pancreas
15: Superior part of duodenum
16: Upper pole of right kidney
17: Body of stomach
18: Splenic flexure of colon
19: Abdominal aorta
20: Spleen
21: Splenic vessels
22: Duodenal "cap" (bulbus)

23: Common hepatic artery
24: Celiac trunk
25: Left suprarenal gland
26: Tail of pancreas
27: Upper pole of left kidney
28: Portal vein behind pancreas
29: Transverse colon
30: Body of pancreas
31: Jejunum with air and barium
32: Descending colon
33: Diaphragm

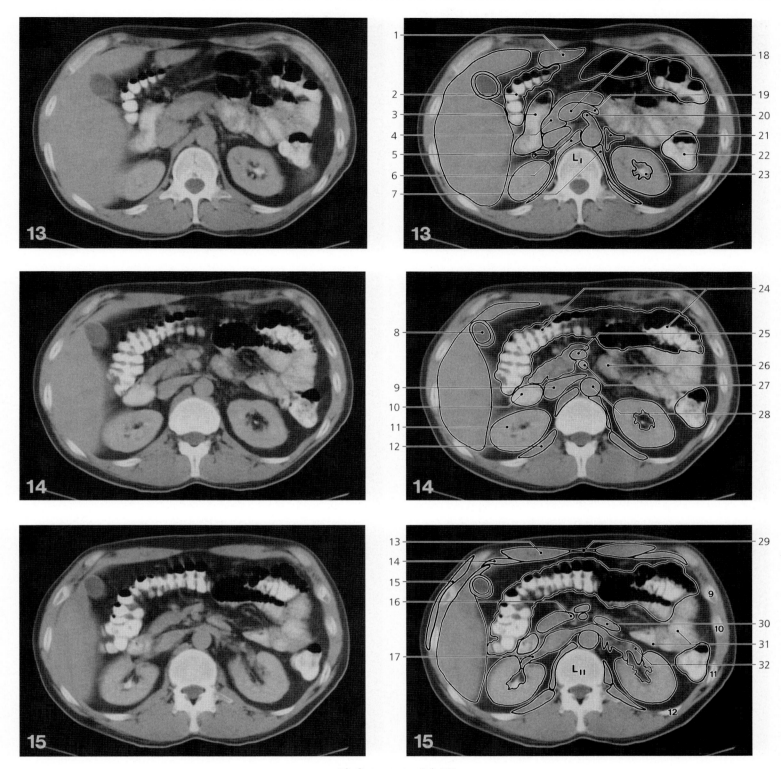

Abdomen, axial CT

Scout view on page 404

1: Left lobe of liver
2: Hepatic flexure of colon
3: Superior part of duodenum
4: Head of pancreas
5: Right suprarenal gland
6: Right crus of diaphragm
7: Left crus of diaphragm
8: Fundus of gall bladder
9: Inferior caval vein
10: Descending part of duodenum
11: Right kidney

12: Quadratus lumborum
13: Rectus abdominis
14: Transversus abdominis
15: Obliquus externus abdominis
16: Uncinate process of pancreas
17: Right renal vein
18: Portal vein
19: Splenic vein
20: Superior mesenteric artery
21: Left suprarenal gland
22: Descending colon

23: Sinus renalis
24: Transverse colon
25: Superior mesenteric vein
26: Duodenojejunal flexure
27: Superior mesenteric artery
28: Abdominal aorta
29: Linea alba
30: Ascending part of duodenum
31: Jejunum
32: Left renal vein

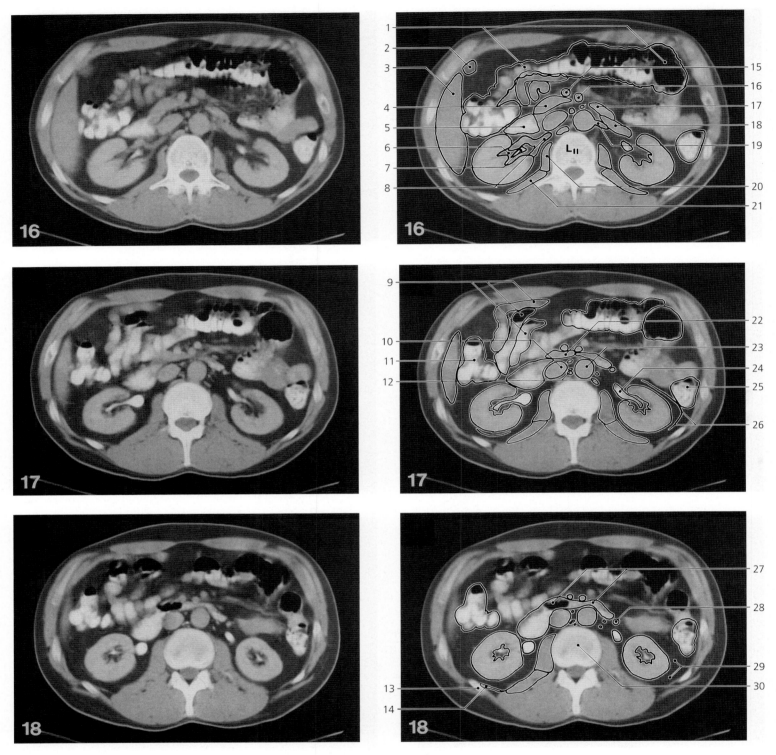

Abdomen, axial CT

Scout view on page 404

1: Transverse colon with air and contrast
2: Fundus of gall bladder
3: Right lobe of liver
4: Head of pancreas
5: Descending part of duodenum
6: Sinus renalis dxt.
7: Pelvis of right kidney
8: Right renal artery
9: Jejunum
10: Inferior caval vein

11: Ascending colon
12: Paraaortic lymph nodes
13: 12th rib
14: Lateral arcuate ligament
15: Superior mesenteric vein
16: Superior mesenteric artery
17: Ascending part of duodenum
18: Left renal vein
19: Left renal artery
20: Psoas major
21: Quadratus lumborum

22: Uncinate process of pancreas
23: Abdominal aorta
24: Pelvis of left kidney
25: Descending colon
26: Renal fascia
27: Horizontal part of duodenum
28: Inferior mesenteric vein
29: Retroperitoneal fat
30: Intervertebral disc L II – L III

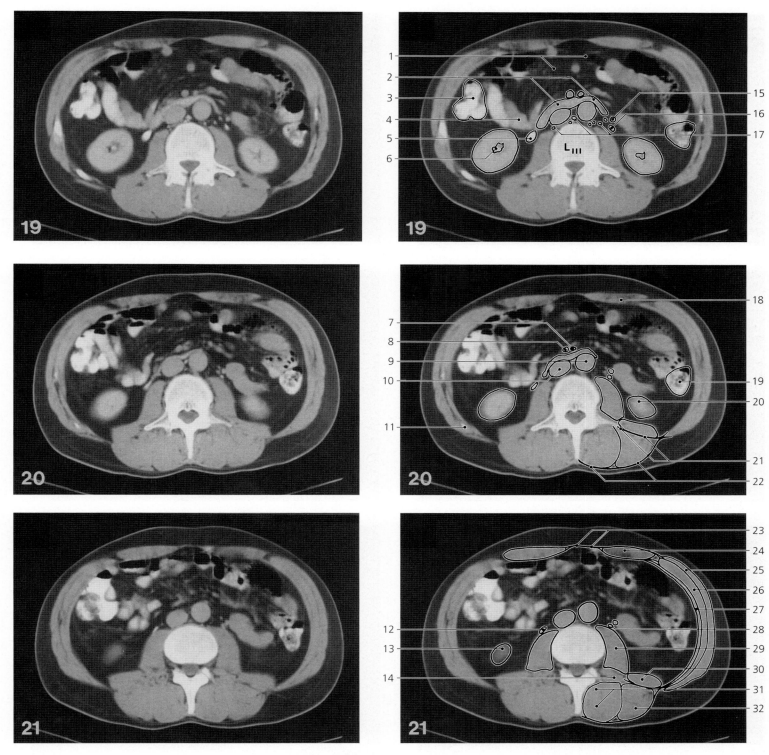

Abdomen, axial CT

Scout view on page 404

1: Mesenterial fat
2: Horizontal part of duodenum
3: Ascending colon
4: Jejunum
5: Pelvis of right kidney
6: Sinus renalis dxt.
7: Superior mesenteric artery
8: Superior mesenteric vein
9: Abdominal aorta
10: Inferior caval vein
11: 12th rib (tip)
12: Right ureter

13: Lower pole of right kidney
14: Intertransversarius muscle
15: Inferior mesenteric vein
16: Pelvis of left kidney
17: Lumbar lymph nodes
18: Tendinous intersection in rectus abdominis
19: Descending colon
20: Lower pole of left kidney
21: Lumbar aponeurosis
22: Thoracolumbar fascia
23: Linea alba

24: Rectus abdominis
25: Obliquus externus abdominis
26: Obliquus internus abdominis
27: Transversus abdominis
28: Left ureter
29: Psoas major
30: Quadratus lumborum
31: Transversospinal muscles
32: Iliocostalis lumborum, and longissimus thoracis

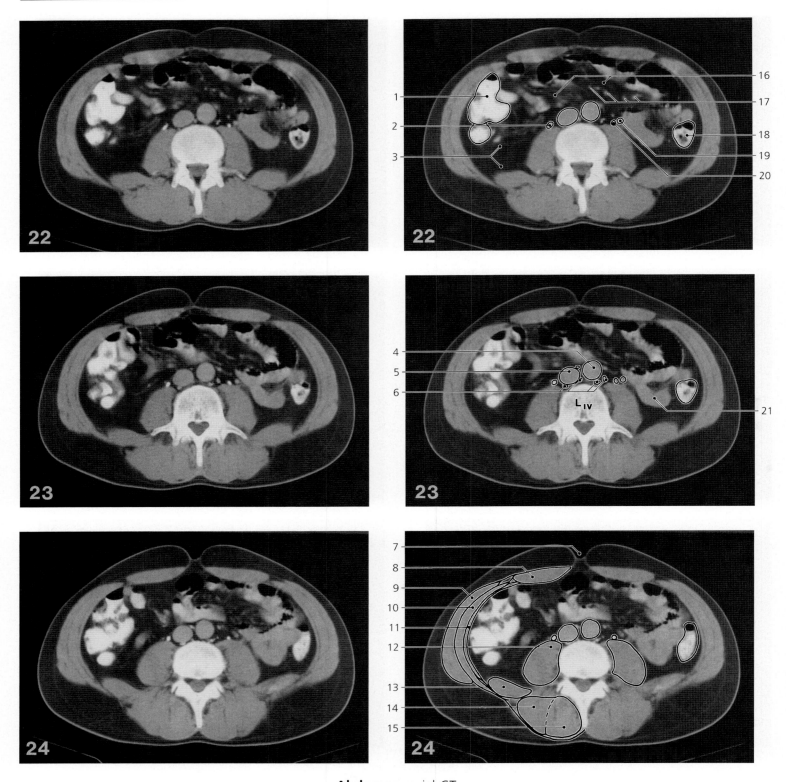

Abdomen, axial CT

Scout view on page 404

1: Ascending colon
2: Right ureter
3: Retroperitoneal fat
4: Abdominal aorta
5: Inferior caval vein
6: Paraaortic lymph nodes
7: Umbilicus
8: Rectus abdominis

9: Obliquus externus abdominis
10: Obliquus internus abdominis
11: Transversus abdominis
12: Psoas major
13: Quadratus lumborum
14: Erector spinae
15: Transversospinal muscles (mostly multifidi)

16: Mesenterial fat
17: Mesenterial vessels
18: Descending colon
19: Inferior mesenteric vein
20: Left ureter
21: Small intestinal loop

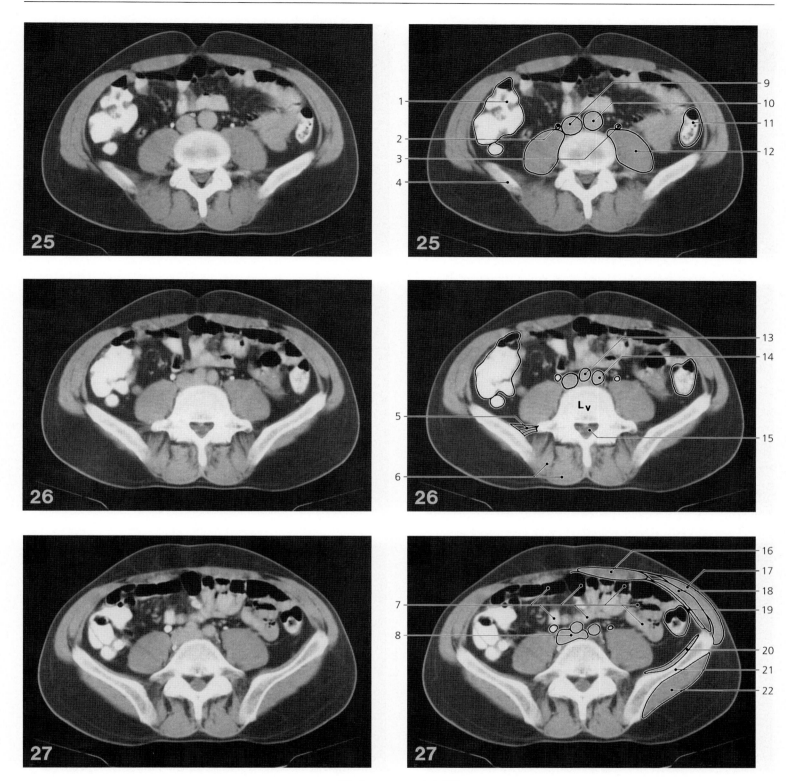

Abdomen, axial CT

Scout view on page 404

1: Ascending colon
2: Right ureter
3: Left ureter
4: Iliac crest
5: Iliolumbar ligament
6: Erector spinae
7: Small intestine with barium and air
8: Inferior caval vein (bifurcation)

9: Inferior caval vein
10: Abdominal aorta
11: Descending colon
12: Psoas major
13: Right common iliac artery
14: Left common iliac artery
15: Cauda equina
16: Rectus abdominis

17: Obliquus externus abdominis
18: Obliquus internus abdominis
19: Transversus abdominis
20: Iliacus
21: Wing of ilium
22: Gluteus medius

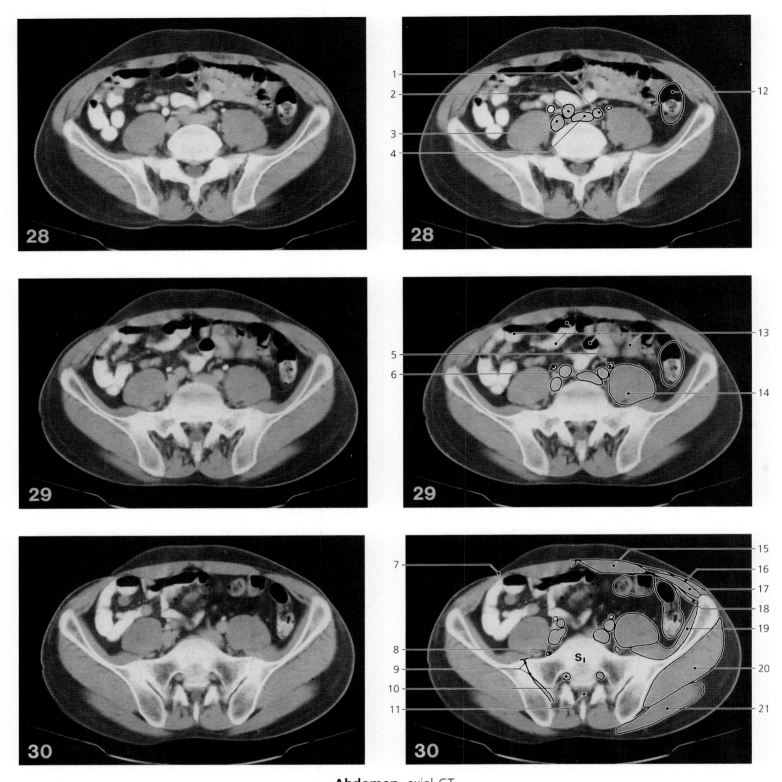

Abdomen, axial CT

Scout view on page 404

1: Left common iliac artery
2: Right common iliac artery
3: Right common iliac vein
4: Left common iliac vein
5: Left ureter
6: Right ureter
7: Appendectomy scar

8: Lumbosacral trunk
9: Sacro-iliac joint
10: Spinal nerve root S I
11: Cauda equina in sacral canal
12: Descending colon
13: Small intestine
14: Psoas major

15: Rectus abdominis
16: Obliquus externus abdominis
17: Obliquus internus abdominis
18: Transversus abdominis
19: Iliacus
20: Gluteus medius
21: Gluteus maximus

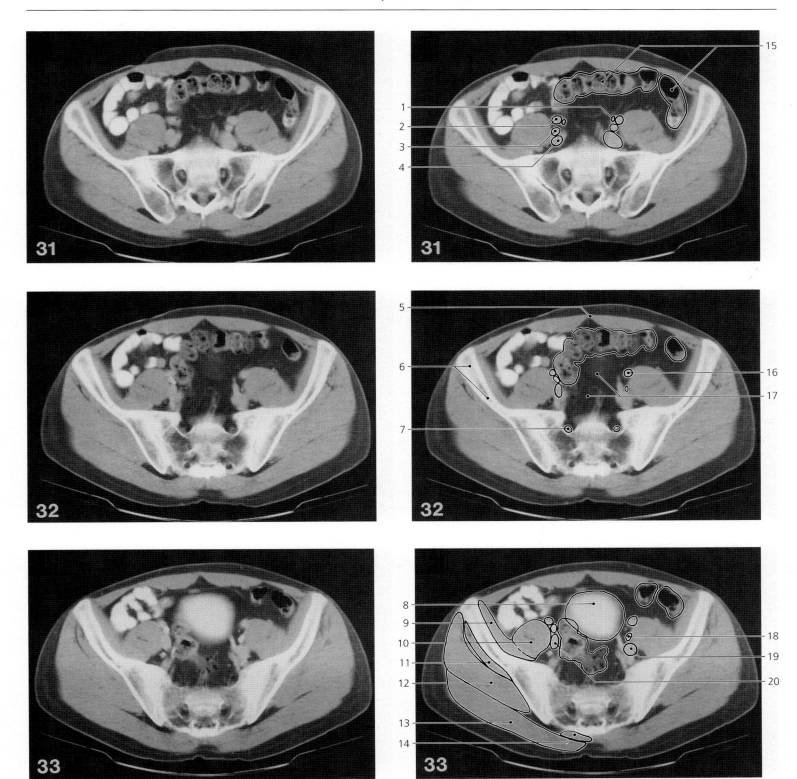

Abdomen, axial CT

Scout view on page 404

1: Left ureter
2: Right external iliac artery
3: Right internal iliac artery
4: Right common iliac vein
5: Linea alba
6: Ilium (wing)
7: Spinal nerve S I in pelvic sacral foramen

8: Urinary bladder
9: Iliacus
10: Psoas major
11: Gluteus minimus
12: Gluteus medius
13: Gluteus maximus
14: Erector spinae (origin)
15: Sigmoid colon

16: Left external iliac artery
17: Mesenterial fat
18: Left ureter
19: Left external iliac vein
20: Right external iliac vein

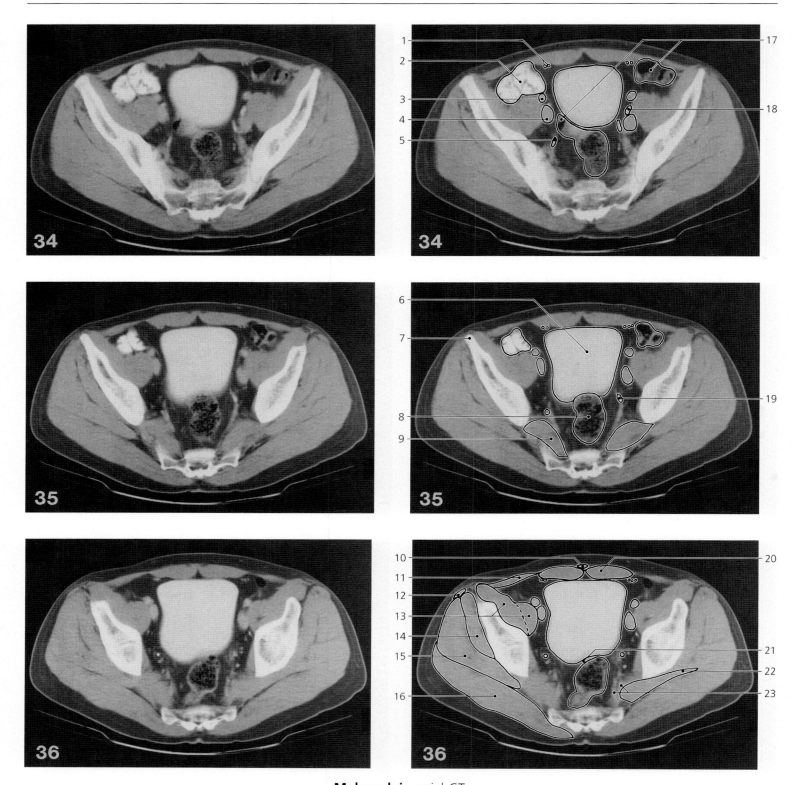

Male pelvis, axial CT

Scout view on page 404

1: Inferior epigastric artery and vein
2: Cecum
3: Right external iliac artery
4: Right external iliac vein
5: Right ureter
6: Urinary bladder
7: Anterior superior iliac spine
8: Rectum
9: Piriformis

10: Pyramidalis muscle
11: Obliquus externus, - internus, and transversus abdominis
12: Tensor fasciae latae (origin)
13: Iliopsoas
14: Gluteus minimus
15: Gluteus medius
16: Gluteus maximus
17: Sigmoid colon

18: External iliac lymph node with contrast medium
19: Left ureter
20: Rectus abdominis
21: Rectovesical fold
22: Piriformis (tendon)
23: Sacral plexus

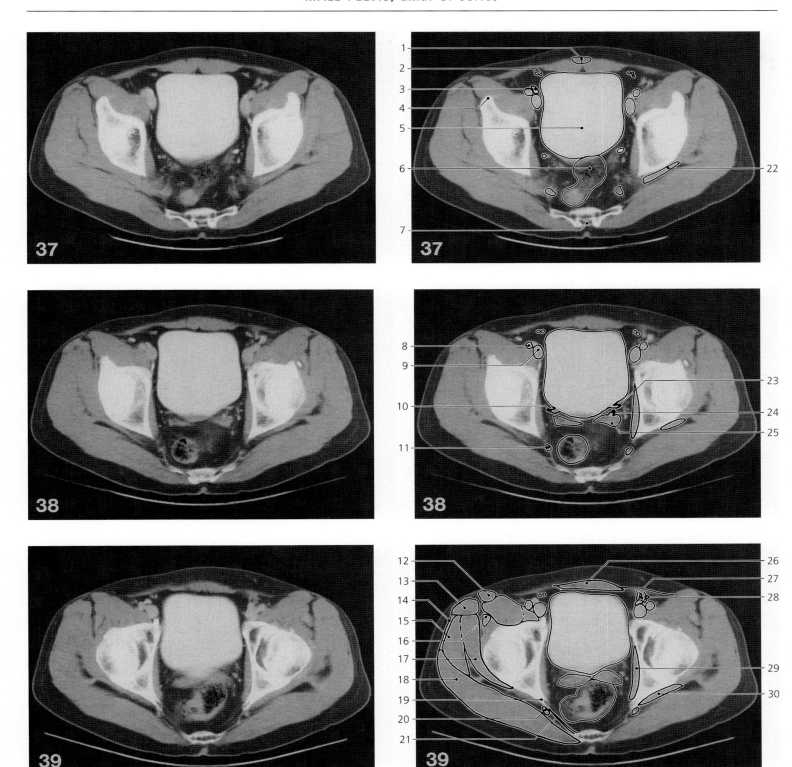

Male pelvis, axial CT

Scout view on page 404

1: Pyramidalis muscle
2: Inferior epigastric artery and vein
3: Lymph node with contrast medium
4: Anterior inferior iliac spine
5: Urinary bladder
6: Rectum
7: Hiatus sacralis
8: Right external iliac artery
9: Right external iliac vein
10: Right ureter
11: Sciatic nerve in infrapiriform foramen

12: Sartorius
13: Tensor fasciae latae
14: Iliotibial tract
15: Gluteus medius
16: Rectus femoris
17: Gluteus minimus
18: Gluteus maximus
19: Ischial spine
20: Sciatic nerve
21: Sacrospinous ligament
22: Piriformis (tendon)

23: Left ureter
24: Ductus deferens
25: Seminal vesicle
26: Rectus abdominis
27: Obliquus externus abdominis (aponeurosis)
28: Inferior epigastric vessels, testicular vessels and deferent duct
29: Obturatorius internus
30: Gemellus superior

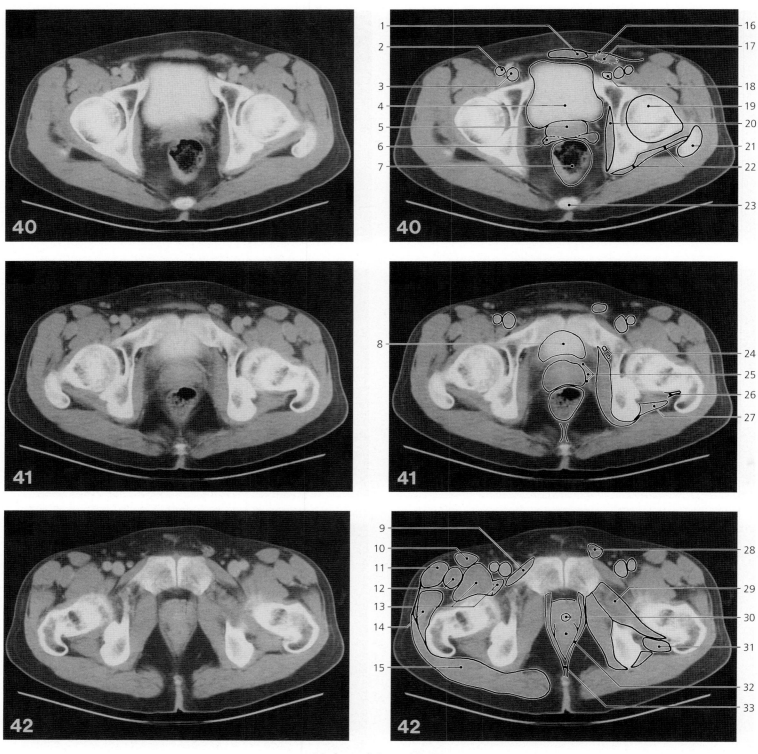

Male pelvis, axial CT

Scout view on page 404

1: Rectus abdominis (tendon)
2: Right external iliac artery
3: Right external iliac vein
4: Urinary bladder
5: Prostate
6: Seminal vesicle
7: Rectum
8: Fundus of urinary bladder
9: Pectineus
10: Sartorius
11: Tensor fasciae latae
12: Rectus femoris

13: Iliopsoas
14: Gluteus medius and minimus
15: Gluteus maximus
16: Superficial inguinal anulus
17: Spermatic cord
18: Deep inguinal lymph node
19: Head of femur
20: Obturatorius internus
21: Greater trochanter
22: Gemellus superior and obturatorius internus (tendon)
23: Coccyx

24: Obturator artery and nerve in obturator canal
25: Prostatic venous plexus
26: Obturatorius externus (tendon)
27: Gemellus inferior
28: Spermatic cord (removed on right side)
29: Obturatorius externus
30: Prostatic part of urethra
31: Quadratus femoris
32: Levator ani
33: Anococcygeal ligament

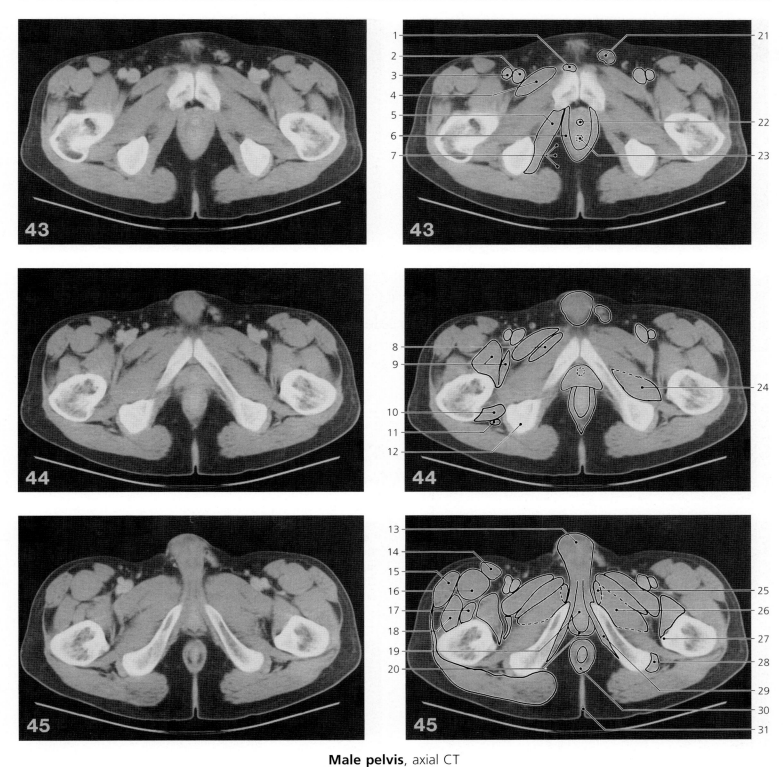

Male pelvis, axial CT

Scout view on page 404

1: Adductor longus (origin)
2: Femoral vein
3: Femoral artery
4: Pectineus
5: Obturatorius internus
6: Puborectalis
7: Ischiorectal fossa
8: Adductor longus
9: Iliopsoas
10: Quadratus femoris
11: Sciatic nerve

12: Ischial tuberosity
13: Penis
14: Sartorius
15: Tensor fasciae latae
16: Rectus femoris
17: Vastus intermedius
18: Vastus lateralis
19: Bulb of penis
20: Bulbocavernosus
21: Spermatic cord (removed on right side)

22: Prostatic part of urethra
23: Anal canal
24: Obturatorius externus
25: Gracilis
26: Adductor brevis
27: Lesser trochanter
28: Biceps femoris (origin)
29: Crus penis and ischiocavernosus
30: Anal sphincter muscles
31: Crena ani

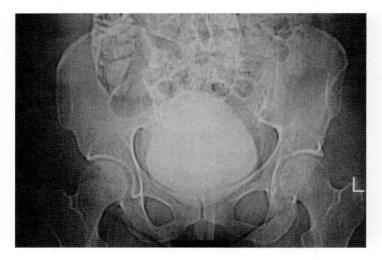
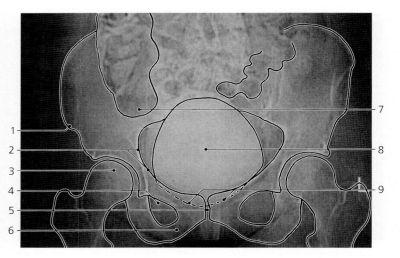

Scout view

1: Anterior superior iliac spine
2: Linea terminalis
3: Head of femur

4: Obturator foramen
5: Symphysis pubis
6: Inferior ramus of pubis

7: Cecum
8: Urinary bladder
9: Fundus of bladder

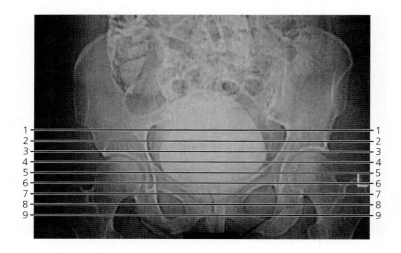

Scout view

Lines #1–9 indicate positions of sections in the following CT series.
Consecutive sections, 10 mm thick.
The gastrointestinal tract is outlined by peroral contrast medium.
The urinary tract is outlined by excretion of intravenous watersoluble contrast medium.

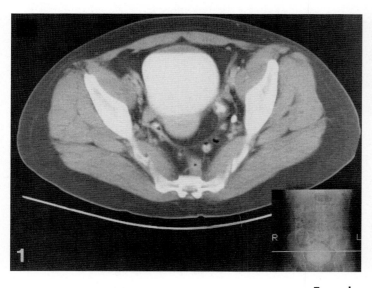
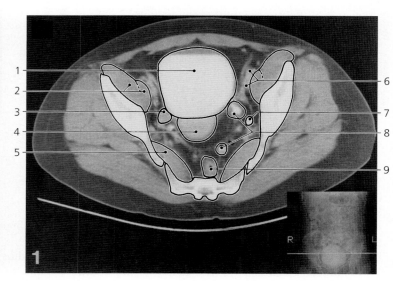

Female pelvis, axial CT

Scout view above

1: Urinary bladder
2: Iliopsoas
3: Right ovary

4: Corpus uteri
5: Piriformis
6: External iliac artery and vein

7: Left ureter
8: Sigmoid colon
9: Rectum

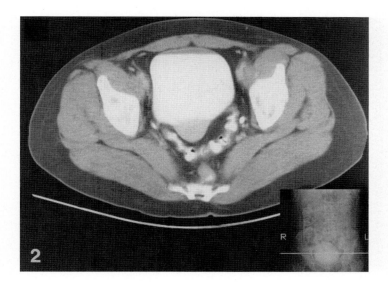

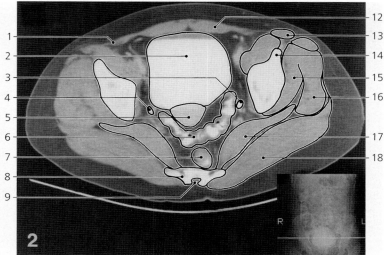

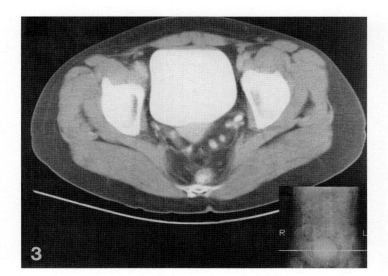

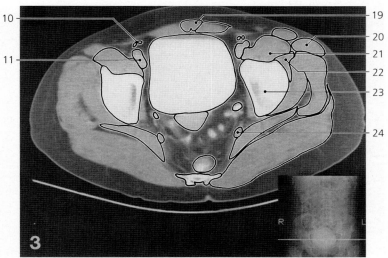

Female pelvis, axial CT

Scout view on page 420

1: Inguinal ligament
2: Urinary bladder
3: Left ureter
4: Right ureter
5: Corpus uteri
6: Sigmoid colon
7: Rectum
8: Sacrum

9: Hiatus sacralis
10: Inferior epigastric artery and vein
11: External iliac artery and vein
12: Rectus abdominis
13: Sartorius
14: Anterior inferior iliac spine
15: Gluteus minimus
16: Gluteus medius

17: Piriformis
18: Gluteus maximus
19: Pyramidalis muscle
20: Tensor fasciae latae
21: Iliopsoas
22: Rectus femoris
23: Body of ilium
24: Sciatic nerve

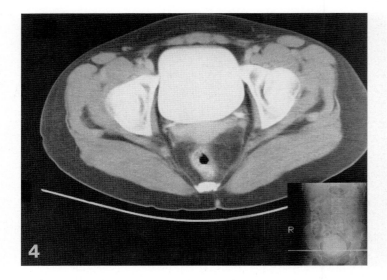

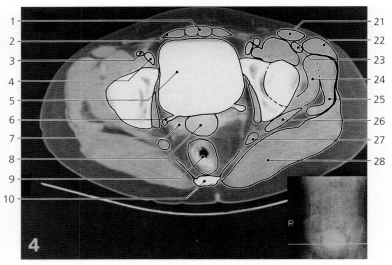

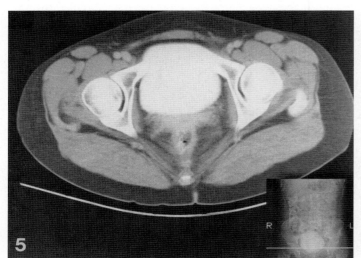

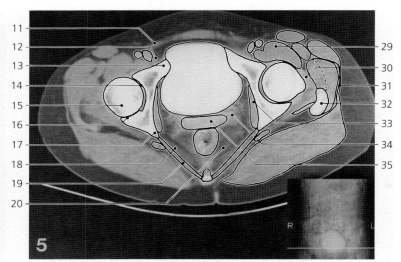

Female pelvis, axial CT

Scout view on page 420

1: Pyramidalis
2: Rectus abdominis
3: External iliac artery
4: External iliac vein
5: Urinary bladder
6: Right ureter
7: Parametrium
8: Cervix uteri
9: Rectum
10: Coccyx
11: Inguinal ligament
12: Deep inguinal lymph node

13: Superior ramus of pubis
14: Acetabular fossa
15: Head of femur
16: Lunate surface
17: Ischial spine
18: Coccygeus muscle
19: Sacrospinous ligament
20: Levator ani
21: Sartorius
22: Tensor fasciae latae
23: Rectus femoris
24: Gluteus minimus

25: Gluteus medius
26: Piriformis
27: Sciatic nerve
28: Gluteus maximus
29: Iliopsoas
30: Iliofemoral ligament
31: Iliotibial tract
32: Greater trochanter
33: Obturatorius internus
34: Vaginal venous plexus
35: Vagina

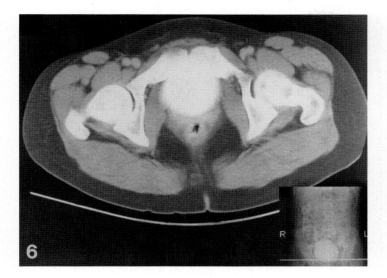

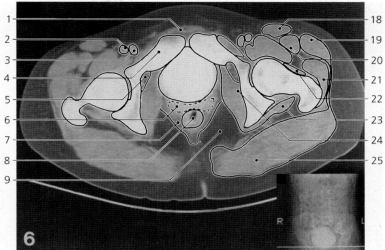

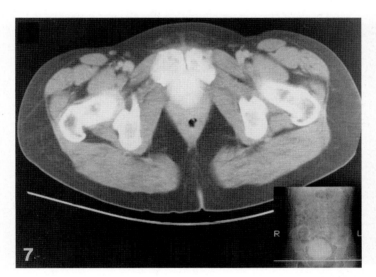

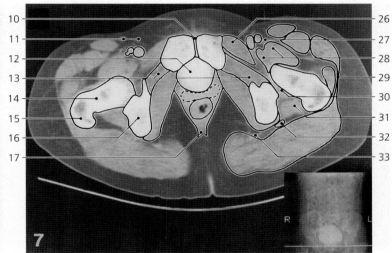

Female pelvis, axial CT

Scout view on page 420

1: Rectus abdominis, and pyramidalis
2: Femoral artery
3: Femoral vein
4: Superior ramus of pubis
5: Obturator canal
6: Vagina
7: Levator ani
8: Rectum
9: Ischiorectal fossa
10: Symphysis pubica
11: Superficial inguinal lymph nodes
12: Fundus of urinary bladder

13: Obturatorius externus
14: Neck of femur
15: Greater trochanter
16: Body of ischium
17: Anococcygeal ligament
18: Sartorius
19: Tensor fasciae latae
20: Rectus femoris
21: Gluteus medius and minimus
22: Iliofemoral ligament
23: Gemelli and tendon of obturatorius internus

24: Obturatorius internus
25: Gluteus maximus
26: Pectineus
27: Femoral nerve
28: Iliopsoas
29: Iliotibial tract
30: Ischiofemoral ligament
31: Quadratus femoris
32: Sciatic nerve
33: Sacrotuberal ligament

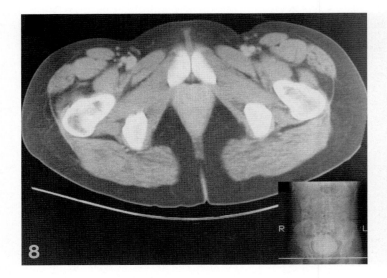

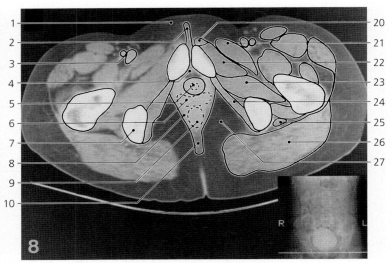

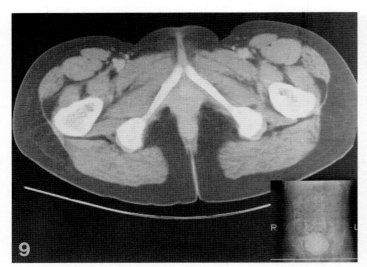

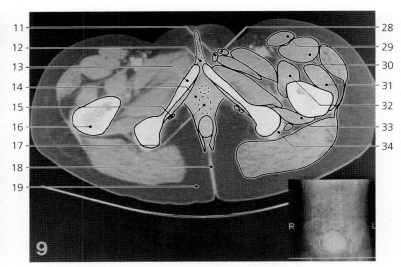

Female pelvis, axial CT

Scout view on page 420

1: Mons pubis (Veneris)
2: Rima pudendi
3: Femoral artery and vein
4: Subarcuate lacuna
5: Urethra feminina, and sphinchter urethrae externa
6: Vagina
7: Ischial tuberosity
8: Levator ani
9: Anal canal
10: Anococcygeal ligament
11: Gracilis
12: Clitoris

13: Inferior ramus of pubis
14: Bulb of vestibule
15: Internal pudendal artery and vein, and pudendal nerve
16: Femur
17: Vestibule of vagina
18: Crena ani
19: Subcutaneous fat
20: Adductor longus (origin)
21: Pectineus
22: Adductor brevis
23: Obturatorius externus
24: Obturatorius internus

25: Sciatic nerve
26: Gluteus maximus
27: Ischiorectal fossa
28: Adductor longus (tendon)
29: Sartorius
30: Rectus femoris
31: Vastus lateralis
32: Iliopsoas
33: Quadratus femoris
34: Common origin of semimembranosus, semitendinosus, and biceps femoris

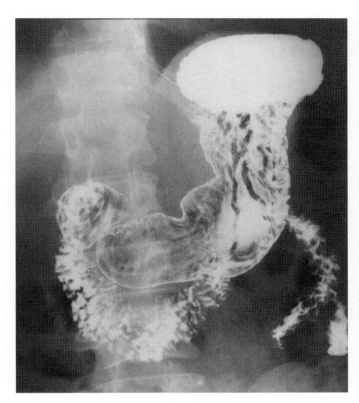
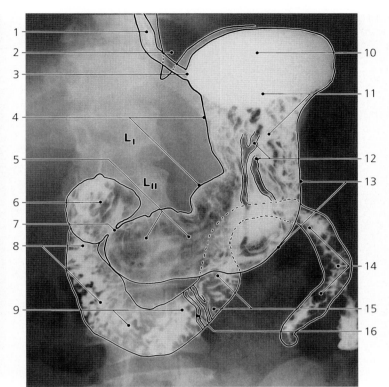

Stomach and duodenum, oblique X-ray, barium meal, double contrast

1: Esophagus
2: Left lung
3: Cardia
4: Lesser curvature of stomach
5: Pyloric antrum
6: Duodenal "cap" (bulbus)

7: Pyloric orifice
8: Descending part of duodenum
9: Horizontal part of duodenum
10: Fundus of stomach
11: Body of stomach
12: Rugae gastricae

13: Greater curvature of stomach
14: Jejunum
15: Ascending part of duodenum
16: Circular folds (Kerckring)

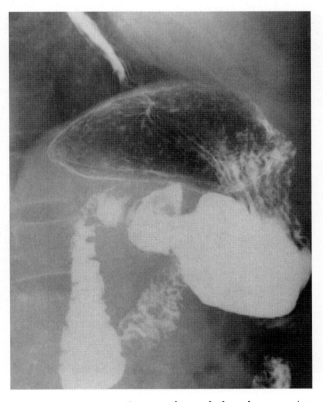
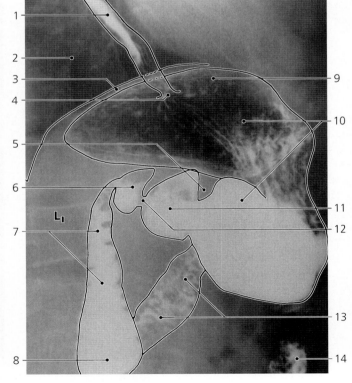

Stomach and duodenum, lateral X-ray, barium meal, double contrast

1: Esophagus
2: Lung
3: Diaphragm and gastric wall
4: Cardia
5: Contraction furrow

6: Duodenal "cap" (bulbus)
7: Descending part of duodenum
8: Horizontal part of duodenum
9: Fundus of stomach
10: Body of stomach

11: Pyloric antrum
12: Pyloric orifice
13: Ascending part of duodenum
14: Jejunum

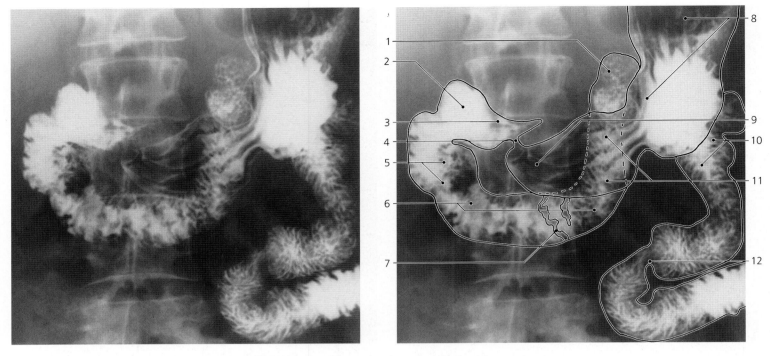

Duodenum, a-p X-ray, barium meal, double contrast

1: Duodenojejunal flexure
2: Superior part of duodenum
3: Duodenal cap (bulbus)
4: Pyloric canal

5: Descending part of duodenum
6: Horizontal part of duodenum
7: Circular folds (Kerckring)
8: Body of stomach

9: Pyloric antrum
10: Jejunum
11: Ascending part of duodenum
12: Peristaltic contraction in jejunum

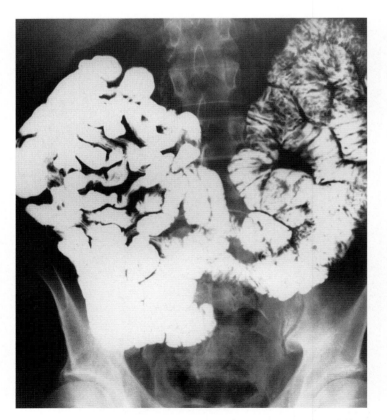
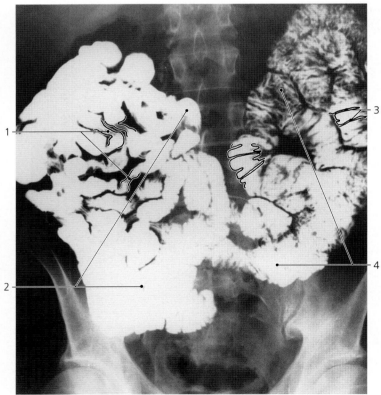

Jejunum and ileum, a-p X-ray, barium meal

1: Peristaltic contractions in ileum
2: Ileum

3: Circular folds in jejunum
4: Jejunum

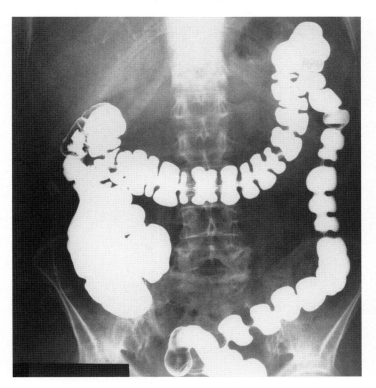
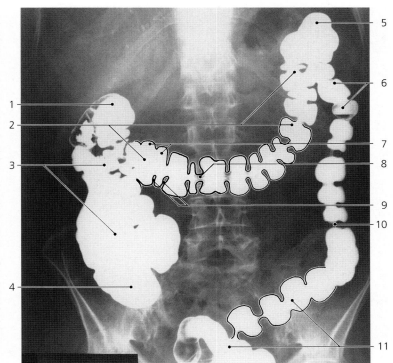

Colon, a-p X-ray, barium enema, single contrast

1: Hepatic flexure of colon
2: Transverse colon
3: Ascending colon
4: Cecum

5: Splenic flexure of colon
6: Descending colon
7: Haustra
8: Peristaltic contraction

9: Semilunar folds
10: Peristaltic contraction
11: Sigmoid colon

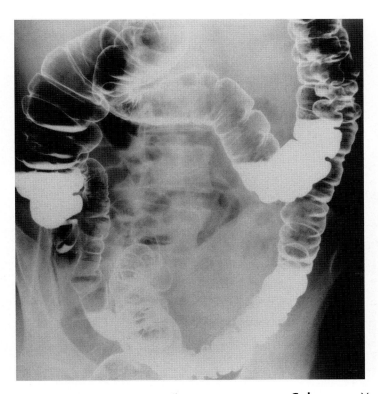
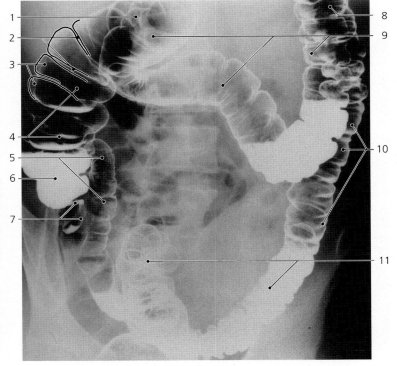

Colon, a-p X-ray, double contrast

1: Hepatic flexure of colon
2: Semilunar folds
3: Haustra
4: Ascending colon

5: Terminal ileum
6: Cecum
7: Vermiform appendix
8: Splenic flexure of colon

9: Transverse colon
10: Descending colon
11: Sigmoid colon

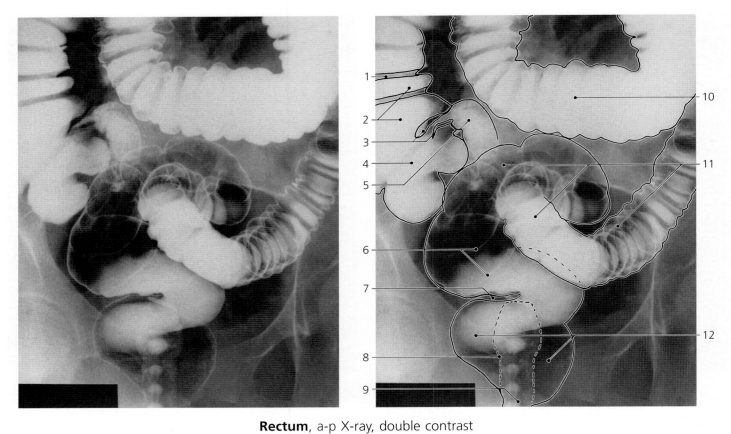

Rectum, a-p X-ray, double contrast

1: Semilunar fold
2: Ascending colon
3: Ileocaecal valve
4: Cecum

5: Terminal ileum
6: Rectum
7: Transverse fold of rectum
8: Tube

9: Anal canal
10: Transverse colon
11: Sigmoid colon
12: Rectal ampulla

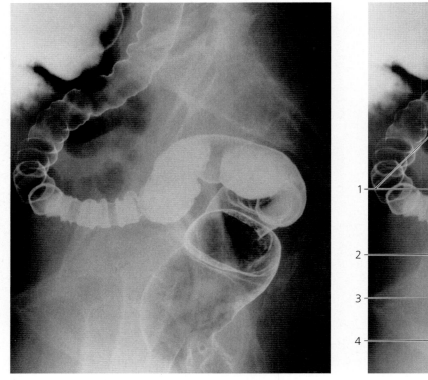

Rectum, lateral X-ray, double contrast

1: Sigmoid colon
2: Transverse fold of rectum
3: Rectal ampulla

4: Tube
5: Sacrum
6: Sacral flexure of rectum

7: Coccyx
8: Perineal flexure of rectum

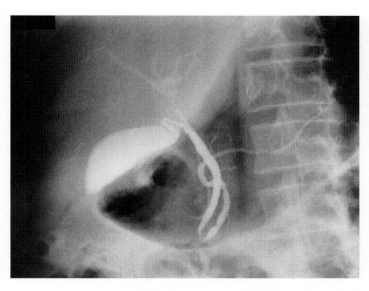
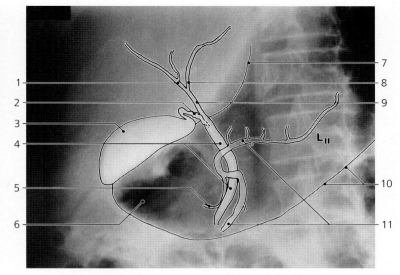

Biliary tract, a-p X-ray, endoscopic retrograde cholangio-pancreatography (ERCP)

1: Right hepatic duct
2: Cystic duct
3: Gall bladder
4: Bile duct (choledochus)

5: Accessory pancreatic duct (Santorini)
6: Pyloric antrum (air-filled)
7: Lesser curvature of stomach
8: Left hepatic duct

9: Common hepatic duct
10: Greater curvature of stomach
11: Pancreatic duct (Wirsung)

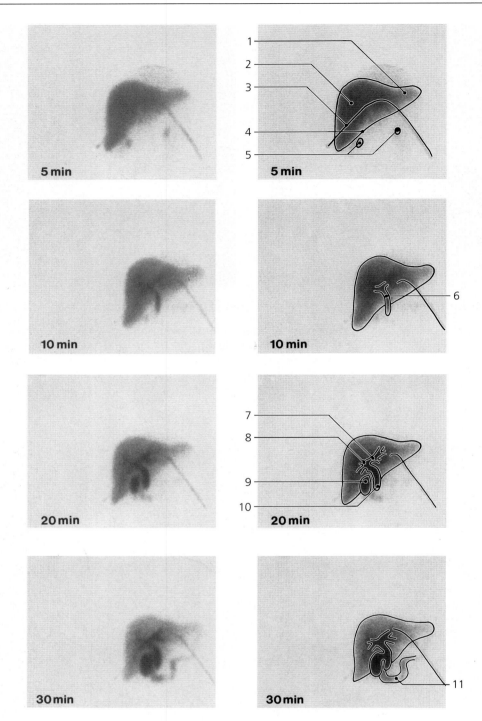

Biliary tract, ^{99m}Tc-HIDA, scintigraphy, anterior view

Biliary excretion of HIDA, 5, 10, 20 and 30 minutes after i.v. injection

1: Left lobe of liver
2: Right lobe of liver
3: Mark on rib curvature
4: Inferior margin of liver

5: Right and left renal pelvis
6: Common hepatic duct
7: Left hepatic duct
8: Right hepatic duct

9: Gall bladder
10: Bile duct (choledochus)
11: Duodenum

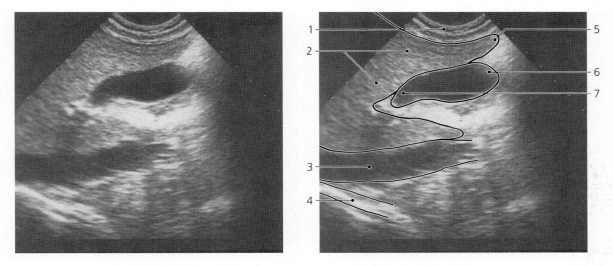

Gall bladder, subcostal sagittal section, US, deep inspiration

1: Anterior abdominal wall
2: Liver
3: Inferior caval vein

4: Diaphragm
5: Inferior margin of liver

6: Fundus of gall bladder
7: Neck of gall bladder

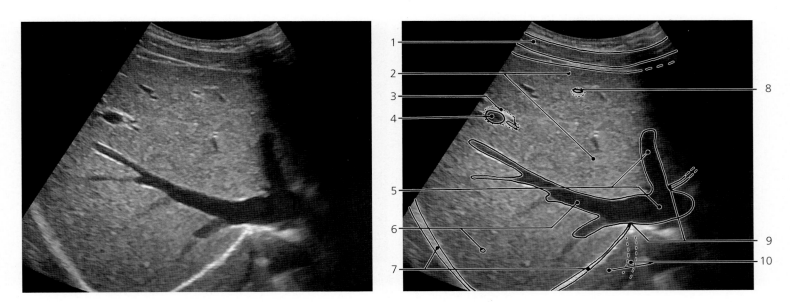

Liver, subcostal, tilted transverse section, US

1: Abdominal wall muscles
2: Right liver lobe
3: Periportal connective tissue
4: Portal vein (large branch)

5: Inferior caval vein and middle hepatic vein
6: Right hepatic vein and small hepatic vein

7: Diaphragm
8: Portal vein (small branch)
9: Caval opening in diaphragm
10: Mirror artefact

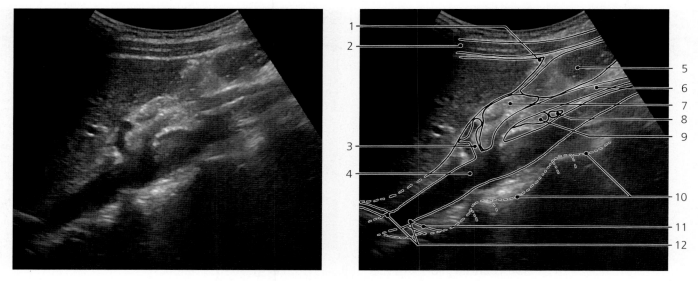

Upper abdomen, midline sagittal section, US

1: Inferior margin of liver
2: Abdominal muscles
3: Celiac trunk
4: Aorta

5: Stomach
6: Superior mesenteric artery
7: Pancreas (body)
8: Left renal vein

9: Pancreas (uncinate process)
10: Vertebral column
11: Diaphragm
12: Aortic hiatus

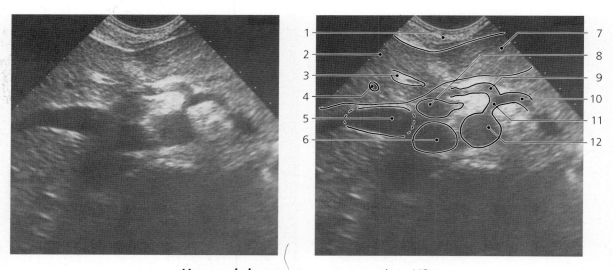

Upper abdomen, transverse section, US

1: Anterior abdominal wall
2: Right lobe of liver
3: Portal tract
4: Hepatic vein

5: Gall bladder
6: Inferior caval vein
7: Left lobe of liver
8: Portal vein

9: Common hepatic artery
10: Splenic artery
11: Celiac trunk
12: Abdominal aorta

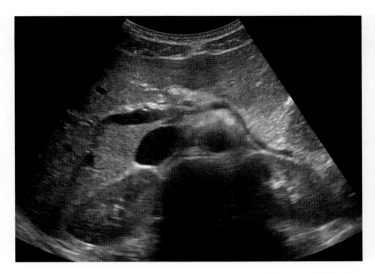
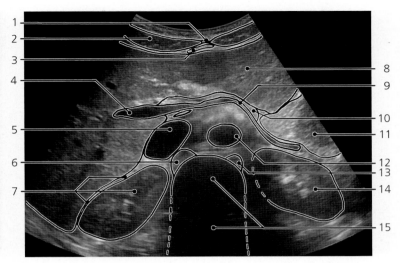

Upper abdomen, transverse section, US

1: Linea alba
2: Rectus abdominis
3: Falciform ligament of liver
4: Portal vein
5: Inferior caval vein
6: Diaphragm (right crus)

7: Right kidney and hepatorenal recess (Morrison's pouch)
8: Left lobe of liver
9: Splenic vein
10: Pancreas (tail)
11: Stomach

12: Aorta
13: Diaphragm (left crus)
14: Left kidney
15: Vertebral body (with acoustic shadow)

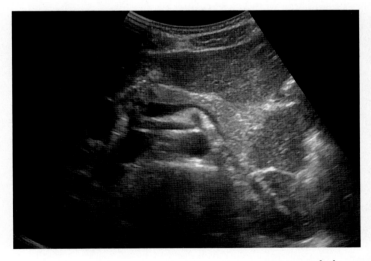
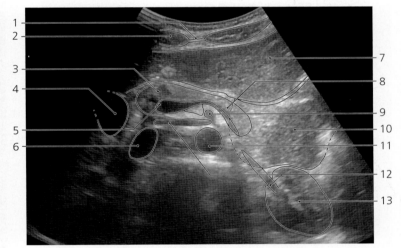

Upper abdomen, transverse section, US

1: Linea alba
2: Rectus abdominis
3: Pancreas (head)
4: Gall bladder
5: Portal vein

6: Inferior caval vein
7: Left lobe of liver
8: Pancreas (tail)
9: Superior mesenteric artery
10: Stomach

11: Aorta
12: Left renal vein
13: Left kidney

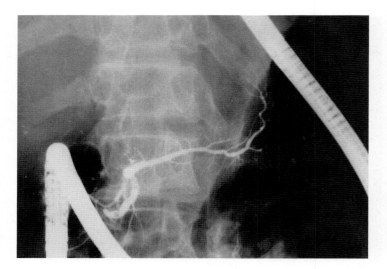
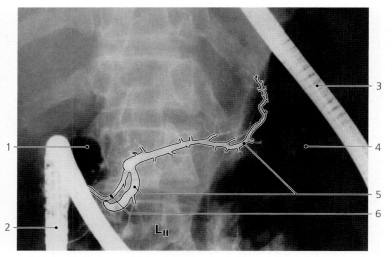

Pancreatic ducts, a-p X-ray, endoscopic retrograde pancreatography

1: Duodenal "cap" (with air)
2: Endoscope in descending part of duodenum

3: Endoscope in stomach
4: Body of stomach (inflated)
5: Pancreatic duct (Wirsung)

6: Accessory pancreatic duct (Santorini)

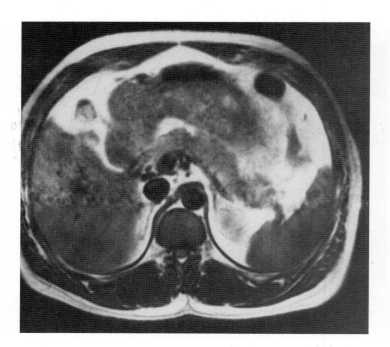
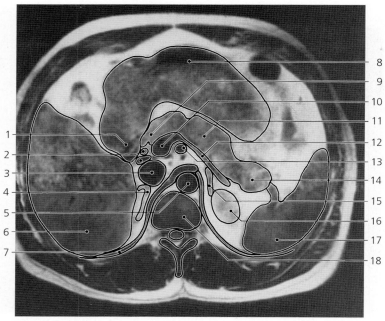

Upper abdomen with pancreas, axial MR

1: Duodenum
2: Bile duct and hepatic artery proper
3: Inferior caval vein
4: Right suprarenal gland
5: Aorta in aortic aperture of diaphragm
6: Liver

7: Lumbar part of diaphragm
8: Stomach
9: Head of pancreas
10: Portal vein
11: Body of pancreas
12: Splenic vein

13: Superior mesenteric artery
14: Tail of pancreas
15: Left suprarenal gland
16: Upper pole of left kidney
17: Spleen
18: Intervertebral disc Th XII – L I

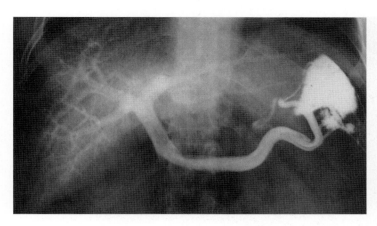
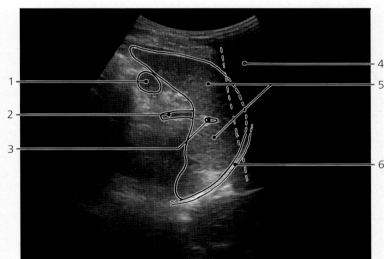

Spleen and liver, a-p X-ray, spleno-portography

1: **Left branch of portal vein**
2: **Right branch of portal vein**
3: **Portal vein**
4: **Superior mesenteric vein (entrance)**
5: **Inferior mesenteric vein (entrance)**
6: **Portal branch in left lobe of liver**
7: **Spleen**
8: **Splenic vein**

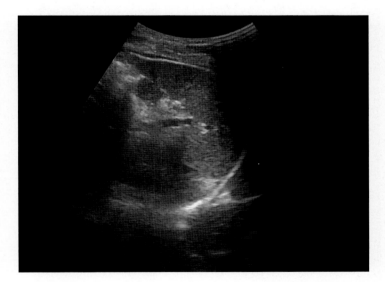

Spleen, transverse intercostal section, US

1: **Accessory spleen**
2: **Splenic vein**
3: **Splenic vessel**
4: **Acoustic shadow of rib**
5: **Spleen**
6: **Diaphragm**

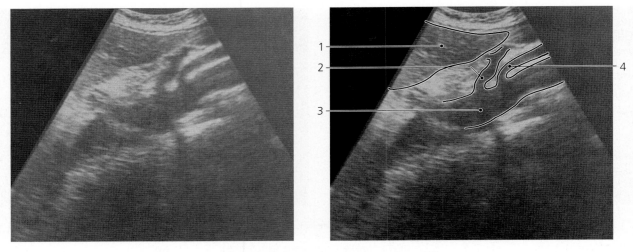

Abdominal aorta, sagittal section, US

1: Liver
2: Celiac trunk

3: Abdominal aorta
4: Superior mesenteric artery

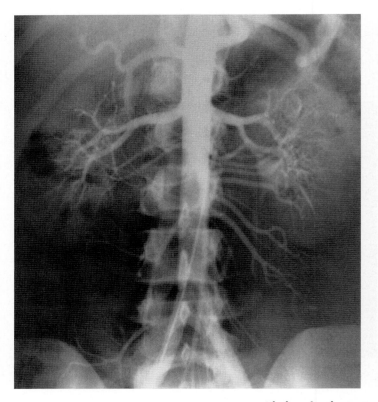
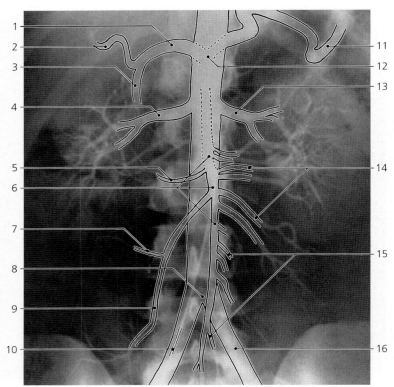

Abdominal aorta, a-p X-ray, aortography

1: Common hepatic artery
2: Hepatic artery proper
3: Gastroduodenal artery
4: Right renal artery
5: Middle colic artery
6: Superior mesenteric artery

7: Right colic artery
8: Aortic bifurcation
9: Iliocolic artery
10: Catheter
11: Splenic artery
12: Celiac trunk

13: Left renal artery
14: Jejunal arteries
15: Ileal arteries
16: Left common iliac artery

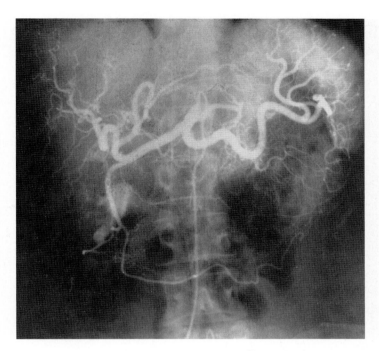
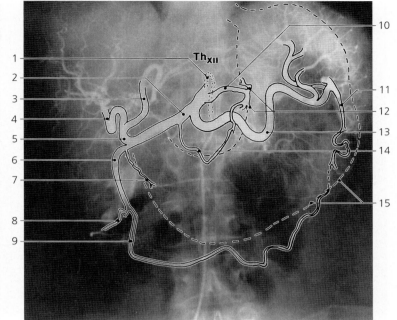

Celiac trunk, a-p X-ray, arteriography (arterial phase)

1: Catheter tip in celiac trunk
2: Common hepatic artery
3: Left branch of hepatic artery
4: Right branch of hepatic artery
5: Hepatic artery proper
6: Gastroduodenal artery
7: Supraduodenal artery
8: Superior pancreatico-duodenal artery
9: Right gastro-omental artery
10: Left gastric artery
11: Left gastro-omental artery
12: Branches of left gastric artery
13: Splenic artery
14: Right gastric artery
15: Contour of ventricle (stippled)

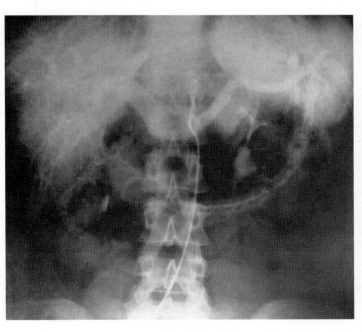
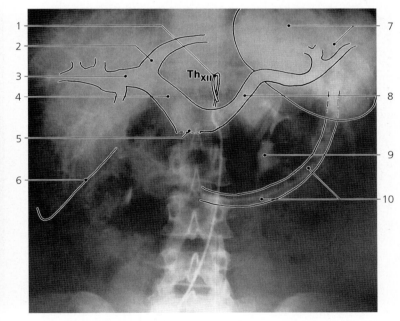

Portal vein, a-p X-ray, venous phase of celiac arteriography (see above)

1: Catheter in celiac trunk
2: Left branch of portal vein
3: Right branch of portal vein
4: Portal vein
5: Superior mesenteric vein (entrance)
6: Lower margin of liver
7: Spleen
8: Splenic vein
9: Pelvis of left kidney
10: Gastric wall (greater curvature)

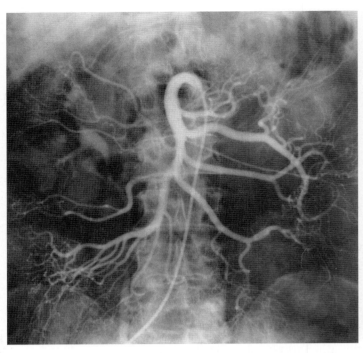

Superior mesenteric artery, a-p X-ray, arteriography

1: Superior mesenteric artery
2: Middle colic artery
3: Right colic artery

4: Ileocolic artery
5: Catheter

6: Jejunal arteries
7: Ileal arteries

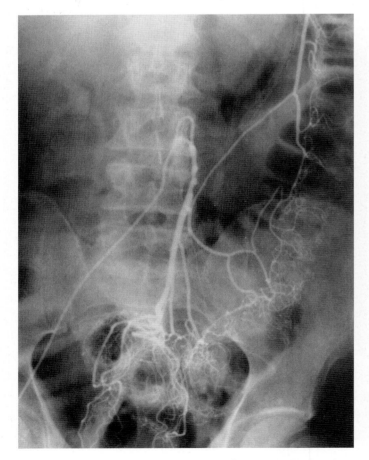
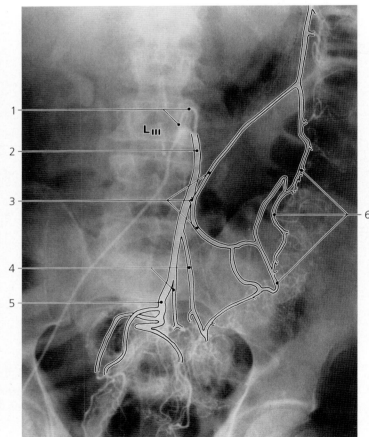

Inferior mesenteric artery, a-p X-ray, arteriography

1: Catheter
2: Inferior mesenteric artery

3: Left colic artery
4: Sigmoid arteries

5: Superior rectal artery
6: Marginal artery

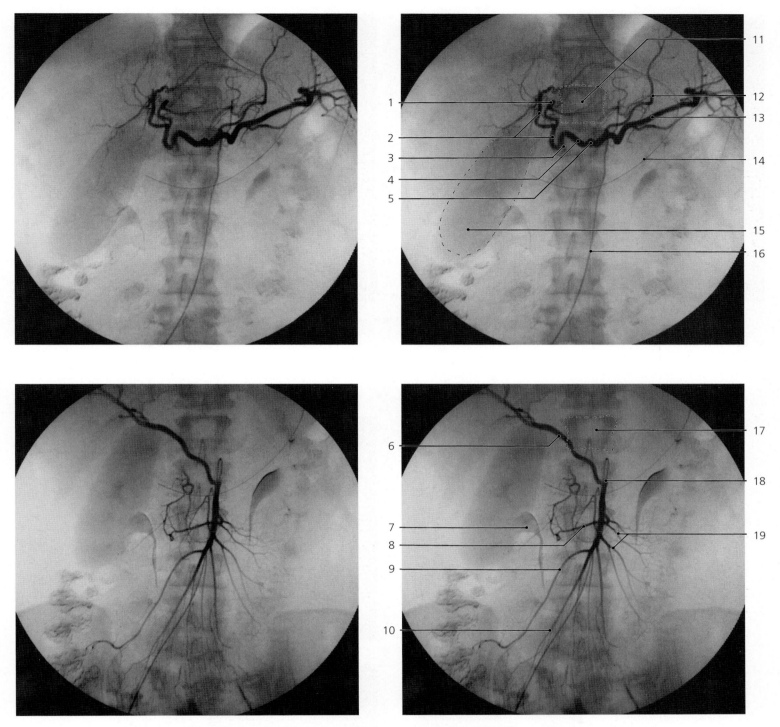

Celiac trunk and superior mesenteric artery, variation (15%), a-p X-ray, arteriography

Right hepatic artery originating from superior mesenteric artery

1: Right gastric artery
2: Left hepatic artery
3: Gastroduodenal artery
4: Common hepatic artery
5: Celiac trunk
6: Right hepatic artery
7: Renal pelvis
8: Middle colic artery
9: Right colic artery
10: Iliocolic artery
11: First lumbar vertebra
12: Left gastric artery
13: Splenic artery
14: Catheter in stomach
15: Gall bladder
16: Catheter in aorta
17: First lumbar vertebra
18: Superior mesenteric artery
19: Jejunal arteries

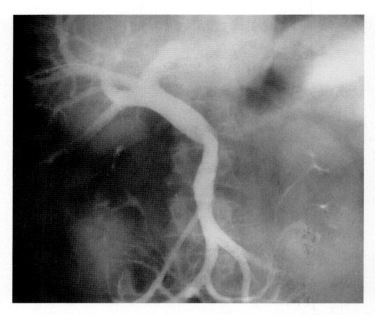

Superior mesenteric vein, a-p X-ray, transhepatic phlebography

1: Left branch of portal vein	4: Portal vein	7: Splenic vein (entrance)
2: Transhepatic catheter	5: Superior mesenteric vein	8: Pelvis of left kidney (duplex)
3: Right branch of portal vein	6: Middle colic vein	9: Jejunal veins

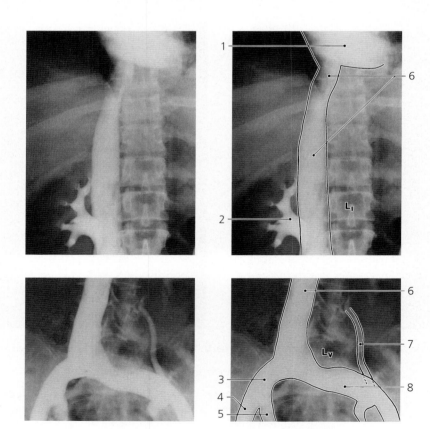

Inferior caval vein, a-p X-ray, phlebography

1: Right atrium	4: Right external iliac vein	7: Left ureter
2: Pelvis of right kidney	5: Right internal iliac vein	8: Left common iliac vein
3: Right common iliac vein	6: Inferior caval vein	

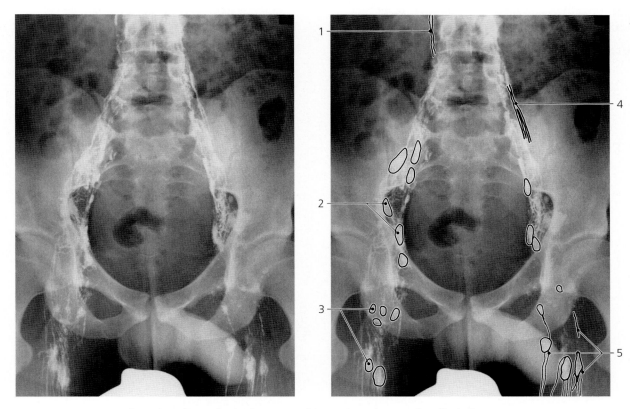

Lumbar lymph system, a-p X-ray, lymphography, first day

Bilateral infusion of contrast medium via lymphatic vessels on feet

1: Right lumbar trunk
2: External iliac lymph nodes

3: Superficial inguinal lymph nodes
4: Major iliolumbar lymphatic vessels

5: Afferent and efferent lymphatic vessels
   of superficial inguinal lymph nodes

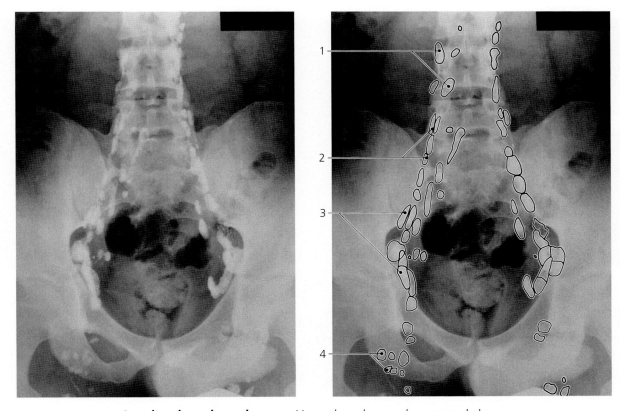

Lumbar lymph nodes, a-p X-ray, lymphography, second day

1: Lumbar (paraaortic) lymph nodes
2: Common iliac lymph nodes

3: External iliac lymph nodes

4: Superficial inguinal lymph nodes

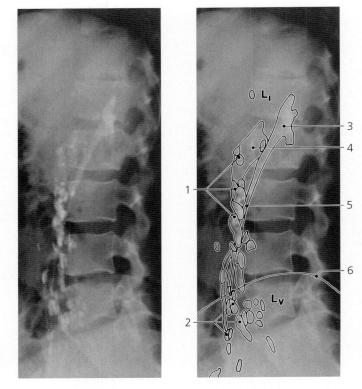

Lumbar lymph nodes, lateral X-ray, lymphography (second day), and intravenous urography

1: Lumbar (paraaortic) lymph nodes   3: Pelvis of left kidney   5: Left ureter
2: Common iliac lymph nodes   4: Pelvis of right kidney   6: Iliac crest

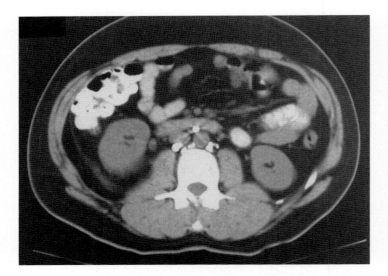 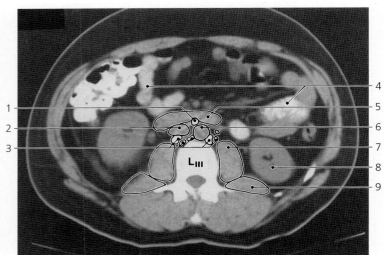

Lumbar lymph nodes, axial CT, after lymphography and peroral contrast

1: Lumbar (preaortic) lymph node   4: Small intestine   7: Psoas major
2: Inferior caval vein   5: Horizontal part of duodenum   8: Left kidney
3: Lumbar (paraaortic) lymph nodes   6: Abdominal aorta   9: Quadratus lumborum

Urogenital System

Kidney

Urinary bladder and urethra

Male genital organs

Female genital organs/embryo

Fetus

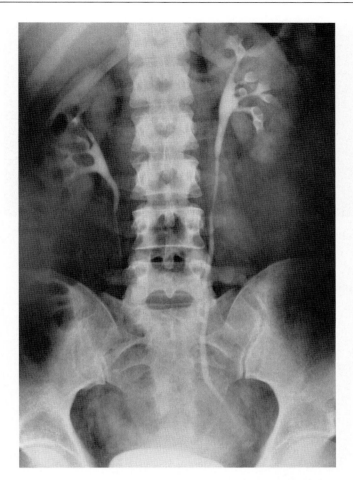

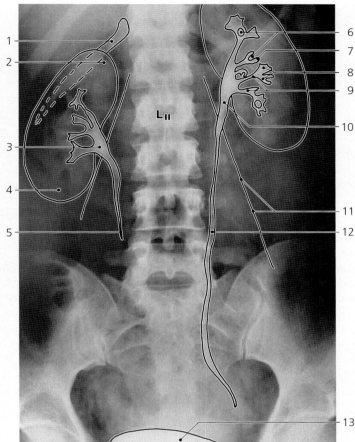

Urinary tract, a-p X-ray, i.v. urography

15 min after intravenous contrast

1: 12th rib
2: Upper pole of right kidney
3: Pelvis of right kidney
4: Lower pole of right kidney
5: Right ureter

6: Renal papillae
7: Fornix of minor calyx
8: Minor calices
9: Major calices
10: Pelvis of left kidney

11: Psoas major (lateral contour)
12: Left ureter
13: Urinary bladder

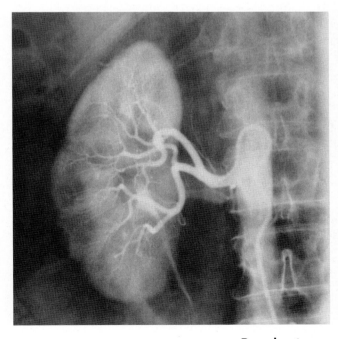

Renal artery, a-p X-ray, arteriography

1: Arcuate arteries
2: Interlobular arteries
3: Interlobar arteries

4: Inferior suprarenal artery
5: Right renal artery

6: Segmental arteries
7: Right ureter

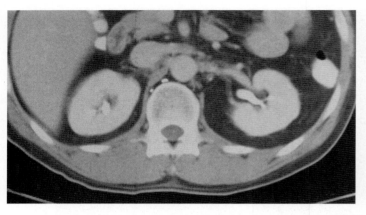
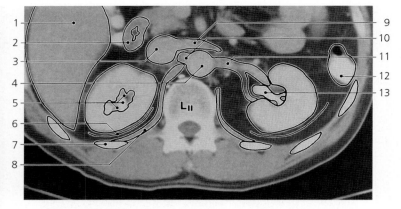

Kidneys, axial CT, after intravenous and peroral contrast

1: Liver
2: Descending part of duodenum
3: Inferior caval vein
4: Abdominal aorta
5: Renal sinus

6: Renal fascia
7: 12th rib
8: Lumbar part of diaphragm
9: Left renal vein
10: Right renal artery

11: Left renal artery
12: Descending colon
13: Pelvis of left kidney

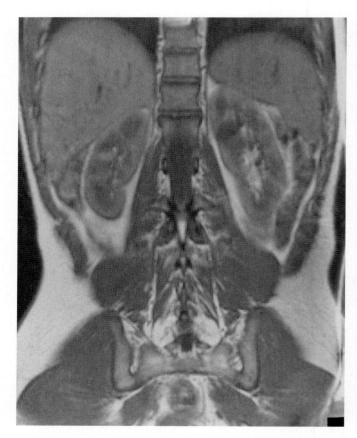
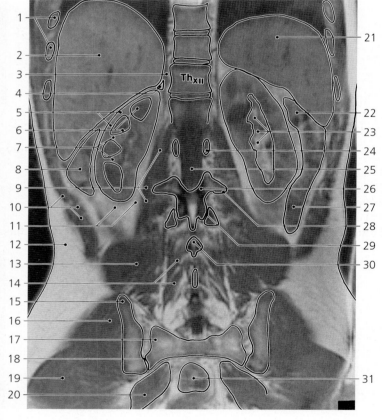

Kidneys, coronal MR, T1 weighted recording

1: Ribs
2: Liver
3: Lumbar part of diaphragm
4: Right suprarenal gland
5: Renal cortex
6: Renal pyramids
7: Renal columns
8: Ascending colon
9: Psoas major
10: Abdominal wall muscles
11: Perirenal fat

12: Subcutaneous fat
13: Quadratus lumborum
14: Transversospinal muscles
15: Iliac crest
16: Gluteus medius
17: Ala of sacrum
18: Sacro-iliac joint
19: Gluteus maximus
20: Piriformis
21: Spleen
22: Splenic flexure of colon

23: Renal sinus
24: Pedicle of vertebral arch L II
25: Vertebral canal
26: Lamina of vertebral arch L III
27: Descending colon
28: Transverse process of L III
29: Zygapophysial (facet) joint L III – L IV
30: Spinous process of L IV
31: Rectum

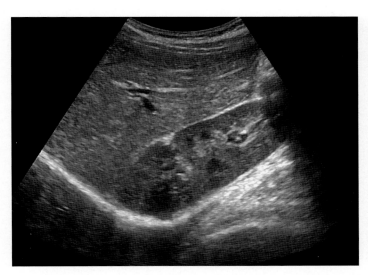
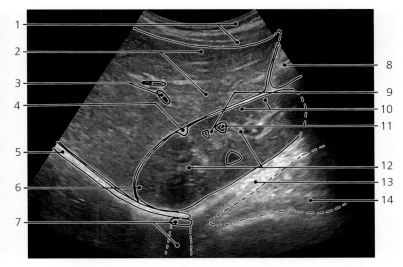

Kidney, longitudinal section, US

1: Abdominal wall muscles
2: Right liver lobe
3: Portal vein branches
4: Residue of fetal lobulation
5: Diaphragm

6: Upper pole of right kidney
7: 12th rib with acoustic shadow
8: Transverse colon
9: Renal column
10: Renal cortex

11: Renal pyramid
12: Renal sinus
13: Pararenal fat
14: Psoas major

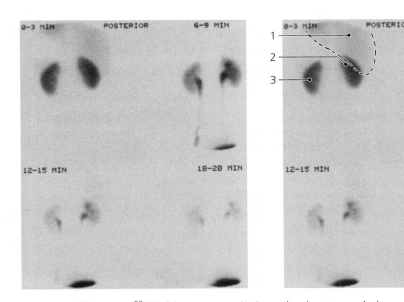

Kidneys, ^{99m}Tc-hippuran, scintigraphy (renography), posterior view

Four samplings at intervals indicated after i.v. injection of ^{99m}Tc-hippurate

1: Liver
2: Right kidney

3: Left kidney (usually more cranial than the right)
4: Renal pelvis

5: Ureter
6: Urinary bladder

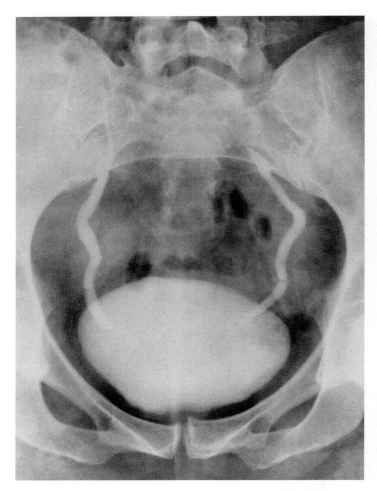
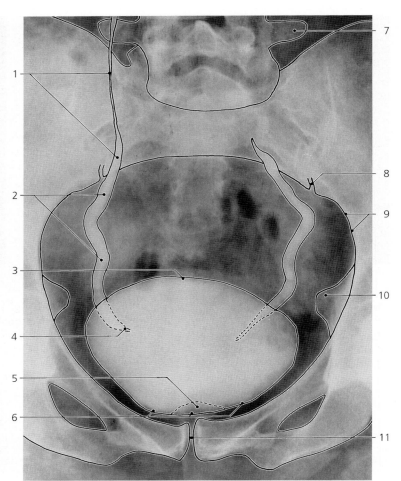

Urinary bladder, male, a-p, tilted X-ray, i.v. urography

20 min after intravenous contrast

1: Abdominal part of ureter	5: Impression of prostate	9: Linea arcuata
2: Pelvic part of ureter	6: Fundus of urinary bladder	10: Ischial spine
3: Apex of urinary bladder	7: Transverse process of L V	11: Pubic symphysis
4: Intramural part of ureter	8: Sacro-iliac joint	

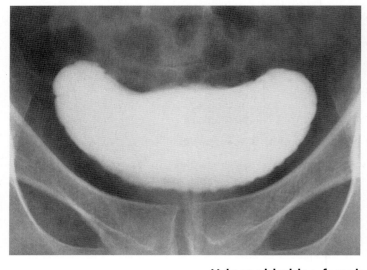
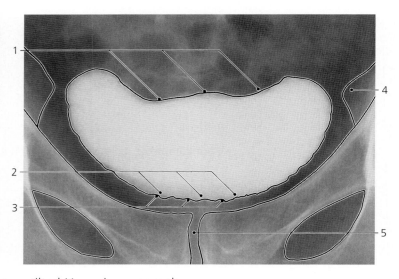

Urinary bladder, female, a-p, tilted X-ray, i.v. urography

1: Impression of uterus	3: Contours of trabecular muscle in	4: Ischial spine
2: Fundus of urinary bladder	bladder wall	5: Pubic symphysis

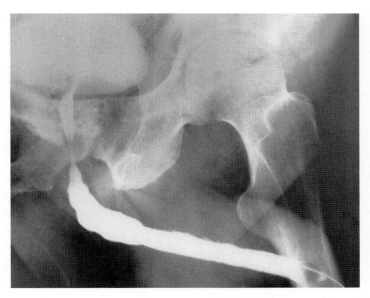
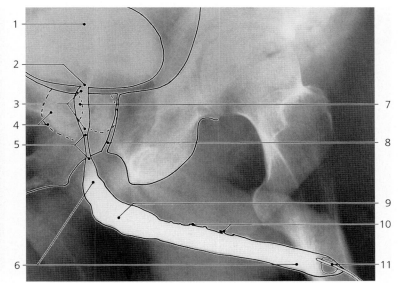

Urethra, male, oblique X-ray, urethrography

1: Urinary bladder
2: Internal urethral orifice
3: Prostatic part of urethra
4: Overflow of contrast medium into prostatic glands
5: Membranous part of urethra
6: Spongiose part of urethra
7: Site of colliculus seminalis (verumontanum)
8: Pubic symphysis
9: Urethral bulb
10: Urethral lacunae
11: Balloon catheter in navicular fossa

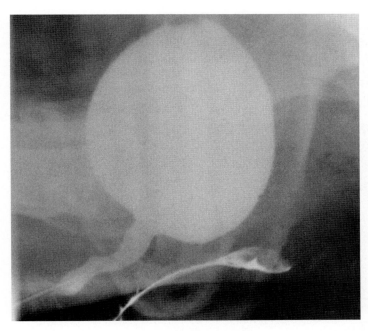
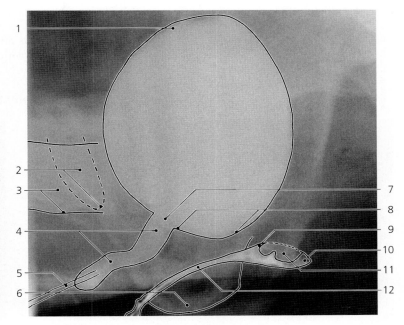

Urethra, female, lateral X-ray, kolpo-cysto-urethrography (KCU), micturating

1: Apex of urinary bladder
2: Pubic symphysis
3: Femoral bone
4: Urethra
5: Catheter
6: Ischial tuberosity
7: Internal urethral orifice
8: Trigone of bladder
9: Anterior fornix of vagina
10: Posterior fornix of vagina
11: Vaginal part of cervix uteri
12: Vagina

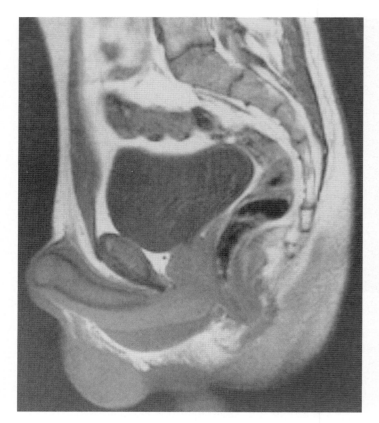
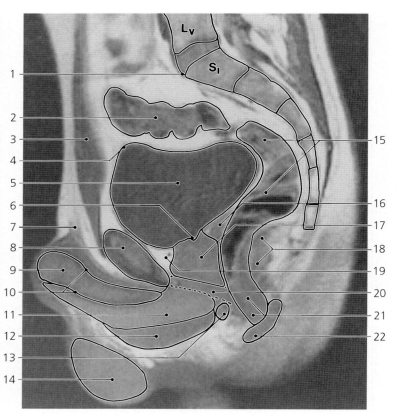

Male pelvis, median MR

T1 weighted recording

1: Promontory
2: Sigmoid colon
3: Rectus abdominis
4: Apex of urinary bladder
5: Urinary bladder
6: Internal orifice of urethra
7: Fundiform ligament of penis
8: Pubic symphysis

9: Corpus cavernosum
10: Tunica albuginea
11: Bulb of penis
12: Bulbospongiosus muscle
13: Bulbo-urethral gland (Cowper)
14: Testis
15: Rectum
16: Ampulla of deferent duct

17: Prostate
18: Levator ani
19: Retropubic space (cavum Retzii)
20: Urogenital diaphragm
21: Anal canal
22: Sphinchter ani externus,
    subcutaneous part

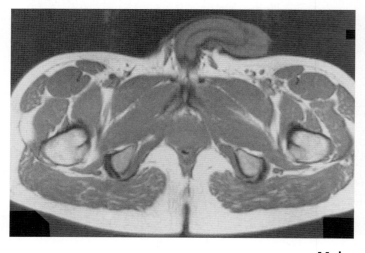
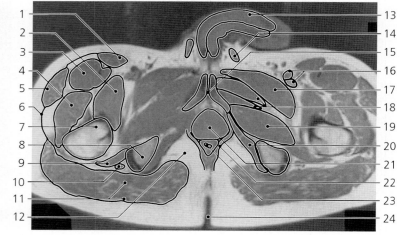

Male pelvis, axial MR

T1 weighted recording

1: Sartorius
2: Iliopsoas
3: Rectus femoris
4: Vastus lateralis
5: Tensor fasciae latae
6: Iliotibial tract
7: Femoral bone
8: Ischial tuberosity

9: Quadratus femoris
10: Sciatic nerve
11: Gluteus maximus
12: Ischiorectal fossa
13: Corpus cavernosum
14: Spermatic cord
15: Pubic symphysis
16: Femoral artery and vein

17: Pectineus
18: Adductor longus and brevis
19: Obturatorius externus
20: Obturatorius internus
21: Prostate
22: Levator ani
23: Rectum
24: Crena ani

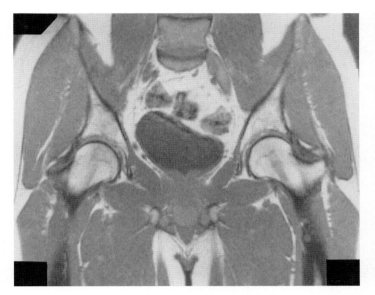
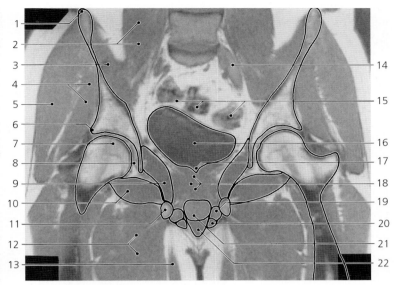

Male pelvis, coronal MR

T1 weighted recording

1: Iliac crest
2: Psoas major
3: Iliacus
4: Gluteus minimus
5: Gluteus medius
6: Acetabular rim
7: Femoral head
8: Acetabular fossa

9: Obturatorius internus
10: Obturatorius externus
11: Inferior ramus of pubis
12: Adductor muscles
13: Gracilis
14: Left common iliac vein
15: Sigmoid colon
16: Urinary bladder

17: Internal orifice of urethra
18: Prostate
19: Crus penis
20: Ischiocavernosus muscle
21: Bulb of penis
22: Bulbospongiosus muscle

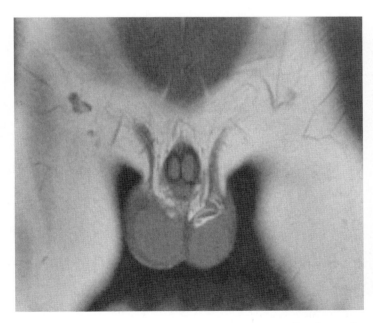
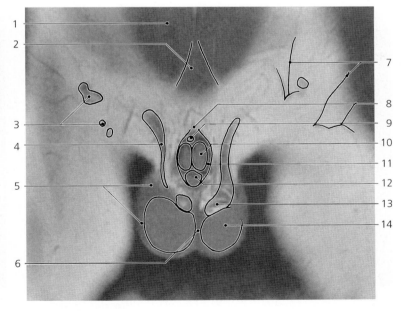

Penis and scrotum, coronal MR

T1 weighted recording

1: Rectus abdominis
2: Pyramidalis muscle
3: Superficial inguinal lymph nodes
4: Spermatic cord
5: Scrotum

6: Septum of scrotum
7: Superficial vessels
8: Suspensory ligament of penis
9: Deep dorsal vein of penis
10: Corpus cavernosum

11: Deep fascia of penis
12: Corpus spongiosum
13: Epididymis
14: Testis

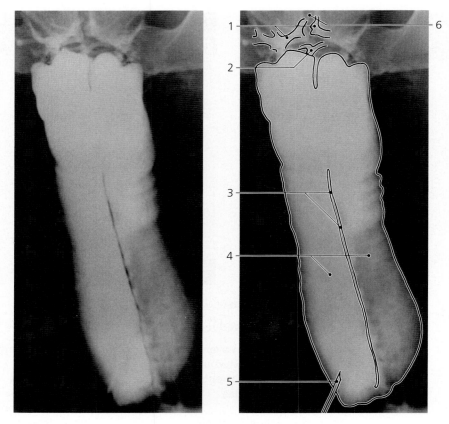

Penis, a-p X-ray, cavernosography

1: Prostatic venous plexus
2: Deep dorsal vein of penis

3: Septum of penis
4: Corpora cavernosa

5: Injection site
6: Pubic symphysis

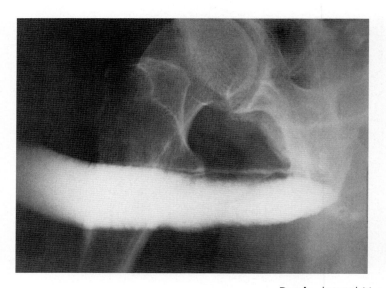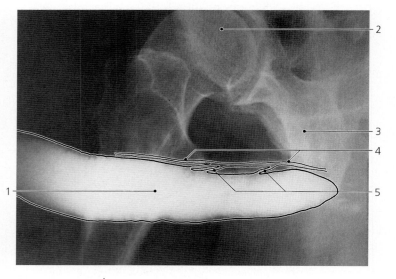

Penis, lateral X-ray, cavernosography

1: Corpus cavernosum
2: Femoral head

3: Pubic symphysis
4: Deep dorsal vein of penis

5: Emissary veins of penis

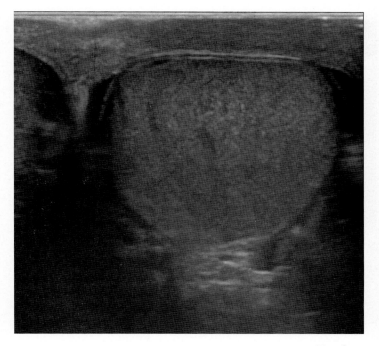
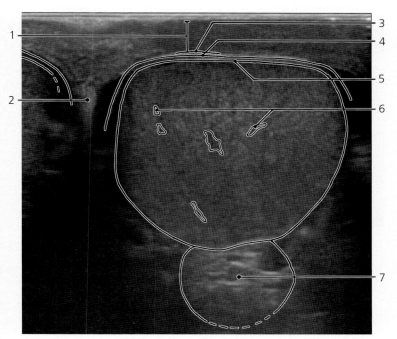

Testis, cross-section, US

1: Dartos fascia, external spermatic fascia and cremasteric fascia
2: Septum of scrotum
3: Internal spermatic fascia
4: Tunica vaginalis (parietal layer)
5: Tunica albuginea
6: Testicular vessels
7: Epididymis

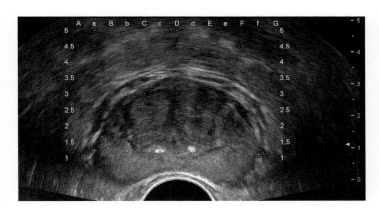
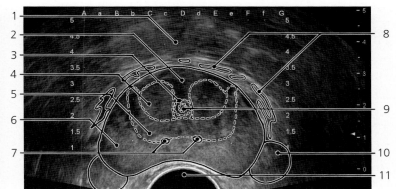

Prostate, transverse section, US

A grid used for planning of biopsies is superimposed on the image

1: Bladder wall
2: Fibromuscular zone of prostate
3: Periurethral zone
4: Transitional zone
5: Central zone
6: Peripheral zone
7: Calcifications
8: Prostatic venous plexus
9: Urethra
10: Seminal vesicle
11: Transducer in rectum

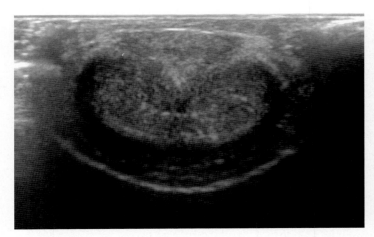

Penis, cross-section, US

1: Corpus spongiosum
2: Corona glandis

3: Corpora cavernosa (connected anteriorly)

4: Urethra
5: Prepuce (retracted)

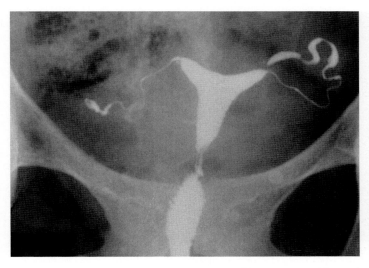
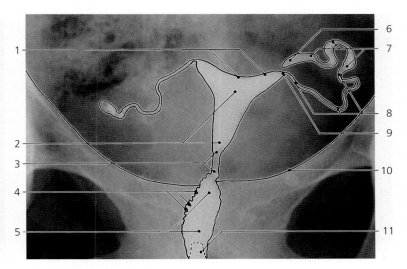

Uterus, a-p X-ray, hysterosalpingography (HSG)

1: Fundus of uterine cavity
2: Uterine cavity
3: Isthmus ("lower uterine segment")
4: Palmate folds of cervix

5: Canal of cervix (dilated and stretched)
6: Infundibulum of uterine tube
7: Ampulla of uterine tube
8: Isthmus of uterine tube

9: Uterine ostium of uterine tube
10: Pecten of pubis
11: Tube

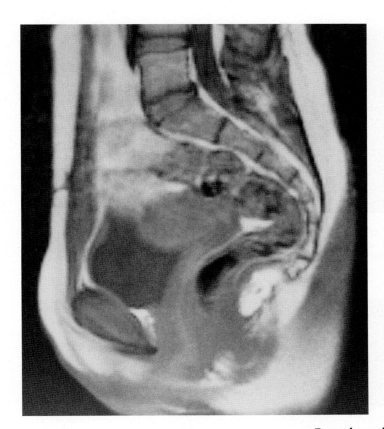
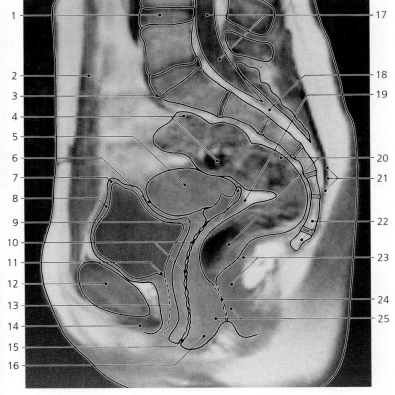

Female pelvis, median MR

T1 weighted recording

1: Intervertebral disc
2: Rectus abdominis
3: Promontory
4: Sigmoid colon
5: Uterus
6: Vesico-uterine pouch
7: Apex of urinary bladder
8: Wall of urinary bladder
9: Posterior fornix of vagina

10: Vagina
11: Internal orifice of urethra
12: Pubic symphysis
13: Urethra
14: Clitoris
15: Vaginal orifice
16: Perineum
17: Dural sac with cauda equina
18: Sacral canal

19: Recto-uterine pouch (fossa Douglasi)
20: Rectum
21: Lumbar aponeurosis covering sacral hiatus
22: Coccyx
23: Levator ani
24: Anal canal
25: Sphinchter ani externus

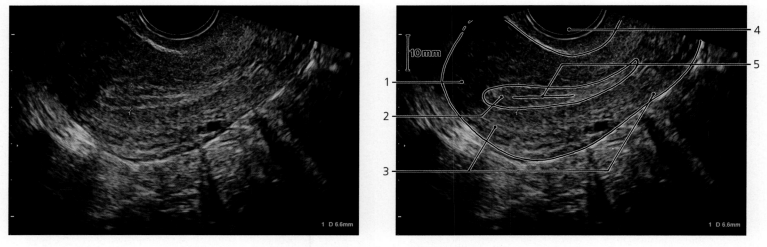

Uterus, sagittal section, US. Endometrial thickness (D): 2 × 3.3 mm

1: Uterus (fundus)
2: Endometrium in late proliferative
   phase (time of ovulation)

3: Body of uterus (myometrium)
4: Transducer in anterior fornix
   of vagina

5: Uterine cavity

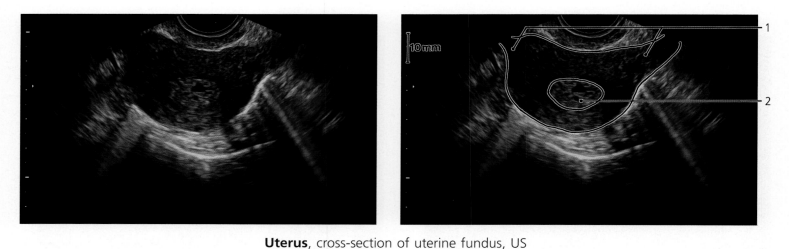

Uterus, cross-section of uterine fundus, US

1: Uterine horns

2: Endometrium in secretory (luteal) phase

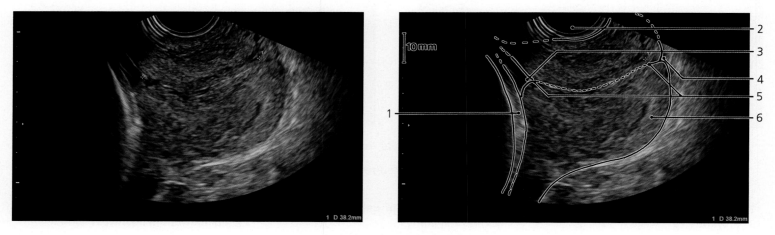

Uterus, pregnant

Sagittal section, US. Length of cervical canal (D): 38 mm

1: Calvaria of fetus
2: Transducer in fornix of vagina

3: Internal ostium of cervix
4: Cervix of uterus (external ostium)

5: Cervical canal
6: Vaginal part of cervix

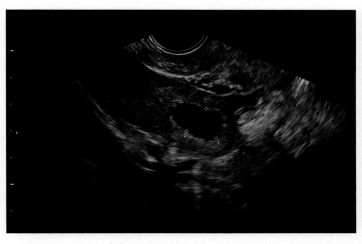
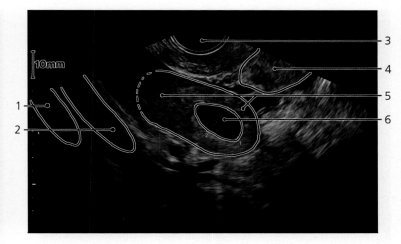

Ovary, US

1: External iliac artery
2: External iliac vein

3: Transducer in anterior vaginal fornix
4: Uterus

5: Ovary
6: Tertiary follicle (11 × 19 mm)

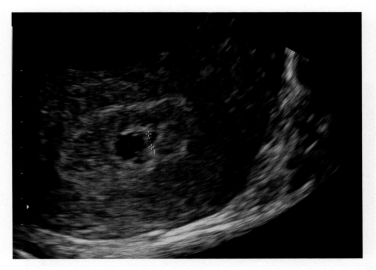
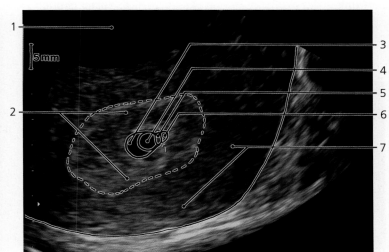

Embryo

Gestational age (GA): 3w6d

1: Transducer in vagina
2: Decidua reaction in endometrium

3: Chorionic cavity
4: Primary yolk sac
5: Embryon (length 2.6 mm)

6: Amniotic cavity
7: Myometrium

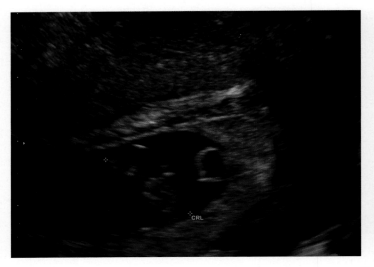

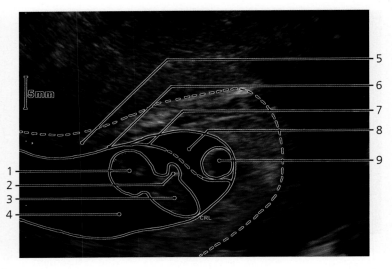

Embryo

GA: 7w6d, crown–rump length (CRL): 15 mm

1: Head
2: Upper extremity
3: Trunk

4: Amniotic cavity
5: Endometrium (decidua)
6: Fused chorion and amnion

7: Amnion
8: Chorionic cavity
9: Secundary yolk sac (remnant)

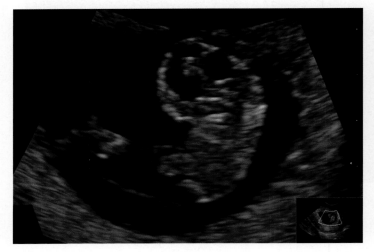

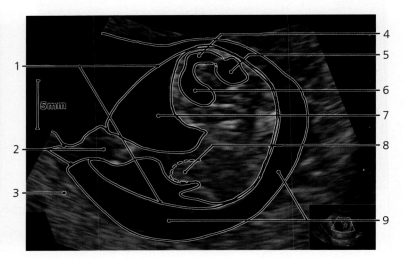

Embryo

GA: 8w2d

1: Amnion
2: Umbilical cord and placental insertion
3: Placenta

4: Cerebral aqueduct/mesencephalon
5: Fourth ventricle/rhombencephalon
6: Third ventricle/diencephalon
7: Amniotic cavity

8: Physiological herniation of midgut into umbilical cord
9: Chorionic cavity

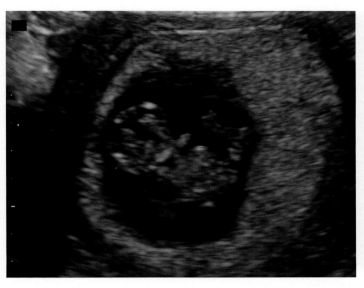

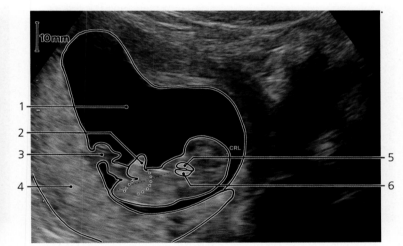

GA: 9w4d, CRL: 23 mm

1: **Decidua capsularis**
2: **Head**
3: **Arm**

4: **Amniotic cavity**
5: **Placenta**

6: **Umbilical cord (placental insertion)**
7: **Legs**

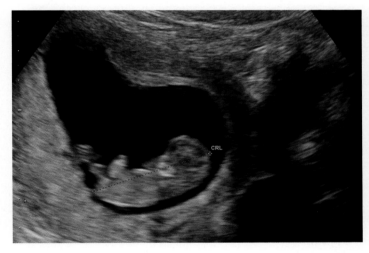

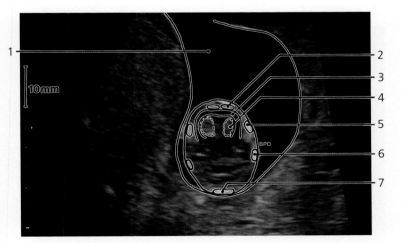

GA: 10w5d, CRL: 40 mm

1: **Amniotic cavity**
2: **Leg**

3: **Umbilical cord**
4: **Placenta**

5: **Maxilla**
6: **Mandibula**

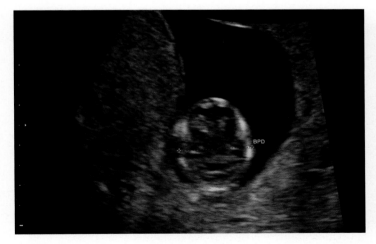

GA: 11w4d, head transverse

1: **Amniotic cavity**
2: **Frontal bone**
3: **Cerebral cortex**

4: **Choroid plexus in lateral ventricle**
5: **Temporal bone**

6: **Parietal bone**
7: **Occipital bone**

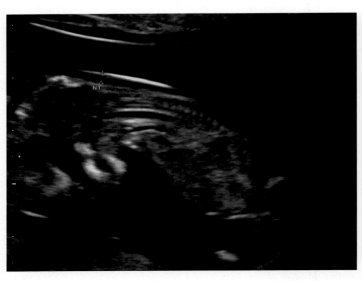
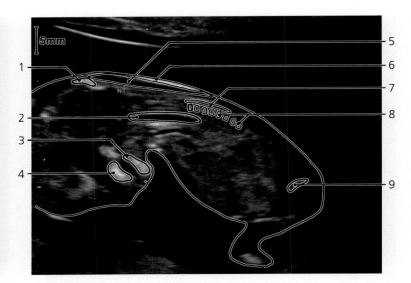

GA: 12w3d, neck, nuchal translucency, sagittal

1: Occipital bone
2: Aorta
3: Mandibula
4: Maxilla

5: Nuchal translucency ("nuchal fold," subcutaneous edema), NF 1.9 mm. (Normal for this GA is up to 2.4 mm)
6: Reflection from skin

7: Vertebral canal
8: Vertebral bodies with ossification centers
9: Ilium

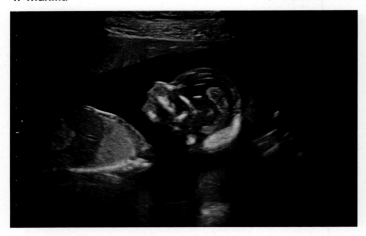
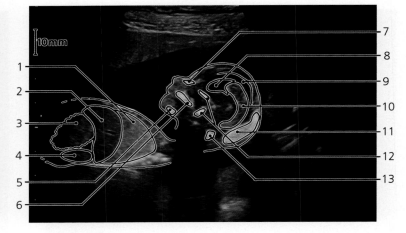

GA: 14w5d, head, sagittal

1: Lung
2: Liver
3: Gut
4: Kidney
5: Mandibula

6: Maxilla and palate
7: Nasal bone
8: Lateral ventricle
9: Cerebral cortex
10: Choroid plexus

11: Occipital bone
12: Sphenoid bone
13: Atlas and axis

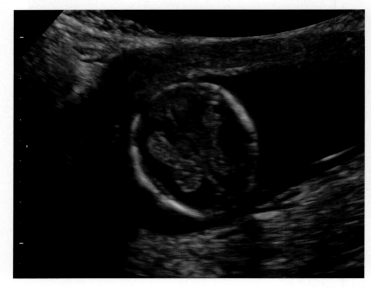
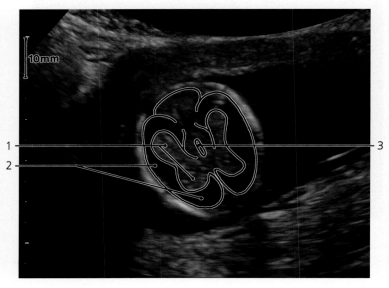

GA: 14w5d, brain, transverse

1: Choroid plexus in lateral ventricle

2: Cerebral cortex

3: Third ventricle

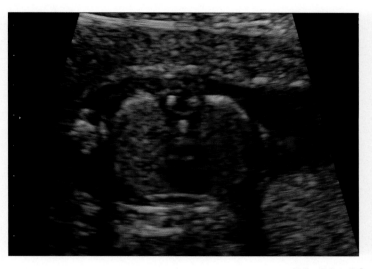
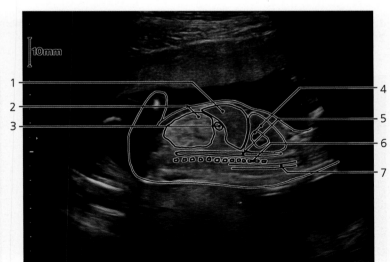

GA: 14w6d, thorax, transverse

1: Arm
2: Heart
3: Rib

4: Ossification centers in vertebral arch
5: Vertebral canal

6: Ossification center in vertebral body
7: Lungs

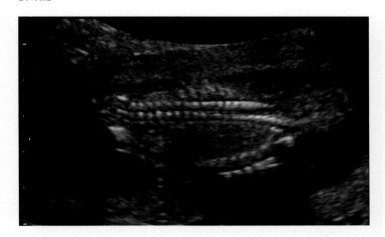
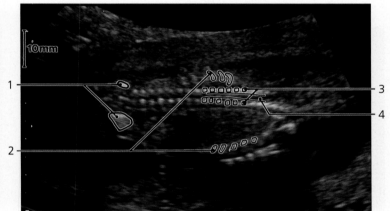

GA: 15w0d, spine, frontal

1: Coxae
2: Ribs

3: Ossification centers in vertebral arch (thoracic)

4: Vertebral canal

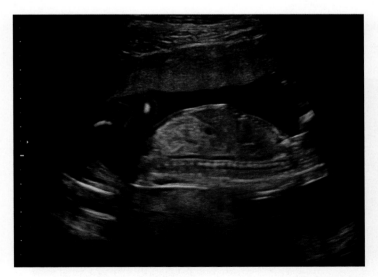

GA: 15w0d, spine, mid-sagittal

1: Liver
2: Gut
3: Stomach

4: Heart and lung
5: Aorta

6: Vertebral bodies
7: Vertebral canal

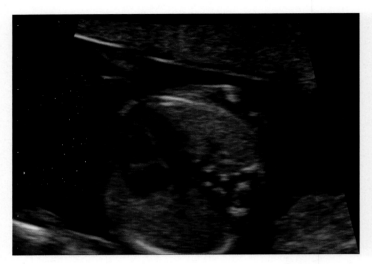

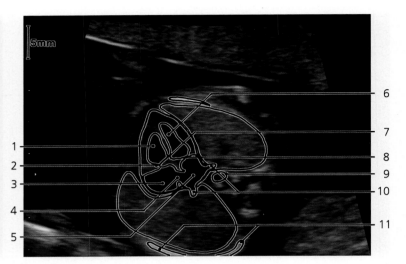

GA: 15w2d, four chamber view of heart

1: **Right ventricle**
2: **Tricuspid valve**
3: **Right atrium**
4: **Oval foramen**

5: **Left atrium**
6: **Left ventricle**
7: **Crux cordis**
8: **Mitral valve**

9: **Aorta**
10: **Pulmonary veins**
11: **Rib**

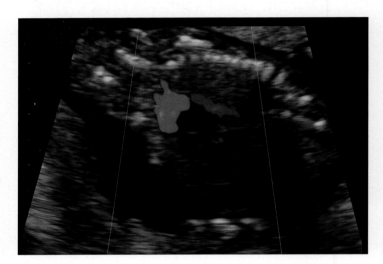

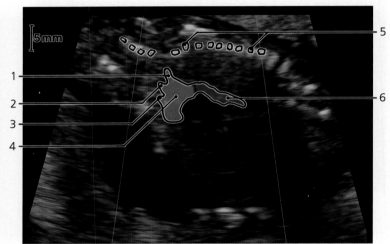

GA: 15w2d, aortic arch. Color-flow Doppler imaging

1: **Left subclavian artery**
2: **Left common carotid artery**

3: **Brachiocephalic trunk**
4: **Aortic arch**

5: **Vertebral column**
6: **Descending aorta**

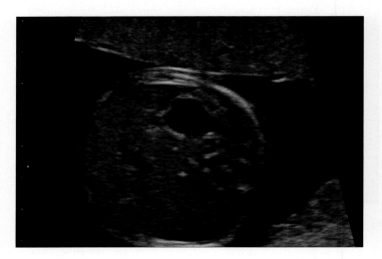

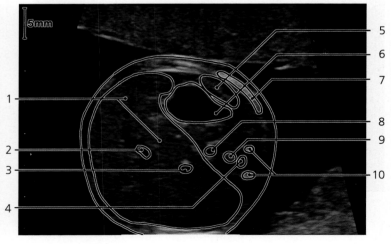

GA: 15w2d, upper abdomen, transverse

1: **Liver**
2: **Umbilical vein**
3: **Inferior caval vein**
4: **Vertebral canal**

5: **Spleen**
6: **Stomach**
7: **Rib**
8: **Aorta**

9: **Ossification center of vertebral body**
10: **Ossification centers of vertebral arch**

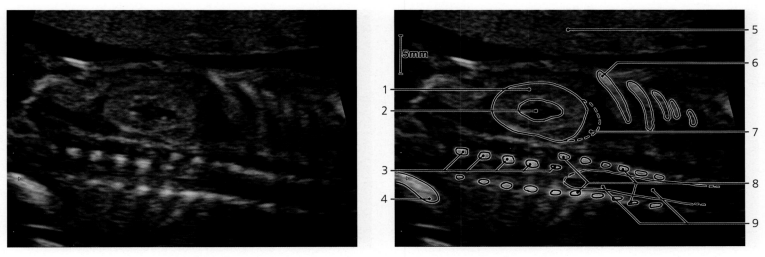

GA: 15w2d, spine, frontal. The shift between 3 and 8 is due to rotation

1: **Renal parenchyma**
2: **Renal sinus**
3: **Ossification centers in vertebral bodies**
4: **Ilium**
5: **Placenta**
6: **Rib**
7: **Suprarenal gland**
8: **Ossification centers in vertebral arches**
9: **Vertebral canal**

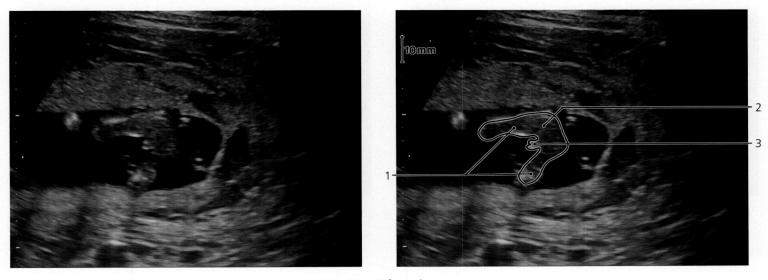

GA: 15w0d, male sex

1: **Legs**
2: **Buttock**
3: **Male genitals**

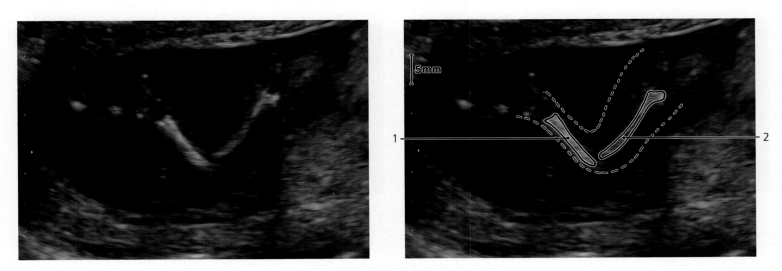

GA: 14w3d, leg

1: **Tibia**
2: **Femur**

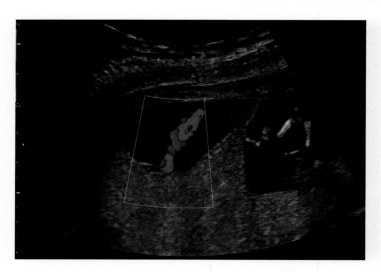

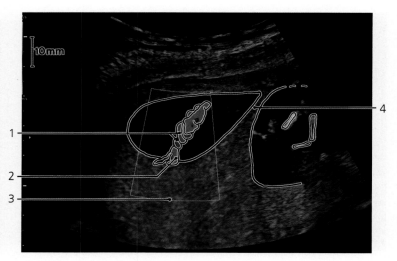

Fetus, dichorionic twins. Color-flow Doppler imaging

1: **Umbilical arteries**
2: **Umbilical vein**

3: **Placenta**

4: **Chorionic septum (2 fused leafs of chorion leave)**

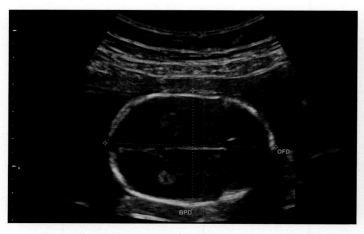

GA: 19w1d, brain, transverse. Biparietal diameter (BPD): 43 mm, occipitofrontal diameter (OFD): 61 mm

1: **Sutures**
2: **Choroid plexus in atrium of lateral ventricle**

3: **Falx cerebri**

4: **Reflection from medial wall in frontal horn of lateral ventricle**

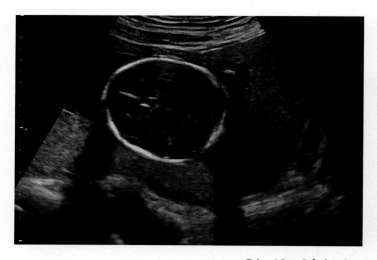

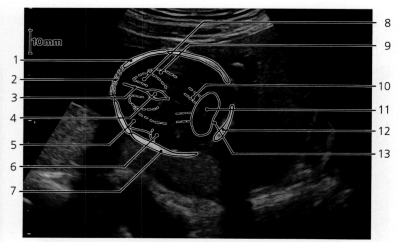

GA: 19w6d, brain, transverse, "Cerebellar view"

1: **Frontal bone**
2: **Anterior fontanelle**
3: **Falx cerebri**
4: **Cave of septum pellucidum**
5: **Frontal cortex**

6: **Temporal cortex**
7: **Parietal bone**
8: **Frontal horn of lateral ventricle**
9: **Choroid plexus**
10: **Cerebral crus**

11: **Cerebellum**
12: **Occipital bone**
13: **Cisterna magna**

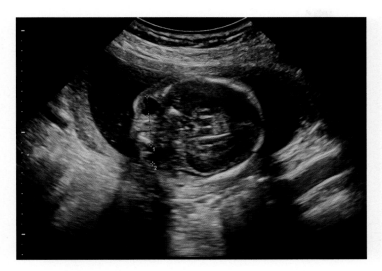

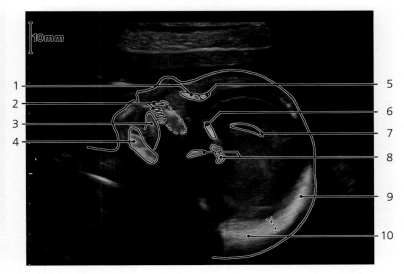

GA: 22w0d, brain and eyes, transverse, "Thalamic view." Interorbital distance: 14 mm, extraorbital distance: 33 mm

1: Eyeball
2: Lens
3: Nasal septum

4: Nasal bone
5: Thalamus
6: Falx cerebri

7: Occipital lobe
8: Choroid plexus
9: Temporal lobe

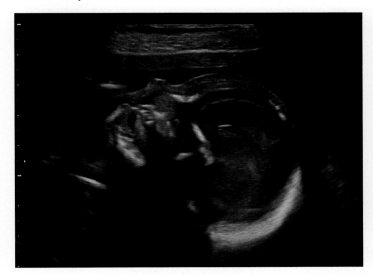

GA: 21w1d, face, sagittal

1: Nasal bone
2: Teeth in maxilla
3: Tongue
4: Mandible with teeth

5: Frontal bone
6: Minor wing of sphenoid
7: Frontal horn of lateral ventricle

8: Sphenoid
9: Parietal bone
10: Occipital bone

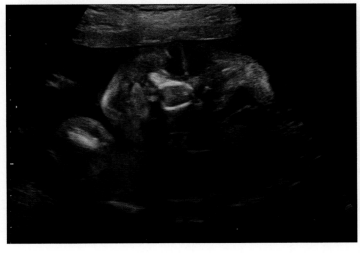

GA: 21w1d, face, frontal

1: Lips
2: Mandible (gnathion)
3: Humerus

4: Eyelids
5: Maxilla

6: Nasal bones
7: Philtrum

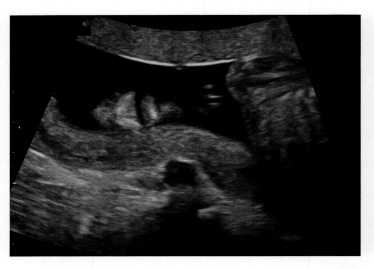
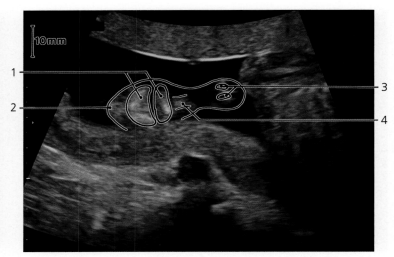

GA: 20w3d, lips, frontal

1: Lips	**3: Nostrils**
2: Gnathion	**4: Philtrum**

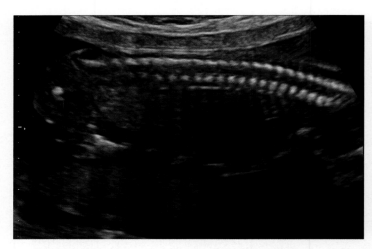
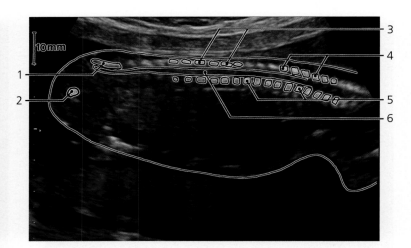

GA: 19w0d, spine, sagittal. Rotation between 3 and 4

1: Sacrum	**3: Laminae of vertebral arches**	**5: Bodies of vertebrae**
2: Ischium	**4: Spinous processes of vertebrae**	**6: Vertebral canal**

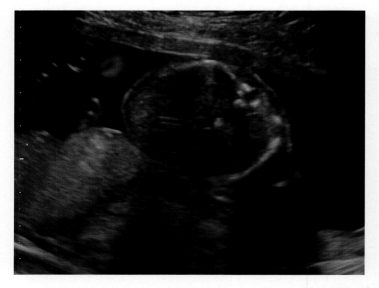
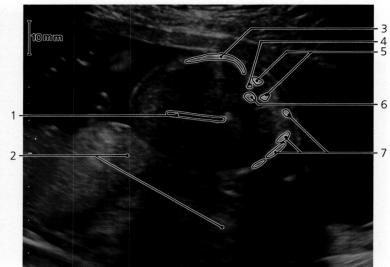

GA: 19w4d, trunk, transverse

1: Umbilical vein	**4: Head of rib**	**6: Body of vertebra**
2: Placenta	**5: Vertebral arch**	**7: Ribs**
3: Rib		

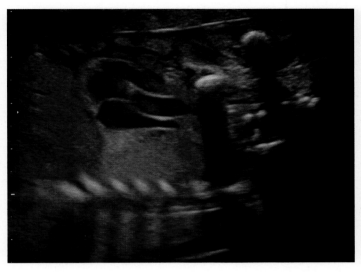
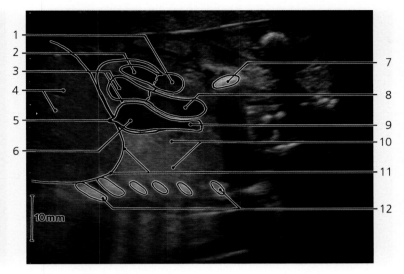

GA: 21w0d, heart and great vessels, oblique

1: **Pulmonary trunk**
2: **Right ventricle and interventricular septum**
3: **Left ventricle**
4: **Liver**

5: **Inferior caval vein**
6: **Right atrium**
7: **Clavicle**
8: **Aorta**

9: **Superior caval vein**
10: **Lung**
11: **Diaphragm**
12: **Ribs**

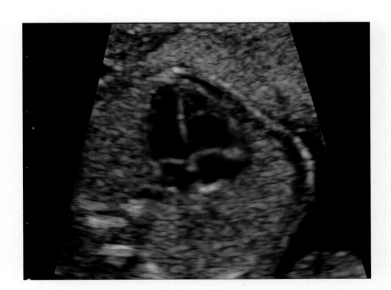
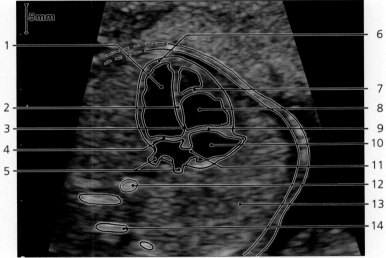

GA: 19w5d, heart, four chamber view

1: **Left ventricle**
2: **Interventricular septum (muscular part)**
3: **Interventricular septum (membranous part, "crux cordis")**
4: **Mitral valve (bicuspid valve)**

5: **Pulmonary veins**
6: **Apex of heart**
7: **Septomarginal trabecula ("moderator band")**
8: **Right ventricle**
9: **Tricuspid valve**

10: **Right atrium**
11: **Oval foramen**
12: **Spine**
13: **Right lung**
14: **Rib**

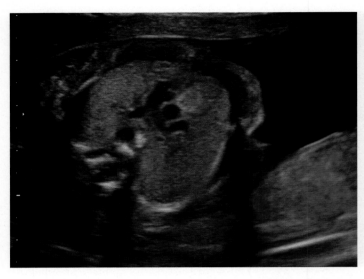
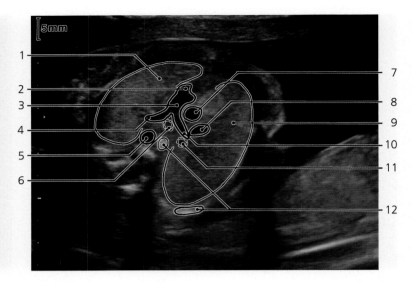

GA: 21w4d, thorax and great vessels, transverse

1: Left lung
2: Outlet tract of right ventricle
3: Pulmonary trunk
4: Left pulmonary artery

5: Descending aorta
6: Left main bronchus
7: Ascending aorta
8: Superior caval vein

9: Right lung
10: Right pulmonary artery
11: Right main bronchus
12: Rib and vertebral body

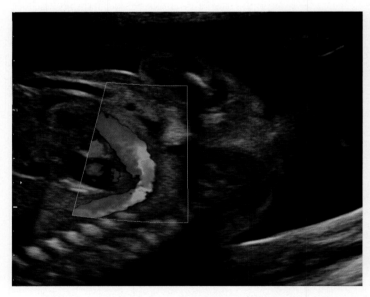
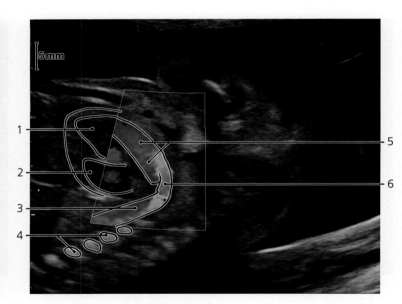

GA: 21w1d, heart and ductus arteriosus. Color-flow Doppler imaging

1: Right ventricle
2: Left ventricle

3: Descending aorta
4: Vertebral bodies

5: Pulmonary trunk
6: Ductus arteriosus

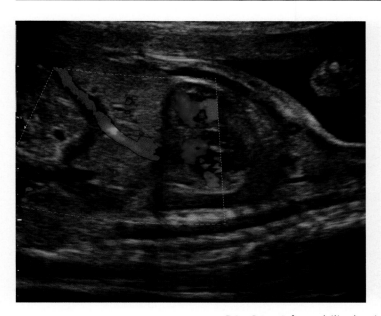

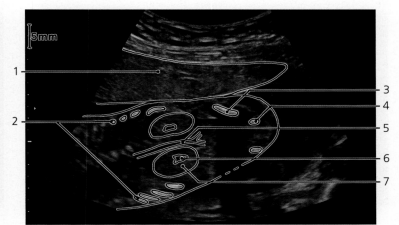

GA: 21w1d, umbilical vein. Color-flow Doppler imaging

1: Umbilical vein	4: Right ventricle	7: Vertebral canal
2: Liver	5: Left ventricle	8: Body of vertebra
3: Gut	6: Aorta	

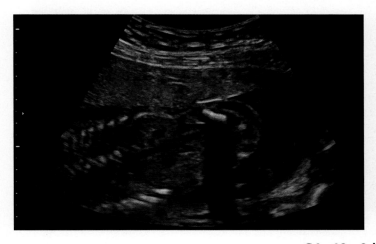

GA: 19w0d, kidneys, frontal

1: Placenta	4: Ischium	6: Renal sinus
2: Ribs	5: Aorta	7: Renal parenchyma
3: Ilium		

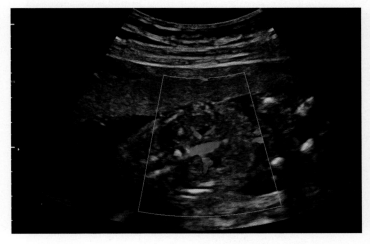

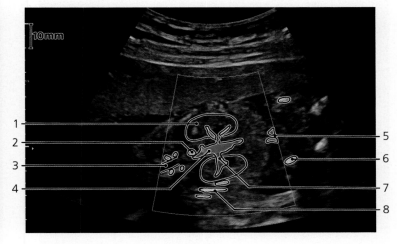

GA: 19w0d, kidney arteries, frontal. Color-flow Doppler imaging

1: Kidney	4: Aorta	7: Renal artery
2: Vertebral body	5: Internal iliac vessels	8: Rib
3: Vertebral canal	6: Ischium	

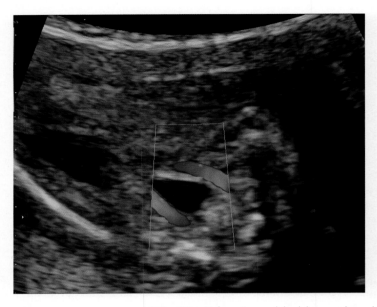
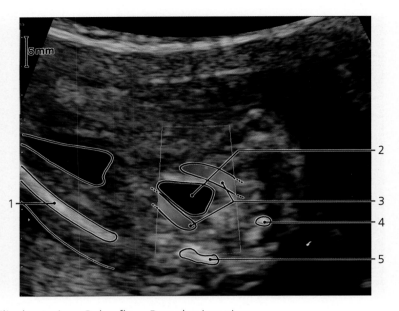

GA: 19w6d, urinary bladder and umbilical arteries. Color-flow Doppler imaging

1: Femur
2: Urinary bladder

3: Umbilical arteries
4: Promontory

5: Coxae

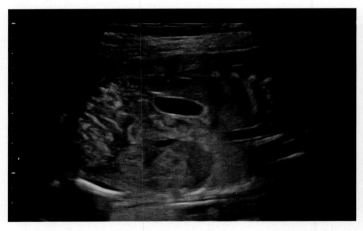

GA: 21w1d, abdomen, frontal

1: Spleen
2: Stomach
3: Gut

4: Ribs (with acoustic shadows)
5: Aorta

6: Lung
7: Liver (right lobe)

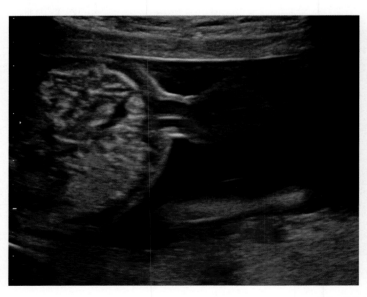
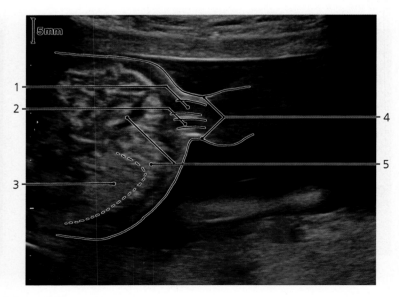

GA: 21w1d, umbilicus

1: Umbilical vein
2: Umbilical artery

3: Liver
4: Umbilical cord

5: Gut

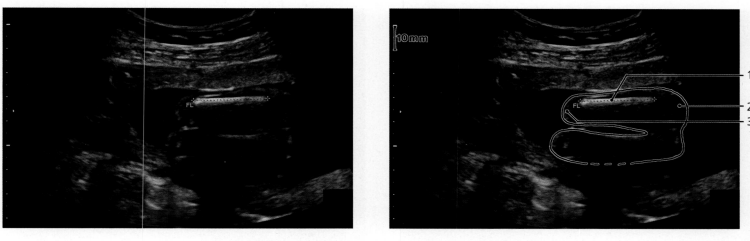

GA: 18w6d, femur length (FL), ossified shaft: 30 mm

1: Femur   2: Buttock   3: Knee

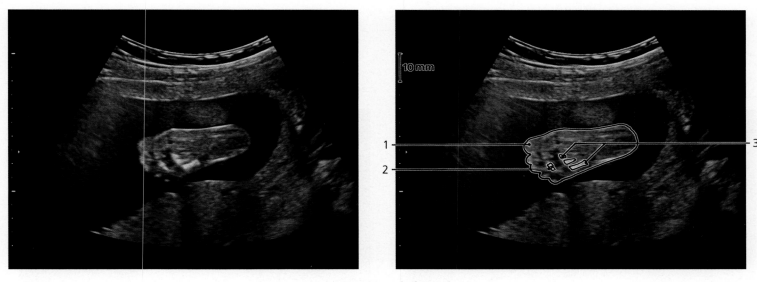

GA: 22w2d, foot

1: Great toe   2: Proximal phalanges   3: Metatarsals

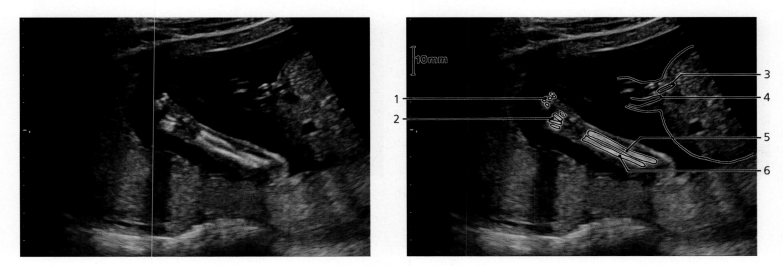

GA: 19w6d, forearm

1: Phalanges   3: Umbilical artery   5: Ulna
2: Metacarpals   4: Umbilical vein   6: Radius

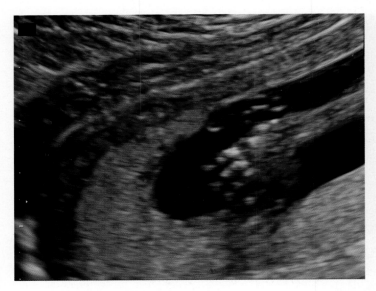
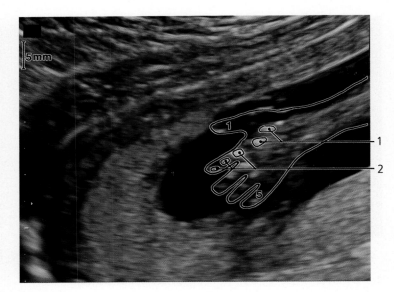

GA: 16w0d, hand

1: **Metacarpals**   2: **Phalanges**

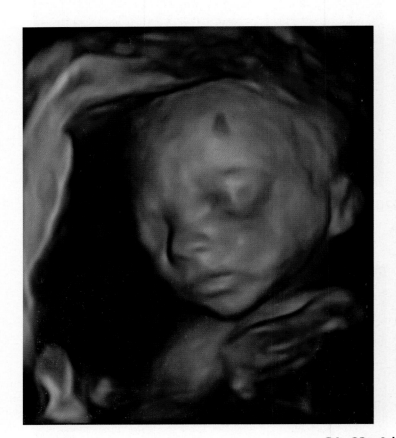
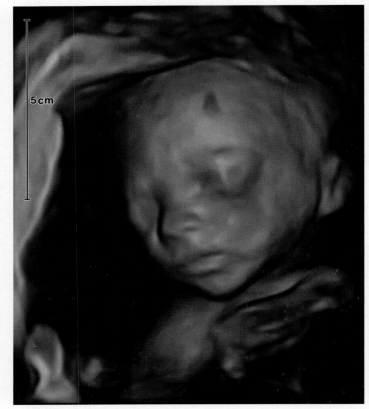

GA: 23w0d, 3D imaging

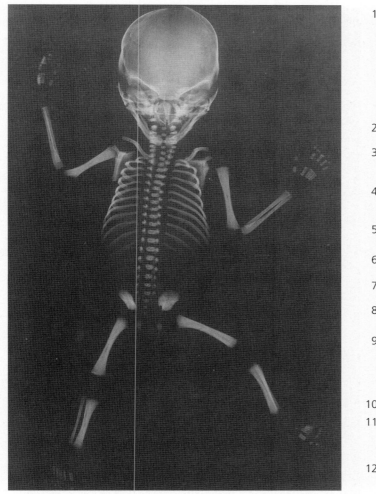
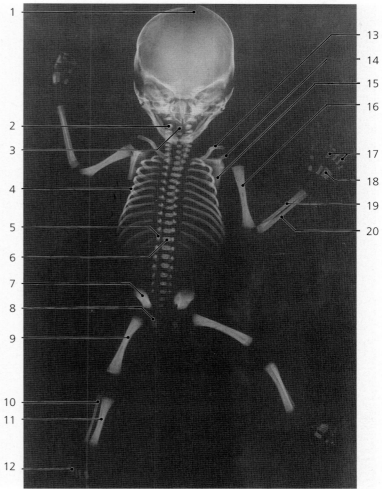

Fetus, 18 weeks, CRL = 140 mm, stillborn, a-p X-ray

1: Anterior fontanelle
2: Arch of second cervical vertebra
   (ossification center)
3: Body of second cervical vertebra
   (ossification center)
4: Fifth rib
5: Arch of 12th thoracic vertebra
   (ossification center)

6: Body of 12th thoracic vertebra
   (ossification center)
7: Ilium
8: Pubis
9: Femur (diaphysis)
10: Fibula
11: Tibia (diaphysis)
12: Metatarsals

13: Clavicle
14: Coracoid process
15: Scapula
16: Humerus (diaphysis)
17: Phalanges
18: Metacarpals
19: Radius
20: Ulna

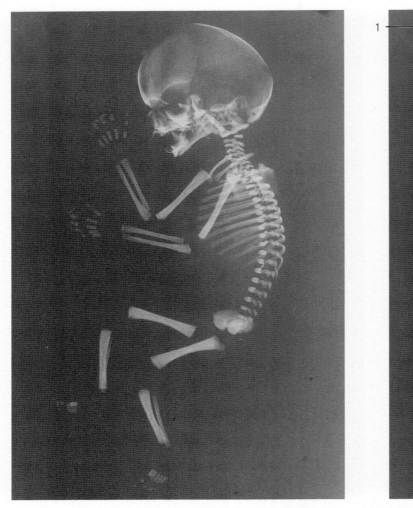
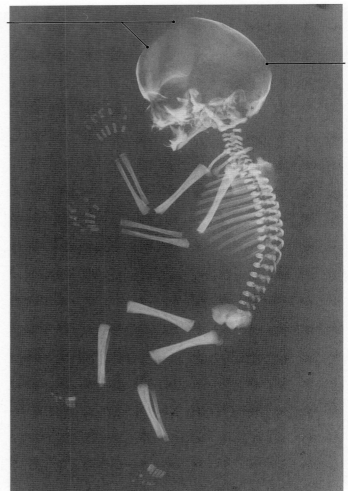

Fetus, 18 weeks, CRL = 140 mm, stillborn, lateral X-ray

1: Anterior fontanelle   **2: Posterior fontanelle**

Short dictionary of examination procedures and concepts in diagnostic imaging

angiocardiography X-ray examination of the heart and the adjacent great vessels. Contrast medium is usually injected into the right ventricle through a catheter introduced via the femoral vein by the Seldinger technique. The passage of contrast is recorded on a rapid sequence of images (cineradiography). See p. 387–8.

angiography Imaging by conventional X-ray, CT, MR or ultrasound of vessels: arteries (arteriography, q.v.), veins (phlebography, q.v.) or lymphatics (lymphography, q.v.).

antegrade pyelography X-ray examination of the urinary tract after puncture and injection of contrast medium into the renal pelvis, often guided by ultrasound.

aortography X-ray, CT or MR examination of the aorta and its branches. Water-soluble contrast medium is injected through a catheter, usually introduced by the Seldinger technique (q.v.) via the femoral artery (transfemoral aortography). The abdominal aorta can also be punctured directly (lumbar aortography). See p. 386, 436.

arteriography Imaging of arteries. Water-soluble contrast medium is injected through a cannula inserted by direct puncture of an artery or by the Seldinger technique, q.v. A rapid sequence of single radiographs or a cineradiographic recording is taken in order to image the passage of contrast medium through the arterial branches. The latest exposures taken, when the contrast medium collects on the venous side, are denoted the *venous phase*, see p. 437.

arthrography Examination of a joint after injection of water-soluble contrast medium or air, often both (double contrast), into the synovial cavity.

axial In or along the axis (midline) of the body. The term is used in conventional X-ray examinations for a positioning where the X-rays pass along, and the film is positioned perpendicular to the long axis of the body. Used in computed tomography and magnetic resonance imaging to denote a cross-section (i.e., transverse section) of the body, an "axial section".

B-mode imaging "Brightness" mode of ultrasound imaging. See p. 37.

barium A suspension of barium sulfate in a watery medium. Used as a contrast medium to visualize the digestive tract. See p. 425–8.

barium enema X-ray examination of the colon and the rectum after introduction of barium through the anus. The colon is cleaned before the examination by laxatives and/or a cleaning enema. See p. 427–8.

barium meal X-ray examination of the upper gastrointestinal tract after ingestion of barium. See p. 425–6.

barium swallow X-ray examination of the esophagus while swallowing barium. See p. 334, 396.

biliary tree scintigraphy Cholecysto-scintigraphy, q.v.

biparietal diameter (BPD) The maximum distance between surface of the parietal bones of the skull, measured perpendicular to the falx cerebri. Used in ultrasonography to determine the age of a fetus. See p. 459, 464.

bite-wing radiography Intra-oral dental X-ray film. The patient bites over a wing which projects from the film packing. See p. 340.

bone mineral content (BMC) See p. 12.

bone mineral density (BMD) See p. 12.

BPD Biparietal diameter, q.v.

bronchography X-ray imaging of the bronchial tree after introduction of contrast medium, often through a catheter placed in a main bronchus. Now replaced by direct endoscopy or virtual CT endoscopy.

cardioangiography Angiocardiography, q.v.

CAT Computed axial tomography. CT scanning where the sections are perpendicular to the long axis of the body.

cavernosography X-ray examination of the cavernous bodies of the penis after direct injection of contrast medium. The venous drainage is also visualized. See p. 452.

cavography Angiographic X-ray examination of the caval vein. Contrast is usually injected simultaneously in both femoral veins. See p. 440.

cholangiogram X-ray imaging of the gall bladder and bile ducts.

cholangiography Imaging of the biliary tree with a contrast medium. Formerly given intravenously (intravenous cholangiography), now directly into a bile duct. This can be performed percutaneously (percutaneous transhepatic cholangiography, q.v.) or through an endoscope (endoscopic retrograde cholangiography) or through a tube inserted in a bile duct during surgery (preoperative or postoperative cholangiography). Imaging may be by X-ray, CT or MRI.

cholecysto-scintigraphy Imaging the biliary tree and the gall bladder by isotopes. Often performed with ^{99m}Tc labeled iminodiacetic acid derivatives, for example ^{99m}Tc-HIDA. See p. 430.

cineangiography Examination of arteries using cineradiography during intravascular injection of contrast medium.

cineradiography Recording of the live image from the X-ray fluorescent screen on film or videotape.

colloid scintigraphy Scintigraphic imaging after intravenous injection of colloid particles labeled with a radioisotope, often ^{99m}Tc. The colloid will be taken up by macrophages. Especially the liver and the spleen can be visualized.

color-flow Doppler imaging An ultrasonographic technique in which a color-coded image of flow directions, determined by Doppler shifts, is superimposed on an ordinary gray-tone ultrasonogram. Used especially for cardiovascular examinations. See p. 39, 470.

computed tomography (CT) CT scanning. Tomographic X-ray imaging technique. See p. 12.

contrast media Compounds used to improve imaging of organs or cavities. See p. 17.

coronal section Term used in radiology to denote a tomographic image of a frontal section.

coronary arteriography Imaging of the coronary arteries by selective injection of contrast medium. Usually performed by the Seldinger technique (q.v.) through the femoral artery or through the brachial artery.

CT Computed tomography, q.v.

CT angiography See p. 324.

CT number Hounsfield unit, q.v.

cystography Examination of the urinary bladder using a water-soluble contrast medium.

cystourethrography X-ray examination of the bladder and the urethra. Water-soluble contrast medium is instilled into the bladder, and the bladder and the urethra are studied during voiding.

dacryocystography or dacryography X-ray examination of the lacrimal canaliculi, -sac, and -canal after cannulation and injection of contrast medium into the two lacrimal points.

diffusion weighted imaging MR imaging mode where the contrast in the image arises from differences in the diffusional mobility of protons. See p. 30.

digital subtraction angiography (DSA) Angiography using digital subtraction. Computer image processing technique for improved imaging of vessels after injection of contrast medium. The image contrast is improved by subtraction of images taken just before and during contrast injection, whereby image details common to both images cancel out. See p. 11–12.

Doppler shifts The apparent change in frequency of a sound wave as a result of changing the relative velocity of the signal source and the receiver. The frequency increases when the source and the receiver move towards each other and decreases when moving away from each other. This phenomenon is used to measure direction and velocity of flowing blood. See p. 39.

Doppler scanning Ultrasound examination with analysis of Doppler shifts.

double-contrast examination Use of positive and negative contrast media in combination, often barium and air. Particularly used for examination of the colon where a barium enema is followed by insufflation of air. See p. 425–7.

DSA Digital subtraction angiography, q.v.

dual energy subtraction Subtraction of two X-ray images, the one exposed at a low kVp setting, the other at a high.

The contrast of bone may be enhanced or reduced by the subtraction. See p. 12.

ductography X-ray examination of a duct, for example in the breast. Contrast is injected through the opening of the duct.

duplex scanning Ultrasound imaging combined with simultaneous measurement of flow velocity by Doppler shifts at a selected site in the image. See p. 39–40.

DXA/DEXA scanning See p. 12.

"echo" (jargon) Synonymous with ultrasonography, q.v.

echogenicity The ability of a tissue/structure to produce echoes by ultrasonography.

echocardiography (ultrasonic cardiography) Ultrasound examination of the heart. The real-time live image is often supplemented with one-dimensional scanning (M-mode), to give quantitative information on the motion of the cardiac walls and valves. Duplex scanning and color flow Doppler imaging yield additional information on velocities and directions of blood flow.

endoluminal ultrasound scanning Examination in which the ultrasound generator and receiver (the probe) is placed in the lumen of a vessel or an organ, for example transesophageal echocardiography or transvaginal scanning of the uterus, or transrectal scanning of the prostate.

endoscopic retrograde cholangio-pancreatography (ERCP) X-ray examination during retrograde injection of contrast medium into the biliary tract (cholangio-) and the pancreatic duct (pancreato-). A catheter is passed into the ampulla Vateri via an endoscope placed in the duodenum. See p. 429, 434.

endoscopy Direct visual examination of an organ by viewing through a tube-shaped optical instrument. The tube is often constructed with fiber optics. Commonly used for examination of the respiratory tract, the gastrointestinal tract, the peritoneal and pleural cavity, the urinary bladder, the reproductive system and joint cavities.

ERCP Endoscopic retrograde cholangio-pancreatography, q.v.

excretory urography Urography, q.v.

FLASH Fast low angle shot. MR imaging method that shortens the data acquisition time by the use of gradient echoes. See p. 28.

flat panel detector Electronic detector of X-rays used analogous to photographic X-ray films. See p. 11.

fluoroscopy X-ray imaging on a screen coated with a thin layer of a material that fluoresces proportional to the intensity of incident X-rays. The screen is positioned instead of the photographic film and is viewed directly or via a video camera. See p. 387.

gadolinium Strongly chelated gadolinium with a high renal clearance used as contrast medium in magnetic resonance imaging. See p. 26.

galactography Mammary ductography. X-ray examination of mammary ducts after injection of contrast into the duct system. See p. 398.

gestational age The age of a pregnancy defined from the first day of the last menstruation.

gradient echoes Method to evoke radio signals from spinning protons in MR imaging. See p. 24.

helical CT scanning "Spiral scanning". CT scanning where the patient couch is moved at a constant speed during the scanning. Scanning times are thereby reduced. Combined with multislice scan (q.v.), the time for a whole body CT scan can be considerably reduced (seconds). See p. 13.

HIDA scintigraphy Cholecysto-scintigraphy, q.v.

hippuran scintigraphy Radiosotope examination of the urinary tract using radioisotope labeled hippuran, which is excreted by the kidneys. See p. 447.

Hounsfield unit (CT number) Unit of X-ray attenuation, expressed relative to water and air. See p. 14.

HSG Hysterosalpingography, q.v.

hyperdense Term used in CT scanning to describe a tissue/structure that attenuates the X-rays more than its surroundings.

hyperechoic Term used in ultrasonography to describe a tissue/structure that produces more echoes than its surroundings.

hyperintense Term used in MRI to describe a tissue/structure that produces more MR radio signals than its surroundings.

hypodense Term used in CT scanning to describe a tissue/structure that attenuates the X-rays less than its surroundings.

hypoechoic Term used in ultrasonography to describe a tissue/structure that produces less echoes than its surroundings.

hypointense Term used in MRI to describe a tissue/structure that produces less MR radio signals than its surroundings.

hysterosalpingography (HSG) X-ray examination where iodine contrast medium is injected through the external uterine orifice and passed through the uterus and the salpinges into the peritoneal cavity.

imaging plate Device for recording X-ray images based on storage of the latent image in a compound that can be read by red laser light and regenerated for subsequent exposures. Otherwise handled like classical photographic X-ray films. See p. 11.

intravenous urography Urography, q.v.

isotope scintigraphy Examination using γ-emitting radioisotopes targeted to specific organs or tissues. The time-dependent accumulation and/or wash-out in a particular organ is recorded and visualized with a gamma camera. See p. 41.

IVP Intravenous pyelography, that is, urography, q.v.

kolpo-cysto-urethrography (KCU) X-ray examination of the female bladder, urethra, and vagina during rest, coughing, and voiding. Contrast medium is introduced in the bladder and vagina via a catheter. Now seldom used. See p. 449.

left anterior oblique(LAO) Oblique X-ray projection with the left antero-lateral side of the patient nearest to the film/image recorder.

left lateral Lateral projection with the left side of the patient nearest to the film/image recorder.

lung perfusion scintigraphy Radioisotope examination of the blood perfusion of the lungs after intravenous injection of a tracer (often ^{99m}Tc-labeled albumin).

lung ventilation scintigraphy Radioisotope examination of the ventilation of the lungs after inhalation of a radioactive gas (often ^{133}Xe or ^{81m}Kr). See p. 349.

lymphangiography Lymphography, q.v.

lymphography X-ray examination of lymphatic vessels and lymph nodes after injection of an oil-based contrast medium containing iodine. Inguinal, external iliac and lumbar nodes are visualized after injection of contrast in a lymph vessel on both feet. Axillary nodes are similarly visualized after injec-

tion on the hand. X-rays taken a few hours after the injection (the early phase) show lymphatic vessels. X-rays taken the next day or later show only the lymph nodes. Yields excellent imaging of lymphatics and lymph nodes, but is now seldom performed. Replaced by MRI. See p. 441–2.

M-mode "Motion" mode of ultrasound scanning. See p. 37.

magnetic resonance imaging That is, MRI, MR, NMR imaging. See p. 19.

mammography X-ray examination of the breast at low kV (20–30 kV) to obtain good differentiation in soft tissue imaging. See p. 397.

maximum intensity projection (MIP) Imaging mode where an operator-chosen imaginary slab of an organ, contained in a stack of CT images, is projected by parallel imaginary "rays" to produce a 2D image, where only the voxel with the highest CT number passed by each "ray" is allowed to contribute to the projected image. The technique is mostly used in CT angiography. See p. 17.

MDP-scintigraphy Methylene diphosphonate scintigraphy, q.v.

median Midsagittal, q.v.

methylene diphosphonate scintigraphy (MDP scintigraphy). Radioisotope examination of bone using ^{99m}Tc-labeled methylene diphosphonate, which concentrates in calcifying tissue in proportion to the mineral metabolism in the tissue. Thus, it concentrates especially around growth plates of the long bones. See pp. 51, 93, 100, 121, 144, 204.

micturating cystography X-ray examination of the urinary bladder during voiding. Now seldom performed. See p. 449.

midsagittal Median. Sagittal section in the midline of the body.

MIP Maximum intensity projection, q.v.

MRA Magnetic resonance angiography. See p. 29.

MRI Magnetic resonance imaging. See p. 19.

multislice scanning Simultaneous recording of many tomographic sections in CT and MR scanning. See p. 13.

myelography Imaging of the spinal cord. Water-soluble contrast medium is injected into the subarachnoid space either by lumbar or by suboccipital injection. The subarachnoid space is subsequently imaged by X-ray or computed tomography (computed myelography).

orthopantomography Panoramic radiograph, q.v.

panoramic radiograph (panorama) X-ray examination of the teeth and the adjacent bone by a special tomographic technique, which produces a curved "slice" through the dental arches.

percutaneous transhepatic cholangiography (PTC) X-ray contrast examination of the biliary tract after percutaneous cannulation of a biliary duct in the liver.

percutaneous transhepatic portography X-ray contrast examination of the portal vein and/or its branches after cannulation of a portal branch by percutaneous liver puncture. The vein is cannulated by the Seldinger technique, q.v.

perfusion lung scanning Lung perfusion scintigraphy, q.v.

PET Positron emission tomography, q.v.

phlebography Imaging of veins. Contrast medium is usually injected by direct puncture of a peripheral vein distal to the region imaged on X-ray. Selective phlebography can also be performed by Seldinger technique, q.v.

pixel The smallest element in a digital image. See also voxel.

plain film radiography Projectional radiography. X-ray examination without use of contrast media. Plain films of the abdomen are usually taken in both supine and upright position to observe changes in the distribution of gases in the abdominal viscera. See p. 403.

portal phlebography X-ray examination of the portal vein. Can be performed after injection of contrast medium into the spleen (splenic phlebography, splenoportography); during the venous phase of splenic arteriography (arterioportography), or after catheterization of the portal vein by percutaneous liver puncture.

portography Portal phlebography, q.v.

positron emission tomography (PET) Radioisotope imaging technique utilizing positron-emitting isotopes. Often combined with CT (PET-CT). See pp. 42–4.

proton spin density weighted imaging MR imaging mode in which the contrast in the image approximately reflects the concentration of protons in soft tissues. See p. 29.

PTC Percutaneous transhepatic cholangiography, q.v.

pyelography X-ray examination of the renal pelvis. Can be performed by percutaneous injection of contrast media into the renal pelvis, or indirectly by retrograde pyelography, q.v.

radiculography X-ray examination of spinal nerve roots after injection of water-soluble contrast medium into the subarachnoid space.

radiogram Radiograph. A conventional X-ray image.

radioisotope imaging Scintigraphy, q.v.

radiolucent Material or structure that is easily penetrated by X-rays, such an object appears dark when imaged.

radionuclide Radioactive isotope.

radiopaque Material or structure that absorbs and scatters X-rays. Such an object appears light when imaged.

renal arteriography Selective arteriography of the renal artery and its branches using Seldinger technique, q.v.

renography Scintigraphic and quantitative examination of the renal excretion of a radiolabeled pharmaceutical, for example hippuran labeled with ^{99m}Tc.

retrograde urethrography Urethrography, q.v.

retrograde pyelography X-ray examination of the renal pelvis, calyces, and ureter after injection of water-soluble contrast medium, through a catheter positioned in the ureter via a cystoscope.

right anterior oblique (RAO) Oblique projection with the right antero-lateral side of the patient nearest to the film/image recorder.

right lateral Lateral projection with the right side of the patient nearest to the film/image recorder.

roentgenogram An X-ray film.

roentgenography Imaging by X-ray.

sagittal section Section parallel to the median plane of the body.

salpingogram Hystero-salpingography, q.v.

scintigraphy Imaging of the intensity and distribution of radioactivity in organs and tissues after administration of a radioactive tracer substance. See p. 41.

scout view Survey image used for orientation in CT and MR scanning. See p. 13.

Seldinger technique Method for introducing a fine tube (catheter) into a blood vessel. After puncture of, for example, an artery by a cannula, a flexible guide wire is introduced through the cannula, which is then withdrawn. A radio-paque catheter is placed over the wire, which guides it into the artery. A catheter inserted in this way may subsequently be guided into smaller vessels aided by fluoroscopic observation of the catheter. This technique permits selective catheterization of small vessels and other narrow hollow structures.

selective arteriography X-ray examination of a selected artery, often performed by placing a tube (catheter) into a small artery by the Seldinger technique, q.v.

sialography Imaging of a salivary gland and its ducts, often performed by dilatation of the external orifice of the duct, followed by catheterization and injection of contrast medium.

single contrast X-ray examination using either a positive or a negative contrast medium.

small bowel enema X-ray imaging of the small bowel after infusion of contrast through a tube placed in the duodenum.

sonography Ultrasonography, q.v.

SPECT Single photon emission computed tomography. Often combined with CT scanning (SPECT-CT). See p. 44.

spin echoes Method to evoke radio signals in MR imaging. See p. 24.

subtraction imaging Photographic or digital method for improving the contrast in diagnostic X-ray imaging, for example removing bone shadows from arteriography images (see digital subtraction angiography).

surface rendering Image processing method where only those voxels located along steep gradients in signal density within a selected range of densities are allowed to contribute to the image. See p. 17.

T1 weighted imaging MR imaging mode where the contrast in the image represents differences in the T1 relaxation time of protons in the tissues. See p. 22.

T2 weighted imaging MR imaging mode where the contrast in the image represents differences in the T2 relaxation time of protons in the tissue. See p. 22.

tomography Imaging an imaginary section or slice at a pre-determined level in the body. In conventional X-ray performed by simultaneous and opposite motion of the X-ray tube and film during the period of exposure. See p. 9. See also computed tomography and magnetic resonance imaging, pp. 13 and 26.

transhepatic catheterization Percutaneous transhepatic portography or cholangiography, q.v.

transesophageal Examination performed via the esophagus.

transrectal Examination performed via the rectum.

transvaginal Examination performed via the vagina.

ultrasonography (sonography) Imaging based on reflection of high-frequency sound waves. See p. 34.

urethrography X-ray examination of the urethra. Water-soluble contrast medium is injected through the external orifice, or the urethra is examined during voiding of contrast medium introduced into the bladder. See also cysto-urethro-graphy.

urography Intravenous urography. Intravenous pyelography (IVP). X-ray examination of the kidneys, the ureters and the bladder after intravenous injection of a water-soluble contrast medium, which is excreted by the kidneys. The contrast medium is concentrated in the urine and visualizes the kidney parenchyma, calyces, pelvis, ureters and bladder, in that order. Besides providing images of the urinary tract, the examination provides information on the renal excretory function. See p. 445.

venography Phlebography, q.v.

venous arteriography Vizualizing arteries after intravenous injection of contrast medium, especially used for imaging with digital subtraction and computed tomography.

ventilation scintigraphy Lung ventilation scintigraphy, q.v.

ventriculography (1) Examination by X-rays or ultrasonography of the cardiac ventricles with contrast medium injected through a catheter. See p. 390. (2) X-ray of the brain after introduction of contrast medium in the cerebral ventricles (obsolete).

vesiculography X-ray examination of the male seminal vesicles and deferent ducts after injection of contrast medium into the ejaculatory ducts.

volume rendering Image processing method where only voxels within one or more selected ranges of densities are allowed to contribute to the image. See p. 17–18.

voxel In CT or MR scanning, the smallest volume element whose average X-ray attenuation or MR radio signal intensity has been determined. A voxel is represented in a 2D image as a pixel. See p. 12.

xeroradiography A special process formerly used for soft tissue X-ray images using metal plates coated with a semi-conductor, such as selenium, analogous to xerographic photocopying.

Index

Entries in English according to *Terminologia Anatomica*. Stuttgart/New York: Thieme 1998.

The index is systematical which means that arteries, fascia, ligaments, veins, etc. are grouped together; the exception to this is bones, which are indexed individually. Each major organ system or bone is also fully sub-indexed with the anatomical features associated with it.

Anatomy in Diagnostic Imaging, Third Edition. Peter Fleckenstein and Jørgen Tranum-Jensen.
© 2014 Peter Fleckenstein, Jørgen Tranum-Jensen and Peter Sand Myschetzky. Published 2104 by John Wiley & Sons, Ltd.